PEDIATRIC
CLINICAL METHODS

<u>Sixth Edition</u>

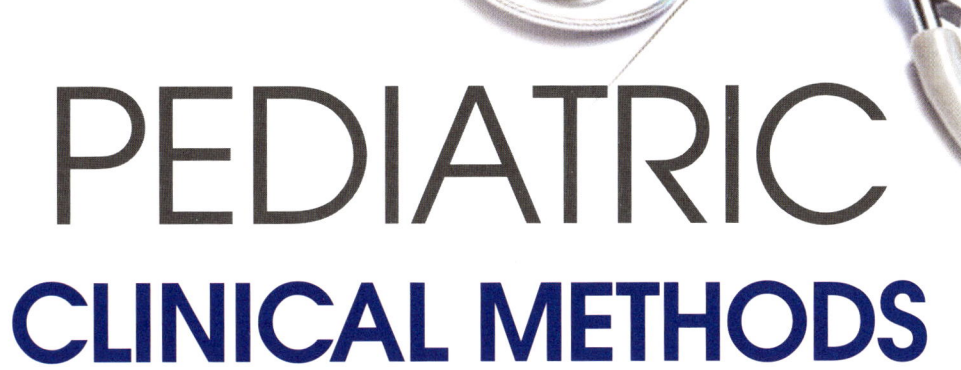

PEDIATRIC
CLINICAL METHODS

Sixth Edition

Meharban Singh
MD, FAMS, FIAP, FIMSA, FNNF, Hony. FAAP

Former Professor and Head
Department of Pediatrics and Neonatal Division
WHO Collaborating Center for Training and
Research in Newborn Care
All India Institute of Medical Sciences
New Delhi

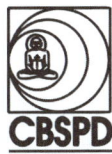

CBSPD

CBS Publishers & Distributors Pvt Ltd

New Delhi • Bengaluru • Chennai • Kochi • Kolkata • Lucknow • Mumbai
Hyderabad • Jharkhand • Nagpur • Patna • Pune • Uttarakhand

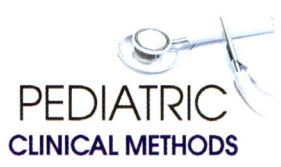

PEDIATRIC CLINICAL METHODS
Sixth Edition

Disclaimer

Science and technology are constantly changing fields. New research and experience broaden the scope of information and knowledge. The author has tried his best in giving information available to him while preparing the material for this book. Although all efforts have been made to ensure optimum accuracy of the material, yet it is quite possible some errors might have been left uncorrected. The publisher, the printer and the author will not be held responsible for any inadvertent errors, omissions or inaccuracies.

ISBN: 978-93-89261-75-2

Copyright © Meharban Singh

Sixth Edition: 2020
  Reprint: 2021, 2023, 2024, **2025**
First Edition: August 1992
  Reprint: March 1995
Second Edition: January 2000
Third Edition: August 2005
Fourth Edition: January 2011
  CBS Reprints: 2015
Fifth Edition: August 2016

All rights reserved. No part of this book may be reproduced or transmitted in any form or by any means, electronic or mechanical, including photocopying, recording, or any information storage and retrieval system without permission, in writing, from the author and the publisher.

Published by **Satish Kumar Jain** and produced by **Varun Jain** for

CBS Publishers & Distributors Pvt Ltd
4819/XI Prahlad Street, 24 Ansari Road, Daryaganj, New Delhi 110 002, India.
Ph: 011-23289259, 23266838 Website: www.cbspd.com
 e-mail: delhi@cbspd.com
Corporate Office: 204 FIE, Industrial Area, Patparganj, Delhi 110 092
Ph: 011-49344934 Fax: 011-49344935 e-mail: publishing@cbspd.com; publicity@cbspd.com

Branches

- **Bengaluru:** Seema House 2975, 17th Cross, K.R. Road, Banasankari 2nd Stage, Bengaluru 560 070, Karnataka, India
  Ph: +91-80-26771678/79   Fax: +91-80-26771680   e-mail: bangalore@cbspd.com
- **Chennai:** 7, Subbaraya Street, Shenoy Nagar, Chennai 600 030, Tamil Nadu, India
  Ph: +91-44-26680620, 26681266   Fax: +91-44-42032115   e-mail: chennai@cbspd.com
- **Kochi:** 42/1325, 1326, Power House Road, Opp KSEB, Ernakulum, Kochi 682 018, Kerala, India
  Ph: +91-484-4059061-65,67   Fax: +91-484-4059065   e-mail: kochi@cbspd.com
- **Kolkata:** 147, Hind Ceramics Compound, 1st Floor, Nilgunj Road, Belghoria, Kolkata-700056, West Bengal, India
  Ph: 033-25633055/56   e-mail: kolkata@cbspd.com
- **Lucknow:** Basement, Khushnuma Complex, 7 Meerabai Marg (Behind Jawahar Bhawan), Lucknow-226001, UP, India
  Ph: +91-522-4000032   e-mail: tiwari.lucknow@cbspd.com
- **Mumbai:** PWD Shed, Gala no 25/26, Ramchandra Bhatt Marg, Next to JJ Hospital Gate no. 2, Opp. Union Bank of India, Noorbaug, Mumbai-400009, Maharashtra, India
  Ph: +91-22-66661880/89   e-mail: mumbai@cbspd.com

Representatives

- **Hyderabad** 0-9885175004   • **Jharkhand** 0-9811541605   • **Nagpur** 0-8692091830
- **Patna** 0-9334159340   • **Pune** 0-9664372571   • **Uttarakhand** 0-9716462459

Printed at Goyal Offset Works Pvt. Ltd. Haryana, India

to
my wife Kaushal
for her courage and compassion
and
to our children Sonia and Manik

The Oaths and Codes for Medical Practitioners

MANU'S CODE OF CONDUCT FOR PHYSICIANS (200 BCE)

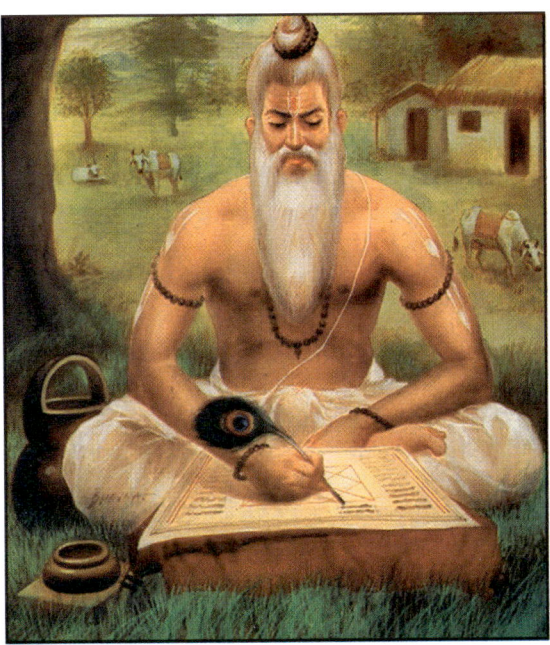

"Dedicate yourself entirely to helping the sick, even though this may be at the cost of your own life. Never harm the sick, not even in thought. Endeavor always to perfect your knowledge. Treat no woman except in the presence of their husbands. The physician should observe all the rules of good dress and good conduct. As soon as he is with a patient, he should concern himself in word and thought, with nothing but the sufferer's cause.

He must not speak outside the house of anything that takes place in the patient's house. He must not speak to a patient of his possible death, if by doing so he hurts the patient or anyone else. In the sights of gods, you are to pledge yourself to this. May the gods help you, if you follow this rule. Otherwise, may the gods be against you".

HIPPOCRATIC OATH (460–370 BCE)

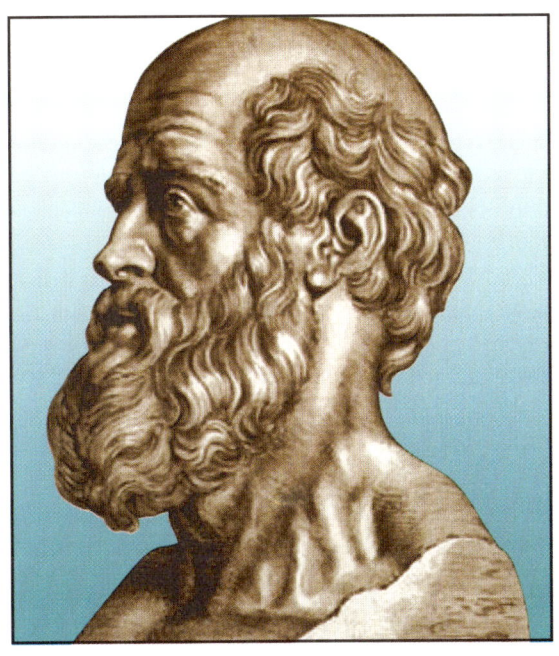

"I swear by Apollo, the Healer, by Asclepius, by Hygieia and by Panacea and by all the gods and goddesses, making them my witnesses, that I will carry out according to my ability and judgement this oath and this indenture.

To hold my teacher in this art equal to my own parents; to make him partner in my livelihood; when he is in need of money to share mine with him; to consider his family as my own brothers, and to teach them this art, if they want to learn it, without fee or indenture; to impart precept, oral instructions, and all other instructions to my own sons, the sons of my teacher, and to indentured pupils who have taken the physician's oath, but to nobody else.

I will use treatment to help the sick according to my ability and judgement but never with a view to injury and wrong-doing. Neither will I administer a poison to anybody when asked to do so, nor will

I suggest such a course. Similarly I will not give to a woman a pessary to cause abortion. But I will keep pure and holy both my life and my art. I will not use the knife, not even verily, on sufferers from stone, but I will give place to such as are craftsmen therein.

Into whatsoever houses I enter, I will enter to help the sick, and I will abstain from all intentional wrong-doing and harm, especially from abusing the bodies of man or woman, bond or free. And whatsoever I shall see or hear in the course of my profession, as well as outside my profession in my intercourse with men, if it be what should not be published abroad, I will never divulge, holding such things to be holy secrets.

Now if I carry out this oath and break it not, may I gain forever reputation among all men for my life and for my art; but if I transgress it and forswear myself, may the opposite befall me."

(Translated from Greek by James Loeb)

CHARAKA OATH (300–200 BCE)

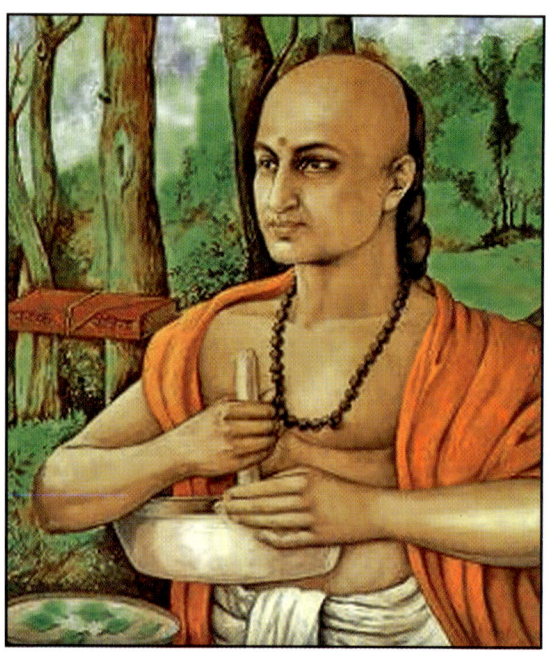

Charaka Samhita contains an Anushasana, the Atreya Anushasana (7th century BCE), predating the famous Hippocratic Oath by two centuries. This oath bears testimony to the high level of professional ethics in ancient India. Charaka revised the 8th century BCE Encyclopedic Treatise of Agnivesa.

1. The teacher then should instruct the disciple in the presence of the sacred fire, Brahamanas (Brahmins) and physicians.
2. Thou shalt lead the life of a celebate, grow thy hair and beard, speak only the truth, eat no meat, eat only pure articles of food, be free from envy and carry no arms.
3. There shalt be nothing that thou should not do at my behest except hating the king, causing another's death, or committing an act of great unrighteousness or acts leading to calamity.
4. Thou shalt dedicate thyself to me and regard me as thy chief. Thou shalt be subject to me and conduct thyself for ever for my welfare and pleasure. Thou shall serve and dwell with me like a son or a slave or a supplicant. Thou shalt behave and act without arrogance, with care and attention and with undistracted mind, humility, constant reflection and ungrudging obedience. Acting either at my behest or otherwise, thou shalt conduct thyself for the achievement of thy teacher's purpose alone, to the best of thy abilities.
5. If thou desirest success, wealth and fame as a physician and heaven after death, thou shalt pray for the welfare of all creatures beginning with the cows and Brahamanas.
6. Day and night, however, thou mayest be engaged, thou shalt endeavor for the relief of patients with all thy heart and soul. Thou shalt not desert or injure thy patient for the sake of thy life or thy living. Thou shalt not commit adultery even in thought. Even so, thou shalt not covert other's possessions. Thou shalt be modest in thy attire and appearance. Thou shouldst not be a drunkard or a sinful man nor shouldst thou associate with the abettors of crimes. Thou shouldst speak words that are gentle, pure and righteous, pleasing, worthy, true, wholesome, and moderate. Thy behavior must be in

consideration of time and place and heedful of past experience. Thou shall act always with a view to the acquisition of knowledge and fullness of equipment.

7. No person, who are hated by the king or who are haters of the king or who are hated by the public, shall receive treatment. Similarly, those who are extremely abnormal, wicked, and of miserable character and conduct, those who have not vindicated their honor, those who are on the point of death, and similarly women who are unattended by their husbands or guardians shall not receive treatment.

8. No offering of presents by a woman without the behest of her husband or guardian shall be accepted by thee. While entering the patient's house, thou shalt be accompanied by a man who is known to the patient and who has his permission to enter; and thou shalt he well-clad, bent of head, self-possessed, and conduct thyself only after repeated consideration. Thou shalt thus properly make thy entry. Having entered, thy speech, mind, intellect and senses shall be entirely devoted to no other thought than that of being helpful to the patient and things concerning only him. The peculiar customs of the patients' household shall not be made public. Even knowing that the patients' span of life has come to its close, it shall not be mentioned by thee there, where if so done, it would cause shock to the patient or others. Though possessed of knowledge, one should not boast very much of one's knowledge. Most people are offended by the boastfulness of even those who are otherwise good and authoritative.

9. There is no limit to the Science of Life Medicine. So thou shouldst apply thyself to it with diligence. This is how you thouldst act. Also thou shouldst learn the skill of practice from another without carping. The entire world is the teacher to intelligent and foe to the unintelligent. Hence knowing this well, thou shouldst listen and act according to the words of instruction of even an unfriendly person, when his words are worthy and of a kind as to bring to you fame, long life, strength and prosperity.

10. Thereafter the teacher should say this—"thou shouldst conduct thyself properly with the gods, sacred fire, Brahamanas, the guru, the aged, the scholars and preceptors. If thou has conducted thyself well with them, the precious stones, the grains and the gods become well disposed towards thee. If thou shouldst conduct thyself otherwise, they become unfavorable to thee." To the teacher that has spoken thus, the disciple should say, 'Amen'.

(Charaka Samhita 7 volumes translated from Sanskrit to English by Ramkaran Sharma and Bhagwan Das)

Abridged Charaka Oath Administered at AIIMS Graduation Ceremony

"… Not for the self, not for the fulfilment of any worldly material desire or gain, but solely for the good of humanity, I will treat my patients and excell all …"

MOSES BEN MOIMONIDES OATH (1135–1204 ACE)

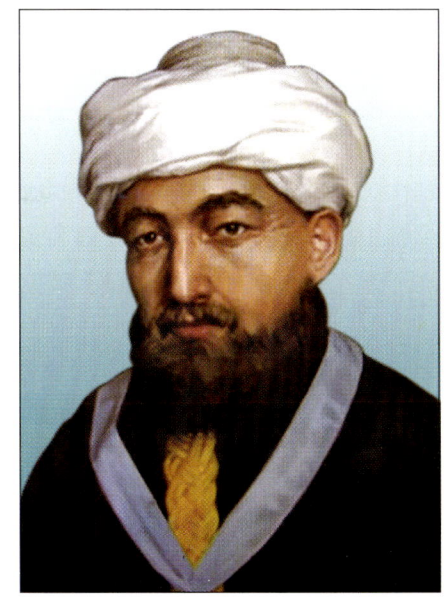

"The eternal providence has appointed me to watch over life and health of thy creatures. May the love of my art actuate me at all time. May neither avarice or miserliness, nor thirst for glory or for a great reputation engage my mind, for the enemies of truth and philanthropy could easily deceive me and make me forgetful of my lofty aim of doing good to thy children. May I never see the patient anything but a fellow creature in pain. Grant me the strength, time and opportunity always to correct what I have acquired, always to extend its domain, for knowledge is immense and spirit of man can extend indefinitely to enrich itself daily with new requirements.

Today thou can discover the errors of yesterday and tomorrow. Thou can obtain a new light on what you think yourself sure of today. Oh God, thou has appointed me to watch over life and death of thy creatures, here I am ready for my vocation and now I turn into my calling."

THE DECLARATION OF GENEVA PROPOUNDED BY THE WORLD MEDICAL ASSOCIATION (1968)

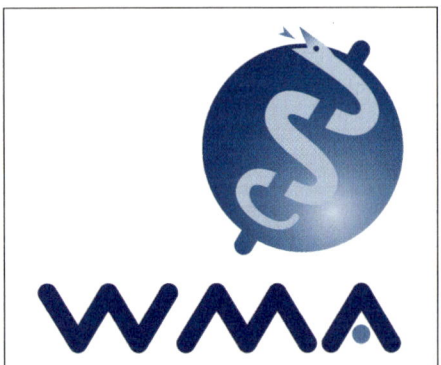

"I solemnly pledge myself to consecrate my life to the service of humanity; I will give my teachers the respect and gratitude which is their due; I will practice my profession with conscience and dignity. The health of my patients will be my first consideration. I will respect secrets that have been confided in me, even after the patient has died. I will maintain by all the means in my power the honor and noble traditions of the medical profession; my colleagues will be my sisters and brothers. I will not permit considerations of age, gender, religion, nationality, race, party politics or social standing to intervene between my duty and my patient. I will maintain the utmost respect for human life from the time of conception. Even under threat I will not use my medical knowledge contrary to the laws of humanity. I make these promises solemnly, freely and upon my honor."

CODE OF MEDICAL ETHICS BY MEDICAL COUNCIL OF INDIA

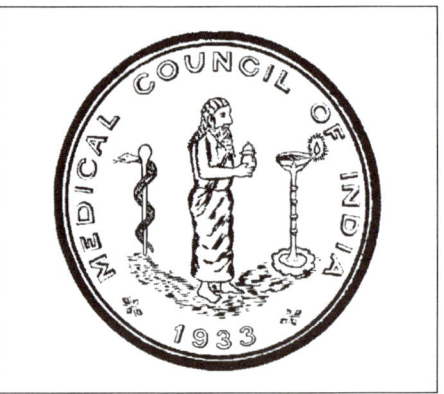

"…… I solemnly pledge myself to consecrate my life to the service of humanity. Even under the threat, I will not use my medical knowledge contrary to the laws of humanity. I will maintain the utmost respect for the human life from the time of conception. The health of my patients will be my first consideration. I will not permit consideration of religion, nationality, race, party-politics or social standing to intervene between my duty and my patient. I will practice my profession with conscience and dignity. I will respect the secrets which are confided in me. I will give my teachers the respect and gratitude which is their due. I will maintain by all means in my power, the honor and noble traditions of medical profession. My colleagues will be my brothers. I make these promises solemnly, freely and upon my honor".

INTERNATIONAL CODE OF MEDICAL ETHICS 1949 AMENDED BY 57th WORLD MEDICAL ASSEMBLY, SOUTH AFRICA 2006

Duties of Physicians in General

- To exercise independent professional judgement and maintain highest standards of professional conduct.
- To honor the right of patient to accept or refuse the treatment.
- Should not allow his/her judgement to be influenced by personal profit or unfair means.
- To be dedicated to provide competent medical services with full professional and moral independence, compassion and respect for human diginity.
- To do deal honestly with patients and colleagues and report to the appropriate authorities those physicians who practice unethically or incompetently, or who engage in fraud and deception.
- Should not receive any financial benefits or other incentives solely for referring patients or prescribing specific medicines and products.
- Should recognize his/her important role in educating the public but should use due caution in divulging discoveries or new techniques or drugs through non-professional lay channels.
- Should not issue any false medical certificate and certify only that which has been personally verified.
- Should strive to use health care resources in the best way to benefit patients and their community.
- Should seek appropriate care and attention, if he/she suffers from any mental and physical illness.
- Should respect the local and national codes of medical ethics.

Duties of Physicians towards Patients

- Always bear in mind the obligation to respect human life.
- Should provide medical care with complete loyalty with all the scientific resources available to his/her command.
- Should respect the patients' right to confidentiality. However, it is ethical to disclose confidential information when the patient consents to it or when there is genuine threat of harm to the patient or others and this threat can only be removed by a breach of confidentiality.
- Should provide emergency care as a humanitarian duty unless he/she is assured that sound and reliable emergency care is available from other resources.
- When a physician is unable to provide rational and reliable treatment, he/she must consult with or refer to another physician who has the necessary ability.
- In a situation when a physician is acting on behalf of a third party, he/she should ensure that the patient has full knowledge of that situation.
- Should never enter into a sexual relationship or any other abusive or exploitative relationship with his/her patient.

Duties of Physicians towards Professional Colleagues

- Should behave towards colleagues as she/he would have them behave towards her/him.
- Should never undermine the patient–physician relationship of colleagues in order to attract patients.
- Should communicate with professional colleagues for the benefit of patients by maintaining due confidentiality.
- The physician must observe the principles of the Declaration of Geneva.

Avoidance of Unethical Practices

- Any self-advertisement except as expressly authorized in a national code of conduct.
- Receiving any cuts or kickbacks for referral of patients and doing laboratory investigations.
- Doing unnecessary investigations, procedures and surgical interventions or needless hospital admissions for monetary gain.
- Collaboration in any form of medical services in which the physician does not have the professional independence.

- Receipt of any gratification for services rendered to a patient other than a proper professional fee, even if the patient is aware of it.

The Physician's Pledge by the World Medical Association (Amended by the 68th WMA General Assembly, Chicago, United States, October 14, 2017)

As a member of medical profession:

- I solemnly pledge to dedicate my life to the service of humanity;
- The health and well-being of my patient will be my first consideration;
- I will respect the autonomy and dignity of my patient;
- I will maintain the utmost respect for human life;
- I will not permit consideration of age, disease or disability, creed, ethnic origin, gender, nationality, political affiliation, race, sexual orientation, social standing or any other factor to intervene between my duty and my patient;
- I will respect the secrets that are confided in me, even after the patient has died;
- I will practice my profession with conscience and dignity and in accordance with good medical practice;
- I will foster the honor and noble traditions of the medical profession;
- I will give my teachers, colleagues and students the respect and gratitude that is their due;
- I will attend to my own health, well-being, and abilities in order to provide care of the highest standard;
- I will not use my medical knowledge to violate human rights and civil liberties, even under threat,
- I make these promises solemnly, freely, and upon my honor.

Reviews Galore

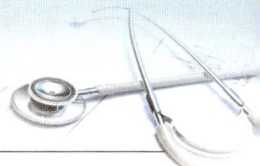

Review of first edition of Pediatric Clinical Methods published in Indian Pediatrics 1993, 30:123

This is a book, which many would have liked to write, but few would have managed to do it so well. Prof. Meharban Singh in his inimitable style has conveyed the essence of Pediatric Clinical Methods within a span of 238 pages. Besides traditional systematic examination, there are chapters on developmental assessment, anthropometry, examination of a newborn baby and special aspects of pediatric physical examination. Each chapter is followed by a summary for ease of presentation. Special tables are presented against a grey outline. The book is well illustrated. Barring a few printer's devils, there is hardly any deficiency to point out. The book is superb, whichever angle it is considered from, viz. production, contents, illustrations and finally the price. It is sure to become a compulsory reading for any one taking any examination in pediatrics.

BNS Walia MD
Emeritus Professor of Pediatrics
Former Director,
Post Graduate Institute of
Medical Education and Research,
Chandigarh-160 012

Review of fourth edition of Pediatric Clinical Methods published in Indian Journal of Pediatrics 2011, 78(10):1301

"Pediatric Clinical Methods" written by Prof. Meharban Singh is an excellent book on clinical examination and the interpretation of the findings in pediatric practice. Prof. Mcharban Singh with his vast experience in the field of pediatrics has used his clinical acumen and writing skills to compile this valuable book. The book contains the art and science of pediatric history taking, clinical examination and diagnosis. The book contains beautiful illustrations, algorithmic approach to diagnosis and photographs indicating the methods of examination. The importance of holistic approach in the clinical examination of a pediatric patient has been aptly emphasized in the book. The book contains important information, like immunization schedule, important developmental milestones and some important clinical photographs for ease of understanding for the clinicians.

Pediatric history taking and examination is different from adults and has been excellently conveyed by Prof. Meharban Singh with his simple and easily understandable language. The book reflects Prof. Singh's highest level of caliber, excellent clinical acumen and understanding of the subject. The abnormal physical signs and their interpretation in arriving at clinical diagnosis shall be a bonus for practicing pediatricians and resident doctors. The historical aspects of oaths and codes for medical practitioners are important and interesting collection which should be known to all medical personnel. The chapter on "Ethical and Legal Issues in Clinical Practice" is of immense value for all medical practitioners. In the era of Consumer Protection Act, the book highlights guidelines for making ethical decisions and ensuring sound professional qualities, duties and attributes of a pediatrician. The book contains WHO growth charts on weight, height, weight-for-height, and head circumference which can be used as excellent ready reckoner. The book also highlights important key points in boxes in each chapter.

I am sure the book would be of immense help to all medical graduates, postgraduates in pediatrics and practicing pediatricians and should be kept on their desktop.

Ashok Kumar Dutta MD
Professor and Head
Department of Pediatrics
Lady Harding Medical College and
Kalawati Saran Children Hospital
New Delhi

Preface to the Sixth Edition

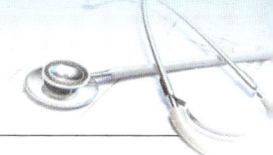

I am amazed at the overwhelming response accorded to the fifth edition of **Pediatric Clinical Methods** both by the undergraduate and postgraduate medical students. I am delighted that the book has admirably served the felt needs of upcoming pediatricians by emphasizing a logical stepwise approach in taking a detailed history, conducting clinical examination of children, elicitation of abnormal physical findings and their interpretation. The feedback received from a large number of my students, residents and pediatricians inspired me to bring out a more comprehensive sixth edition.

Despite advances in diagnostic technology, it must be remembered that communication and clinical skills are the hallmarks of a good physician and they are crucial for building a trustworthy doctor–patient and doctor–parent relationship, faith and credibility to catalyze the process of healing. The systematic approach pursued for making clinical diagnosis is indeed more complicated than solving a crossword puzzle and demands a unique understanding of science and art of clinical pediatrics. The chapter on *The Art and Science of Pediatric Diagnosis* has been further expanded and should be read as the core essence of the book to imbibe the philosophy and wisdom of holistic clinical approach towards sick children.

All the chapters have been revised, rewritten and updated. The cardinal and fundamental pediatric orientation of the book has been further reinforced by including a detailed description of common dysmorphic syndromes, failure to thrive and short stature which are common clinical problems in day-to-day practice. The scope of differential diagnosis of a large number of abnormal physical findings has been greatly enhanced and the book would now serve as a useful manual of pediatric diagnosis. A number of new illustrations and clinical photographs have been included. The contents are summarized and amplified by a large number of tables, boxes and medical quotations. It is hoped that the systematic clinical approach emphasized in the book would be useful to the pediatricians to optimally utilize the available diagnostic plethora of tests more rationally and with greater safety and cost-effectiveness to their patients.

I would like to take this opportunity to thank Mr YN Arjuna, Mrs Ritu Chawla, Mr Tarun Rajput for composing and inserting the manuscript in the word processor and to my friend Shri Satish Kumar Jain for his enthusiasm and commitment to publish the revised book in an improved style and format.

I greatly appreciate the inputs and suggestions made by a number of my former postgraduate students and colleagues. My special thanks are due to Rakesh Lodha for his suggestions which have been incorporated. He was instrumental in seeking inputs from a number of pediatric residents which have been inserted in the text. Our grand daughter Ishita has taken the photographs of several clinical procedures in my ambulatory clinic. I am confident that **Pediatric Clinical Methods** would continue to enthuse and inspire upcoming pediatricians to imbibe the art and science of clinical examination of children with a sense of compassion and concern to provide holistic and rational care to children.

26th January, 2020 **Meharban Singh** MD
Child Care Center
625, Arun Vihar, Sector 37
Noida 201 301
Tel: 0120-4346451, 9818888772
e-mail: drmbsk@gmail.com

Preface to the First Edition

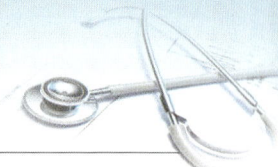

The foundation of this book was laid in Afghanistan where the author in his capacity as Director, Indira Gandhi Institute of Child Health, Kabul, Afghanistan had the onerous task of taking bedside clinics and tutorials of students of Diploma in Child Health who had relatively scant core information and limited clinical experience. It is a sad reality that there is a gradual rusting of clinical acumen and lack of interest for bedside teaching among physicians due to ready availability of modern diagnostic technology. The patients are often viewed as systems and organs and art of medicine is being sacrificed at the altar of scientific and technological revolution. The book has been written to provide a simplified clinical approach to children with medical disorders. The focus is entirely on clinical methods to elicit physical symptoms and signs. It is not intended to be a comprehensive manual for pediatric diagnosis because interpretation of clinical findings and laboratory investigations have not been covered. The book is, therefore, complementary to Hutchison's Clinical Methods that must be read by all the medical students before making efforts to develop skills to handle children.

The chapter on *The Art and Science of Pediatric Diagnosis* provides knowledge, skills and philosophy to handle children and their parents with concern and compassion. Anthropometry and developmental assessment have been covered in depth in view of the importance of growth and development of children in health and disease. Specific differences regarding approach and interpretation of physical findings between children and adults have been highlighted. The chapter on *Differential Diagnosis of Common Abnormal Physical Signs* would assist the pediatricians to make logical deductions to arrive at the most likely diagnosis. The unstructured approach to clinical examination of children have been emphasised in order to elicit maximum co-operation during systemic examination. A summary has been provided at the end of all chapters to highlight a uniform scheme of recording and presentation. In view of unique health problems of neonates and a different approach for their clinical evaluation, a separate chapter has been devoted to provide comprehensive coverage.

I am indebted to my colleagues Vinod K Paul, Ashok K Deorari, Arvind Bagga, and S Bhushan for their assistance and help in preparing photographs and appendices. My special thanks are due to Shri Sanjay Sehrawat and Shri Raju Tandon for typing the manuscript. I have continued to associate myself with Sagar Publications because of the special consideration and all out cooperation extended to me by the proprietor Shri Narinder Sagar to publish the book. I am confident that **Pediatric Clinical Methods** shall fill the much felt void and serve the felt needs of medical graduates, pediatric residents and pediatricians to rejuvenate the dwindling art of clinical pediatrics.

August 15, 1992
All India Institute of Medical Sciences
New Delhi 110 029

Meharban Singh MD

"Learn to see, learn to hear, learn to feel, learn to smell, and know that by practice alone can you become perfect. Medicine is learnt by the bedside and not in the classroom or library. Let not your conceptions of the manifestations of disease come from words heard in the lecture room or read from the book. See and then reason, analyze and interpret. But see first".

Sir William Osler

Contents

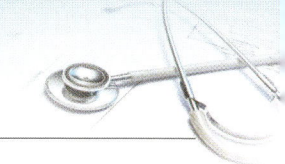

The Oaths and Codes for Medical Practitioners   vii
Preface to the Sixth Edition   xv
Preface to the First Edition   xvi

1. The Art and Science of Pediatric Diagnosis   1
2. History Taking   15
3. General Physical Examination   31
4. Salient Differences between Physical Examination of Children and Adults   58
5. Anthropometry for Assessment of Nutritional Status   62
6. Developmental Assessment   77
7. The Dysmorphic Child   96
8. Differential Diagnosis of Common Abnormal Physical Signs   111
9. The Skin and its Appendages   140
10. The Musculoskeletal System   166
11. The Alimentary System and Abdomen   181
12. The Respiratory System   198
13. The Cardiovascular System   215
14. The Central Nervous System   238
15. Examination of a Newborn Baby   280
16. Ethical and Legal Issues in Clinical Practice   314
17. The Diagnosis of Death   325

    Bibliography   329

    Appendices   331

    Index   375

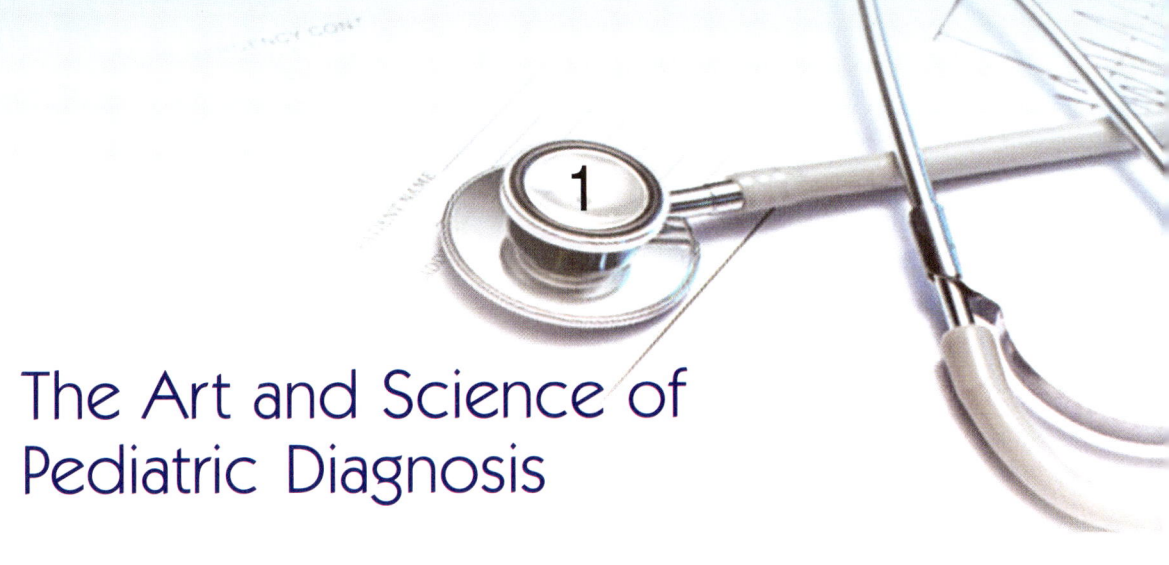

The Art and Science of Pediatric Diagnosis

THE ATTRIBUTES OF A PHYSICIAN

"The medical student must exhibit a calm and generous disposition, besides being virtuous and of a noble mind. He must be tolerant of others and exhibit patience and perseverance in his academic pursuits. Although of sharp intellect, he must be both rational and modest. He should possess a pleasant appearance and good looks, with a well-proportioned body which should be free from physical defects or any obvious diseases. Above all, he must be compassionate. He must exhibit deep interest in the art and science of healing. He must use his intelligence to discuss facts about the disease and to understand the clinical significance of symptoms. Such knowledge he must use not only for his own intellectual enrichment, but also for acquiring requisite skills in practical management. He must be humble and loyal to his teachers and instructors. He should be free from any addictions, greed, arrogance and intolerance."

Charaka Samhita (300–200 BCE)

(The initial encyclopedic medical treatise was written in Sanskrit by Agnivesa under the guidance of the ancient physician Atreya in the 8th century BCE. Charaka revised it and it gained popularity as Charaka Samhita)

The ideal pediatrician must have genuine interest and love for children. The opportunity of nurturing one's own children or grandchildren is a great learning experience for a pediatrician. He must be humane, systematic in his approach and genuinely interested in the welfare of his patients. He should exude confidence, patience and politeness to elicit cooperation of patients and his attendants. These qualities are crucial to generate faith of parents in his capabilities, which is a great healing force. The physician who exhibits evidences of hurry, worry, and indecision is unlikely to inspire any confidence in his patients. *To augment the process of healing, the patient must have faith in his doctor and the doctor must have faith in himself and his medicines.*

The pediatrician should approach children as children (not patients) with tact, gentleness, warmth and genuine concern. He should have a sober and affectionate look so that children are not afraid of him. *Unlike adults, children distrust the man who looks into their eyes.* To seek cooperation, the child should be watched in a sneaky unconcerned manner. He must have scientific bent of mind, use logical systematic steps to arrive at a diagnosis with the help of core knowledge and basic principles. He should not be dogmatic and should be aware of limitations of his own knowledge and of knowledge in general and should never hesitate to say "I don't know". He is a perpetual student, constantly learning and unlearning to transform knowledge into wisdom. The attributes of a pediatrician are listed in ***Box 1.1***. The welfare of the patient must be considered as supreme and should take precedence over all other considerations including his personal pride or commercial gain. Nevertheless, he should not underestimate his own ability to make new and original observations. Above all, though medicine is a profession but life should never be weighed in gold—it is too precious! *According to Mother*

> **Box 1.1 The attributes of a pediatrician**
> - Good physical and mental health
> - Knowledge, clinical and communication skills
> - Wisdom
> - Confidence and imperturbability
> - Patience
> - Politeness
> - Humility and integrity
> - Common sense
> - Pleasant demeanor and bedside manners
> - Experience and expertise
> - Tactful and good listener
> - Caring and compassionate
> - Kind and affectionate look with a smile
> - Love for children
> - Intuition
> - Healing touch
> - Good human being

Teresa, medicine must be viewed as a mission and it should not be downgraded as a profession or business.

Children are afraid of hospitals, doctors and needles and they should never be blackmailed through threats of injections to modify their behavior. It is controversial whether pediatricians should wear white coats or not, while it appears immaterial to me. The white coat does complement the professional attitude and inculcates a sense of discipline and decorum. The pediatrician must conduct himself with dignity, seriousness and respect towards parents regardless of how deviant their behavior may appear at times of distress. He should establish a warm and cordial interpersonal relationship with patients, their parents and his team members by virtue of qualities of his head and heart. He must demonstrate impeccable bedside manners and serve as a role model to his students. He should not merely be a healer but truly serve as a teacher, philosopher and guide to his patients, parents and students. Remember, that the academic title doctor, originates from the Latin word "*docere*" which means "to teach" and physicians must spend adequate time to teach their students, patients and their attendants or caretakers.

THE APPROACH TO DIAGNOSIS

"The patients should not be viewed as systems, organs, tissues, cells and DNA. They must be viewed in totality (body, mind, heart and soul) and that too not in isolation but in context with the dynamics of ecology, family, friends and society."

Meharban Singh

The methods of physicians are like those of a detective, one seeking to explain the disease, other a crime. There are no short cuts for making a physical diagnosis. It is learnt only by practice, not a dull, dreary monotonous practice but practice with all the five senses alert. The astute physician is endowed with sharp and sensitive special senses (especially keen observation) and must harness the skills of a lawyer, detective and a judge. During the last two decades, a revolution in imaging technology by introduction of ultrasound, CT scanning, magnetic resonance imaging, and positron emission tomography has eroded the confidence and enthusiasm of clinicians. It is a sad reality that physicians are becoming more of technocrats and they are losing the art of medicine. The patient is being fragmented into systems, organs, tissues, cells and even DNA! It is crucial that we should not lose sight of totality of the patient and his interactions with social and ecological milieu. Instead of causing disuse atrophy of clinical judgement, the newer technology should be fully exploited and harnessed to improve clinical judgement and enhance the understanding of pathogenetic mechanisms underlying the disease process. The correct diagnosis of the underlying disorder and its probable etiology are crucial for rational management and prognostication. The diagnosis is based on elicitation of correct evidence and its analysis and interpretation of findings and observations in the light of core knowledge, wisdom and experience of the pediatrician (Figure 1.1).

THE EVIDENCE

Just as evidence is crucial for a detective to identify the culprit, similarly sound evidence as collected by history, physical examination and investigations

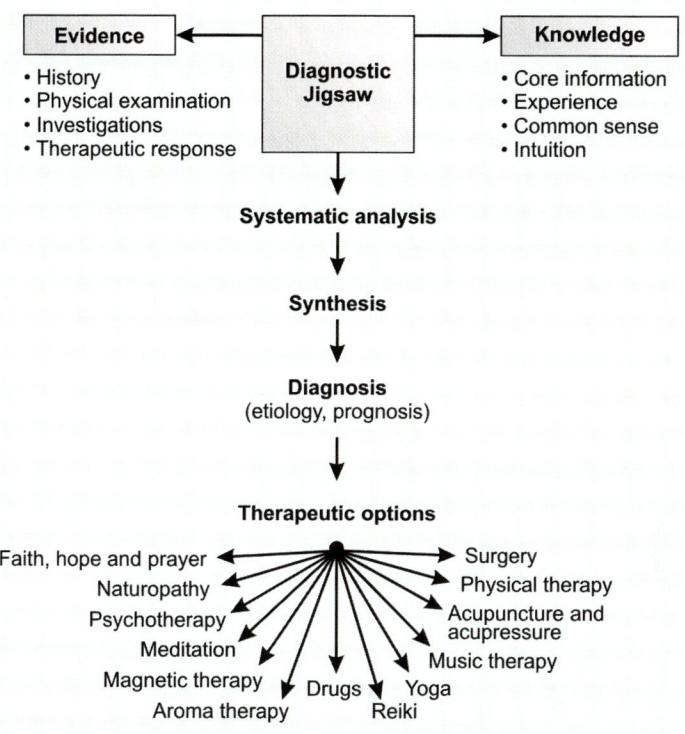

Figure 1.1 The key elements to solve the diagnostic puzzle. The correct diagnosis is crucial to institute rational therapy.

is of fundamental importance to solve the diagnostic dilemma.

History

Symptoms are cries of the diseased body organs and they provide an alert or warning to seek medical help. Good history taking is an art and it needs inquisitiveness, persistence and tact. You must emphasize the important, minimize unimportant and suppress irrelevant information. The history should be sifted off undue parental anxiety and concern in order to obtain a lucid chronological story with a special emphasis on the onset and evolution of the disease process. Through a process of detailed review of various symptoms and systems, an attempt should be made to identify the organ(s) affected by the disease process. Identify whether a single system is affected or one is dealing with a multisystem disorder. Attempt should be made to identify whether a disorder is acute, subacute and chronic or insidious and classify it into static, resolving or progressive in nature.

The psychological, social, ethnic, geographical, ecological and genetic factors influencing the disease process should be identified. Sir William Osler rightly said, *"Medicine is about sick people, not about diseases"*. Therefore, our focus should be the patient and not his disease. Race and ethnicity play an important role in the expression of disease. In addition to genetic factors, individuals with similar ethnic backgrounds share cultural, nutritional, environmental, economic, and social characteristics that influence the disease.

An experienced pediatrician is able to emphasize the important, minimize unimportant and suppress irrelevant information in the history. It must be remembered that over 75% of diagnoses can be correctly made by virtue of good history alone. It is important that no observation of the mother, whether apparently trivial or unimportant, should be ignored or set aside, even when it fails to fit into the tentative diagnosis. Indeed, it may be the most important clue or hint to unravel the diagnostic puzzle.

Physical Examination

"A great part, I believe, of the art of medicine is the ability to observe. Leave nothing, to chance, combine contradictory observations and allow yourself enough time."
— **Hippocrates**

The history tells of events which have led to the present condition of the patient while examination reveals the status of the patient at a given moment. Accuracy of history depends upon the education, memory, intelligence and concern of the attendant while yield of physical examination depends upon the experience, skills and thoroughness of the pediatrician. *Most errors in medicine are made by making cursory incomplete examination and not due to lack of knowledge and skills.*

The approach during examination of children is determined by the age, development status and level of understanding of the child. The clinical examination should be unstructured and made a fun to relieve the anxiety of the child. The pediatrician must have inherent fondness and love for children and examine them with warm hands and warm heart. The examination chamber should be warm, familiar, well lighted and stocked with soft toys. Deep yellow or blue-colored curtains should be avoided in the examination chamber because they may interfere with evaluation of jaundice and cyanosis. *The children must be treated as children and not patients and examination should be conducted in an unstructured playful manner.* Patients must be handled with utmost care and reverence as they are the real books of physicians. The maximum time should be devoted to observation of the child and to the system or organ which appears to be predominantly affected on the basis of history.

"To study the phenomena of disease without books is to sail an uncharted sea, while to study books without patients is not to go to the sea at all ..."
— **Sir William Osler**

Physicians must sharpen their observation skills by enhancing the capabilities of their special senses. Pediatrics deals with children from birth to adolescence, varying in size from less than 1.0 kg to over 50 kg and having different grades of functional maturation of various body organs. Pediatrics has been likened to a flying bird which deals with dynamic, evolving and changing size and maturity of children. The knowledge regarding developmental anatomy, developmental pharmacology, developmental biochemistry and developmental biology in general is crucial for proper evaluation of normal children at different ages for appreciation of abnormalities or deviations due to diseases. You must have information and knowledge regarding normal variations at different ages before you can pick up the abnormalities. The developmental or functional status of the child affects the incidence and expression of various diseases and conversely diseases may adversely affect the growth and development of children. The lymphoid tissue is physiologically hypertrophied in children leading to development of large tonsils, adenoids, or cervical lymphadenopathy following minor infections.

Laboratory Investigations

They are useful to assess the degree of organ dysfunction, assist in confirming the diagnosis, help in management, prognostication and follow-up. *There is no justification to undertake routine investigations in every patient.* Instead, appropriate and relevant investigations should be ordered depending upon the diagnostic possibilities entertained on the basis of a detailed clinical evaluation. The pediatrician should be aware of limitations of all laboratory tests and follow the philosophy to use the laboratory as a slave and not as a master.

Physicians must have faith in their clinical acumen and use laboratory as an aid for confirmation of diagnosis in order to provide effective and rational management to the patient. *The approach should be to treat the patient and not his laboratory reports.* Nevertheless, the diagnosis should not be delayed by deferring to undertake essential investigations. Timely laparotomy may be life-saving in a child with acute abdomen, undiagnosed lump and for differentiation between neonatal hepatitis and extrahepatic biliary atresia. The children with cervical lymphadenitis should not be given a trial of antitubercular therapy unless the diagnosis is confirmed by fine needle aspiration cytology or lymph node biopsy.

THE CORE KNOWLEDGE

The evidence generated by painstaking history, physical examination and investigations should be viewed in the light of available knowledge and experience of the pediatrician. Every pediatrician should be aware of the essential features and criteria for making the diagnosis of common childhood disorders. It must be remembered that no symptom or sign has a 100% frequency or specificity in a disorder because no two patients are alike. In general, the manifestations of diseases are rather atypical among neonates and infants. You must have an up-to-date knowledge pertaining to the current state-of-the-art for diagnosis and management of common pediatric problems otherwise you will get rusted and outmoded.

A large number of diseases in children can be diagnosed on the basis of typical facies or facial dysmorphism. The physician must be equipped with some core knowledge because chance favors only the prepared mind. *It is well known that what mind knows, it is more likely to explore and unravel in the patient.* The diagnosis of acute post-streptococcal glomeruloncphritis can only be made, if one knows that it is characterized by acute onset of puffiness and edema feet, oliguria and smoky urine (microscopic hematuria), hypertension and azotemia following two weeks later after an inadequately treated or missed attack of acute streptococcal pharyngitis.

THE ART OF DIAGNOSIS

"Oh God, let my mind be ever clear and enlightened. By the bedside of the patient, let no alien thought deflect it. Let everything that experience and scholarship have taught it be present in it and hinder it not in its tranquil work. For great and noble are those scientific judgements that serve the purpose of preserving health and lives of thy creatures......."

Moses ben Maimonides

The diagnostic process is one of the greatest challenges in medicine. The patient should be viewed as a jigsaw puzzle and physician should be calm, relaxed and methodical to solve the dilemma. The evidence (demography, epidemiology, symptoms, signs, investigations) pertaining to the patient should be sifted and analyzed through a process of logical thinking in the light of core knowledge, experience and clinical judgement of the pediatrician to arrive at plausible diagnostic possibilities. All the points in favor and against a particular diagnosis should be listed and carefully sifted to arrive at a final diagnosis. The physician should have thorough understanding of basic principles to solve the diagnostic puzzle and be aware of limitations of his own knowledge to avoid dogmatism. There is no place for expressions, such as NEVER and ALWAYS in medicine. The greater the ignorance, greater is the dogmatism. Be humble and don't have "know all" attitude. It is wiser to confess ignorance than to "beat about the bush" or give silly explanations. *We must keep in mind that our knowledge in matters of health and disease is like a pond while our ignorance is Atlantic.* The following principles are useful to keep in mind while making a diagnosis.

1. The psychogenic label is the commonest refuge of the inexperienced physician lacking in diagnostic skills. The functional disorder should be diagnosed both by exclusion of an organic disorder and by the presence of positive evidences of a psychogenic disturbance. The attention must be paid to the whole child along with his environment rather than merely to his body organs. The focus should be the child and not his disease. Ask the mother how the index child differs or compares with other siblings. The behavior and personality disorder in a child is a reflection of parental discord and the child should be considered as a barometer of the family's emotional health. The psychological symptoms in a child is a signal to implore us, "please help my family."

2. It is important to keep in mind that common diseases occur more commonly. *The rare manifestations of a common disorder are more common than the common manifestations of a rare disorder.* When a symptom or a sign is commonly found in a large number of diseases, its absence is more significant than its presence for making a specific diagnosis.
3. Give due credence to the diagnosis made by the previous physician but do not accept it as a gospel truth. You should make your own decision regarding the likely diagnosis based on the sequence of events, course of the disease, leads obtained on investigations and therapeutic response to medications.
4. Efforts should be made to fit the total clinical picture into a single diagnostic entity. This is more often possible in a child as compared to an adult. No diagnosis should be taken for granted, even when it is attributed to a reliable physician or a renowned medical institution, unless it is based on a sound evidence and logic.
5. Avoid masking symptoms and signs by giving drugs to a patient with an evolving disease process. Do not instil mydriatics into the eyes for examination of fundus or give sedatives to a child with head injury because this would compromise the diagnostic utility of pupillary size and level of consciousness. In a case of undiagnosed acute abdomen or head injury, strong analgesics and sedatives should be avoided.
6. Do not delay the surgical diagnostic procedure or a laparotomy whenever it is indicated.
7. The diagnosis of a curable disease should not be overlooked. When clinical picture is compatible both with tuberculosis and Hodgkin's disease, it is preferable to confirm the diagnosis by a lymph node biopsy before starting the treatment.
8. Do not allow the social position of the patient or family to limit your examination. Undress the child completely whenever necessary. Incomplete or cursory examination is the most important cause of diagnostic misadventures.
9. Be confident but don't be biased or dogmatic in your approach. Be humble with due empathy and consideration.
10. The diagnosis may be made in stages and do not hesitate to revise your diagnosis after a period of observation. The appearance of new symptoms and signs, as the disease evolves, may offer additional diagnostic clues. Sir Robert Hutchison, the legendary clinician, has enunciated several don'ts for the diagnosticians *(Box 1.2)*.

Box 1.2 Don'ts for diagnosticians
- Don't be too clever
- Don't diagnose rarities
- Don't be in a hurry
- Don't be faddy
- Don't mistake a label for diagnosis
- Don't diagnose two diseases simultaneously
- Don't be too cocksure
- Don't be biased
- Don't hesitate to revise your diagnosis
- Don't be dogmatic
- Don't be arrogant
- Don't ignore your intuition and common sense

THE DIAGNOSTIC POSSIBILITIES

In allopathic system of medicine, most diseases can be classified into eight broad etiologic groups (Table 1.1). Infections account for over 75% of all diseases. In children, protein-calorie malnutrition and deficiency of micronutrients (vitamins and minerals) constitutes the core health problem which makes children susceptible to develop infective disorders which are likely to run a relatively protracted and fulminant course. Overnutrition and obesity are emerging as public health problems among adolescent children belonging to affluent or well-to-do families. Most genetic (inborn errors of metabolism), chromosomal and developmental abnormalities manifest during childhood. The degenerative disorders due to aging are uncommon

TABLE 1.1 The spectrum of diagnostic possibilities

Etiology	Spectrum of diseases
Infections	Viral, bacterial, spirochetal, fungal and parasitic
Exogenous toxins and injuries	Drugs, chemicals, foreign body, trauma, burns, and electric shock
Deficiency states or disorders of abundance*	Hypoxia, dehydration, protein-calorie malnutrition, deficiency of vitamins, minerals, and hormones
Developmental disorders	Genetic diseases, or inborn errors of metabolism, chromosomal disorders and congenital malformations
Neoplasms	Benign or malignant
Allergic, hypersensitivity, or autoimmune disorders	Allergic diathesis, atopy, bronchial asthma, post-infectious disorders, collagen vascular or connective tissue disorders, etc.
Degenerative disorders	Atherosclerosis, progeria, degenerative disorders of central nervous system
Psychogenic and psycho-somatic disorders	Breath-holding spells, nocturnal enuresis, recurrent abdominal pain, anxiety, conversion reaction, conduct disorders, behavior disorders, depression, autism spectrum disorders, attention deficit hyperactivity disorder, substance abuse, learning disability, etc.

*For example, hyperoxia (retinopathy of prematurity), over hydration (over infusion, low oncotic pressure, capillary damage), obesity, hypervitaminosis, excessive release of hormones (thyrotoxicosis, gigantism, hypercorticism, insulinoma).

in children but there is a need to identify various clinical and laboratory markers for these disorders so that preventive strategies can be instituted during childhood to reduce the burden of these diseases during adult life. *We must remember that seeds of most adult diseases, like obesity, hypertension, type 2 diabetes mellitus and coronary artery disease, are sown in childhood.* After clinical assessment, a tentative diagnosis should be made and various differential diagnostic possibilities in the order of their probability should be listed before ordering laboratory investigations.

It is essential to make a complete diagnosis including the *primary condition and likely cause, associated complications,* like intercurrent infections, and *concomitant disorders.* For example; protein-calorie malnutrition, marasmic type, faulty feeding and weaning practices, recurrent diarrhea, hypothermia, nutritional anemia, zinc deficiency, primary pulmonary complex and scabies.

In systemic disorders, the clinical diagnosis should indicate the site of disease *(anatomy), physiologic basis, pathology, etiology, predisposing or risk factors, complications* and *associated disorders.* The examples of clinical diagnoses in various systemic disorders are given below.

Alimentary System and Abdomen

1. A case of cirrhosis (pathology) following viral hepatitis (etiology) with portal hypertension, anemia, hepatocellular failure, and hematemesis (complications) and a past history of blood transfusion at the age of 3 years (risk factor).
2. A case of failure to thrive with recurrent episodes of diarrhea (malabsorption) due to fibrocystic disease of pancreas (pathology) with iron deficiency anemia, rickets and rectal prolapse (complications).

Respiratory System

1. A case of right upper lobe (anatomy) consolidation (pathology) probably due to bacterial pneumonia (etiology) with empyema (complication) following pyoderma and protein-energy malnutrition (risk factors).
2. A case of left-sided (anatomy) pleural effusion (pathology) probably because of tuberculous origin (etiology) with history of primary pulmonary complex at 2 years of age (risk factor).

Cardiovascular System

1. A case of mitral (anatomy) stenosis (physiology) of rheumatic origin (etiology) without any congestive heart failure or rheumatic activity and the patient is in sinus rhythm at present.
2. A case of mitral stenosis and aortic (anatomy) incompetence (physiology) of rheumatic origin (etiology) with bacterial endocarditis, cardiac failure and atrial fibrillations (complications).

Central Nervous System

1. A case of spastic paraparesis in extension (deficit or physiology) due to compressive myelopathy caused by caries spine (etiology) and the lesion is at the level of T10 segment of the spinal cord (anatomy or site of lesion) with urinary retention and urinary tract infection (complications).
2. A case of left-sided complete hemiplegia (deficit or physiology) due to cerebral thrombosis involving lenticostriate branch of middle cerebral artery (etiology) and site of lesion is in the right internal capsule (anatomy or site of lesion) with protein-energy malnutrition and impetigo (associated conditions).

THE RATIONAL MANAGEMENT

The purpose of making a correct diagnosis is to institute rational therapy and provide prognostic guidelines to the family. It is preferable to use a single most appropriate therapeutic agent, which should be administered in an optimal dose through the most convenient route, instead of instituting a "shot gun" therapy with half a dozen drugs. Avoid administration of unnecessary medicines. The most experienced physician gives the least number of medicines. Most diseases recover spontaneously and no drug is entirely safe. Virtually every drug has side effects including a placebo! It is desirable to use familiar drugs which have withstood the test of time. The newer drugs or procedures are not necessarily better. The discomfort and pain of the patient must be relieved by appropriate and safe medicines with due regard for their comfort and wellbeing.

"A person may have learnt a great deal and still be an exceedingly unskillful physician, who awakens little confidence in his powers....... The manner of dealing with patients, art of winning their confidence, soothing and consoling them, or drawing their attention to serious matters ...... all this cannot be learnt from books ...."
John Apley

We must provide global health care to the child rather than mere cure against a disease process. A comprehensive advice regarding diet, personal hygiene and immunizations should be given to all children irrespective of the underlying disease process. The medical systems should not be fragmented into watertight compartments and instead all systems including complementary and alternative systems (CAS) should be exploited and harnessed to provide relief. The Government of India has introduced the concept of AYUSH by providing a kit to primary health care providers, which contains **A**yurvedic, **U**nani, **S**iddha and **H**omeopathic medicines, apart from medicines belonging to the modern or Allopathic system. However, it is illogical to treat a patient simultaneously with a homeopathic as well as allopathic medicines because the former is supposed to expel out the disease while the latter tries to suppress it. The physician must establish a rapport with the child and his parents to provide them emotional support and win their confidence.

The pediatrician who is likely to exhibit evidences of hurry, worry, and indecision is unlikely to inspire confidence in his patients. The skillful physician knows when to sedate with drugs, when to soothe with words, when to treat aggressively for cure, palliatively for relief and consolingly for comfort. What we don't say and what we do say, how we say it and when we say it, makes all the difference between helping and not helping our patients. These attributes and skills cannot be learnt from books but by emulating the example of one's model teachers which are unfortunately a dwindling tribe in the modern commercialized society.

The patients and attendants have emotional feelings and one should avoid saying "nothing can be done" (because something can always be done), "there is nothing wrong" (even when it is a functional disorder), "don't worry", "it is all right", etc. The *world needs caring and concerned physicians, and not merely curing and commercial robots who lack compassion and deny the healing virtues of hope and human touch.* Identify the major worries and fears of the child and his parents. Relieve their anxiety, reassure them and restore their confidence so that the will to fight is never dulled or extinguished. Nevertheless, we should be honest and pragmatic towards our patients. There is hardly any place for use of injections in ambulatory pediatric practice except for the administration of vaccines and treatment of anaphylactoid reaction.

The news regarding the incurable or serious disease in a child should preferably be disclosed to both the parents simultaneously by the consultant with due concern, empathy and compassion. The dialogue should be unhurried and parents should be encouraged to express their feelings, fears and concerns by asking questions. It has been rightly said by Bernie Siegel that "Our power to heal people and their lives seems to have diminished as dramatically as our power to cure diseases has increased by the technology boom". In the maze of scientific advances, we seem to have lost the human dimension. There is a need to resurrect the art of medicine. *There is no doubt that we should make sincere efforts not only to become knowledgeable and skillful physicians but we should strive to evolve as effective healers and above all good human beings.* These virtues of physicians are extolled in Charak Samhita "...Though shall behave and act without arrogance and with undistracted mind, humility and constant reflection, though shalt pray for the welfare of all creatures..." When we look at our patients with a smiling, kind and caring eyes, the act of looking becomes a prayer, a meditation and a way of healing. And when we perceive outside world with calmness and clarity, our inner self reflects positive energy, which is endowed with great healing potential.

The principles of rational management of diseases and art of medicine have been beautifully summed up by Sir Robert Hutchison in the following quote:

> *"From inability to let well alone, from too much zeal for the new and contempt for what is old; from putting knowledge before wisdom, science before art and cleverness before common sense, treating patients as cases, from making the cure of the disease more grievous than endurance of the same, good Lord deliver us"*
> **Sir Robert Hutchison**

In order to avoid therapeutic misadventures, there are five messages or pearls of wisdom encapsulated in the aforementioned quote.

1. Most diseases are self-limiting and they recover spontaneously without any drugs. Nature, time and patience are the three great physicians.
2. We should not be enamoured and fascinated or carried away to use newer drugs which have not withstood the test of time and we should remember the well-known dictum that "old is gold".
3. Art of medicine should not be sacrificed at the altar of technology.
4. Patients should not be viewed as systems or organs but in their totality—body, mind, heart, soul and society. A good physician treats the disease, the great physician treats the patient who has the disease.
5. Medicines should be used only when indicated and they should not cause more harm to the patient than the disease itself for which they are prescribed.

We must use those medicines which have withstood the test of time with an assured efficacy and safety track record. It is important to remember that no medicine is entirely safe and it has been cynically summed up by Oliver Wendell Holmes, *"If the whole materia medica as being used now, could be sunk to the bottom of the sea, it would be better for all the mankind – but all the worse for the fishes."*

Integrated Management of Neonatal and Childhood Illnesses (IMNCIs)

WHO and UNICEF in collaboration with many other agencies have adopted an integrated management of neonatal and childhood illnesses strategy to provide comprehensive or holistic approach for welfare and survival of children. Algorithms have been developed to diagnose and manage common childhood diseases. Apart from rational management of common diseases, health workers promote breastfeeding, provide immunizations, health and nutrition education. The emphasis has shifted from purely curative services to a package of comprehensive health preventive, and promotive services at each contact of the health worker with the consumers. The IMNCI strategy is being implemented in a phased manner for teaching of undergraduate medical and nursing students throughout the country.

The Components of IMNCI

The IMNCI guidelines for case management of common diseases have been divided into two age categories, i.e. infants from birth to 2 months and children above 2 months to 5 years of age. The salient guidelines of IMNCI are listed below.

1. The frontline workers, accredited social health activists (ASHAs) and Anganwadi workers (AWWs), after completing their IMNCI training, are required to visit newborns at their households three times during the first week of life. During their visits, the workers assess newborns, promote healthy practices, manage simple problems and refer those with a serious illness to healthcare facilities.
2. All sick infants up to 2 months of age should be assessed for "possible infection and jaundice" and they must be routinely evaluated for the major symptom of "diarrhea".
3. All sick children between 2 months and 5 years should be examined for "general danger signs" which indicate the need for immediate referral or admission to the hospital. They should be routinely assessed for major symptoms, like fever, cough, difficult or rapid breathing, diarrhea and ear problems.
4. All sick under-5 children should be routinely assessed for nutritional and immunization status, feeding problems and other common day-to-day problems.
5. A limited number of carefully selected clinical signs are used, based on their sensitivity and specificity, to diagnose the disease. These signs were selected considering the conditions and ground realities prevalent at the first-level healthcare facilities.
6. On the basis of a combination of various signs, the child is classified into various groups (instead of a diagnoses) and further divided into color-coded triage as *pink* which requires urgent referral or admission to a hospital, *yellow* when specific treatment is required through the outpatient health facility and *green* which calls for home management (Figure 1.2).
7. The IMNCI guidelines address most but not all the major reasons for which a sick infant or child is brought to the clinic. The guidelines, for example, do not describe the management of trauma or other acute emergencies due to various accidents or injuries and also do not cover resuscitation and care of the baby at birth.
8. The management procedures outlined in the IMNCI protocols use a limited number of essential drugs and encourage active participation by caretakers in the treatment of sick infants and children.
9. In order to promote local health traditions and indigenous medicines, village health care workers and ASHAs are provided with a kit of medicines containing AYUSH (Ayurvedic, Unani, Siddha and Homeopathy) and allopathic or modern medicines to treat common day-to-day illnesses.
10. An essential component of the IMNCI guidelines lays emphasis on providing counseling and guidance to caretakers about home care, feeding, administration of fluids, immunizations, healthy lifestyle, etc. and guidelines to return back to health care facility for further management and follow-up.

THE ART OF HEALING

"The best six doctors are sunshine, clean air, safe water, sound sleep, exercise and nutritious diet. These six will attend you only if you are willing, your mind they will mend. And charge you not a shilling."
— **Wayne Fields**

The art of healing comes from nature and physician must exploit the natural forces with an open mind.

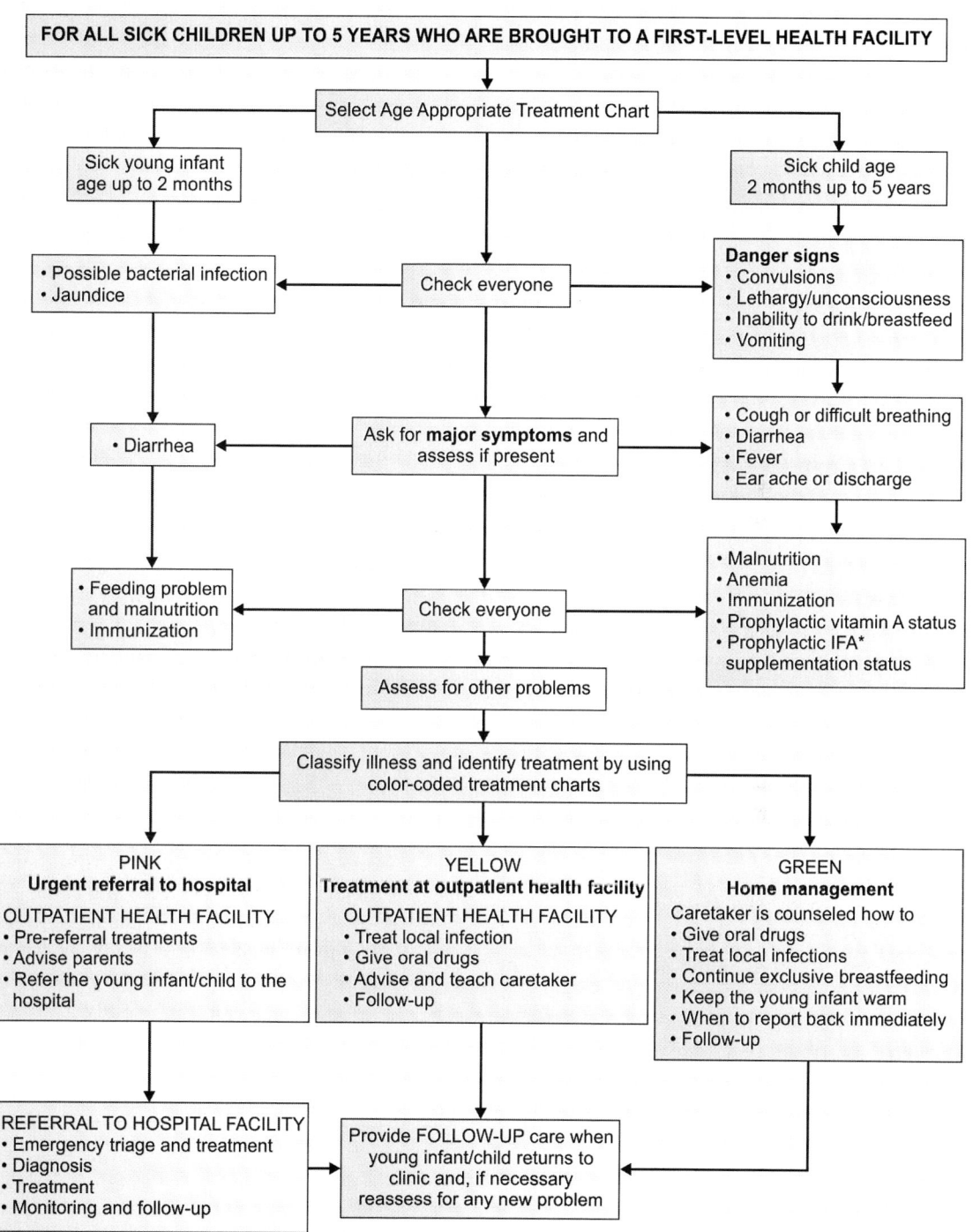

Figure 1.2 IMNCI case management process

The best "doctors" to maintain and promote good health are sunshine, clear air, safe water, sound sleep, exercise, nutritious diet and healthy lifestyle.

Physicians should not underestimate the healing power of touch, smile, a kind word, listening ear, an honest compliment and a genuine act of caring and compassion. The spiritual components of healing include power of touch, divine spirit, human mind, prayer, faith and hope. *The patients should not be merely treated with your head alone but also with your heart.* There is scientific evidence to suggest that the electromagnetic field generated by the human heart is for more powerful than the one created by the human mind. When a physician looks at a patient with a smiling, kind and caring eyes, the act of looking becomes a healing force.

Modern medicine is dominated by the doctrine that the disease is caused by external agents or environment, thus ignoring the importance of host or genome and body-mind integrity or importance of psycho-neuro-immuno-endocrinal interactions. The master controls of our body are nervous system, immune system and endocrine system and the process of healing depends upon their balance and integrity. Physicians treat patients by giving medications but healing originates from within. Several studies have shown that patients and attendants who have a positive attitude, trust their doctor and surrender themselves to his care are more likely to recover than those who approach medicine with distrust, fear and antagonism. According to Bernie Siegel, our healing capabilities are mobilized by love, faith and hope. Anything that offers hope has the potential to heal including positive thoughts, suggestions, symbols and placebos. The physicians must be careful about their body language, how they look at, touch and talk with their patients and attendants. They should not be merely concerned with diseases but with patients as human beings. In order to augment the process of healing, the patient and their attendants must have faith in their doctor and the doctor must have faith in himself and his medicines. According to Hippocrates, the critically sick patients are likely to recover simply through the goodness, concern and capability of their physicians.

> *"The technical and diagnostic skills of a physician are no substitute for his bedside manners"*
> **Meharban Singh**

Medical schools teach everything we need to know about writing prescriptions but nothing about understanding people and our patients. Because of rapid advances in medical technology, the physicians are becoming more of technocrats and less of human beings or healers. It is desirable that doctors should understand their holistic role as health *care* providers and not merely health *cure* providers. The world need caring, concerned and compassionate physicians and not merely curing and commercialized robots. Doctors who believe that they can cure the disease without caring for the patient may be excellent technicians but they are incomplete doctors. It is unfortunate that medicine is getting more and more dehumanized and patients are being touched mostly by the machines and sparingly by the physicians. It should be kept in mind that touching the patient with compassion and concern has great healing capabilities. Medicine and spirituality are complementary to each other in catalyzing the process of healing. The healing forces can be augmented through spiritually guided life forces like activation of body chakras and reiki for balancing the life energy field. According to our scriptures, physicians should see and visualize God in every human being (*Aham Brahman Asmi*) and feel honored that they have been given the supreme responsibility to serve Him. When they follow this celestial principle, their work becomes worship and they become true healers.

PROGNOSIS

> *"Parents (and attendants) have emotional feelings. Never say "nothing can be done", because something can always be done. Never give a hopeless prognosis in order to avoid neglect and sustain the will to fight. Nevertheless be pragmatic and honest"*
> **Meharban Singh**

Most parents and attendants are worried and concerned about the outcome of the disease. They commonly ask "will the child become alright" and "how soon he is likely to recover"? The outcome depends upon the nature and severity of disease process and the type of the host or victim which is afflicted with the disease. Every patient is unique, a treatment method or an educational plan that works in one child, may not work for another. Nevertheless, one common denominator for recovery is early intervention before the disease process is advanced or becomes irreversible. The disease with an acute and sudden onset is likely to have either a dramatic recovery or a deadly outcome.

Most diseases are self-limiting and they recover on supportive management without any medications. Faith, will power, positive thinking and sound genetic constitution are great healers. A true healer cannot simply rely on technology, there must be a spiritual bond between the patient and physician. To augment the process of healing, the patient must have faith in his doctor and doctor must have faith in himself and his medicines. Infants below 3 months and children having protein-energy malnutrition or obesity, immunodeficiency state and defective genome are likely to have poor outcome.

The parents should be handled with due compassion and told about the likely outcome of the disease and possible side effects of the medications. They should be explained about the expected course of the disease. For example, most viral infections are usually self-limiting and likely to take 3–5 days for recovery. The acute onset of vomiting is usually followed by diarrhea after 12–24 hours, and a child with typhoid fever is likely take 4–5 days to settle even after start of specific antimicrobial therapy. The physician must establish a rapport with the child and his parents to provide them emotional support and win their faith, trust and confidence.

When a child is suffering from a chronic or incurable disease or an affliction with a lifelong disability, the parents are likely to respond with disbelief, anger and shock. The news about a disabling or deadly disease should preferably be given to both the parents simultaneously with due concern, compassion and empathy. The facts should be explained in a simple language without any medical jargon. The physician should allow the parents to ventilate their feelings and concerns, and try to answer their queries in an honest and unambiguous manner. Physician should be pragmatic but not pessimistic. It is important to remain positive and hopeful, which is a great healing force. Hope is the greatest healer and we should give a guarded but not a hopeless prognosis. It is important to remember that nature is supreme and miracles do happen.

We should be careful and diplomatic in conveying the nature of the disease without hurting parental feelings. Instead of bluntly saying, "your child is mentally retarded", it is better to say that the child is rather "slow" or having "developmental delay". In Indian society, giving a spiritual context to parents of "special children" is useful to buffer their anxiety and feeling of hopelessness. *For example, you can say that "God has chosen you to provide care and comfort to this special child because you are so compassionate, caring and sensitive human being."* The family should be encouraged to join Self Help Association of Parents to share their mutual concerns and difficulties, and ensure effective utilization of available specialized services.

End-of-Life Issues

"Death is certain for the born and rebirth is inevitable for the dead. You should not, therefore, grieve over the inevitable."

Bhagavad Gita

During their career, physicians are likely to face several "end-of-life" situations. *Despite all the technological advances, medicine can never achieve immortality!* It is as natural to die as to be born. When faced with a critically sick or dying child, physician should allow the parents to express their feelings and concerns and try to answer their queries in an honest and unambiguous manner. In this situation, we should follow the well-known dictum—"talk less and listen more." The coping of death of a child in the hospital is a painful and challenging experience for everybody concerned with the care of the child.

Death deflates our ego and teaches us humility and provides strength to handle the greatest reality of life with equanimity, composure and confidence. During the care of critically sick children in the intensive care unit, it is important to show due concern, care and compassion (but in a detached manner) to the parents/attendants, and keep them duly informed about the condition of their child. *It is important that the physician should not only provide state-of-the-art care to the child but also make the parents and attendants preceive that whatever was humanely possible, it was done for their child.* The family should be emotionally and spiritually prepared before declaration of death. The news of death should be conveyed with utmost compassion but in no unmistakable terms that the child has died despite our best intents and efforts. When a child is conscious and dying, the parents should be at his bedside holding his hand and talking with him to allay his fears and provide him emotional support, for his journey to the unknown.

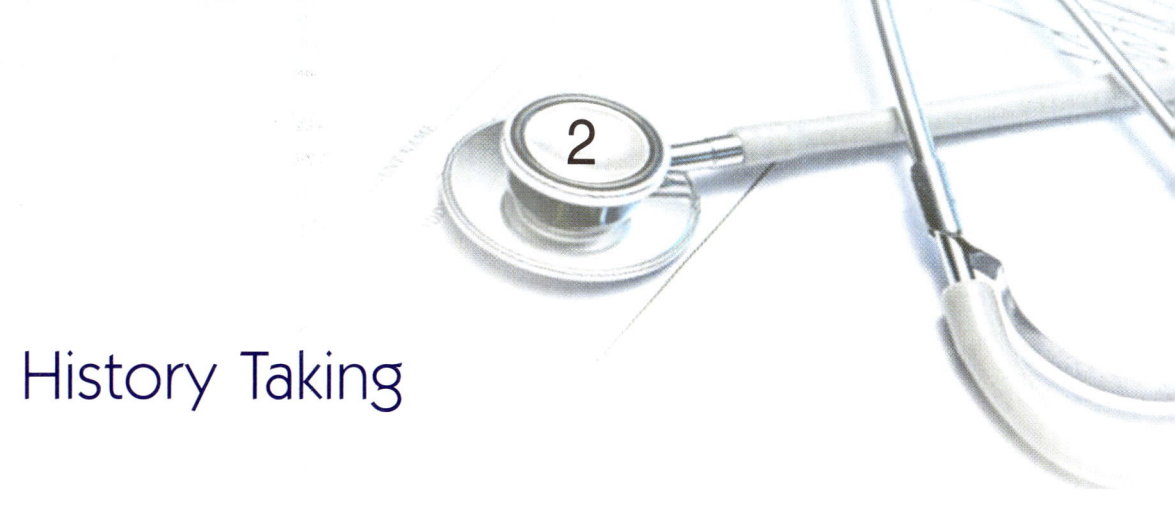

History Taking

"Methods of physicians are like those of a detective, one seeking to explain the disease, other a crime".
Arthur Conan Doyle

History taking is an art and demands skills of a lawyer, detective and judge. It requires inquisitiveness, persistence and tact. The physician should strive to obtain a lucid chronological story of child's illness with special emphasis on mode of onset, course of events and evolution of disease process. Pediatrics has been likened to veterinary medicine because young children cannot express their symptoms. The symptomatology in young children is often "colored" by the perceptions of "caregivers" or the parents. An intelligent and observant mother can provide satisfactory story of illness but at times may exaggerate facts due to her anxiety and concern. Father spends little time with the child and is generally ill-informed about child's problems. Schoolgoing children can give a fair account of their physical difficulties and should always be encouraged to talk and explain their symptoms.

The physician must exhibit humility, concern and politeness while recording the history. He should be gentle, sympathetic, gracious and kind in his approach but alert and attentive. During history taking, provide positive non-verbal cues to enhance doctor–patient/parent communication. You should lean forward, listen attentively with interest, maintain eye contact, nod appropriately, do not cross your arms or exhibit any sense of superiority or arrogance.

The clinician should maintain a friendly, warm, relaxed, unhurried and informal atmosphere throughout the interaction with the family. Always keep your mind open and receptive—even an experienced physician can learn something new from his patients and their attendants. There is a popular saying, that *"a smart mother or grandmother can make a better diagnosis than a dull doctor"*. Physician must remember that the patient is his honored client and he should relieve the anxiety of the parents and instil confidence in them towards himself during the interview. However, he should not behave like an enthusiastic salesman by dramatizing the illness of the child. It is often forgotten that while you are taking history and assessing the attendant and child, you are also being assessed by them on the basis of your behavior and approach. Your facial expression, tone of the voice, body language and attitude of impatience, arrogance, disbelief and reproach can all affect the outcome of communication between the doctor and patient/parents.

History taking is the beginning of the most crucial doctor–patient (parent) relationship, which is essential for developing mutual trust and confidence. The doctor must know his or her own personality, recognize weaknesses and develop strengths and abilities to improve his or her communication skills. Assess the quality of parent–child and parent–parent relationship while recording history and conducting physical examination. Unsatisfactory parent–child or mother–father interaction may lead to emotional deprivation or psychosocial and behavior disorder in the child.

The consultation room should be well lighted, comfortable, quiet and decorated with toys and pictures to allay the anxiety of the child (Figure 2.1). There should be no distractions and disturbing sounds, the mobiles should be kept on silent mode. Infants and young children should be offered a soft squeaky toy or a rattle to establish rapport while taking history. Schoolgoing children feel at ease when they are directly asked their name, details about school, hobbies and health problems. While taking history, the child should be observed "sneakily" for facial appearance, discomfort, distress and dyspnea (Figure 2.2). Avoid staring at the child because children are often scared, if you intently look into their eyes. Watch him without yourself being watched by the child. The child must visualize the physician as the friend of the mother and not a frightening figure who prescribes painful pricks and pungent potions.

It must be remembered that most common diseases can be diagnosed by good history alone. Elicitation of history should continue during physical examination to seek additional information especially when unexpected abnormal physical findings are detected. History and physical examination should be viewed in continuum and one should influence the other. The leads obtained on history should encourage the pediatrician to pay special attention to certain organ(s) on physical examination. The presence of positive physical findings should encourage the pediatrician to seek more detailed review of the symptoms pertaining to the involved system. To gain the confidence of parents and child, the pediatrician should maintain a friendly, warm, unhurried, courteous, informal and relaxed attitude throughout the assessment. You must put the parent or attendant at ease and encourage him or her to talk freely. Never judge or belittle the mother, instead encourage and support her. You should provide positive non-verbal cues to

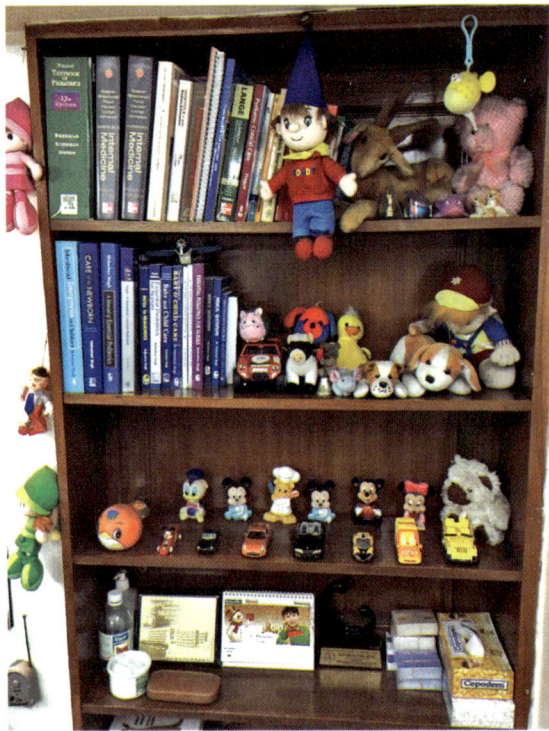

Figure 2.1 Ambulatory clinic stocked with toys to create a child-friendly ambience.

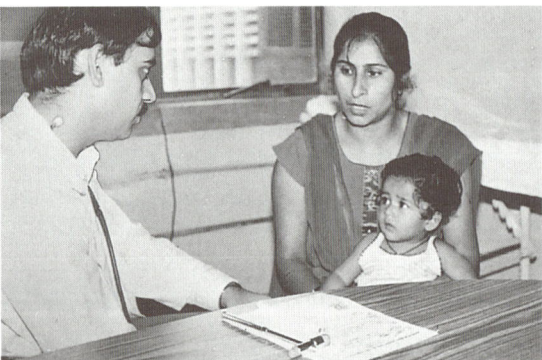

Figure 2.2 The cordial atmosphere is crucial while recording history. The pediatrician is watching the child sneakily while child is "evaluating" the pediatrician during history taking. In this situation, the child is likely to cooperate during examination.

the family. Your behavior should not be influenced by the social and educational status of the parents. Instead you must visualize God in every human being and feel honored that you have been given the responsibility to serve Him.

BASIC INFORMATION

The salient components of history taking are summarized in *Box 2.1*. Informant (mother, father, relative, child, etc.), name, age (preferably date of birth) and sex of the patient should be enquired. Parent's name, age, address, telephone number, income, occupation, education and religion should be recorded. The history may be unreliable due to informant's poor memory, intelligence or education. The origin and ethnic background of the family is important in some genetic diseases. Thalassemia trait and disease are common among migrants from west Pakistan. Glucose-6-phosphate dehydrogenase deficiency is common among Parsis and north Indians while sickle cell disease is seen among tribal population.

Box 2.1 Key points for taking history

- Personal and demographic details
- Presenting complaints
- History of present illness
- Onset
  - Symptom review
  - System review
  - Medications received
- Course of events
- Past history
  - Perinatal events
  - Significant illnesses and accidents
  - Physical growth and developmental milestones
- Family history
  - Genetic diagram
- Social history and lifestyle of the family
- Feeding history
- Immunization status

PRESENTING COMPLAINTS

The chief complaints for which the patient has been brought to the hospital should be recorded in a chronological order in accordance with sequence of events, e.g. fever 5 days, headache 3 days, vomiting 3 days, convulsions 1 day and loss of consciousness 12 hours. The key symptoms obtained on history should initiate a cascade of logical reasoning, based on the experience and knowledge of the physician to consider plausible diagnostic possibilities or hypotheses for further probing.

HISTORY OF PRESENT ILLNESS

The informant should be encouraged to give details of sequence of events during the course of illness without the help of leading questions. You must put the parent or attendant at ease and encourage him or her to talk freely. The mode of onset, course of disease and details of treatment already received must be recorded in all cases. The parents are very keen to tell you what the previous doctor(s) thought about the child's illness and often use terms like rheumatism, weak liver, acidity, tonsils, migraine, etc. You should not brush them aside but assure them that you shall see all the documents and reports but "let me first understand or grasp the problem". A detailed information pertaining to various symptoms manifested by the patient should be elicited (symptom review). The symptoms referable to various body systems should be reviewed in order to identify the site of the disease (system review). The history should provide information whether the disease is localized to a specific body system or is generalized by involving several body organs and systems. The purpose of detailed review of symptoms is to identify the anatomical site(s) and etiology of disease process. The clinical characteristics and morphology of common symptoms are given below.

Cry

Cry is the "language" of the child and an important signal of discomfort, boredom or hunger. The intelligent mother can differentiate between the cry of a well baby (hunger, wet napkin, sleepiness and boredom) from that of a sick baby. Infants with painful conditions, like intestinal colic, acute otitis media, inflammatory or traumatic conditions of bones and joints, torsion of testis, etc., are likely to have incessant unconsolable crying and they cannot be pacified by cuddling or feeding. Cry is an important symptom of hypoxia in infants with lower respiratory tract infection and obstructive airway disease. A high-pitched shrill cry is a characteristic feature of cerebral irritation and raised intracranial tension (meningitis) and tetanus neonatorum. In some conditions, like arthritis, osteomyelitis, periosteitis, abscess, peritonitis, etc., the crying becomes worse when child is picked up. These children are relatively more comfortable when undisturbed. Hoarse cry is a feature of "excessive crying", cretinism, laryngitis, laryngotracheobronchitis and paralysis of left recurrent laryngeal nerve due to compression by dilated main pulmonary trunk. Crying due to temper tantrum or fussiness in healthy pre-school children (6 months – 3 years) may be followed by breath holding spell. The child usually cries or screams loudly, holds the breath in expiration for 20–30 sec and becomes blue (cyanotic) or pale (pallid). Rarely, the child may exhibit seizure like activity with transient loss of consciousness. In a child with tetralogy of Fallot, crying is a feature of cyanotic or tet spell.

Fever

The normal body temperature is maintained within a narrow range of 98.2°F ±0.7°F (36.8°C ±0.4°C). Fever is defined as an elevation of oral temperature above 100°F (>37.8°C). Hyperpyrexia is diagnosed when rectal temperature exceeds 105.8°F (>41.0°C). Onset (acute or insidious), duration, character (continuous, remittent, intermittent, step-ladder type, Pel-Ebstein, etc.), severity, chills and rigors, associated localizing symptoms, etc. should be enquired. Pel-Ebstein relapsing fever is characterized by episodes of fever lasting for 3–10 days followed by afebrile periods of 3–10 days and is a classical feature of Hodgkin disease and other lymphomas. Young children cannot complain of chills (perception of extreme cold) but rigors may be observed by the mother as goose skin, vigorous shaking movements or tremors. When body temperature never touches normal and daily fluctuations are less than 1°C, it is described as continuous fever. When the daily fluctuations exceed 2°C, it is called remittent or hectic fever which is a characteristic feature of septicemia and Kawasaki disease. Evening rise of fever occurs in most infections but is a characteristic feature of tuberculosis and juvenile rheumatoid arthritis.

In intermittent pyrexia, the temperature may touch or remain normal daily (quotidian), every alternate day (tertian) or after every two days (quartan) (Figure 2.3). Quotidian fever occurs due to a number of conditions including juvenile chronic arthritis, tertian fever occurs classically due to *Plasmodium vivax* malaria and quartan fever because of *Plasmodium malariae* malaria. However, because of widespread use of antipyretics and antibiotics, the classical pattern of fever is no longer seen. During therapy, fever may settle down quickly within 6–12 hours with marked sweating (crisis) or slowly over several days (lysis).

Hyperthermia is defined as an alteration of temperature homeostasis because of unregulated rise in heat production (exercise, drugs), decrease in heat dissipation (rise in ambient temperature) or failure of hypothalamic thermoregulation (brain injury).

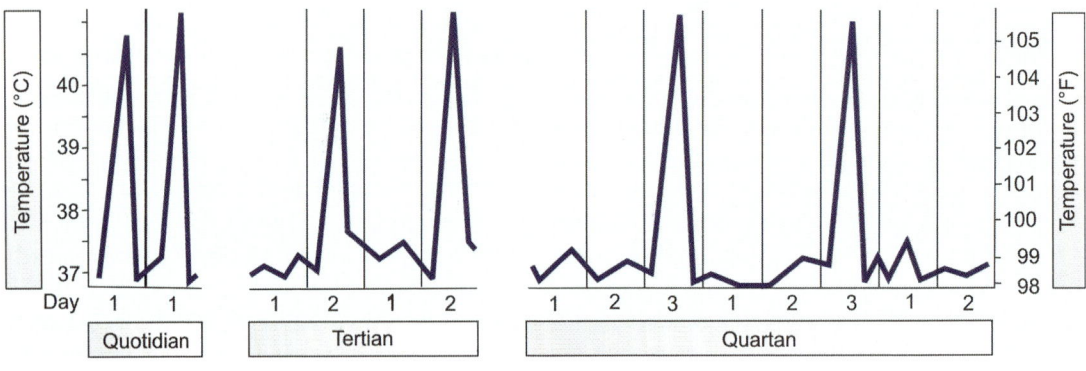

Figure 2.3 Types of intermittent fever.

Cough

The duration, frequency, character (hacking, brassy, barking, paroxysmal cough) followed by long and deep noisy inspiration ('whoop'), should be looked for. Ask whether cough is dry or productive, postural relationship, diurnal variations and associated features. In children with bronchitis, wheezing and congestive heart failure, cough is worse on lying down and during sleep. Cough is worse at night and early morning in children with bronchial asthma. Infants do not expectorate but they swallow the phlegm and may vomit it out. History of inhalation of a foreign body should always be enquired in any child with sudden onset of choking and cough with breathlessness and in children with recurrent or persistent pulmonary suppuration. Many a times clinical morphology of cough provides more useful information than findings on auscultation of chest. The characteristic nature of various types of cough and the likely underlying causes are listed in Table 2.1.

TABLE 2.1 Differential diagnosis of a child with cough

Type of cough	Likely cause/s
Dry hacking cough	Throat irritation due to pharyngitis, sour or spicy food
Productive or "chesty" cough	Bronchiolitis or bronchitis, bronchial asthma, bronchopneumonia, and bronchiectasis
"Throat-clearing" cough	Post-nasal drip, sinusitis, enlarged adenoids, and psychological cough
Hoarseness with "croupy" or barking cough	Laryngitis and tracheitis
Paroxysmal cough with or without vomiting*	Pertussis, bronchial asthma, foreign body inhalation, and endobronchial tuberculosis
Nocturnal and early morning cough	Bronchitis, bronchial asthma, left ventricular failure, bronchiectasis, and mucoviscidosis
Cough after exercise or cold water bath	Exercise or cold-triggered asthma

*Phlegm is passed in the vomitus which is followed by relief of cough.

Vomiting

Regurgitation of feeds (possetting) is a common symptom in infants due to swallowing of air while feeding or crying (aerophagy). Some children are very vulnerable to vomit following a bout of cough or when food is forced or medicine is given. Ask the duration, severity and frequency of vomiting and whether it is associated with nausea or anorexia. The presence of bile or fecal matter in the vomitus is suggestive of intestinal obstruction. Blood-tinged phlegm or vomitus is a common correlate of epistaxis. Frankly bloody vomiting (hematemesis) is a medical emergency. Aggravating factors and associated symptoms often provide useful clues to the diagnosis. Association of vomiting with fever, headache, neck rigidity and alteration in consciousness are suggestive of meningitis. The presence of abdominal distension and absolute constipation with nonpassage of flatus is diagnostic of intestinal obstruction. When vomiting is followed by development of diarrhea it is indicative of acute gastroenteritis or food poisoning. Episodes of vomiting with fever, ketosis and acidosis are suggestive of diabetic ketoacidosis. Cyclical vomiting may occur due to autonomic dysfunction or visceral epilepsy. Ask for symptoms of dehydration, such as excessive thirst, absence of sweating or tears, reduced frequency of passing urine or anuria.

Diarrhea

Some infants may pass stools after each feed, due to exaggerated gastrocolic reflex, and it should not be mistaken with diarrhea. Diarrheal episodes are common in bottle- or sipper-fed children due to intake of contaminated or infected feeds. Ask for history of duration, severity and frequency (purge-rate) of diarrhea and associated symptoms, like fever, vomiting and colicky abdominal pain. Assess the bulk (small or bulky), consistency (watery, rice-water, semiloose or semisolid), contents (undigested food particles, steatorrhea, froth, mucus, pus, blood), color (yellow, pale, green) and odor (foul smelling, rancid) of stools. Dysentery is characterized by passage of blood and mucus in the stools, tenesmus (frequent urge to defecate but with little evacuation) and rectal prolapse. Ask for symptoms and correlates of dehydration, like inadequate intake of fluids, excessive crying due to thirst, absence of sweat or tears, cold extremities, oliguria and anuria.

Pain Abdomen

> "The further away the chronic abdominal pain in a child is from the umbilicus, it is more likely to have an organic cause."
>
> *John Apley*

Duration, frequency, timing, site (vague, precise, localized, diffuse), severity (mild, moderate, severe, excruciating), character (burning, piercing, boring, colicky), radiation, precipitating, aggravating and relieving factors, and associated symptoms should be asked and recorded.

The characteristics of pain can be remembered by an acronym SOCRATES which stands for **S**ite, **O**nset, **C**haracter, **R**adiation, **A**ssociated symptoms, **T**iming, **E**xacerbating and relieving factors and **S**everity. The child with recurrent abdominal pain, if puts his whole hand vaguely in an unconcerned manner over the navel or whole of abdomen to indicate the site of pain, is most likely having a functional or psychogenic disorder. When pain abdomen is associated with pain at multiple body sites, like headache, chest pain and body aches, it is likely to be functional rather than organic. Episodes of momentary abdominal pain which occur at home and in relation to intake of food, are usually due to attention seeking behavior, or food fussiness. When pain occurs in school or during play activity or child wakes up with pain at night, the site of pain is away from umbilicus, it is likely to be due to organic causes.

Common Symptoms due to Involvement of Various Body Systems

The common symptoms referrable to various body systems are listed in Table 2.2. It is important to give due credit to all observations of the parents, even if they do not fit into your line of thinking or diagnosis. Parents often confuse between pallor and jaundice, hematemesis and hemoptysis, rigors and seizures, breath-holding spells and seizures, pus

TABLE 2.2 Review of systems

General features
- Fever
- Crying, irritability and lethargy
- Loss of appetite
- Body aches
- Pallor
- Lassitude, "off color", fatigue, lack of vigor or interest in play activity
- Failure to thrive

Gastrointestinal system and abdomen
- Pain abdomen
- Dysphagia
- Vomiting
- Diarrhea or constipation
- Bulky or oily stool
- Dyspepsia and gastroesophageal reflux
- Anorexia or excessive appetite
- Distension or "wind"
- Jaundice
- Hematemesis and hematochezia
- Anal itching
- Rectal prolapse
- Failure to thrive

Genitourinary system
- Pain abdomen
- Tight prepuce
- Dysuria
- Frequency of micturition
- Nocturnal enuresis
- Hematuria or tea-colored urine
- Oliguria or anuria
- Puffiness of face and swelling of feet
- Inguinoscrotal swelling or genital anomaly
- Sexual maturity
- Failure to thrive

Respiratory system
- Cough
- Coryza
- Sneezing
- Nasal congestion
- Breathing difficulty
- Wheezing
- Cyanosis and clubbing
- Vomiting preceded by bouts of cough
- Chest pain

Cardiovascular system
- Tachypnea and dyspnea
- Palpitations
- Feeding difficulties

(contd.)

TABLE 2.2 Review of systems (*contd.*)

- Puffiness of face and swelling of feet
- Cough and breathing difficulty in supine position (orthopnea)
- Cyanosis and clubbing
- Chest pain

Hematologic system
- Lassitude, irritability, fatigue, and exertional dyspnea
- Pica
- Petechiae and blood loss
- Bone pains
- Enlarged glands or swellings in neck, axillae and groins
- Dietary and drug history

Central nervous system
- Slow or delayed neuromotor development
- High-pitched crying, irritability, alterations in sleep, behavior and consciousness
- Learning disability
- Syncope
- Vertigo
- Abnormalities in the size of head and any spinal defects
- Symptoms suggestive of raised intracranial tension and meningeal irritation: Headache, vomiting, photophobia, neck or spinal stiffness, bradycardia
- Seizures or tremors
- Paralyses
- Incontinence or retention of urine and feces
- Gait abnormalities

and wax in the ears, etc. and you must try to differentiate between them by asking appropriate leading questions.

HISTORY OF MEDICATIONS

History of current medications and their effect on the course of disease process should be enquired. Ask whether child is receiving any long-term medications, or nutritional supplements from any system of medicine. Ask if patient is taking any medications from the complementary and alternative systems. Take note of diagnosis already made or medications being taken but never say a slighting word or talk ill of the prior practitioner colleague. History of any adverse or allergic reactions to any medications in the past should be asked and recorded. Enquire if child is known to be suffering from any genetic disorder (like G-6-PD deficiency, inborn error of metabolism or enzymopathy) which increases the risk of adverse reactions to certain medications. Assess the likely compliance and commitment of the family to administer the medications in a dose, frequency and duration as recommended by the physician.

HISTORY OF PAST ILLNESSES

Ask for past history of common childhood diseases (recurrent upper respiratory tract infections, asthmatic bronchitis, diarrheal episodes, exanthemata, pertussis) and whether they ran a normal, complicated or a protracted course. Details of perinatal history, birth asphyxia, severe neonatal jaundice, and meningitis are important in a child with developmental retardation or seizures. Delayed cry at birth if associated with seizures having onset within first 36 hours of life, abnormal neurological behavior and difficulties in self-feeding are suggestive of significant birth asphyxia. In children suffering from asthma, epilepsy, nephrotic syndrome, arthritis, eczema, etc., enquiry should be made regarding history of similar attacks and their frequency in the past. Specific enquiries should be made regarding previous illnesses which may be related to the present symptoms or illness, e.g. past history of jaundice in a child with cirrhosis, joint pains in a child who is suspected to have rheumatic heart disease, recurrent chest infections in a patient with left-to-right shunt so on and so forth. Ask for any known allergies against environmental pollutants, foods and drugs. Record any previous hospital admissions with dates and diagnosis.

PERINATAL HISTORY

It is pertinent to ask perinatal history when dealing with neonates or infants but may be ignored in older children with normal development and cognition. Ask for history of maternal diseases or medications during pregnancy (especially during first trimester), presentation, mode and place of delivery, first cry after birth, and Apgar score if known. Ask for gestation, birth weight, respiratory distress, feeding difficulties, seizures, sepsis and jaundice during first week of life. Record if baby needed NICU care and assisted ventilation.

DEVELOPMENTAL HISTORY

In children suspected to have delayed development or CNS disorder, a detailed developmental history should be asked. Precise timing of social smile, head control, rolling over, sitting, standing, walking, self-feeding and dressing, bladder and bowel control and speech should be enquired. It is useful to compare the development of the index child with other normal siblings. It is easier for the mother to recall differences in the development of index child as compared to other siblings rather than absolute ages for attaining various milestones of development. Identify whether it is a global developmental retardation, or retardation is present in a specific field, e.g. delayed speech in the presence of normal motor development is indicative of deaf-mutism, while delayed standing and walking with normal social and adaptive development is indicative of protein-energy malnutrition, and congenital dislocation of hips. A detailed assessment of development is discussed in *Chapter 6*.

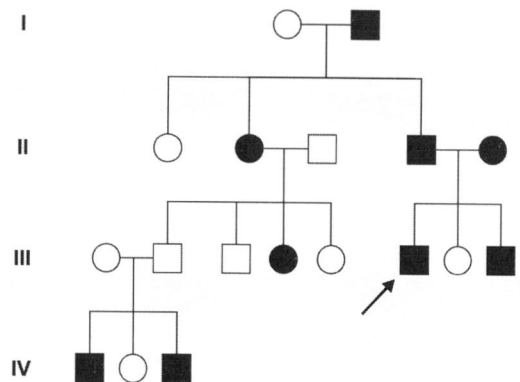

Figure 2.4 Pedigree of four generations of brachydactyly which is inherited as a dominant trait.

FAMILY HISTORY

Family pedigree should be enquired and a genetic diagram or family tree of three or four generations constructed as shown in **Figure 2.4**. Ask information from both the parents and grandparents to identify the nature and mode of inheritance of genetic disorders. The details of symbols used for constructing a pedigree chart are shown in *Box 2.2*. Record whether child is adopted or biological? In an out of family adopted child, it is not possible to ascertain the genetic background.

Consanguinity (blood relationship between parents) refers to kinship of common lineage or ancestory. The offsprings of consanguineous parents are at a greater risk to suffer from certain genetic disorders because of sharing of genes. The closer is the relationship among the parents, greater is the risk of genetic disorder (Table 2.3). The most common consanguineous relationship is first degree cousins, in which the spouses share 1/8 (12.5%) of their genes. According to Ayurveda, marriage within the *Gotra* in Hindu culture is a consanguineous marriage and should be avoided to reduce the burden of genetic disorders. First cousin marriages, are common among Muslims and they have high incidence of genetic disorders.

History of contact with possible infectious illnesses should be sought, e.g. viral fever, tuberculosis, leprosy, childhood infectious diseases, infective hepatitis, typhoid fever, scabies, and pyoderma. The index case may be in the family, neighbourhood, creche or school. History of similar ailment in the family members should be asked when genetic, infective or allergic disorder is strongly suspected. In a child with fever of acute onset, history of fever and coryza among family contacts is highly suggestive of viral infection. Ask for history of consanguinity among parents when a genetic disorder is suspected. In case a particular disease is manifesting only among male siblings, it is suggestive of X-linked inheritance, e.g. hemophilia, pseudohypertrophic muscular dystrophy, G-6-PD deficiency, etc.

SOCIAL HISTORY

Socioeconomic status (SES) is an important determinant of the health and well-being of the family. The useful determinants of social status include education and occupation of the family head and his monthly income. A number of scales are available to objectively assess the SES of the family but Kuppuswamy scale is the most popular. The scale is relevant for urban population and takes

History Taking

Box 2.2 Symbols used for constructing a pedigree chart

Symbol description		Symbol description	
Normal male	□	Affected male	■
Normal female	○	Affected female	●
Sex unknown	◇	Affected but sex unknown	◆ or ?
Adopted	(□)	Proband or propositus	↗■
Mating	□—○	Heterozygous for autosomal gene	◐ ◐
Divorced	□/○	Carrier of X-linked gene	⊡ ⊙
Consanguineous mating	□=○	Deceased	⌀
Woman with children sired from two men	□—○—□ with children	Adopted child	(dashed line to circle)
Dizygotic or fraternal twins	/\ □ ○	Foster child	(dotted line to circle)
Monozygotic or identical twins	/\ with bar	Pregnancy	△
Triplets	/|\	Abortion	▲ crossed
Zygosity uncertain	/\ □?○	Miscarriage	▲ crossed small

Birth order from oldest to youngest is shown from left to right below or to the right of the genogram symbol, or alternatively date of birth or age can be mentioned. In case of death, age at death can be mentioned. Gestational age can be mentioned in case of abortion or stillbirth.

TABLE 2.3 Degrees of consanguinity

Degree of consanguinity	Percentage of shared genes	Relationship
First degree	50%	Parents, children and siblings
Second degree	25%	Grandparents, uncles, aunts, nephews, nieces, and half-siblings
Third degree	12.5%	First degree cousins
	3.1%	Second degree cousins

into account education, occupation and income of the family head. The steady inflation and resultant devaluation of Indian rupee and increase in the consumer price index, necessitates periodic revisions of the income variable. The modified Kuppuswamy SES scale 2016 is shown in Table 2.4. Instead of monthly income of family head, it is more logical to know the total income or per capita income of the family. Other variables, which are ignored in most SES scales, include habitat (rural, urban, semi-urban or slums), type of housing or dwelling conditions, availability of safe drinking water, toilet facilities, and availability of reliable and affordable medical facilities within a reasonable distance.

If mother is working, ask who looks after the child at home when she is away or is the child left in a creche. Ask whether the family is nuclear or joint and whether grandparents are staying with the family or not. Calculate per capita income by dividing total income of the family by the number of family members. Housing conditions, toilet facilities, sewage disposal and water source should be asked. Ethnic background and religion may provide clues to certain genetic disorders. Harmful social and cultural practices regarding child rearing should be identified, e.g. dummy nipple or pacifier, complementary bottle or sipper feeding, use of *kajal, janam ghutti*, etc.

Ask whether child is attending school or not, what is his rank in the class and whether the disease has interfered with his studies or not. Assess the interactive behavior, habits, hobbies, interests, lifestyle and personality of the child and how he differs from other siblings. Ask about the time being spent by the child with mobile, iPad, video games, television, etc. Whether child sleeps in the parents' room or in a separate bedroom. Ask about the eating, sleeping and toilet habits of the child. Adolescent children should be encouraged to talk regarding their worries, anxieties, psychosexual difficulties and substance abuse tendencies. Ask whether any pets and animals are kept at home or courtyard. Enquiry should be made regarding smoking, intake of alcohol or drug abuse by parent(s) which can adversely affect the family dynamics and child rearing practices. In an unexplained fever, ask for any history of travel to an endemic area.

TABLE 2.4 Revised Kuppuswamy socioeconomic status scale (2016)

Parameter	Score
A. Education of family head	
• Professional or honors or postgraduate degree	7
• Graduate	6
• Intermediate or diploma after high school	5
• High school certificate	4
• Middle school certificate	3
• Primary school certificate	2
• Illiterate	1
B. Occupation of family head	
• Legislator, senior official and manager	10
• Professional	9
• Semiprofessional	8
• Clerical, shop owner, farmer	7
• Skilled worker (industry)	6
• Skilled worker (agriculture)	5
• Craft and trade worker	4
• Plant or machine operator	3
• Unskilled worker	2
• Unemployed	1
C. Income of family head per month (INR 2016)	
• ≥40,430	12
• 20,210–40,429	10
• 15,160–20,209	6
• 10,110–15,159	4
• 6,060–10,109	3
• 2,021–6,059	2
• ≤2,020	1

(Real-time update for income categories is *provided at www.scaleupdate.weekly.com*)

Total score (A + B + C)	Socioeconomic class
26–29	Upper (I)
16–25	Upper middle (II)
11–15	Lower middle (III)
5–10	Upper lower (IV)
<5	Lower (V)

FEEDING HISTORY

History of dietary intake is of special importance in children because they need food for activity, growth and development. The energy or caloric requirements of infants per unit body weight are at least 4 times as compared to adults. Ask whether child received breastfeeding or not, whether it was exclusive or complemented with bottle feeding. The frequency, type of schedule (time or demand) duration and reasons for discontinuation of breastfeeding should be recorded. If top fed, age at starting, nature of formula (dried milk or fresh milk), dilution, amount, frequency, mode of feeding (bottle or cup and spoon or *paladay*), should be enquired in detail. Age at weaning, nature and amount of semisolid food or other supplementary foods, vitamins and minerals given to the child should be asked. Ask whether family is vegetarian or non-vegetarian. Assess whether child is having food fussiness and using "black mailing" tactics because of over indulgence by parents and grandparents. Is the child taking a balanced diet or having craving for junk food with poor intake of green leafy vegetables and fruits. Dietary intake just before the onset of illness and during illness should be enquired. Ask in detail the actual food intake during the last 24 hours to calculate approximate caloric and protein intake per day (Tables 2.5 and 2.6).

IMMUNIZATION STATUS

Ask for various immunizations received so far. This information is useful to guide the diagnosis and ensure comprehensive management of the child. Look for scar of BCG vaccination during physical examination. All children must be given advise regarding feeding and immunizations whether they are attending OPD or discharged from the hospital. Table 2.7 outlines the current schedule of immunization recommended by Indian Academy of Pediatrics.

TABLE 2.5 Caloric and protein content of common Indian food stuffs (per 100 g)

Food stuff	Calories (kcal)	Protein (g)
Wheat	350	11.0
Rice	345	6.5
Pulses/legumes	350	20–25
Leafy vegetables	25–50	2.0–5.0
Other vegetables, roots and tubers	50–100	1.0–2.5
Ground nuts	550	25.0
Apple	60	0.2
Banana	120	1.2
Flesh foods	150–200	20
Egg	180	13.0
Cow's milk	67	3.2
Curd	60	3.0
Ghee and oil	900	—
Sugar	400	—

Adapted from Food and Health, VR Murthy, BR Rama Sastri, K Srilakshmi (Eds.). National Institute of Nutrition, Hyderabad, 1979.
1. Standard hen's egg weighs 50–60 g and provides 300 mg cholesterol.
2. *Khichdi* gruel and cooked pulses contain one part of dry food stuff and 4 parts of water. Cooked rice contains one part of rice and one part of water.
3. Common home measures: Teaspoon 5 mL, tablespoon 15 mL, *katori* or cup 150 mL and glass 250 mL.
4. Average sized *chapati* has 30 g wheat flour.

TABLE 2.6 Nutritional values of cooked food items

Food item	Energy (kcal)	Protein (g)
Chapati (small) 20 g	68	2.4
Chapati (medium) 30 g	102	3.6
Parantha (medium) 40 g	200	3.6
Plain rice (medium *katori*) 30 g	100	2.0
Khichdi (medium *katori*)	100	3.5
Dal or *Sambhar* (medium *katori*)	105	7.0
Idli (medium)	50	1.0
Upma (medium *katori*)	150	3.5
Bread slice 20 g	50	1.7
Vegetables (medium *katori*)	50	1.0
Curd (medium *katori*)	90	3.5
Cow's milk 100 g	67	3.2

Adapted from Nutritional values of Indian foods, National Institute of Nutrition, Hyderabad

TABLE 2.7 Recommended immunization schedule

Essential Vaccines

Age	Vaccine	Dose
Birth–4 weeks	BCG OPV HBV	Single dose 1st dose 1st dose
6–8 weeks	DTwP or DTaP + Hib + IPV + HBV OPV	1st dose 2nd dose
10–12 weeks	DTwP or DTaP + Hib + IPV + HBV OPV	2nd dose 3rd dose
14–16 weeks	DTwP or DTaP + Hib + IPV + HBV OPV	3rd dose 4th dose
6–9 months	MMR OPV HBV	1st dose 5th dose 3rd dose (may be given along with 3rd dose of DTP)
10–12 months	Typhoid vaccine[a]	1st dose followed by a booster after 6 months to one year
15–18 months	MMR DTwP or DTaP + Hib + IPV + HBV OPV	2nd dose 1st booster 6th dose
4½–5 years	DTaP or Tdap OPV HBV booster	2nd booster 7th dose[b]
10 years	Tdap or Td or TT booster[c]	Single dose Booster of Td every 10 years

Optional Vaccines (after one-to-one discussion with parents who can afford)

Age	Vaccine	Dose
6–8 weeks	Rotavirus vaccine + PCV 13[d]	1st dose
10–12 weeks	Rotavirus vaccine + PCV 13	2nd dose
14–16 weeks	Rotavirus vaccine + PCV 13	3rd dose
12 months	HAV	[e]Two doses at an interval of 6 months–1 year
15 months	PCV 13	Booster
15–18 months	Chickenpox vaccine	Two doses are given at an interval of 6 months–1 year. A booster dose is being recommended after the age of 5 years
9–13 years (Girls)	[f]HPV two doses at an interval of 6 months	
≥14 years (Girls)	Three doses of HPV are given at 0, 1 or 2 and 6 months	

(contd.)

TABLE 2.7 Recommended immunization schedule (*contd.*)
Additional Vaccines during Special Situations
IPV (injectable or inactivated polio vaccine) is given to immunocompromised or HIV-positive children. It is being administered routinely as a part of post polio eradication policy.
Meningococcal quadrivalent conjugate vaccine (MCV4 or Menactra) is given after 9 months in two doses 8 weeks apart.
Pneumococcal polysaccharide vaccine, i.e. PPV 23 (chronic lung and heart disease, splenectomy, nephrotic syndrome, immunocompromised child) is given in a single dose or maximum of 2 doses.
Influenza cum swine flu vaccine (bronchial asthma, immunocompromised child). Initially 2 doses are given 4 weeks apart in children between 6 months and 9 years, followed by yearly boosters at the onset of winter. In children above 9 years, single primary dose is recommended.
Anti-rabies vaccine "pre-exposure prophylaxis" is given to high-risk individuals (children having pets, hostelers, postmen, veterinary doctors, wildlife or dog handlers) in 3 primary doses 1.0 mL IM on day 0, 7 and 21 or 28. A booster dose is given after one year and then every 5 years or alternatively a booster dose is taken when titer of antibodies falls below 0.5 iu/mL. In immunized subjects, for post-exposure protection, only two doses are given on days 0 and 3. In these subjects, there is no need to administer rabies immune globulins (RIG).
Cholera vaccine (to control epidemics, visitors to *Kumbh Mela,* Haj pilgrims).
Japanese B encephalitis vaccine (endemic areas, and during epidemics) is administered (0.5 mL 1–3 years, 1.0 mL 3–10 years SC) in 2 primary doses 4 weeks apart to children above one year of age. The need for boosters is not determined.
Yellow fever (travelers to South Africa). A single dose of vaccine is given after the age of 6 months. Avoid in pregnant women and infants below 6 months.

[a]Vi capsular polysaccharide *S. typhi* type 2 conjugated to tetanus toxoid (Typbar TCV) can be given during 9–12 months followed by a single booster after 6 months to one year for lifelong protection.
[b]Additional doses of oral polio vaccine given under pulse polio immunization program must be taken by all children below the age of 5 years.
[c]Pregnant women must receive 2 doses of TT or Td at 4 weeks interval. The second dose should be taken at least 4 weeks before delivery.
[d]In older children, single or two primary doses of PCV13 are given.
[e]Live hepatitis A vaccine (Biovac-A) is given in a single or two doses.
[f]Human papillomavirus vaccine for girls. The vaccine is currently being recommended for males as well.
BCG: Bacillus Calmette-Guerin vaccine for TB, HBV: hepatitis B vaccine, DTP: triple antigen containing vaccines against diphtheria, tetanus and pertussis (whooping cough), DTwP (whole cell pertussis), DTap (acellular pertussis), PCV13: 13-valent pneumococcal conjugate vaccine, PPV 23: 23-valent pneumococcal polysaccharide vaccine. OPV: oral polio vaccine, IPV: inactivated polio vaccine, MMR: measles, mumps and rubella vaccine, Tdap: tetanus toxoid with low dose diphtheria and pertussis vaccine, Td: dual vaccine with small dose diphtheria vaccine (5 Lf or 2 i.u.) which can be safely given to adults, TT: tetanus toxoid, Hib: *Haemophilus influenzae* type b, HAV: hepatitis A vaccine

MODERN TRENDS FOR RECORD KEEPING

I. The SOAP Chart

It incorporates baseline conventional data plus system review with detailed list of problems, plan of management for each problem, auditing and computerization of data. It is undergoing modifications and its biggest disadvantage is that it leads to depersonalization.

The acronym of SOAP is used to document problem-oriented medical record where **S** stands for subjective, **O** for objective, **A** for assessment or analysis for differential diagnosis and **P** for plan of action, with the help of a flowchart or algorithm.

Example: Rahul 2 years old boy from Ballabgarh township presented with following complaints:

S
1. History of high grade, continuous fever of one week duration.
2. Semiloose stools without any blood and mucus with a purge rate of 5–6 stools/day, and was treated with concentrated ORS and injectable antibiotics. Urine out put was adequate.
3. Vomitings for 2 days with a frequency of 5–6 times/day.
4. One episode of generalized tonic-clonic seizures 12 hours ago.
5. Altered sensorium for 12 hours.

O
Toxic sick looking semi-comatosed child with stable vital signs. Rectal temperature 40°C. No evidences of dehydration or meningeal irritation. Liver 3 cm and spleen just palpable. Deep tendon jerks were exaggerated with bilateral extensor plantars but no focal neurological signs. Fundus examination was normal.

A
1. *Enteric fever with encephalopathy*: Prolonged fever with diarrhea, splenomegaly and altered sensorium. Seizures may occur but are uncommon.
2. *Shigella encephalopathy*: Fever preceded the onset of diarrhea which was non-invasive in character.
3. *Pyogenic meningitis*: History is rather long and there are no signs of meningeal irritation.
4. *Hypernatremic dehydration*: The onset of dehydration is often delayed and use of concentrated ORS is well known to produce hypernatremia and seizures. However, high grade fever and splenomegaly cannot be explained.
5. *Reye syndrome*: The presence of high grade continuous fever and onset of vomitings later during the course of disease are against this possibility.
6. *Brain abscess*: The absence of any focal neurological signs and lack of any predisposing conditions, like head injury, otitis media and congenital cyanotic heart disease, are against this possibility.

P
1. Complete hemogram, serum electrolytes, blood glucose, liver and kidney function tests, stool microscopic examination and culture, Widal test, blood culture, CSF examination and contrast-enhanced CT scan of head.
2. Administer IV fluids, give appropriate antibiotics and anticonvulsants.

II. Problem-Oriented Medical Record (POMR)

The POMR is a useful method to maintain concise, complete and accurate record of the patient in a problem-solving format. It is a useful legal document of patients' medical record. The salient components of POMR are listed below.

1. ***Data base*** Salient features in history, physical examination and routine laboratorty studies. The problem-oriented diagnosis is based on the cardinal features of the patient to identify the body system involved, the exact organ or part of the system affected, the nature of the lesion and likely cause of the lesion.
2. ***Complete list of problems*** Record all the clinical problems and abnormal findings of laboratory studies. Identify the need for additional laboratory investigations to make a precise diagnosis, severity of the problem and associated complications of the underlying disease process. The status of problems should be categorized into either improving or worsening, dormant or resolving.
3. ***Initial plans*** Based on the tentative diagnosis and differential diagnosis, initial plans for management should be listed. To analyze and manage various problems, a SOAP format should be created for each problem *vide supra*. The initial plan must include three components, i.e. diagnostic plan, therapeutic plan and patient education plan.
4. ***Daily progress notes*** Many physicians object to POMR because of lengthy progress notes. There is no need to list progress of all problems, only evolution and resolution of active problem should be listed. A status report for all active problems should be provided whether they are better, static or worse.

5. *Discharge summary and status at the time of discharge* The status of all the problems as per SOAP format should be listed. All the resolved and any active problems should be listed in the discharge summary. The **S**ubjective data should include brief review of the evolution of systems. The **O**bjective findings should include the course and status of physical abnormalities and laboratory parameters. The **A**ssessment and **P**lan of action should include the likely course during follow-up and define end-points as a guide to duration of therapy. The emphasis of discharge summary should be on the unresolved problems. The problems which have resolved should be documented briefly.

III. Flow Sheet Analysis

It has been proposed to simplify diagnostic approach for community health workers by use of algorithms (**Figure 2.5**).

IV. Diagrammatic Summary

It is useful to ascertain and assimilate the information at a glance (**Figure 2.6**).

Maintain an accurate record of history, physical examination and follow-up both in the hospital and ambulatory practice in view of the increasing incidence of medical litigation following enactment of Consumer Protection Act in 1986.

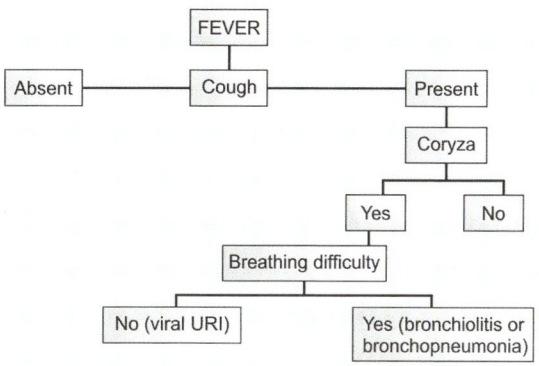

Figure 2.5 Algorithm giving a simplified step-wise approach to a healthcare worker to identify the cause of fever in a child. The presence of cough and coryza are useful clues for localizing infection to upper respiratory tract while breathing difficulty is diagnostic of acute lower respiratory tract infection.

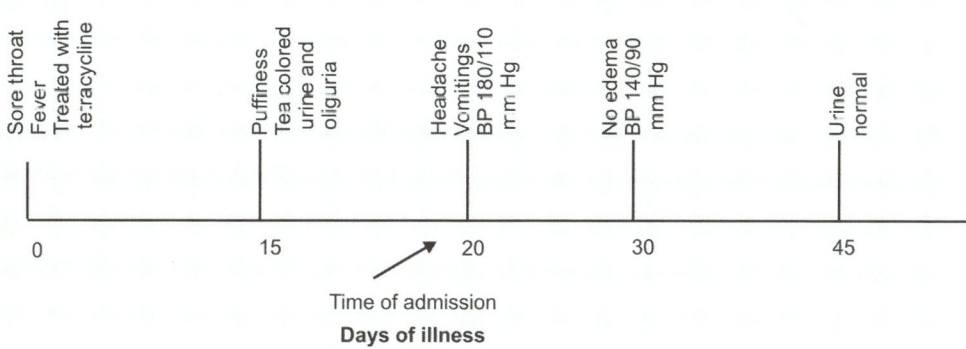

Figure 2.6 Typical diagrammatic summary of a child with post-streptococcal acute glomerulonephritis. Inappropriate treatment of streptococcal pharyngitis with tetracycline may lead to development of classical manifestations of AGN followed by complete recovery.

	Scheme for Presentation
Basic information	Name, age and sex of the child, informant and his/her reliability, socioeconomic status, education, occupation, religion, ethnic and geographic background.
Presenting complaints	The main complaints and concerns which compelled the parents to seek medical aid. They should be recorded in a chronological order.
History of present illness	Present a lucid chronological story with special emphasis on the *onset* and *evolution* of the disease process, and a detailed symptom and system review.
Medication history	Medications taken and their effect on the course of illness, intake of long-term medications and nutritional supplements, adverse drug reactions in the past, compliance and commitment of the family to administer medications.
History of past illnesses	History of common childhood illnesses (exanthemata, pertussis, acute respiratory and gastrointestinal infections), episodes of similar disease in the past, occurrence of other serious or significant diseases in the past, ingestion, inhalation or insertion of foreign bodies.
Perinatal history	Intrauterine and perinatal events constitute important past events and relevant details must be recorded especially in infants and under-five children.
Developmental history	Developmental milestones and differences between the development of the index child as compared to other siblings.
Family history	Family history of infectious, developmental, genetic and chromosomal disorders, family pedigree for three generations to assess the nature of inheritance.
Social history	Socioeconomic and educational background, Kuppuswamy SES score, ecological considerations, child rearing cultural practices, who looks after the child when mother goes to work, creche facilities, schooling, interactive behavior, habits, lifestyle and personality of the child.
Feeding history	Duration of breastfeeding, time and type of weaning, dilution of formula feeds, mode of top feeding, food intake before illness, effect of the disease process on the appetite and dietary intake, vegetarian or non-vegetarian, actual intake of food by recall in the last 24 hours and calculation of approximate caloric and protein intake.
Immunization status	Timing of various primary and booster immunizations received so far, any adverse or unusual reactions, presence of BCG scar.

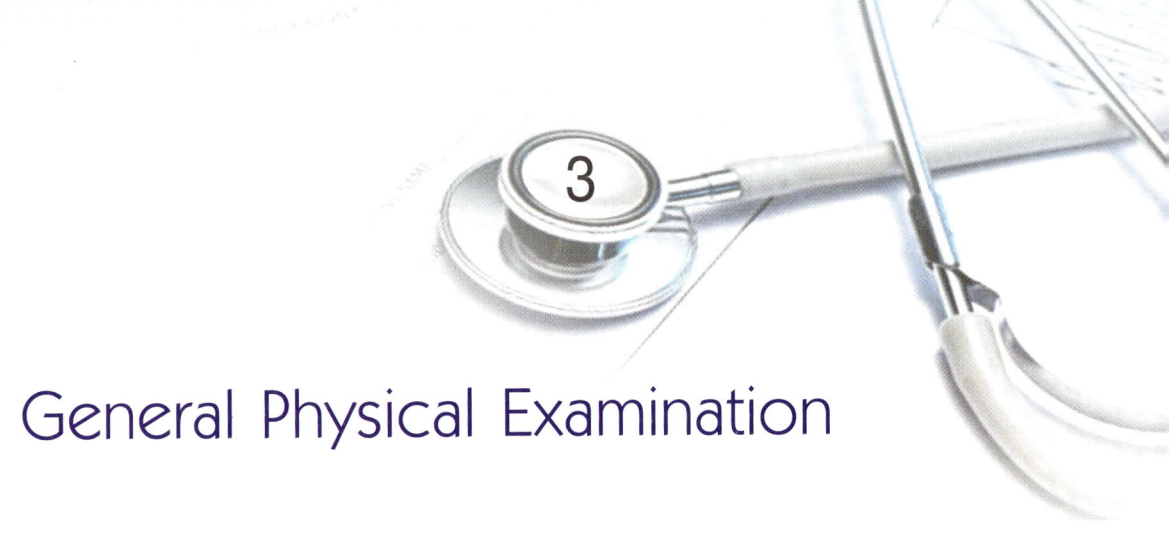

3

General Physical Examination

"There are no short cuts for physical diagnosis. It is learnt only by practice, not a dull, dreary or monotonous practice but practice with all the five senses alert."
Sir Robert Hutchison

PRINCIPLES AND ART OF EXAMINATION OF CHILDREN

Prerequisites

Physical examination is subjective (provides soft data) and its yield depends upon the experience, skills, thoroughness and the time spent by the pediatrician for making the clinical assessment. Eyes, ears, nose and palpating fingers are the real gems of a physician and an analytical brain is the necklace. Sharp, sensitive and well conditioned special senses are mandatory for making correct observations. Sight (sharp and keen observation), hearing (listen, percussion, auscultation), smell (sickness, fetor hepaticus, uremia, ketosis, poisons, pus, metabolic disorders, etc.), taste (least important), touch (gentleness, healing, sensitive and delicate hands with long fingers), perceptive and analytical mind, intuition and common sense are essential attributes of a successful physician.

Essential Tools

Stethoscope, torch, spatula, digital thermometer or aural thermoscan, hand lens, percussion hammer, fiberglass tape measure, white plastic ruler, diagnostic set, sphygmomanometer (with cuffs of different sizes), fingertip pulse oximeter, developmental assessment tools, weighing machine, infantometer for measurement of length and a wall chart or stadiometer for measurement of height should be available (Figure 3.1). The tools of

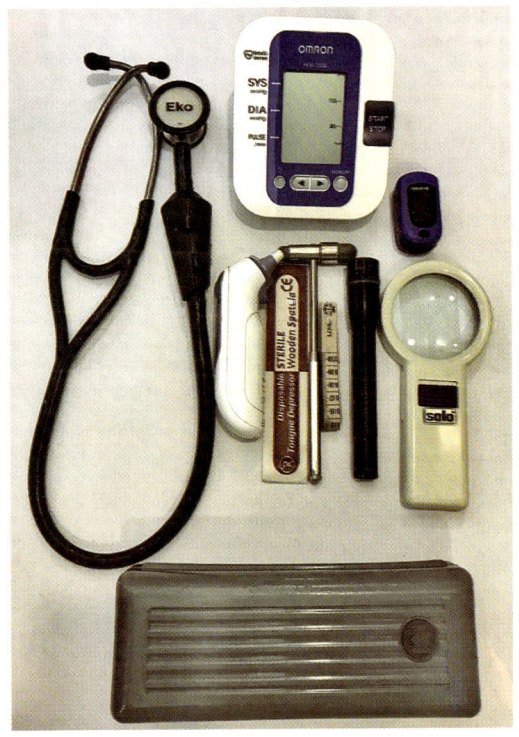

Figure 3.1 Essential tools for conducting physical examination. Hand lens with in-built light is useful to examine skin lesions and dermatoglyphics. Fingertip pulse oximeter provides SpO_2 in critically sick children.

different sizes are required because pediatricians are expected to deal with a preterm baby of under 1.0 kg and an adolescent of over 50 kg.

Setting

Well-lighted, warm, colorful, comfortable room and warm hands are essential. The physical examination is often unsuccessful, if the examiner has cold hands, cold instruments and cold manner. Toys, pictures and cartoons are useful in the consultation chamber to allay apprehension of the child. Avoid deep yellow/blue curtains which may interfere with proper evaluation of jaundice and cyanosis.

Approach

Gentleness, confidence, enthusiasm, patience, tact, compassion, concern, kind look and love for children are essential attributes of a pediatrician. A good pediatrican begins his examination as soon as mother enters the consultation room and while eliciting history. Welcome and greet the child and his family with a smile. During interview "sneaky" observation of the child, offering a small bright object or a soft toy, are useful to make the child comfortable. The "intelligent neglect" of the child and giving mother/attendant due respect and courtesy are useful to gain the confidence of the family and cooperation of the child. *The best way to make friends with children is not to try*! Avoid staring into the eyes of a child because unlike adults, children distrust the man who looks into the eyes. The experienced pediatrician should be able to assess and grade whether child looks well, mildly ill or gravely sick requiring urgent attention.

Cooperation

> "Patients must be handled with utmost care and reverence as they are the real books of physicians."
> — Meharban Singh

Win the confidence of the child with a smile, "intelligent neglect" and distraction. *Children should be treated as children and not patients.* Parents should not spoil the image of the doctor by frightening children with threats of injections. When the family enters the consultation room, they should be greeted with a smile and a friendly demeanor. Smile is the key to unlock an atmosphere of love, acceptance and cooperation. Remember, it takes only 17 muscles to smile and 43 to frown! While recording history, you can offer a toy to the toddler, in an unconcerned manner and without intently staring into his eyes. Let the child touch or play with the physician's instruments, like torch, stethoscope and percussion hammer. You should adopt a play attitude, and follow an unstructured approach. Physical examination of children should be a fun both for the pediatrician as well as the child. The pediatrician should literally come down to the level of the child, both physically and mentally to elicit cooperation. If you are unable to obtain the cooperation of the child, it is usually due to your fault either because of lack of tact or unskillful approach. The experience with earlier physicians, nature of illness, tact of the physician, rearing of the child, unnecessary removal of clothes, and a fixed sequence of examination are useful determinants whether a child is likely to cooperate or not.

Unnecessary and complete undressing of the child is undesirable and it often compromises with cooperation. The undressing should be limited to removal of some clothes at a time to facilitate specific aspects of examination. Postpone examination or examine after sedation, if a child is uncooperative, cranky and fussy. The relatively traumatic examination, like percussion, throat and rectal examination, should be done in the end. The older child may be explained the procedure, if it is unpleasant. The child should be given a firm direction to follow instead of making a meek request which gives him the option to refuse to cooperate.

Position of the Child for Examination

To elicit maximum cooperation, children at different ages are best examined in different positions as shown in **Table 3.1**. It is useful to have a revolving padded armless chair with a back for the mother and/or child to sit during examination

General Physical Examination

TABLE 3.1 Best position for examination at different ages

Age	Position
0–3 months	Examination table
3 months–1 year	Mother's lap
1–3 years	Standing or mother's lap
After 3 years	Examination table
Adolescent girl	Female attendant, mother or nurse should be present at the time of examination

so that the position of the child can be easily changed by rotating the chair. Most children feel comfortable sitting or standing during the examination rather than lying down on a bed. When the child appears friendly and not frightened, he or she can be examined on the examination table.

Observation

"A great part, I believe, of the art of medicine is the ability to observe. Leave nothing to chance. Overlook nothing, combine contradictory observations and allow yourself enough time".

Hippocrates

Spend maximum time on observation because it is the key attribute of a good diagnostician. Keep your eyes and ears open (and mouth shut!) and be aware, alert and alive with an analytical mind. You can observe the whole infant at a time and it is least disturbing to the child and most informative. Attitude and posture (bed-ridden or walking, opisthotonos or emprosthotonos, side posture, orthopneic, motionless, restless, comfortable), should be recorded. The expression and mental state (fully conscious, drowsy, delirious, stuporosed or semicomatosed, coma) should be assessed. Abnormal movements, signs of meningeal irritation, odor and nature of cry should be observed. Be alert for any characteristic odor (breath or urine) of the patient due to ingested poison, acetone (diabetic ketoacidosis), urine-like (azotemia), fruity smell (diphtheria) and a specific odor due to inborn errors of metabolism (like maple syrup or caramel-like, musky or mousy, dried malt and "sweaty" feet).

Never ignore the nonverbal communication of the patient. Pay due attention to the looks and anxiety on the patient's or parents face, the lowering of his eyes, the tremble in his hands and contents of his drawings. Observation is the soul of clinical medicine and physicians must sharpen this capability. We should develop a keen sense of observation during our day-to-day social interactions by comparing different individuals to identify subtle differences in their facial features, phenotype, physique, posture, demeanor, gait, voice, etc. It is a unique characteristic of nature that among millions of people, no two human beings look alike! You can sharpen your observation skills by critically evaluating various characteristics and uniqueness of every person that you meet.

Sequence of Examination

The approach to examination should be unstructured to elicit cooperation and to ensure that maximum time is spent on the most relevant component of examination. The unpleasant examination should be postponed to the end. Auscultation may be done at the beginning in an infant suspected to have a cardiac problem because conventional sequence of examination would lead to crying by the time auscultation is done. This should be followed by inspection, palpation, percussion, recording of blood pressure, elicitation of deep tendon jerks, ENT examination, and rectal examination. The examination of the painful site or limb should be conducted in the end.

Scheme of Recording and Presentation

The presentation of physical findings should be standardized and recorded in accordance with a set pattern although the sequence of examination of children is unstructured *(Box 3.1)*.

Build and Nutrition

Skeletal size, body frame, subcutaneous fat, and muscle mass should be assessed. Is the child tall, short, fat, thin, muscular, asthenic or cachectic? Look for clinical evidences of marasmus, marasmic kwashiorkor and kwashiorkor *(Figures 3.2 and 3.3)*.

Box 3.1 Scheme for recording general physical examination

- General appearance, build and nutrition
- Anthropometry*
- Developmental assessment
- Vital signs
- Head and face
- Eyes
- Ear, nose and throat
- Neck
- Skin and its appendages
- Evidences of any deficiency or over abundance states
- Bones and joints
- Genitals and sexual maturity rating

*Anthropometry should be recorded by the nurse before child enters the physician's cabin

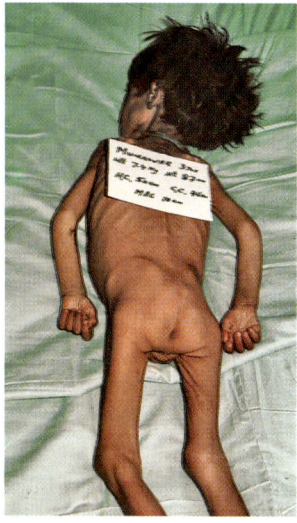

Figure 3.2 3-year-old boy with marasmus. Note wasted extremities, poor muscle mass, loss of subcutaneous fat (skin hangs in folds over buttocks and thighs) and visible bony prominences.

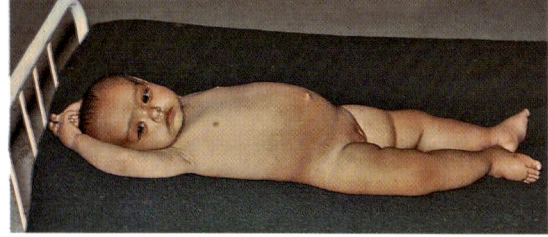

Figure 3.3 1½-year-old girl with kwashiorkor. Note apathy, growth retardation, generalized edema, sparse hair, and crazy-pavement dermatosis over legs. There was hepatomegaly due to fatty infiltration of liver.

Measurements

Detailed anthropometry is conducted to record weight, height (or recumbent length with the help of an infantometer), surface area, body mass index, midarm circumference, stem length (crown rump or sitting height), arm span, upper segment (vertex to pubic symphysis) to lower segment ratio, chest circumference and head circumference is essential for evaluation of children. Refer to Chapter 5 for details regarding anthropometry.

Developmental Examination

Objective assessment of development is required in selected cases. The dates for achieving target milestones should be recorded. Refer to Chapter 6 for details pertaining to formal developmental assessment. Identify and record any behavior disorder like temper tantrums, breath holding spells, food fussiness, thumb sucking, nail biting, pica, enuresis, nightmares, teeth grinding (bruxism), tics, school phobias, etc.

Vital Signs

Temperature, pulse, breathing and blood pressure (Hess capillary test, Trousseau's sign should also be looked for, if indicated) are recorded.

Temperature The conventional thermometers (skin, oral, rectal) usually contain mercury in glass or are digital by using electronic technology. Single-use chemical dot thermometers (Tempor.Dot™) are available to reduce the risk of inter-patient infection in healthcare facilities. Skin temperature (groin and axilla) is recorded in infants and preschool children and is quite reliable. Axilla or groin should be dried with a cloth and bulb of thermometer is placed snugly by tightly holding the arm against chest or flexing thigh over the abdomen. Thermometer should be left in place for at least 2 minutes before reading the temperature. Skin temperature is 0.4°C (0.7°F) lower than the oral temperature, while rectal or eardrum temperature is 0.4°C (0.7°F) higher than oral temperature. In school going children, oral temperature is recorded by placing the thermometer under the tongue and asking the child to breathe through the nose. *Oral temperature is the reference* *temperature and fever is diagnosed when it exceeds 100°F (37.8°C).* Oral temperature should not be taken immediately after intake of a hot or cold drink. Rectal temperature may be recorded in critically sick children but should be avoided as a routine office or domiciliary procedure. Rectal thermometer has a bulbous tip with a red mark compared to the long tip of oral thermometer. While recording rectal temperature, thermometer should be introduced by directing its tip posteriorly towards the back up to a maximum depth of 2.5 cm. The child should be kept in lateral decubitus and buttock kept opposed.

Temperature can also be recorded over the skin of forehead and eardrum by using thermo-phototrophic-crystal strips and infrared technology with the help of thermoscan respectively (Figure 3.4). These methods are quick and convenient but unreliable at times. They are operator dependent and not reliable in infants, and children with wax in the ear canal. In severely malnourished children and neonates, low reading thermometer (30–40°C) should be used to assess the severity of hypothermia. Heads of most infants feel warm to touch due to increased blood flow to the brain and it should not be mistaken for fever. Due to their constitution, some children have warm hands while others may be endowed with relatively cold hands and feet. During episodes of fever, elevation of body temperature is usually associated with peripheral vasoconstriction leading to development of cold extremities. It should be remembered that many normal children have diurnal variations in their body temperature, being lowest in the early morning and highest in the evening around 4 PM. Mild elevation of temperature (oral temperature up to 37.7°C or 99.9°F) in some children especially during the afternoons in summer months is not indicative of any disease process. Avoid unnecessary work up, if child is otherwise well, active, playful, feeding and growing normally.

Pulse The pulse should be recorded when child is at rest or during sleep because crying, anxiety, activity and restlessness are likely to increase the pulse rate. Radial pulse is usually recorded by gently placing the middle and index fingers over the lateral or outside of the anterior surface of the wrist. Rate, volume, rhythm and character of the pulse are noted. Pulse rate should be recorded for full one minute by watch. Pulse can also be recorded from the femoral (groin), carotid (neck), brachial (elbow) and anterior tibial (ankle) arteries. In neonates and infants, radial pulse is difficult to feel and instead apical impulse or heart beats may be recorded by palpation or with the help of a stethoscope. In infants, the radial and femoral pulses should be checked simultaneously. In coarctation of aorta, the femoral pulses are feeble and delayed compared to the radial pulse (brachio-femoral delay).

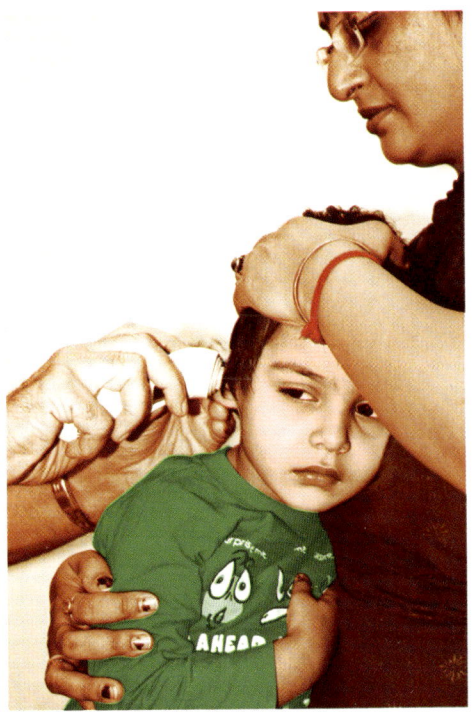

Figure 3.4 Recording temperature of the eardrum with a thermoscan which works on the principle of infrared technology. The ear should be pulled outward in an infant and upward and outward in an older child for proper exposure of eardrum. It is useful in a busy ambulatory clinic because temperature read-out is obtained within one second.

Respiration The breathing should be recorded in a quiet resting child because crying and restlessness are likely to increase the breathing rate. The breathing is usually relaxed and mostly abdominal or abdominothoracic in infants. It becomes predominantly thoracic after the age of 5 years. Record the rate, regularity and depth of breathing (whether normal, shallow or deep). Note whether accessory muscles of respiration and alae nasi are working or not. Look for suprasternal and intercostal retractions. Note the character of voice or cry. A number of audible sounds during breathing provide useful clues. They include stridor, croup, grunting, wheezing and stertorous or bubbly pharyngeal sounds.

Blood pressure It is conventionally recorded in the upper arm at the site of brachial artery. The child should be quiet and lying supine in bed or sitting comfortably with arm kept at the level of heart. Depending upon the age of the child, the appropriate size of the cuff should be used. It should cover two-thirds of the upper arm or its width should be at least 40% of the arm circumference. The recommended cuff size in infants under one year of age is 2.5 cm, 1–4 years: 5 cm, 5–9 years: 9 cm and over 10 years it is 13 cm. *When cuff width is too narrow for the upper arm, it gives an erroneously high blood pressure and when cuff is too wide, the blood pressure recording is likely to be low.* Cuff is wrapped snugly over the upper arm with its lower margin about 2–3 cm above the cubital fossa.

Flush method This method is used in small infants and instead of pulse, flushing or blanching of the hand is used to record systolic blood pressure. This method is time consuming and unreliable and has been replaced by technology-based recording of blood pressure.

Palpatory method Cuff is inflated above the anticipated level of systolic blood pressure of the patient in order to obliterate the radial or brachial pulse. The cuff is gradually and slowly deflated till the radial or brachial pulse can be felt again. This gives only systolic blood pressure of the patient.

Auscultatory method Mercury sphygmomanometer is the gold standard instrument for recording blood pressure in ambulatory patients. It is more reliable than an aneroid instrument or electronic devices. Cuff is inflated to obliterate the arterial pulse. Brachial artery in the cubital fossa (medial or inner side of elbow) is auscultated while gradually and slowly deflating the cuff. The point at which the Korotkoff sounds are first heard gives the systolic blood pressure. The cuff is further deflated slowly while listening to the sound. When the sound becomes muffled, it is taken as diastolic blood pressure. The difference between the systolic and diastolic blood pressure provides the pulse pressure (strength or volume of the pulse).

Blood pressure monitor Doppler system which is based on the principle of oscillometry and sound waves provides an accurate and non-invasive means for recording blood pressure in newborn babies and critically sick children. The ultrasonic waves are picked up by the transducer located in the cuff. The instrument provides continuous digital display of heart rate, systolic, diastolic and mean blood pressure. There is a provision for an alarm or warning signal when blood pressure falls or rises beyond certain preset limits.

Intra-arterial blood pressure Direct arterial blood pressure can be recorded by introducing a transducer into the umbilical artery or a peripheral artery in critically sick newborn babies and infants. The method is accurate but rather invasive and fraught with several complications. The normal range of vital signs at different ages is given in Chapter 4.

Shock

In a critically sick or a drowsy child, shock is diagnosed if any one or more of the following clinical signs are present.
- Cold and mottled extremities.
- Capillary refill time of more than 2 seconds.
- Rapid and thready (low volume) peripheral pulses.
- Systolic blood pressure of less than 5th percentile for the age.
- Urine output of less than 1 mL/kg/hour.

Tourniquet test (Hess capillary resistance test, Rumple-Leede test). Sphygmomanometer cuff is wrapped around upper arm and inflated midway between systolic and diastolic blood pressure for 10 minutes. The skin of the forearm is examined

10 minutes later. The development of more than 15 petechiae over an area of 5 cm diameter circle on the flexor surface of forearm is considered as positive and suggestive of bleeding diathesis because of increased capillary fragility, thrombocytopenia, or thrombasthenia. If the test is negative on one side, it may be repeated on the other arm.

Trousseau's sign The blood pressure cuff is inflated above the systolic blood pressure for 3 minutes. The increase in muscle tone over thenar eminence and adduction of thumb are suggestive of positive Trousseau's sign and is indicative of hypocalcemia. The sign can be elicited by firmly compressing the forearm for one minute (Figure 3.5). Peroneal sign can be elicited by applying the blood pressure cuff over the thigh and keeping the cuff inflated above the systolic blood pressure for 3 minutes.

General Features

Anemia, cyanosis, lymphadenopathy, jaundice and edema are looked for during general physical examination. Look for pallor of pelpebral conjunctiva, tongue and palms as a marker of anemia. Anemia may be over diagnosed in a child with fair complexion.

Cyanosis occurs when level of reduced hemoglobin (deoxygenated hemoglobin) exceeds 5.0 g/dL. Peripheral cyanosis may occur due to shock, exposure to cold and hypothermia. Skin is mottled and cyanosis is limited to the nails and lips. Central cyanosis occurs due to hypoxia because of life-threatening pulmonary or cardiac disorder. Tongue and buccal mucosa become blue colored. Arterial oxygen saturation can be reliably assessed with a hand-held pulse oximeter. SaO_2 or SpO_2 of less than 90% in a neonate and less than 93% in an older child is suggestive of hypoxia.

The peripheral lymph nodes are examined in the neck, axillae, epitrochlear region, groins and popliteal fossae. Axillary nodes are examined by keeping the patient's arm slightly abducted and using fingers of the left hand for right axilla and vice versa. The examination of lymph nodes should include their location or site (Figure 3.6), size, consistency, tenderness, warmth, whether discrete or matted, mobile or fixed to the overlying skin. Matted lymph nodes are characteristically seen in chronic inflammation due to tuberculosis. Discrete rubbery or firm lymph nodes are suggestive of malignancy or Hodgkin's disease (Figure 3.7). There is physiological hyperplasia of lymphoid tissue in children. Cervical lymphadenopathy up to 1.0–1.5 cm diameter, when lymph nodes are discrete, mobile and non-tender is not significant. Cervical lymph nodes readily enlarge in children having pediculosis, pyoderma and recurrent upper respiratory tract infections.

Jaundice is characterized by yellowness of sclera and undersurface of tongue. The patient should be

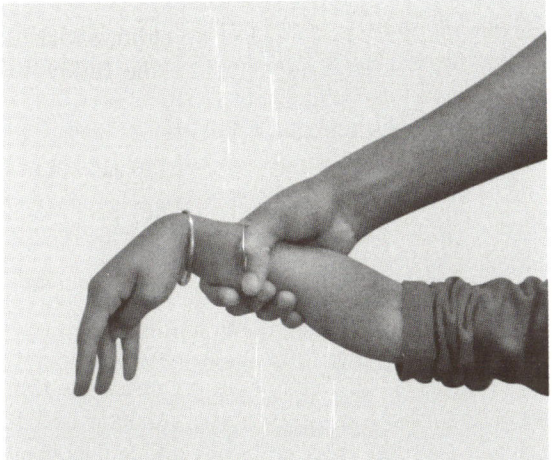

Figure 3.5 Carpopedal spasms in a 6-year-old girl having hypocalcemia because of DiGeorge syndrome.

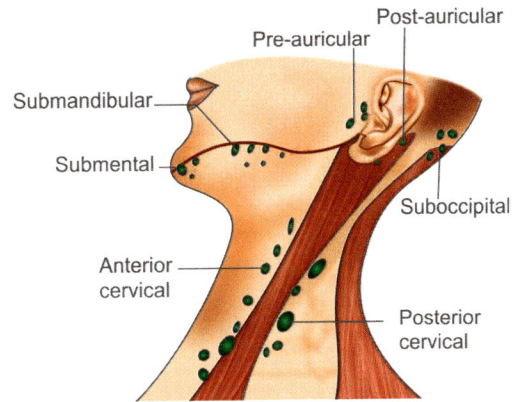

Figure 3.6 The location of lymphatic glands in the neck. The cervical lymph nodes are grouped into horizontal and vertical chains.

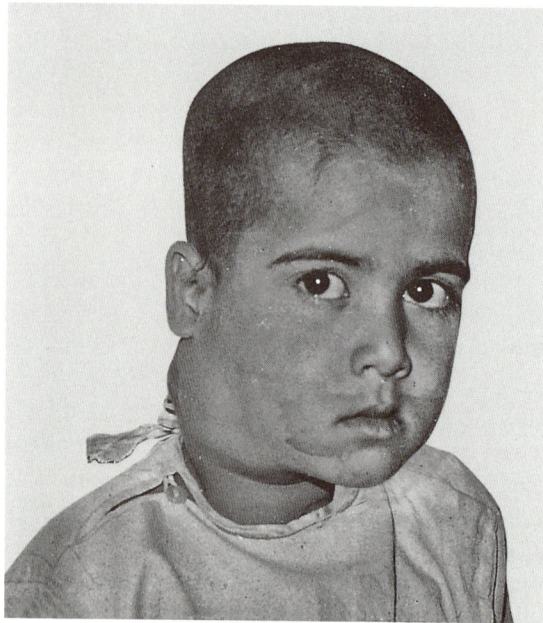

Figure 3.7 Typical appearances of cervical lymphadenopathy in a child with Hodgkin's disease. The glands are mobile, discrete and rubbery in consistency.

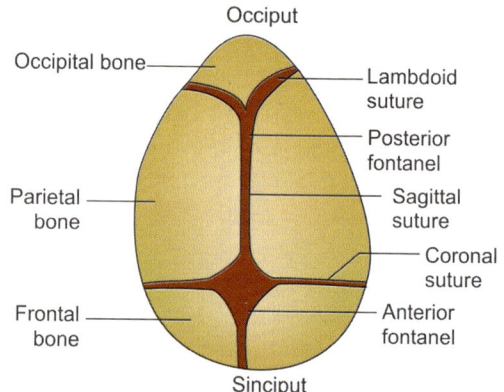

Figure 3.8 Skull bones and sutures as viewed from above.

examined in natural daylight for assessment of jaundice. In neonates and young infants, jaundice may cause yellowness of skin because skin is thin and it lacks pigmentation. Jaundice is usually associated with high colored urine. In obstructive jaundice, the stools may be pale or clay colored.

Edema should be looked for in the dependent parts like feet and legs. Press the medial malleolus or shin for 5 seconds to look for pitting edema. In infants, puffiness and sacral edema are more common because they are not up and about. Edema due to lymphatic obstruction is usually nonpitting. Anasarca or generalized edema is characterized by swelling of face, ascites, hydrothorax and scrotal edema.

Head and Face

Look for size, shape, symmetry, bossing or prominences of cranial bones, anterior fontanel (size and tension) and sutures. There are six fontanels at birth, of which two are large and midline (anterior and posterior fontanels) and four are small and not palpable (two anterolateral and two posterolateral). Figure 3.8 shows the skull bones, sutures and fontanels at birth. The fontanels should be examined when baby is quiet and head is kept upright. Look for the size of anterior fontanel and whether it is depressed, flat or bulging. When intracranial tension is raised, the anterior fontanel starts bulging and feels tense and becomes nonpulsatile. A bulging and pulsatile anterior fontanel in a crying infant is of no significance. The anterior fontanel is depressed or sunken when there is significant dehydration. The posterior fontanel is small at birth and closes by 6 weeks of age while anterior fontanel measures 2.5 × 2.5 cm and usually closes by 10–18 months of age. Auscultation, and transillumination of skull are indicated in infants with unexplained cardiac failure or large head.

Macewen's sign or cracked-pot sound is elicited by percussion of skull. The amplified sound may be listened with the help of a stethoscope (Figure 3.9A and B). The sign is positive when sutures are separated due to raised intracranial tension. It is physiologically present during infancy as long as the anterior fontanel is open. Transillumination of skull is indicated in all infants below one year of age. Flash light equipped with a rubber foam cuff is snugly applied over the frontal and occipital areas in a dark room and rim of translucency is looked for. When translucency extends beyond 2.0–2.5 cm in the frontal area and over 1.0 cm in the occipital region, it is abnormal and is indicative of subdural effusion, subdural hematoma, hydrocephalus,

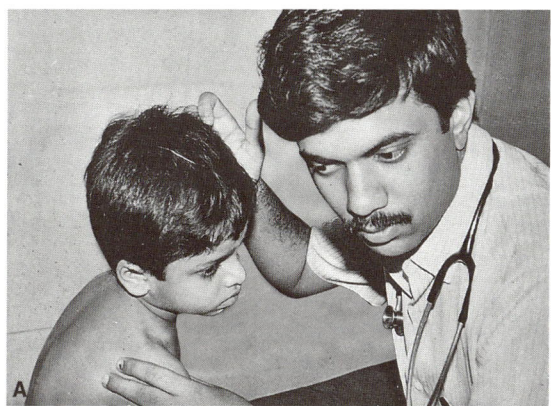

Figure 3.9A Macewen's sign. The cracked-pot sound on percussion of skull is evident to naked ears. It is indicative of separated sutures due to raised intracranial tension but is normally present, if anterior fontanel is open.

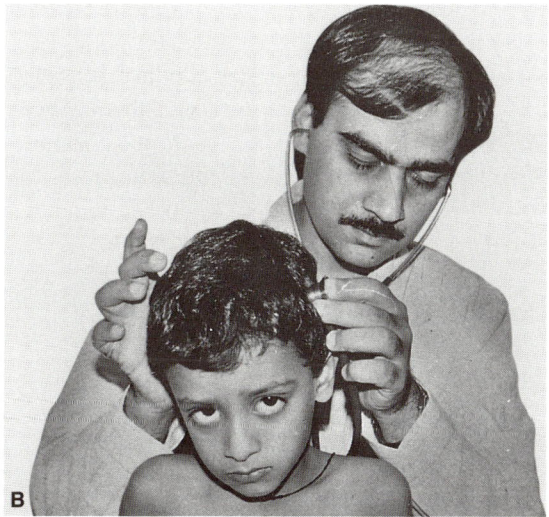

Figure 3.9B Macewen's sign being elicited with the help of a stethoscope.

hydranencephaly, and porencephaly. Intracranial bruit should be looked for in infants with raised intracranial tension and intractable congestive heart failure. It may be heard in 10 to 15% of normal children.

The skull may become odd-shaped due to premature fusion of skull sutures because skull bones grow at right angle to the direction of sutures. The anteroposterior diameter may be increased (dolichocephaly) or decreased (brachycephaly). The skull may appear grossly asymmetrical (plagiocephaly), may grow vertically like a tower (oxycephaly, acrocephaly) or appear like a boat (scaphocephaly). In clover leaf skull, all the cranial sutures are prematurely fused and brain grows through the anterior and temporal or anterolateral fontanels producing projections or bulges at the vertex and temporal areas.

Characteristic facies are diagnostic of Down syndrome, cretinism, gorgoylism, and chromosomal disorders. The evidences of facial dysmorphism, like asymmetry of face, size and position of ears, distance between eyes, alignment of eyes, nasal bridge, lips and chin, etc., should be looked for. Develop a keen sense of observation to identify minor features of dysmorphism. Lips also mirror the abnormalities seen in the oral mucosa. Perleche or angular stomatitis is caused by nutritional deficiency or candida infection. Cheilosis is a form of fissuring and cracking of lips which may occur due to drooling and vitamin B complex deficiency. Rhagades are moist radiating lesions over the philtrum due to persistent nasal discharge in infants with congenital syphilis.

Salivary Glands

Look for swelling of salivary glands and their openings in the oral cavity. The major salivary glands include one pair each of parotids, submandibular and sublingual glands. Parotids are located in front of the angle of the jaw just below the lobule of the ear. The parotid duct (Stenson duct) is located opposite the crown of second upper molar teeth. The swelling of parotid gland lifts the ear lobule laterally which is best seen when child is viewed from behind. Submandibular glands are walnut-sized paired structures located beneath the angle of the jaw under the posterior ramus of the mandible. Their duct is present under the tongue on either side of frenulum. Sublingual glands are located under the tongue and they drain their secretions in the floor of the mouth. Apart from major salivary glands, there are numerous tiny glands called minor salivary glands which are located in the lips, buccal mucosa and throat. They are not visible to the naked eye in normal circumstances. Salivary glands produce saliva, which moistens the oral cavity, tongue, gums and lips. It washes and inactivates bacteria, initiate digestion of food and protect teeth from decay. Examine for any swelling of salivary gland(s), foul breath and dryness of mouth or drooling due to excessive production or poor swallowing of saliva.

Eyes

Eyes are the windows of central nervous system. The palpebral conjunctiva of lower eyelids is examined by pulling down the lower eyelid and asking the child to look upwards. To expose the palpebral conjunctiva of the upper eyelid, ask the child to look downwards and pull the upper eyelid upwards and evert the eyelashes by placing left thumb just below the upper edge of the orbit. Grasp the eyelashes between the forefinger and thumb of the right hand and evert the lid by rotating it around the left thumb. Look for pallor of palpebral conjunctiva (anemia), xerosis and bitot spots over the temporal side of corneoscleral junction (vitamin A deficiency) and circumcorneal vascularization (riboflavin deficiency). Conjunctivitis is common in children and is characterized by redness and chemosis of conjunctiva with purulent discharge and sticky eyelids. Look for any bulging, prominence and proptosis of one or both eyes. Stye or hardeolum is a localized, tender swelling at the edge of eyelid with a yellow punctum due to staphylococcal infection. Chalazion or meibomian cyst is a firm, discrete, nonpainful, flat, erythematous nodule on the bulbar conjunctival aspect of the lid adjacent to the tarsal plate. The presence of lilac or heliotropic discoloration and scaly dermatitis of eyelids with periorbital edema and telangiectasia are pathognomonic of dermatomyositis.

Look for developmental defects, like epicanthic folds, slanting of eyes, ptosis, cataracts, coloboma (partial absence of a part of eye), glaucoma, cloudy cornea, corneal opacity, white reflex (cataract, retinoblastoma), exophthalmos and setting-sun sign. Increased distance between the inner canthi of eyes (hypertelorism) with or without epicanthal folds and slanting of eyes should be looked for (Figure 3.10). Cataract is best examined with the light of an ophthalmoscope wherein red reflex is replaced by leukocoria or white reflex. Examine the eyes through the +10 diopter lens of an ophthalmoscope from a distance of 10 inches from the child's eyes. Coloboma or absence of part of iris (with or without involvement of choroid and retina) may occur in association with dermal hypoplasia, trisomy 13, CHARGE association, and Wolf-Hirschhorn syndrome.

Aniridia or complete absence of iris is rare and may be associated with Wilms' tumor, Rieger syndrome, neoplasms of adrenal cortex and liver. Heterochromia of irides (different colors of the iris of two eyes either partially or completely), may be associated with iridocyclitis of Fuchs, Waardenburg syndrome, Parry-Romberg syndrome, Sturge-Weber syndrome, Hirschsprung's disease, Horner syndrome, and cervical or mediastinal neuroblastoma. It may also occur due to injury or foreign body in the eye and following topical medications for glaucoma (prostaglandin analogue). Kayser-Fleischer ring, golden-brown or golden-green ring

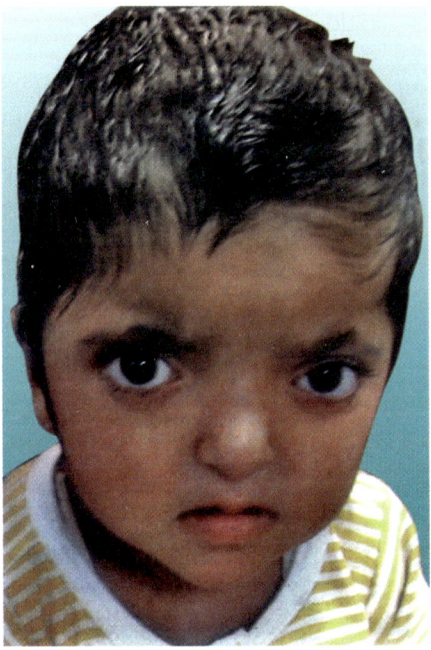

Figure 3.10 Physiologic hypertelorism with normal alignment of eyes. The child also has seborrhea capitis.

at the limbus of cornea, may be seen with a hand lens or slit-lamp examination in patients with Wilson disease, cholestatic syndromes and cholestatic hepatitis. Brushfield spots ("salt and pepper" speckling of iris) may be seen on naked eye or slit-lamp examination in children with Down syndrome. Iridodonesis, a quivering vibrations of iris, may be caused by subluxation of lens in patients with Marfan syndrome and homocystinuria. Examine the eyebrows and eyelashes which may be sparse or absent in children with ectodermal dysplasia (Figure 3.11). Due to unexplained reason, children with protein-energy malnutrition and tuberculosis may have relatively long eyelashes. Long and curly eyelashes with bushy eyebrows which extend to the nasion over the middle of forehead (synophrys) is a characteristic feature of Cornelia de Lange syndrome (Figure 3.12).

Size of pupils and pupillary reflex to light and red reflex in each eye separately and both the eyes simultaneously should be checked in a dark room with the help of a direct ophthalmoscope. Hand lens with an inbuilt light is useful for assessment of pupillary response to light. When indicated, fundus should be examined for papilledema, optic atrophy, cherry-red spot, chorioretinitis, flame-shaped hemorrhages (bacterial endocarditis), leukemic deposits and inflammatory granulomas (tuberculomas, candidemia).

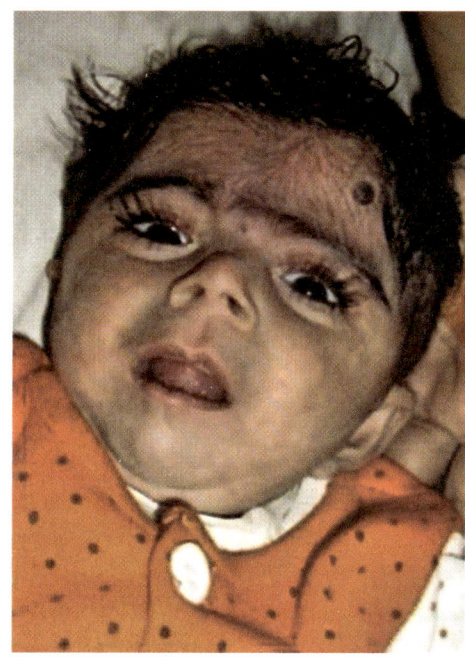

Figure 3.12 Cornelia de Lange syndrome. Note bushy eyebrows meeting in the center (synophrys), long eyelashes and long philtrum.

Squint is checked by shining the torch light on the eyes of the child. When eyes are normally aligned, the light reflex should be visible at an identical position in both the eyes (Figure 3.13). When strabismus is present, cover test is done to assess primary and secondary deviation of eyes. (Figure 3.14). The child is asked to fix on the torch light or a toy held infront of the face. Suddenly cover one eye, the uncovered eye will make some corrective movement (primary deviation) for fixation, if squint is present. Now look at the eye behind the cover while keeping it shielded from the light or object. In concomitant squint, the deviation of shielded eye (secondary deviation) will be equal to primary deviation while in a case of paralytic squint, secondary deviation is more than the primary deviation. Concomitant or non-paralytic squint is more common in children and is characterized by (i) onset before 3 years, (ii) normal movements of eyeballs in all directions, (iii) absence of diplopia or double vision, (iv) primary and secondary deviations are equal and (v) the deviating eye has defective vision or

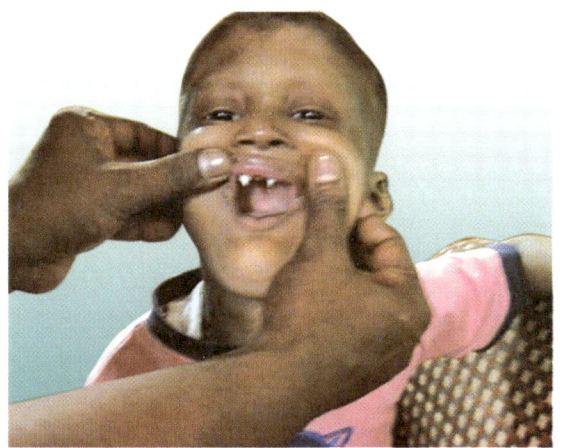

Figure 3.11 Ectodermal dysplasia. Absence of scalp hair, eyebrows and eyelashes with absent or conical teeth.

amblyopia. The concomitant squint may be convergent or divergent, constant or intermittant, may be monocular or affect both eyes alternately.

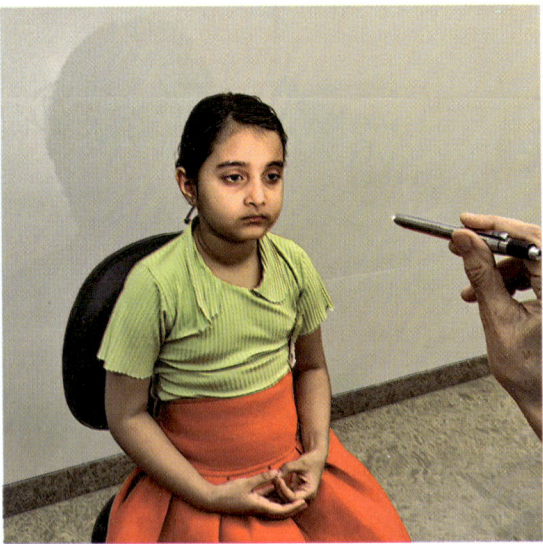

Figure 3.13 Corneal light reflex. The child is asked to see straight and a torch light is thrown in the eyes. The corneal light reflex is asymmetrical when there is strabismus.

Ear, Nose and Throat

Evidences of vitamin B complex deficiency, angular stomatitis, and cheilosis should be looked for. Tongue should be examined whether it is dry or wet, coated or clean, color, papillae, tremors, symmetry, aphthous ulcers, fissuring, etc. Geographic tongue is characterized by irregular red patches of desquamated epithelium and filiform papillae with sharp whitish-yellow border giving an appearance of map over the tongue. The patches may change in size and shape and are of no significance (Figure 3.15). Beefy-red smooth tongue due to atrophy of papillae is a recognized feature of vitamin B complex deficiency. Strawberry tongue is characterized by white, swollen fungiform papillae standing against raw, beefy-red background in children with scarlet fever, Kawasaki disease and toxic shock syndrome (Figure 3.16). Tongue-tie or ankyloglossia is often suspected by the grandmother when child is believed to have delayed speech. It is uncommon and should be suspected, if frenulum is thick and tight causing midline depression over the tip of the tongue. It neither causes difficulty in feeding nor delay in speech.

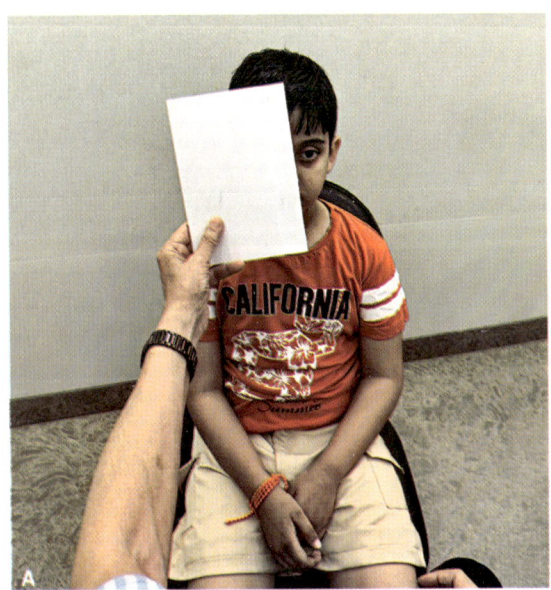
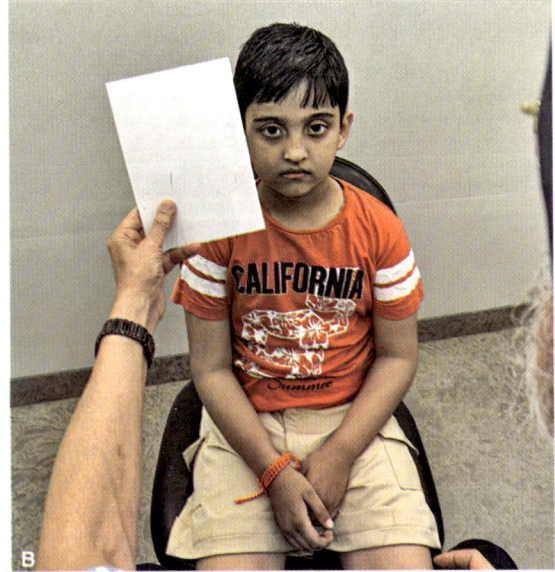

Figure 3.14A and B Cover uncover test. The child is asked to focus on an object or torch light. (A) One eye is suddenly covered. The uncovered eye will make some corrective movement which is called primary deviation; (B) The shield is suddenly removed to look for secondary deviation. *See* the text for details.

General Physical Examination

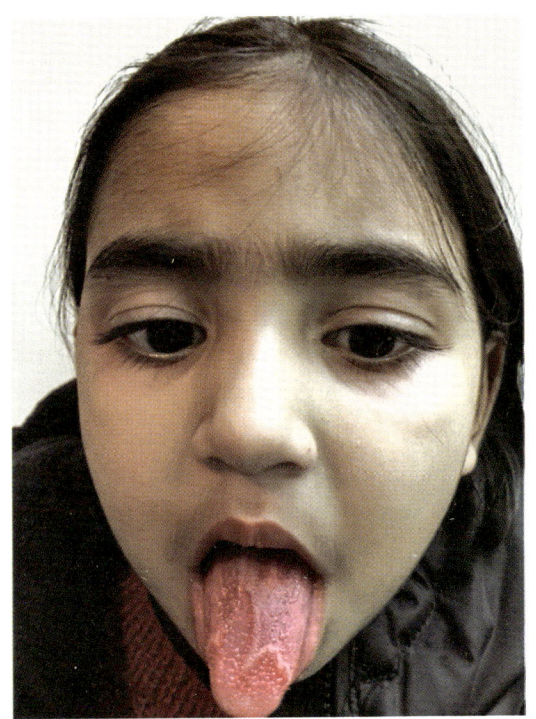

Figure 3.15 Typical appearances of geographical tongue.

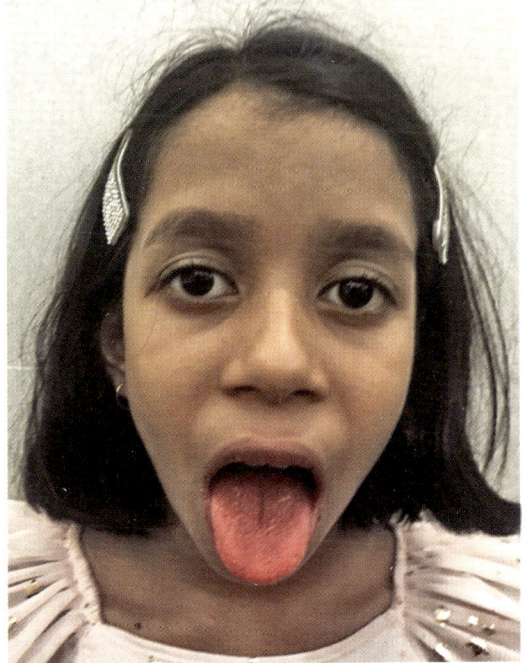

Figure 3.16 Strawberry tongue in a child with scarlet fever.

Teeth and gums should be examined for orodental hygiene, gingival hyperplasia (phenytoin therapy) and bleeding manifestations. A blue line on the gums is diagnostic of lead poisoning. Note how many deciduous or permanent teeth have erupted. The timing or onset of primary dentition is variable (due to genetic or constitutional factors) and is unreliable for assessment of nutritional status. Primary dentition may be delayed up to one year due to constitutional factors. Milk teeth are white in color and have a smooth edge in contrast to permanent teeth, which have an ivory-white or off-white color and have a finely serrated edge. Look for Koplik's spots in all children presenting with upper respiratory tract infection to diagnose measles during the prodromal stage. They are pinhead-sized white spots (like sago) with a red margin and are distributed over the buccal mucosa opposite the molar teeth. In mumps, look for redness and edema around the opening of Stenson's duct (opposite second upper molar).

Examine throat in all children for size of tonsils, evidences of inflammation, follicles, membrane, and petechiae (Figure 3.17A and B). In children above 3 years, throat can be examined without spatula by asking the child to open the mouth and say "aaha...." (Figure 3.18). A number of scales are available to assess the grade of tonsillar enlargement (Table 3.2). Herpangina is an acute febrile illness due to coxsackie viruses A and B, echoviruses and enteroviruses. It is characterized by dysphagia because of development of painful 1–4 mm size papulovesicular lesions surrounded by intense zone of erythema which are located mostly over the anterior tonsillar pillars and soft

TABLE 3.2 Friedman grading for enlargement of tonsils	
Grade	Discription
0	Tonsils barely visible
1	Located within tonsillar fossa
2	Visible beyond anterior pillars
3	Block 75% of airway
4	Two tonsils almost touching each other (Kissing tonsils)

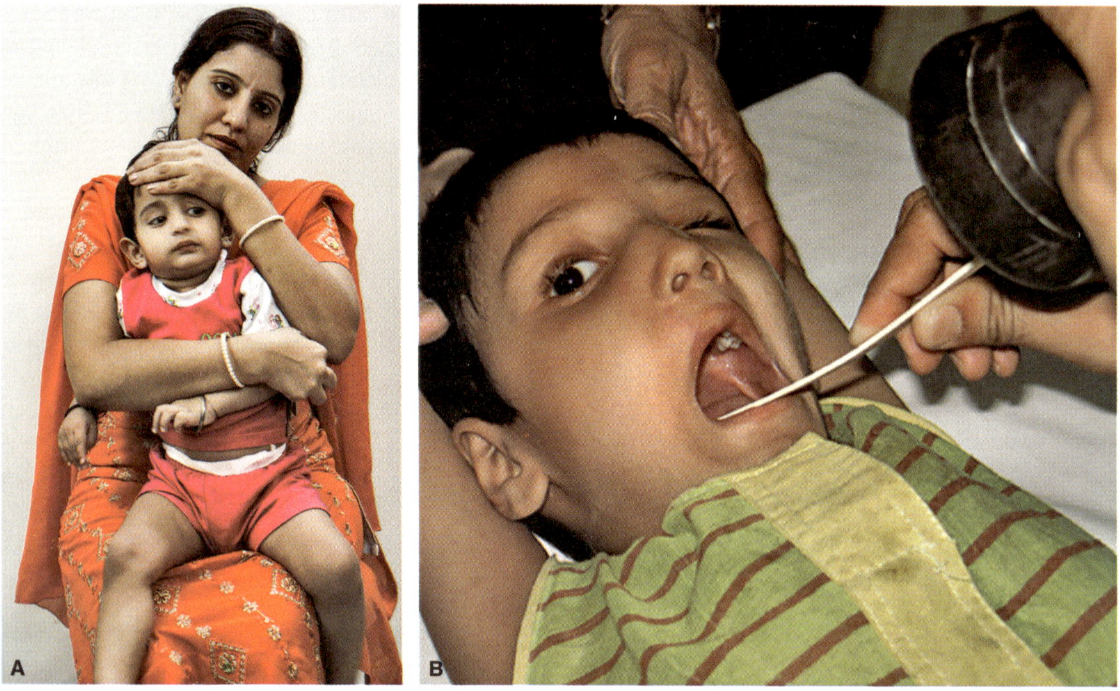

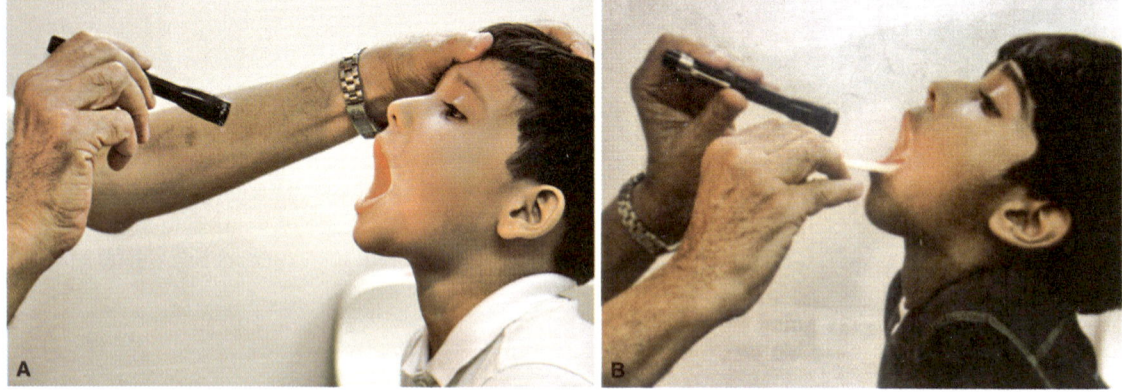

Figure 3.17 A and B The mother or nurse is asked to restrain the child by immobilizing his head and holding both the upper limbs. Throat can be examined both in sitting (A) and supine (B) positions. The neck should be slightly extended and crying actually helps to see the throat. In patients with stridor or suspected epiglottitis, no attempt should be made to examine the throat by inserting a spatula as it may lead to complete airway obstruction.

Figure 3.18A and B Throat being examined without any restraint in a 5-year-old boy. The child is asked to open the mouth widely and say "aaha…". In most cases, throat can be examined without using a spatula.

palate. Aphthous ulcers due to herpetic infection are seen over the anterior aspect of oral cavity involving the gums, buccal mucosa and tongue. In children, tonsils are physiologically large in size and should not be diagnosed as "tonsillitis" unless associated with fever, inflammation and exudates. Small and atrophic tonsils may be seen in children with immunodeficiency disorder or tonsils may be absent because of tonsillectomy. Unilateral enlargement of tonsils may occur due to peritonsillar abscess (quinsy) that develops between the tonsils and the constrictor pharyngeal muscles in school-going children. There is sudden onset of high grade fever, severe throat pain which radiates to ipsilateral ear, marked dysphagia, severe toxicity and torticollis with tilting of head towards the involved side. There is trismus, muffled speech and drooling of saliva. In infants, parapharyngeal abscess may occur. It is characterized by high grade spiking fever, marked toxicity, torticollis, markedly tender swelling in the neck with overlying erythema. Tonsillar lymphoma is rare and should be considered when there is unilateral tonsillar enlargement, painless dysphagia without any features of acute infection. There is characteristic enlargement of cervical lymph nodes and splenomegaly.

Ludwig angina is a potentially life-threatening infection of the mandibular floor. The symptoms begin with signs of dental abscess that rapidly progress to form a tense swelling of the mandibular floor and marked cervical edema resulting in a "bull neck".

Nose should be examined for any discharge (watery or purulent yellow or green), congestion or blockage, erosions or bleeding from Little's area, polyps, deflected nasal septum, snuffles and foreign body. Nasal itching, transverse crease over the bridge of the nose, allergic "shiners" or dark circles under the eyes may be seen in children with allergic rhinitis. Children with enlarged adenoids are likely to have open mouth, drooping of jaw, drooling of saliva, protrusion of teeth and expressionless face. They are uncomfortable at night, sleep with mouth open, and are prone to have snoring, sleep apnea and recurrent episodes of middle ear infection. Infants with respiratory distress are likely to have movements of alae nasi, retractions of intercostal spaces and expiratory grunt.

External ears should be examined for their size, shape, location (normal or low set) and anatomical landmarks (Figure 3.19). Look for pre- and post-auricular skin tags or sinuses which may be associated with renal malformations. Potter facies (squashed face with receding chin, low-set ears and prominent skin folds below the eyes) is a characteristic feature of oligohydramnios due to bilateral renal agenesis.

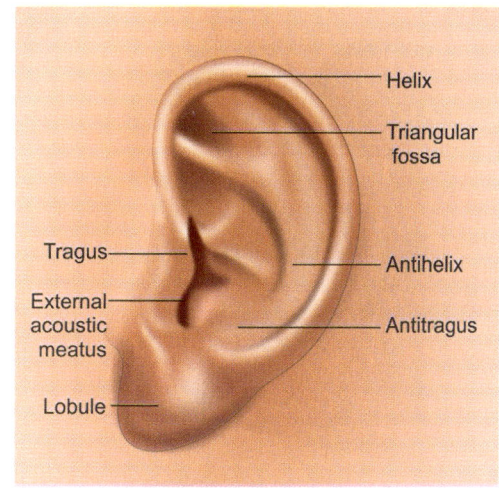

Figure 3.19 Anatomic landmarks of the external ear.

Ear canal and middle ear should be examined in all children with unexplained fever, upper respiratory tract infection, earache or discharging ear. The child should be positioned properly and restrained for ease of examination **(Figure 3.20)**.

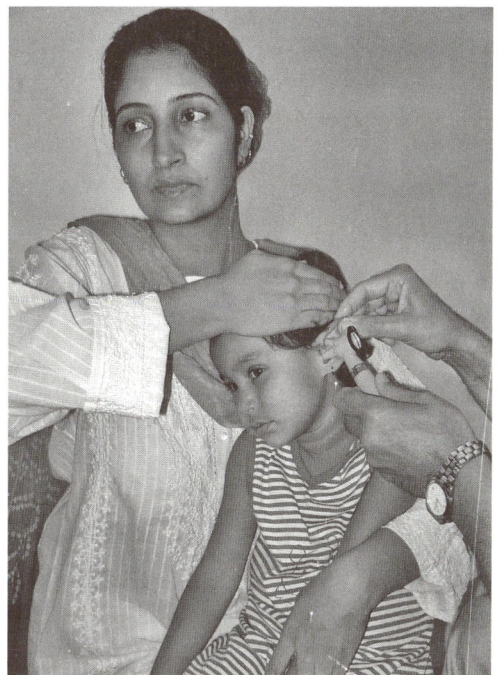

Figure 3.20 Holding and restraining the child for otoscopic examination of the ear. The mother or attendant should be asked to hold the child and restrain the arm firmly to avoid any damage to the ear canal.

In newborn babies and infants, the direction of ear canal is outwards while in older children it runs outwards and upwards. To visualize the tympanic membrane, pull the pinna of the ear with thumb and index finger upward and backwards in older children and outwards or laterally in infants and newborns. Use the largest speculum that will fit the ear canal. The hand holding the otoscope should rest against the cheek or head of the child so that, if child moves, the otoscope moves accordingly without imposing any risk to the child. Look for secretions, wax, foreign body and inflammation in the ear canal. Examine the tympanic membrane for its color, clarity, bulging or retraction, cone of light and perforation (Figure 3.21). Absence of cone of light indicates loss of lustre due to inflammation. The common types of perforations are antero-inferior, subtotal (rather large in size) and attic over the pars flaccida.

Neck

Neck is short in children and should be examined for any swelling, webbing, hair line, jugular venous pressure (JVP), arterial and venous pulsations, thyroid gland, lymph nodes, cysts, and fistulae. Minor enlargement of thyroid is better seen than felt and swelling moves upwards on swallowing. Thyroid gland is best palpated from behind with both hands on either side of the neck. When gland is enlarged, assess whether it is uniform or nodular, soft or hard in consistency. A standard clinical staging protocol is used to assess the size of goiter (Table 3.3). Ultrasonography is useful to assess

TABLE 3.3 Clinical staging of thyroid enlargement

■ Stage 0	No goiter is present
■ Stage 1	Goiter is palpable but not visible even when neck is fully extended
■ Stage 1A	Goiter is palpable and visible even when neck is fully extended
■ Stage 2	Goiter is visible when neck is in normal position
■ Stage 3	Goiter is visible from a distance

the size and nature of goiter more objectively. Physiological goiter is common during adolescence because of increased demands of thyroxine or relative iodine deficiency. Iodine deficiency in endemic areas is the most common cause of goiter. Other causes of euthyroid goiter include puberty goiter, chronic lymphocytic thyroiditis, benign thyroid adenoma, and carcinoma. Goiter with hypothyroidism is commonly seen in children with dyshormonogenesis, iodine deficiency, Hashimoto thyroiditis, intake of antithyroid drugs (iodides, lithium carbonate, and amiodarone), and goitrogens like cruciferous vegetables (broccoli, brussels sprouts, cabbage and cauliflower, mustard, turnips, radish, spinach, etc.), strawberries, peaches, and peanuts. Rarely, goiter may occur because of viral or pyogenic infection, cyst, adenoma, or cancer. In thyrotoxicosis, a bruit is usually heard over the goiter.

The tilting of neck should be differentiated from torticollis by examining the head from behind. In torticollis, the occiput is tilted to one side and chin to the other while in head tilting both occiput and chin are tilted to the same side. Look for cystic swellings like dermoid, thyroglossal cyst and goiter in the midline. Dermoid cyst is attached to the overlying skin while thyroglossal cyst is attached to the underlying structures and it moves upwards when child is asked to protrude the tongue. The swelling in the lateral side of neck usually occurs due to enlargement of lymph nodes, sebaceous cyst, branchial cleft cyst or sinus and lymphatic malformation. Lymphangioma or hygroma of neck is characterized by a soft, boggy, compressible and transilluminant swelling which may extend into upper thorax (Figure 3.22). Branchial cleft cysts

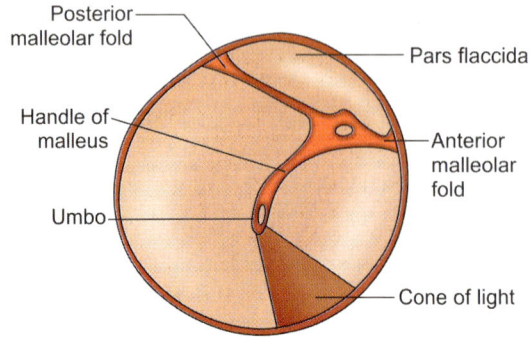

Figure 3.21 The normal anatomy and landmarks on the tympanic membrane of the ear.

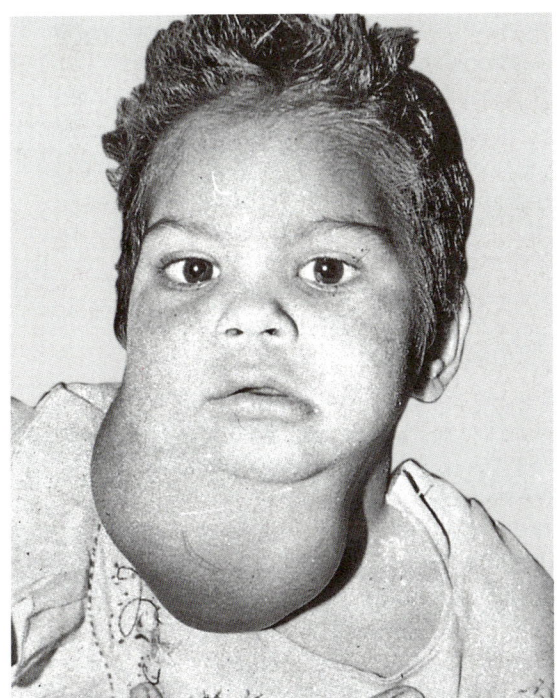

Figure 3.22 Typical location and appearance of hygroma neck. The swelling is soft, compressible and transilluminant.

bullosa, fetal alcohol and phenytoin syndromes. Koilonychia or spooning of nails as a sign of iron deficiency is relatively uncommon in children.

Skin should be examined for color, texture, elasticity/turgor, pigmentation, hemorrhagic spots, erythematous rash (blanches on pressure as opposed to petechiae and ecchymoses), pyoderma, subcutaneous nodules, neuroectodermal dysplasia, nevi, xanthoma, spider nevi, and palmar erythema (Figure 3.23 A and B). Follicular hyperkeratosis or phrynoderma (toad skin) is characteristically seen over extensor surfaces of extremities and buttocks. It is characterized by excessive development of keratin in hair follicles resulting in rough, cone-shaped, elevated papules. It occurs due to nutritional deficiency of vitamin A, and essential fatty acids.

The nature and distribution of skin lesions, whether isolated or generalized, symmetrical or asymmetrical, centrifugal or centripetal, present on flexor or extensor surfaces or areas exposed to sunlight should be looked for. The morphology of skin lesions is described as macules (areas of

may develop in adolescent children just infront of upper third of the anterior border of sternomastoid muscle. They appear as smooth, discrete, movable, tense cystic swelling(s) varying between 1 and 5 cm in size. When cyst ruptures, sticky, clear and mucoid secretions are drained. The position of trachea should be examined, whether it is central or tilted to one side.

Skin and its Appendages

Examine nails of hands and feet for clubbing, koilonychia or flattening, splinter hemorrhages, Osler nodes, brittleness and transluscent bands. Pitting of nails along with thickening and ridging may be seen in psoriasis, fungus infection and atopic dermatitis. White spots (leukonychia) or white lines over the nails may occur due to trauma or acute illness but are usually of no significance. Dystrophic or dysplastic nails may be seen in children with ectodermal dysplasia, nail patella syndrome, dystrophic form of epidermolysis

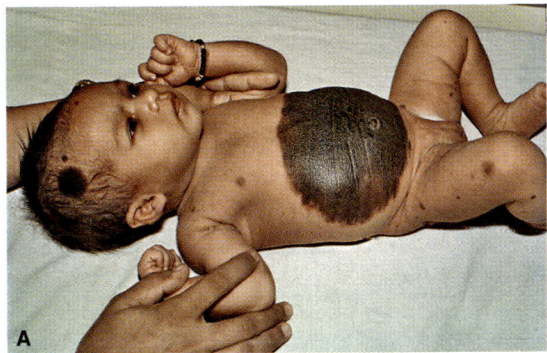

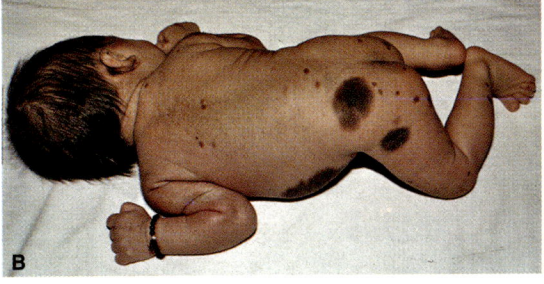

Figure 3.23 A and B Giant pigmented nevus over the abdomen (A). There are smaller pigmented nevi over the face, back and buttocks (B).

discoloration, neither raised nor depressed), papules (elevations up to 5 mm diameter), nodules (larger than papules), vesicles (blisters up to 10 mm diameter), bullae, wheals (pale, flat papules with surrounding erythematous flare as seen in urticaria), scales, burrows (dark brown straight or sinuous elevations in interdigital areas produced by female scabies mite), comedones (blackheads of acne), plaques (circumscribed flat areas of skin either raised, depressed or thickened), ulcerations, erosions or scar formation, etc. Look for distribution, color, texture, brittleness of scalp hair and presence of seborrhea and lice. Rarely hair may show alternate bands of depigmentation producing typical flag-sign in children with chronic malnutrition. For detailed examination of skin and its appendages, refer to Chapter 9.

Hands and Feet

A number of genetic and inflammatory diseases can be diagnosed by clinical examination and imaging studies of hands and feet. Examine the extremities for the size of hands and feet, length, swelling, deformity and mobility of fingers and toes. Look for pallor, cyanosis, jaundice, sweaty or erythematous palms and abnormalities of nails. Sudden appearance of itchy papules and vesicles or wheals over hands and feet is suggestive of hand-foot-mouth disease and mosquito bites. A number of developmental and chromosomal disorders are associated with characteristic abnormalities in the hands and feet (Table 3.4). "Radial ray anomalies" (RRAs), i.e. underdevelopment or complete absence of thumb, defective or deficient radius, triphalangeal thumb, preaxial polydactyly and syndactyly should be looked for.

Dermatoglyphics

The pattern of creases, ridges and mounts over the palms may provide useful information of clinical significance in children. Single horizontal palmar crease or simian crease (due to merging of head and heart lines) is classically seen in children with Down syndrome or as an isolated minor anomaly and it may occur in association with other chromosomal disorders (*Box 3.2*). When there are two transverse creases and the proximal one runs across the entire palm (Sydney line), it is seen in congenital rubella syndrome. Distal triradii are seen over the bases of index (A), middle (B), ring (C) and little (D) fingers while proximal triradius (T) is located on the palm close to the wrist. The ATD angle in normal subjects measures 40°. The ATD angle is obtuse (between 75° and 80° due to

TABLE 3.4 Abnormalities of hands and feet in common genetic disorders	
Disorders	Abnormalities
Down syndrome	Small hands, simian crease, incurved little finger
Ellis-van Creveld syndrome	Polydactyly with extra small digit on the ulnar side
Marfan syndrome	Arachnodactyly with excessively mobile long and thin digit, flexed thumb protrudes beyond the four fingers when fist is made (Steinberg thumb sign
Achondroplasia	"Trident hand deformity" with inability to fully extend the fingers, short middle finger due to shortening of third metacarpal
Nail-patella syndrome	Nails are often absent, hypoplastic or dystrophic
Mucopolysaccharides	"Claw hand", carpal tunnel syndrome, wide phalanges with thickening of subcutaneous tissues
Fibrodysplasia ossificans progressiva	Shortening and valgus deviation of great toes and thumb, painful fibrous nodules over neck, back and shoulders
Pseudo- and pseudo-hypoparathyroidism	Shortening of 4th and 5th metacarpals and metatarsals

Box 3.2 Causes of single transverse crease (Simian crease)

- Down syndrome
- Fetal alcohol syndrome
- Turner syndrome
- Cri du chat syndrome (chromosome 5)
- Klinefelter syndrome
- Wolf-Hirschhorn syndrome
- Noonan syndrome
- Patau syndrome (chromosome 13)
- Edward syndrome (chromosome 18)
- Aarskog–Scott syndrome
- Leukocyte adhesion deficiency-2 (LAD2)
- Poland syndrome
- Idiopathic (mostly unilateral in about 1.5% of general population)

distal location of axial triradius) in children with Down syndrome, Turner syndrome and congenital rubella syndrome (Figure 3.24). There may be abnormalities in the pattern of ridges over finger tips in children with Down syndrome (ulnar loops in all fingers), congenital rubella syndrome (mostly whorls), trisomy-18 (increase in arches) and Klinefelter syndrome (marked reduction in ridge count).

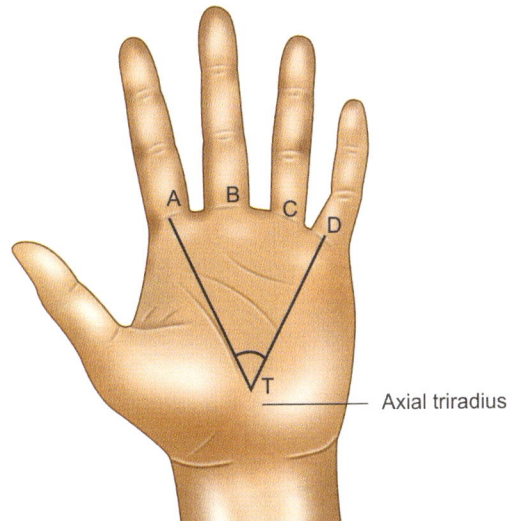

Figure 3.24 Single palmar crease and ATD angle by joining AD distal triradii with axial triradius (T). ATD angle becomes obtuse when axial triradius is shifted distally towards fingers.

Evidences of Deficiency States

When pre-illness weight of the child is known, the severity of dehydration can be assessed accurately by degree of weight loss (Table 3.5). But most of the times accurate pre-illness weight of the child is not known and severity of dehydration is graded as per WHO recommendations (Table 3.6). In marasmic children, skin turgor is impaired due to loss of subcutaneous fat. The severity of dehydration is thus overestimated in malnourished children. They may have sunken eyeballs, flat fontanel and poor skin turgor without any dehydration. You should look for evidences of excessive water loss (vomiting, diarrhea) or poor intake, excessive thirst, dry tongue or buccal mucosa, oliguria/anuria, acidosis and shock (cold extremities, tachycardia, feeble radial pulse, delayed capillary refill time of >2 sec) for making the diagnosis of dehydration in malnourished children. On the other hand, in chubby or obese children, dehydration is likely to be overlooked or underestimated. When child is in the hospital and being weighed daily, sudden weight gain or weight loss are reliable correlates of overhydration (overinfusion and cardiac failure) and dehydration, respectively.

Look for evidences of protein-calorie deficiency (undernutrition, marasmus, marasmic-kwashiorkor, kwashiorkor), deficiency of water-soluble (vitamins B complex and C) and fat-soluble (vitamins A, D, E, K) vitamins (Table 3.7) and deficiencies of various minerals, like iron, calcium, iodine, zinc, copper, magnesium, manganese, molybdenum and selenium (Table 3.8).

Bones and Joints

Look for chest deformity, localized swelling, sternal tenderness, ends of long bones, joint inflammation, swelling, mobility of joints, size and symmetry of limbs (Figure 3.26). Arthralgia (joint pain alone) and arthritis (joint pain with swelling and inflammatory signs) should be differentiated. Migratory or fleeting joint pain is suggestive of acute rheumatic fever and gonococcemia. Examine hands and feet for their size, shape and length of fingers and toes, dermatoglyphics, syndactyly and

TABLE 3.5 Clinical evaluation of severity of dehydration

Degree	Acute weight loss	Signs
Mild	Up to 5%	Irritability, excessive thirst
Moderate	5–10%	Depressed anterior fontanel, sunken eyes, reduced tears and sweat, loss of skin turgor, dry mucosa, and reduced urine output.
Severe	>10%	Extreme loss of skin turgor (Figure 3.25) and absence of tears, drinks poorly or unable to drink, marked oliguria or anuria, tachycardia, cold, clammy and mottled skin, shock, capillary refill >2s, metabolic acidosis*, and alteration in consciousness.

*Renal shutdown is diagnosed, if no urine is passed for 6 hours in an infant and for 12 hours in an older child. In metabolic acidosis, breathing is rapid and deep or sighing (Kussmaul's breathing). In hypernatremic dehydration, mucosa is parchment like, with marked thirst, skin is doughy, shock and renal shut down are delayed. Seizures may occur during rapid correction of hypernatremic dehydration.

TABLE 3.6 WHO criteria for assessment of dehydration

Signs	No dehydration	Some dehydration	Severe dehydration
General appearance	Alert and normal	Restless, irritable	Lethargic or unconscious
Thirst	Normal	Thirsty and drinks eagerly	Drinks poorly or not able to drink
Eyes	Normal	Sunken	Very sunken and dry
Oral mucosa and tongue	Moist	Dry	Dry and parched
Skin pinch*	Goes back quickly	Goes back slowly	Goes back very slowly (>2 sec)
Urine output	Normal	Oliguria may be present	Severe oliguria or anuria (no urine for 6 hr in an infant and 12 hr in older children)

*Pinch and lift the skin of abdomen or chest between the thumb and index finger for 3–4 sec and release. Oliguria is defined as urine output of less than 1 mL/kg/h in infants and <0.5 mL/kg/h in children. Anuria is diagnosed when urine output is less than 100 mL in a day.

polydactyly; whether preaxial (towards the side of thumb) or postaxial (towards the side of little finger). Examine fingers for clinodactyly (deflection of finger) and camptodactyly (fixed flexion of interphalangeal joints producing claw-like appearance). Hands and feet may look short and stubby because of shortening of metacarpals and metatarsals. In children with pseudohypoparathyroidism, index finger may be longer than middle finger because of shortening of all metacarpals except second.

Look for deformities, like club foot (plantar flexion, inversion and adduction of foot) and calcaneovalgus deformity (dorsiflexion and eversion of foot). Bowed legs are normally seen during first two years of life while slight knock knees are common between the ages of 2 to 5 years. The severity of bowed legs is assessed by measuring the distance between the knees when medial malleoli are closely aligned in a supine infant. For assessment of severity of knock knees, the child is asked to stand with knees barely touching each other and distance between medial malleoli at ankles is measured. The physiological severity of bowed legs and knock knees is usually less than 5 cm. The arch of feet is obliterated by a pad of fat during first 2 years of life producing physiological flat feet.

TABLE 3.7 Clinical features of vitamin deficiencies in children

Deficiency state	Symptoms and signs
Vitamin A	Night blindness, bitot spots on scleral conjunctiva (chalky-grey spots on the temporal side of corneoscleral junction), xerophthalmia, and keratomalacia. Toad-like skin due to follicular hyperkeratosis (phrynoderma), faulty epiphyseal bone formation, mucosal alterations leading to frequent respiratory and GI infections, stunting and formation of renal and vesical calculi.
Vitamin B complex	*Thiamine (B_1)*: Dry beri-beri (polyneuritis, ptosis, hoarseness of voice, tenderness of calf muscles, sluggish deep tendon jerks) and wet beri-beri (palpitation, tachycardia, dyspnea, cardiomegaly and edema with low voltage, prolonged QT interval and inversion of T waves on EKG). *Riboflavin (B_2)*: Glossitis (sore, red and glazed tongue), cheilosis and angular stomatitis (cracking of the angles of the mouth), scaly dermatitis at nasolabial folds, photophobia and blurred vision due to circumcorneal vascularization and keratitis. *Niacin (PP factor or B_3)*: Pellagra characterized by diarrhea, dermatitis (over parts of skin exposed to sunlight), and dementia (muscle weakness, loss of memory, depression and lethargy). *Pantothenic acid (B_5)*: Burning sensations in hands and feet, gastrointestinal disturbances, muscle cramps, fatigue and hypoglycemia. *Pyridoxine (B_6)*: Hypochromic anemia, irritability, seizures and peripheral neuritis. *Biotin (B_7)*: Hair loss, scaly erythematous rash around eyes, nose, mouth and genital area. *Folic acid or folate (B_9)*: Megaloblastic anemia, glossitis, pharyngeal ulcers and impaired immunity. *Cyanocobalamin (B_{12})*: Anemia, pigmentation of knuckles, thrombocytopenia, and tremors.
Vitamin C (ascorbic acid)	Scurvy characterized by marked irritability, hemorrhages under the periosteum of long bones (pseudoparalysis with frog-like posture), gums, mucous membranes and skin, and scorbutic rosary (posterior dislocation of sternum). Angulation of "scorbutic beads" is seen unlike rickets where swelling is rounded or dome-shaped. There is increased risk of infections and poor wound healing.
Vitamin D (cholecalciferol)	Rickets characterized by bossing of skull, craniotabes, delayed closure of anterior fontanel, costochondral beading (rachitic rosary which is broad, smooth and dome-shaped), pigeon-shaped chest, Harrison's sulcus* (retractions at lower borders of chest corresponding to the insertion of diaphragm), spinal deformities, widening and enlargement of ends of long bones, bowing of legs, knock knees, coxa vara, pot-belly, etc. Stunting is common and tetany may occur.
Vitamin E (tocopherol)	Hemolytic anemia in preterm babies, progressive neuromyopathy manifesting as ataxia, muscular cramps, and paralysis of extrinsic ocular muscles.
Vitamin K	Early and late-onset hemorrhagic disease of the newborn with bleeding manifestations from different sites.

Vitamins A,D,E and K are fat-soluble while vitamins B complex and C are water-soluble vitamins.
*Harrison's sulcus is also seen in children with obstructive airway disease or enlarged adenoids.

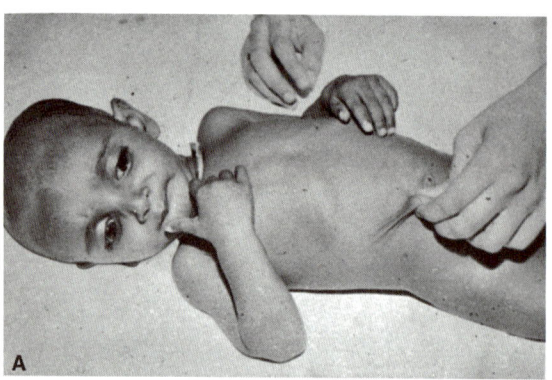 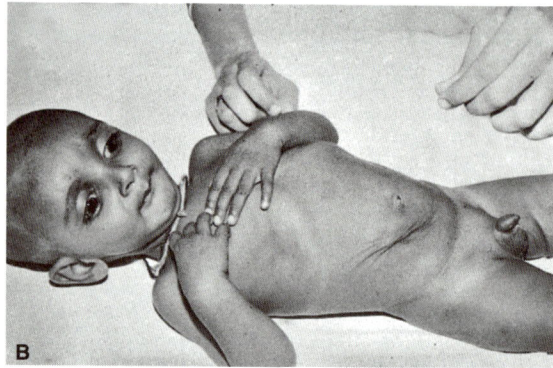

Figure 3.25 A and B Method for elicitation of skin turgor. The abdominal skin is pinched, lifted and released (A). When skin turgor is lost due to dehydration (or marasmus) it takes several seconds before the pinched skin assumes its unwrinkled appearance (B). Note the sunken eyes of the child.

TABLE 3.8 Clinical features due to deficiency of trace minerals	
Deficiency state	Symptoms and signs
Iron	Pica, lethargy, easy fatigability, irritability, impaired physical growth and neuromotor development, reduced work capacity, breathlessness on exertion, pallor (conjunctiva, tongue, palms and soles), koilonychia or flattening of nails.
Calcium	Tetany, carpopedal spasms, muscle cramps, weakness, poor mineralization of bones and teeth, rickets and stunting. EKG may show prolonged QoTc.
Iodine	Simple goiter, stunting, neuromotor retardation, learning disorders, deafness, coarse skin, cold intolerance and constipation.
Zinc	Stunting, acrodermatitis enteropathica (vesiculobullous skin lesions with pigmentation of extremities), psoriasiform ulcerations of mucocutaneous junctions involving perioral and perianal regions, alopecia, white spots over nails, hypogonadism, poor wound healing, recurrent infections due to poor immunity.
Copper	Refractory anemia, osteoporosis, neutropenia, hypopigmentation of skin and hair and ataxia.
Magnesium	Tics, muscle spasms, cramps, anxiety, low energy, sleep problems, abnormalities of cardiac rhythm.
Chromium	Depression, craving for sweets, poor ability to metabolize glucose, decreased protein synthesis, increased production of cholesterol and triglycerides.
Manganese	Impaired growth, poor glucose tolerance, low immunity, osteoporosis, chronic fatigue syndrome.
Molybdenum	Oral mucosa and gum disorders, tachycardia, night blindness and sulfite sensitivity.
Selenium	Fatigue, hair loss, slow mentation, hypothyroidism, goiter, low immunity and Kashin–Beck disease (osteochondropathy).

General Physical Examination

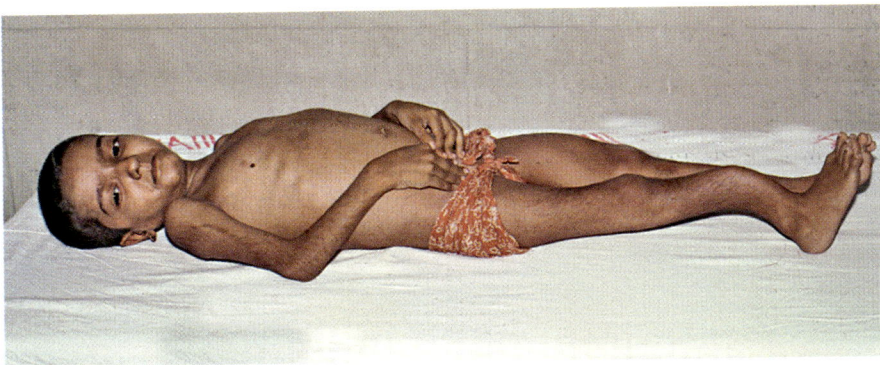

Figure 3.26 Skeletal deformities due to renal rickets in a 10-year-old child. There is failure to thrive, widening of ends of long bones, costochondral beading and marked deformities of bones of lower limbs (saber tibia).

In children with history of arthralgia or arthritis, mobility of joints should be tested in all directions. Limitation of internal rotation is an early sign in many diseases of hip joints particularly slipped epiphysis and Legg-Perthe's disease. Excessive external rotation of hips is a common finding in infants up to 18 months. Curvature (kyphosis, lordosis, scoliosis), swelling, tenderness, and range of movements of spine should be looked for. Spinal deformity may account for displacement of apex beat.

Sexual Maturity Rating

Adolescence extends from 10–16 years in girls and 12–18 years in boys. Adolescence and sexual maturation is earlier by 2 years in girls compared to boys. The age of onset of puberty is variable but usually occurs between 10 and 12 years in girls and 12 and 14 years in boys. Breast development is the first manifestation of sexual development in girls while testicular enlargement heralds the onset of sexual maturity in boys. Prader orchidometer or orchiometer (Beads of different volumes ranging from 1.0 to 25.0 mL) can be used to accurately assess the testicular volume **(Figure 3.27)**. In preadolescent obese boys, penis may be embedded in the pubic fat giving an erroneous impression of hypogonadism. The stages of sexual development or sexual maturity rating are shown in **Table 3.9** and **Figure 3.28 A and B**. Identify whether sexual maturation is advanced, normal or retarded. Puberty is considered as delayed, if no secondary sex characters (budding of breasts) are seen by 14 years in the girls and 16 years in boys (increase in the volume of testes). Precocious puberty is diagnosed in girls when breast development occurs before 8 years and menarche before 10 years of age and in boys when testicular enlargement occurs before 9 years of age.

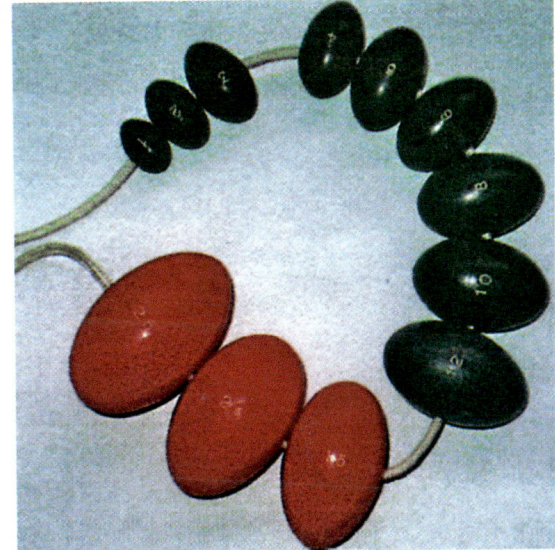

Figure 3.27 Prader orchidometer for assessment of testicular volume.

During assessment of sexual maturity, look for any abnormalities in the external genitalia, inguinal hernia, hydrocele, undescended testes, developmental defects, posthitis, balanitis, cysts, tight prepuce, etc.

TABLE 3.9 Stages of sexual development

GIRLS

Age (yr)	SMR*stage	Pubic hair	Breasts
<10	1	None	Preadolescent, no breast growth
10–12	2	Sparse, lightly pigmented over medial border of labia	Breast and papilla elevated to form a mound, areolar diameter is increased
12–13	3	Darker and coarse, beginning to curl on mons pubis	Breast and areola enlarged, no contour separation
13–14	4	Coarse, curly, and abundant	Areola and papilla elevated beyond the contour of the breast to form a secondary mound
14–16	5	Adult feminine triangle, spread to inner sides of thighs	Nipple projects, areola part of general breast contour

BOYS

Age (yr)	SMR*stage	Pubic hair	Scrotum and testes	Penis
<12	1	None	Preadolescent (<4 mL)	Preadolescent
12.5–14.5	2	Scanty light-colored over the base of penis	Enlarged scrotum, pink in color with altered texture. Testes 4–10 mL	Slight increase
13–15	3	Darker, beginning to curl and spread laterally	Larger scrotum, testes 10–15 mL	Longer
13.5–15.5	4	Adult type, black and coarse	Larger with dark scrotum, testes 15–20 mL	Larger with increase in the size of glans and width of penis
16–18	5	Spread to medial surfaces of thighs	Adult size of scrotum and testes measuring 4.5 cm × 3.5 cm × 2.0 cm with an average volume of about 20 mL	Adult size with average flaccid length of 9.16 cm and girth of 9.31 cm

*Sexual maturity rating
Note: Axillary hair appear after 2 years of onset of pubic hair and coincides with development of facial hair in boys.

Assessment of Severity of Illness

It is important to assess whether an acutely sick child can be managed on an ambulatory basis or should be admitted to the hospital. The presence of following clinical features suggests that the child is critically sick:

- Age < 3 months with a body temperature ≥39°C (102.2°F) in the absence of cough and cold due to viral infection.
- Anxious, dull and expressionless toxic look.
- Altered sensorium, moaning or groaning sounds, absence of cry, or inconsolable, shrieking and high pitched cry, lack of any response to parental overtures, bulging anterior fontanel or neck rigidity.
- Refusal to drink or eat.
- Abdominal distension or marked tenderness of abdomen.
- Seizures without any past history of epilepsy or febrile convulsions.
- Hyperpyrexia (despite adequate antipyretic therapy and cold sponging) or hypothermia.
- Marked respiratory distress with intercostal recessions, grunting and stridor or slow gasping breathing.

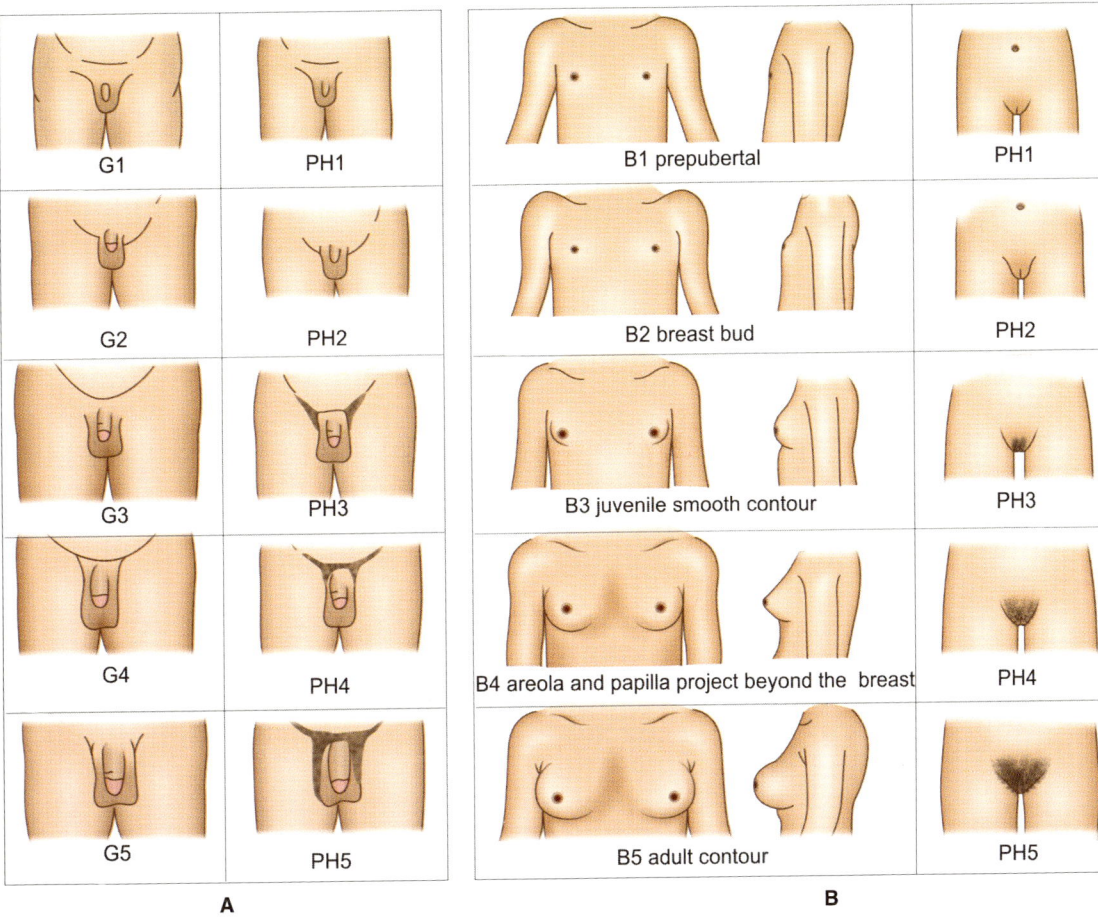

Figure 3.28A and B Diagrammatic representation of stages of sexual maturity in boys (A) and girls (B). B1–B5, breast development, G1–G5, male genitals, PH1–PH5, pubic hair.

- Central cyanosis (in the absence of cyanotic heart disease), ashen-grey pallor, mottling of skin, cold and clammy (wet) extremities, slow capillary refill, hypotension and shock.
- Evidences of moderate to severe dehydration or acidosis (Kussmaul's breathing), oliguria or anuria (lack of urination for more than 6 hours in an infant and 12 hours in an older child).
- Ecchymoses, petechiae and bleeding manifestations.

Objectivized Structured Clinical Examination (OSCE)

In order to eliminate subjectivity and cover a wide-spectrum of skills for teaching and assessment of medical graduate and postgraduate students, OSCE has been introduced. In a short period, the students can be taught or assessed for a large number of skills and use of diagnostic tools. Instead of coventional long case and short case allocations for clinical examination, a number of clinical stations are created to assess a wide range of clinical skills of the students. The station may have a live patient or vignettes of case scenarios, laboratory reports and assessment of various skills and procedures. Each station is allocated a time slot and student is asked to do a task and record his or her observations on a pre-coded questionnaire. Apart from assessment of a wide range of skills and allocation of identical case material to all students, OSCE also eliminates the subjective bias of the examiners. However, creation of OSCE stations is time consuming and labor-intensive for the examiners. Depending upon the available clinical cases and skills to be tested, a wide range of OSCE stations can be created as mentioned in following examples:

1. Assess muscle tone of this one-year-old infant. *5 min*
2. Assess the developmental quotient of this girl with a corrected age of 18 months. *7 min*
3. Assess the vital signs including blood pressure in both the upper as well as lower limbs. *7 min*
4. Do the relevant physical examination in this child with history of partial seizures on the right side. *5 min*
5. Do examination of the heart on this 3-year-old boy. *7 min*
6. Record anthropometric measurements of this 6-month-old infant. *5 min*
7. Conduct abdominal examination in this 5-year-old boy. *5 min*
8. Assess the primitive or automatic reflexes in this 2-week-old infant. *5 min*
9. Examine the chest in this 10-year-old boy with history of fever and cough for one month. *7 min*
10. Examine the cranial nerves in this 5-year-old girl. *7 min*

General Physical Examination

	Scheme for Presentation
General	Attitude, posture, appearance, cry, comfortable or irritable, gravely sick, toxic, restless, dyspneic, orthopneic, grunting, stridor, level of consciousness, and evidences of cerebral and spinal meningeal irritation.
Build and nutrition	Skeletal size, body frame, muscle mass, subcutaneous fat, average build, tall, short, fat, thin or cachectic.
Anthropometry	Weight, height (or length in infants below 2 years), mid-arm circumference (for children between 1 and 5 years), head circumference, chest circumference, upper segment to lower segment body ratio and arm span. State the weight age, height age, percentile placement of measurements on the standard growth charts, body mass index (BMI), weight-for-age, weight-for-height and degree of malnutrition.
Developmental assessment	Is development normal, globally retarded or retarded in a specific field, developmental age and developmental quotient.
Vital signs	Temperature, pulse, respiration, blood pressure.
General features	Anemia, cyanosis, jaundice, edema, lymphadenopathy.
Head and face	Head size, shape, bossing, fontanels, sutures, Macewen's sign, characteristic facies, facial dysmorphism, abnormalities in the eyes, ears, nose, mouth, lips, chin, etc.
Eyes	Ptosis, corneal opacity, bitot spots, cataract, glaucoma, white reflex, strabismus, proptosis and fundus examination.
ENT examination	Orodental hygiene, teeth, gums, tongue, tonsils, buccal mucosa, examination of ears, nose and throat.
Neck	Hair line, webbing, JVP, arterial and venous pulsations, thyroid gland, trachea, cysts, fistulae, lymph glands, etc.
Hands and feet	Size of hands and feet, any swelling, deformity and limitations of movements of fingers and toes. Excessive sweating, erythema of palms and soles, itchy papules or vesicles over the hands and feet and radial ray anomalies.
Skin and its appendages	*Skin*: Color, texture, turgor and elasticity, skin rash, nodules, purpura, ecchymoses, pigmentation, pyoderma, eczema, neuroectodermal dysplasia, nevi, xanthoma, spider angioma and palmar erythema. *Hair*: Distribution, hair loss, color, texture, brittleness, dandruff, pityriasis scalp, lice, nits, eyebrows, eyelashes, and hirsutism. *Nails*: Clubbing, flattening or koilonychia, dystrophy, color, translucent bands, white spots, and splinter hemorrhages.
Evidences of deficiency states	Evidences of hypoxia, dehydration, protein-energy malnutrition, deficiencies of vitamins, minerals and trace elements.
Bones and joints	Gait, deformities of long bones, thorax, spine, hands and feet, evidences of arthritis, bony tenderness, rickets, etc.
Genitals and sexual maturity stage	Are genitals normal or ambiguous, sexual maturity stage: Normal, retarded or advanced (precocious). Look for inguinal hernia, hydrocele, undescended testis, developmental defects, posthitis, balanitis, cysts of glans penis, tight prepuce, etc.

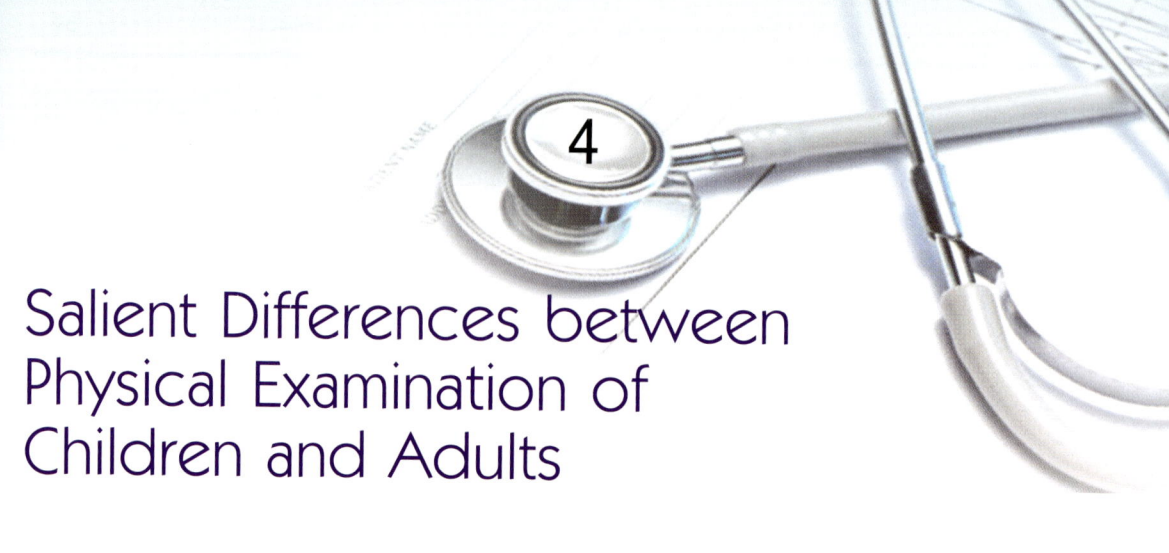

4
Salient Differences between Physical Examination of Children and Adults

PHYSIOLOGICAL HANDICAPS

Children are not mini-adults and they are poorly equipped to maintain homeostasis. There are important anatomic and physiological differences between children and adults. They have a large surface area compared to the body weight with an increased risk to develop hypothermia and excessive insensible water losses. They are equipped with immature and unstable mechanisms to control body temperature. Children have a higher metabolic rate, increased oxygen (minute ventilation of 600 liters/kg/day in an infant versus 200 liters/kg/day in an adult) and caloric need (120 Kcal/kg in infants compared to 40 Kcal/kg in adults). They have a poor ability to excrete carbon dioxide and are more susceptible to develop metabolic acidosis. Children are more vulnerable to develop dehydration because of excessive insensible water losses, poor ability to concentrate urine and rapid daily turnover of body water (15% in children compared to 5% in adults). Because of small blood volume, children are more vulnerable to develop shock due to blood loss. Above all, children are completely dependent and at the mercy of their parents and caretakers to satisfy their basic needs for rearing, protection, calories, nutrients and fluids. Nutritional disorders are far more common in children compared to adults.

GENERAL DIFFERENCES

1. History is often imprecise because children cannot express or explain their problems. The accuracy of history depends upon the intelligence, education, observational ability and concern of the mother, father or attendant.
2. Dietary and immunization history is of special significance among children. Children are more prone to develop protein-energy malnutrition and deficiency of micronutrients because they are at the mercy of their caretakers. Perinatal events, growth and developmental history should be enquired and recorded, especially in preschool children.
3. There is general lack of cooperation by young children during examination. Observation is most contributory or informative in children and should be accorded maximum importance.
4. The approach during clinical examination does not follow any set sequence but is unstructured. The unpleasant components of physical examination is postponed to the end. *Children must be handled as children and not as patients.*
5. Childhood period is characterized by rapid physical growth and neuromotor development. A pediatrician, therefore, deals with subjects varying in weight from 1.0 to 50 kg and in different stages of neuromotor development and maturation of various body organs. The examination tools of different sizes are needed

depending upon the age of the child, e.g. size of the stethoscope, ear specula, cuff of blood pressure apparatus, weighing scales, little finger for rectal examination so on and so forth.
6. Developmental defects, chromosomal disorders and inborn errors of metabolism, by and large, produce their manifestations during childhood and should be looked for.

GENERAL PHYSICAL EXAMINATION

1. Anthropometry is of particular importance and of special significance in children. Availability of electronic weighing scales for infants and children and infantometer for infants and stadiometer for older children is mandatory.
2. Developmental assessment is mandatory and peculiar to children.
3. Disorders of head size and shape are limited to children because of open sutures and fontanels.
4. Infants with cardiac failure or low oncotic pressure are more likely to have sacral edema and puffiness of face instead of pedal edema.
5. Peculiar and diagnostic facies (dysmorphism) and developmental disorders are, by and large, limited to children.
6. Nutritional deficiency states are far more common among children because of greater caloric and nutritional needs per unit body weight, reduced dietary intake because of food fussiness and "blackmailing tactics" and their dependence on caretakers to meet their nutritional requirements. Some deficiency states produce different manifestations among children as compared to adults, e.g. rickets vs osteomalacia.
7. Signs of meningeal irritation may be minimal or absent during first year of life (especially first 3 months) and in malnourished children.
8. There is marked hyperplasia of lymphoid tissues during preschool period, leading to adenoidal hypertrophy, enlargement of tonsils and cervical lymph nodes.
9. Iron deficiency is common but koilonychia is rare among children.
10. The norms for vital signs are different in children of different ages (Table 4.1). Heart rate (pulse rate) and breathing rates should be recorded for one minute when child is quiet, resting or asleep.

SYSTEMIC EXAMINATION

Alimentary System

1. Abdomen is protuberant (pot-belly) and soft in infants. Divarication of recti, umbilical hernia and hydrocele are very common.
2. Palpation of abdomen in infants is best achieved during feeding.
3. Palpable liver up to 2 cm with soft consistency is normal throughout childhood while spleen tip may be normally felt during first 3 months of life.

TABLE 4.1 Normal range of vital signs at different ages*

Age	Heart rate (beats/min)	Respiration rate (breaths/min)	Blood pressure (systolic/diastolic mm Hg)
Neonate (<28 d)	100–165	40–70	60–85/45–55
Infant (1 mo–1 y)	100–150	30–55	80–100/55–65
Toddler (1–2 y)	70–110	20–30	90–105/55–70
Pre-school age (3–5 y)	65–110	20–25	95–107/60–71
School age (6–11 y)	60–95	14–22	95–110/60–73
Adolescent (12–15 y)	55–85	12–18	110–124/70–79

*Vital signs should be recorded when child is quiet and resting
Note: Temperature is 37 ±0.2°C at all ages. In a newborn baby, breathing rate and heart rate are double of an adult while blood pressure is one-half of the adult.
Source: Kliegman RM, et al. Nelson Textbook of Pediatrics, 20th edition, Philadelphia, PA: Elsevier, 2015

4. Genital area should be routinely examined to look for congenital malformations, inguinal hernia, hydrocele and undescended testis.

Respiratory System

1. The breathing is rapid and abdominothoracic in infants. Tidal volume is proportional to body weight (7–10 mL/kg). The normal rhythm of breathing is inspiration–expiration–pause. It gets reversed to expiratory grunt–inspiration–pause in respiratory distress syndrome and pneumonia. Intercostal and suprasternal recessions are common because of soft ribs.
2. Chest deformities (pigeon chest and funnel-shaped chest) and Harrison's sulcus are common in children with rickets and recurrent respiratory infections and obstructive airway disease.
3. Tongue is relatively large while narrow air passages predispose to frequent development of stridor, croup, wheezing and atelectasis.
4. The larynx in children is located opposite the level of 1st or 2nd cervical vertebrae compared to adult larynx which is located at the level of 4th or 5th cervical vertebrae.
5. Percussion may be impaired over the manubrium sterni due to enlarged thymus. The chest is more resonant in children as compared to adults because of thin chest wall.
6. The normal breath sounds are hollow and peurile or harsh vesicular in children. Because of small thorax, the adventitious sounds from one side may be conducted to the opposite side.

Cardiovascular System

1. Pulse is rapid and difficult to feel among infants due to small size of the wrist and decreased vagal tone. Sinus arrhythmia, i.e. increase in heart rate during inspiration and bradycardia on expiration, is common in children.
2. Jugular venous pressure is difficult to evaluate in infants because of short and obese neck.
3. It is preferable to auscultate the heart of an infant first before he starts crying because of palpation and percussion.
4. Precordial bulge may occur as a sign of long-standing cardiac enlargement because of soft rib cage.
5. Apex beat is located in the 4th intercostal space at or slightly outside the midclavicular line.
6. Splitting of second heart sound is common. P_2 is louder than A_2 in infants up to 6 months of age. Heart sounds are better audible due to thin chest.
7. Functional systolic murmurs and venous hum are common in children.
8. Right ventricular hypertrophy is seen in newborn babies while left ventricular preponderance occurs in adults.
9. Blood pressure is lower in children and proper cuff size (to cover two-thirds of upper arm) is essential for recording it. Doppler system is used to record blood pressure in infants and critically sick children.
10. Most congenital cardiac defects produce their clinical manifestations during early childhood while rheumatic heart disease is unlikely below the age of 3 years.

Central Nervous System

1. Cooperation for proper CNS examination of children is exceedingly difficult. Several tricks or play attitude may have to be adopted for thorough CNS assessment. Sensations are most difficult to assess.
2. Head is relatively large, fontanels and sutures are open in infants with increased incidence of development of hydrocephalus.
3. The likelihood of neurological symptoms, like alteration in consciousness and seizures, being due to a disease outside the CNS (because of toxins and metabolic disorder)

is more likely in children than adults. Febrile seizures are limited to children between 6 months and 5 years of age.

4. Several primitive or automatic reflexes (Moro reflex, palmar grasp, neck tonic reflex) are present at birth and they disappear by the age of 4 to 5 months. Their persistence is indicative of brain damage.

5. Developmental screening is a part of CNS evaluation in children. Delay in appearance of social smile, persistence of automatic reflexes, neck tonic posture, clenched fists, increase in muscle tone, inability to follow light/red ball and delay in achieving motor skills are useful early markers of cerebral palsy.

6. Deep tendon jerks are normally brisk during infancy. When knee jerk is elicited on one side, crossed adductor response may be seen in normal infants. Cremasteric response is also exaggerated in infants and may be preserved even when there are other evidences of pyramidal involvement. It may be lost in a child with torsion of testis.

7. Plantars may be normally extensor on both sides in infants up to 2 years of age. The presence of unilateral extensor plantar reflex is more significant at this age.

8. Fundus examination reveals that optic disc is normally pale in infants. Papilledema due to raised intracranial pressure appears only after 2 to 3 years of age when sutures have closed.

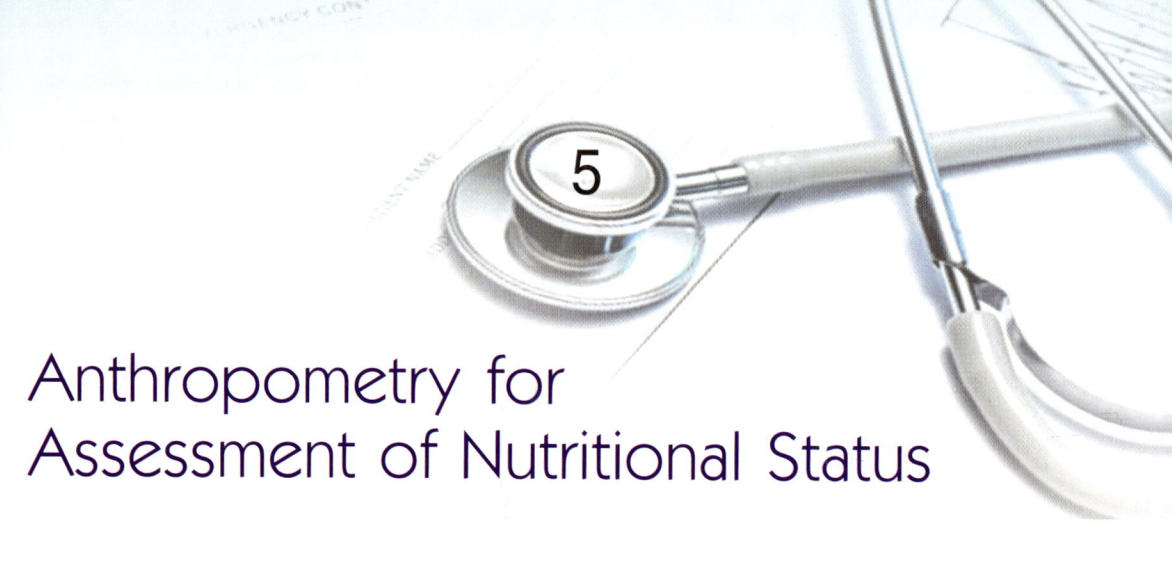

5
Anthropometry for Assessment of Nutritional Status

Growth and neuromotor development are the most distinctive attributes of children which distinguish them from adults. Physical growth is influenced by many factors, including overall health, genome, gender, environmental factors like safe drinking water and adequacy of nutrition and freedom from developmental defects. The anatomical characteristics and functional maturity of various organs at different ages affect the incidence and manifestations of diseases in children and childhood disorders can adversely affect the growth and development of children. Protein-energy malnutrition is the core health problem in children which makes them vulnerable to develop a variety of infectious diseases perpetuating a vicious cycle of disease and debility.

Corrected Age

In prematurely born babies, corrected or conceptional age should be used for assessment of growth and development. For example, if a child is born on April 2, 1999 while his expected date of delivery was June 2, 1999, this means his gestational age at birth was 32 weeks. He will be zero day old on June 2, 1999. Therefore, the corrected post-natal age of this child on August 2, would be only 2 months (not 4 months). His physical growth and mental development on August 2, 1999 would correspond to a normal 2 months old child. The concept of corrected age is used for assessment of growth and development at least during the first year of life.

WEIGHT

The measurement of weight is a simple and most reliable criterion for assessment of health and nutritional status of children. Birth weight depends upon the health, nutrition and well-being of the mother during pregnancy. The physical growth after birth depends upon the interaction between genetic endowment and environmental influences, especially dietary intake and occurrence or absence of infectious diseases. Weight is a measure of total body mass and is sensitive to changes in body fluids, fat, muscle mass, skeleton and body organs. The weight can be recorded on a beam type weighing scale (Detecto scale with an accuracy of ±20 g). The scale should be frequently calibrated with standard weights and zero error must be adjusted before weighing. Electronic weighing scales for infants (±5–10 g) and children (±100 g) are available and should be preferred for their accuracy and convenience (Figures 5.1 to 5.4). It is ideal to record nude weight in infants but in clinical practice it is acceptable and convenient to record weight with minimal or identical clothes each time. The bathroom type of mechanical scale is unreliable for monitoring weight of children and should not be used. In field conditions, Salter spring machine is quite satisfactory because it is convenient to carry (Figure 5.5). The balance is hung from a hook or held by an attendant and baby is placed on the sling attached to the bottom hook. The periodic weight record on a Road-to-Health chart is essential for monitoring the growth of under-5 children (Figure 5.6).

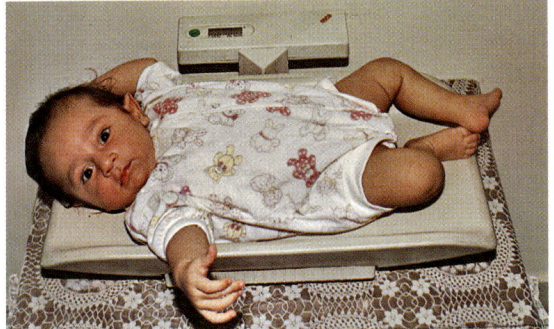

Figure 5.1 Weighing the infant on an electronic weighing scale having a resolution of ±5 g.

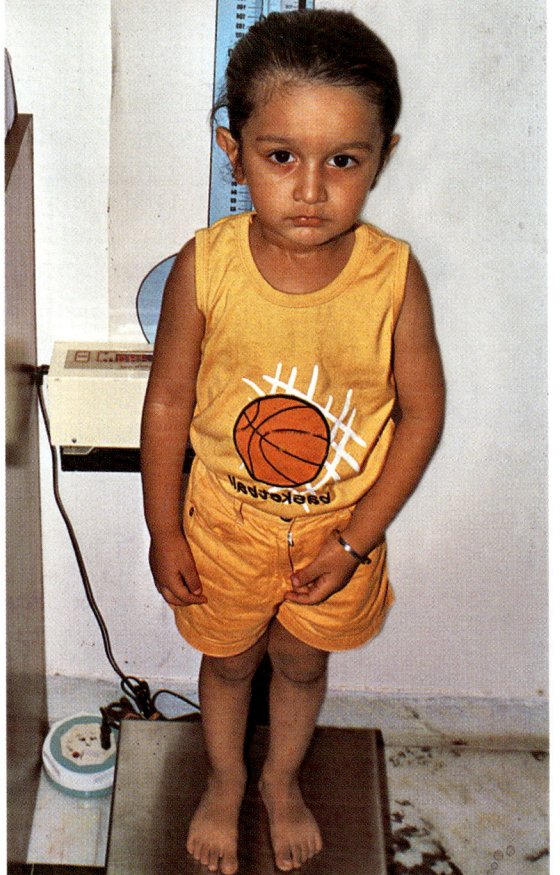

Figure 5.2 The child is being weighed on an electronic weighing scale (range 10–100 kg) with a resolution of ±100 g. Zero reading is obtained by pressing the tare knob.

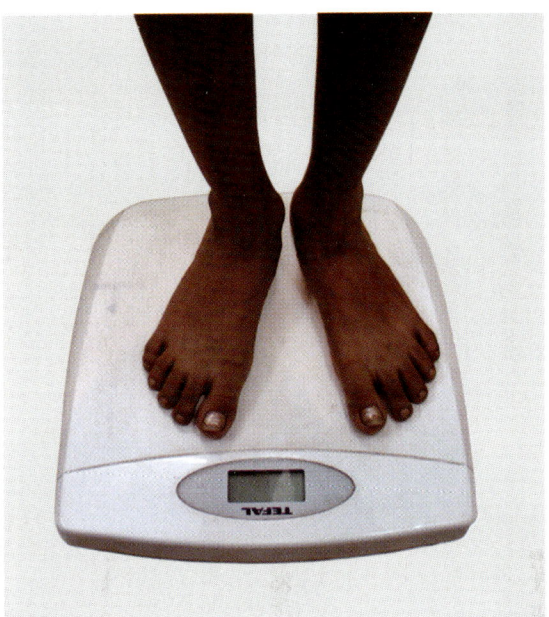

Figure 5.3 Weighing the child on an electronic digital readout type of weighing scale with a resolution of ±100 g.

The National Center for Health Statistics (NCHS) and WHO reference data and growth charts are recommended for use throughout the world for sake of uniformity. However, the use of a single international reference standard assumes that all children have the identical genetic potential for growth which is not true. It would, therefore, be more logical to use reference growth charts prepared from healthy Indian children belonging to higher socioeconomic group without any developmental, environmental or nutritional constraints. Isolated weight record does not provide any information regarding growth velocity or pattern of growth. The average growth velocity during childhood is shown in Table 5.1. The boys generally weigh more than the girls up to the age of 12 years. During 12 to 14 years, the girls weigh more than the boys because of early pubertal growth spurt. Depending upon the actual weight of the child, weight age should be expressed by consulting the standard growth chart.

The weight-for-age is a reliable index of the nutritional status of a child. The IAP classification of malnutrition based on weight-for-age is given

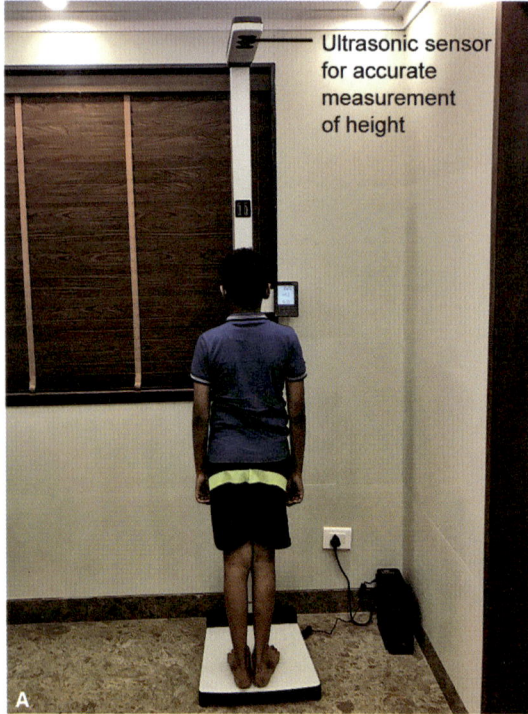
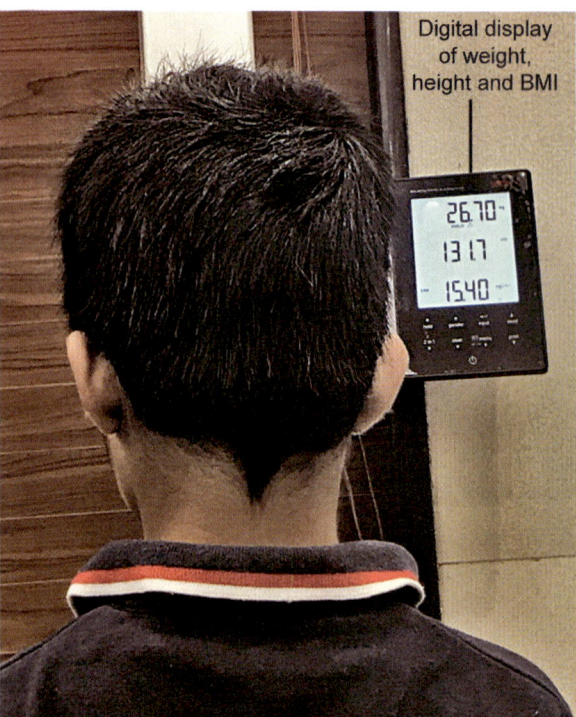

Figure 5.4A and B High precision Seca 286 electronic measuring station provides weight (resolution ±50 g), ultrasonic sensor-based height (resolution ±0.5 cm) and body mass index (kg/m^2). It has a facility for zero hold to weight an uncooperative or crying toddler in mother's lap. (A) The child stands erect with minimal clothes. (B) It is equipped with a speaker to provide audible as well as digital display of weight, height and body mass index.

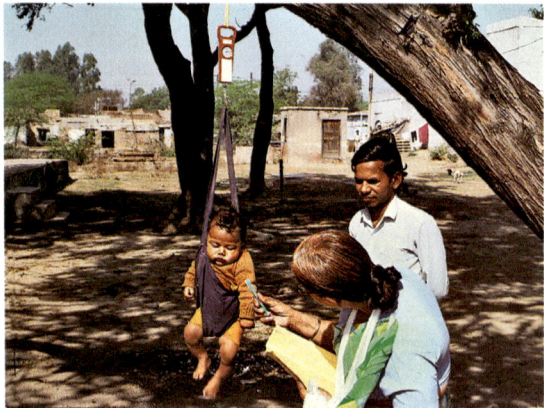

Figure 5.5 Spring balance with a hamper sling for recording weight of neonates and infants by community health workers.

in Table 5.2. In under-5 children, a weight-for height/length of <–3 Z-scores of WHO growth standard is suggestive of severe acute malnutrition.

The growth parameters and charts of healthy Indian children are available at site: http//iapindia.org/Revised–IAP–Growth–Charts–2015.php.

LENGTH OR HEIGHT

Up to 2 years of age recumbent length is measured with the help of an infantometer while in older children standing height or stature is recorded. Accurate recording of length is difficult and often unreliable although it is a better index of physical growth. The infant is placed supine on the infantometer. Assistant or mother is asked to keep the vertex or top of the head snugly touching the fixed vertical plank, so that external auditory meatus and lower margins of orbits are aligned perpendicular to the table. The legs are fully extended by pressing over the knees, and feet are kept vertical at 90°. The movable pedal plank of the infantometer is snuggly apposed against the

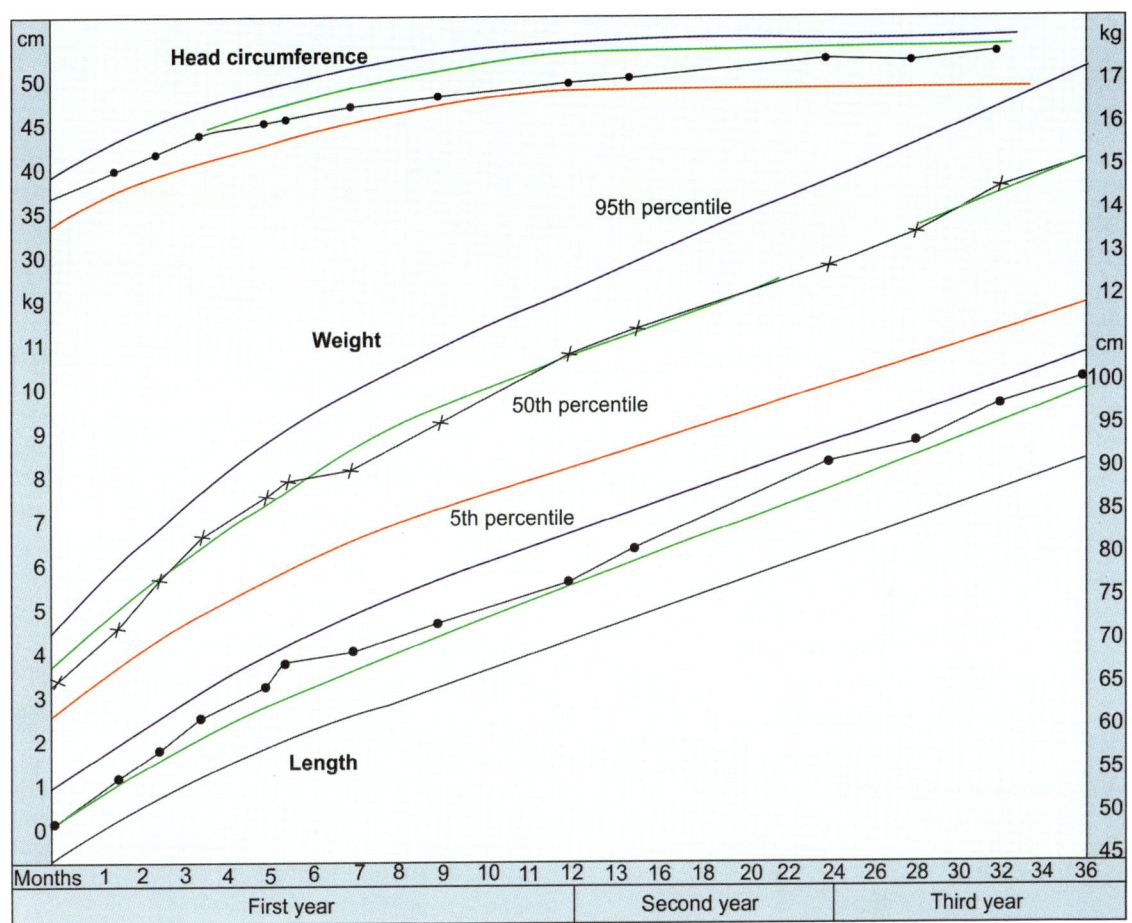

Figure 5.6 Road-to-Health card for monitoring the growth of under-five children. It is recommended to record growth parameters once a month (during visits for vaccinations) during first year, every 2 months during second year and every 3 months subsequently. The card also gives simple messages for immunizations, feeding and developmental milestones on the reverse. The mother should be explained the importance of growth monitoring and given the responsibility to keep the card in her safe custody. The periodic weight record provides valuable information regarding growth velocity of the child as opposed to an isolated weight record. The trend or slope of the weight curve is more important than its location on the chart. The satisfactory growth curve is directed upward and lies parallel to the thick lines on the chart. If the growth curve is flat or directed downward, the child needs urgent attention to identify the cause and reverse the trend. During early infancy, weight gain depends upon the gestational age, birth weight, health and well-being of the mother and adequacy of breastfeeding. By 1 to 2 years of age, most children would find their constitutional or genetic growth curve and maintain their growth velocity along their genetically appropriate growth curve. The growth chart serves as a useful tool to promote nutrition education and interaction between the health worker and mother.

soles and length is read from the scale to the nearest 0.1 cm. In practice, it is difficult to extend both the legs while it is convenient and satisfactory to extend only one leg to record the length (Figure 5.7). It is more convenient to externally rotate the leg because complete extension at the knee is not possible due to physiological hypertonia in infants. It is difficult to measure recumbent length or standing height in children between the ages of 2 and 4 years.

TABLE 5.1 Growth velocity and expected estimates for weight-for-age

A.		
	0–3 months	1.0 kg/month (30 g/day)
	3–6 months	0.75 kg/month (20 g/day)
	6–9 months	0.50 kg/month (15 g/day)
	9–12 months	0.25 kg/month (10 g/day)
	1–3 years	3.0 kg/yr
	4–12 years	2.0 kg/yr
	Adolescence	
	Girls 12–16 years	3.0–4.0 kg/yr
	Boys 14–18 years	6.0–7.0 kg/yr
B.	Weight at 4–5 months	2 × birth weight
	Weight at 1 year	3 × birth weight
	Weight at 2 years	4 × birth weight
	Weight at 3 years	5 × birth weight
	Weight at 7 years	7 × birth weight
	Weight at 10 years	10 × birth weight
C.	Weech's weight-for-age formulae	
	<1 year = (age in months + 9) ÷ 2	
	1–6 years = (2 × age in years) + 8	
	7–12 years = (7 × age in years − 5) ÷ 2	
D.	APLS* formula: (age in years + 4) × 2	
	Revised APLS formula:	
	1–12 months: (0.5 × age in months) + 4	
	1–5 years: (2 × age in years) + 8	
	6–12 years: (3 × age in years) + 7	

Based on National Center for Health Statistics (NCHS) Standards.
APLS: Advanced Pediatric Life Support.

TABLE 5.2 Weight-for-age classification of malnutrition by Indian Academy of Pediatrics

Weight-for-age*	Grade of malnutrition
>80%	Normal
71–80%	Grade I (mild)
61–70%	Grade II (moderate)
51–60%	Grade III (severe)
<50%	Grade IV (very severe)

*50th percentile or median of NCHS or WHO data

$$\text{Weight-for-age (\%)} = \frac{\text{Weight of child (kg)}}{\text{Weight of normal child of same age (kg)}} \times 100$$

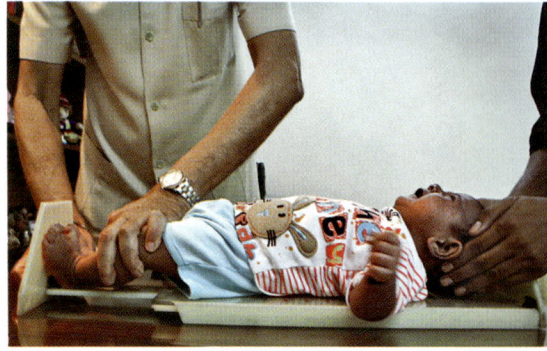

Figure 5.7 Method for recording length on an infantometer. Length is marginally longer than the height.

In older children who can stand, height can be measured by the rod attached to the lever type machine or by a stadiometer or simply asking the child to stand against a wall on which a measuring scale is inscribed. The child should stand with bare feet on a flat floor against a wall with feet parallel and with heels, buttocks, shoulders and occiput touching the wall. The head should be held erect with eyes aligned horizontally and ears vertically without any tilt. The child should be asked to stand erect and try to make himself "as tall as possible" without lifting the heels from the ground. With the help of a wooden spatula or plastic ruler, the topmost point of the vertex is identified on the wall (Figure 5.8). It is convenient to use an in-built stadiometer affixed on the wall which provides a direct read out of height with an accuracy of +0.1 cm (Figure 5.9). The linear growth (stature or height) ceases after fusion of epiphyses when puberty or sexual maturation is achieved. However, several body organs and tissues, like hair, skin, nails, lining of gastrointestinal tract and immune cells, go through a continuous process of degeneration, regeneration and growth throughout life.

Nutritional deprivation over a period of time (generally over 6 months) affects the stature or linear growth of the child while acute starvation is associated with weight loss due to wasting or loss of subcutaneous tissue and muscle mass. Depending upon the actual height of the child, the height age should be expressed by consulting the standard height chart. The average length or height velocity during childhood is shown in Table 5.3.

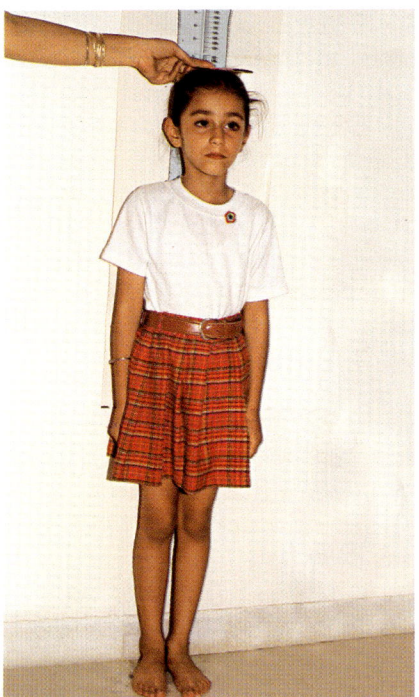

Figure 5.8 Method for recording height against a chart affixed on the wall. Refer to details in the text.

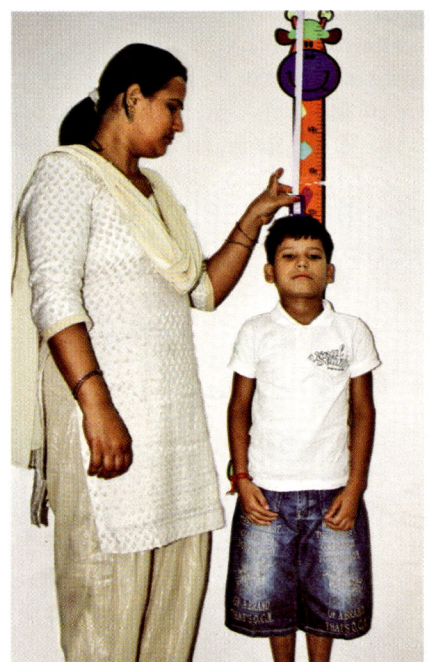

Figure 5.9 Method of recording height with a stadiometer. Note the erect posture with perfect alignment of eyes and ears of the child.

TABLE 5.3 Length or height velocity	
At birth	20 inches (50 cm)
Gain during 1st year	10 inches (25 cm)
Gain during 2nd year	5 inches (12.5 cm)
Gain during 3rd year	3–4 inches (7.5–10 cm)
Gain during 3–12 years*	2–3 inches (5.0–7.5 cm)/year
Adolescence	
Girls 12–16 years	8 cm/year
Boys 14–18 years	10 cm/year

*During a period of observation of at least 6 months, if the growth velocity is less than 5 cm per year after the age of 4 years, it is suggestive of growth failure or poor linear growth.

During adolescence, 20% of body stature and 50% of adult bone mass is laid down. Adolescent growth spurt continues for a period of 2.5 to 3.0 years and occurs mostly during the sexual maturity stages 2–5. In girls, adolescent growth spurt becomes minimal or stops after the onset of menstruation while it continues up to 18 years in boys. Adolescent growth is more in boys as compared to girls for all body measurements except hip width. The average adult height of males is about 13 cm (5 inches) greater than that of females.

Calculation of expected height up to 12 years

Length or height (inches)
= Age in years × 2.5 + 30

Length or height (cm)
= Age in years × 6 + 77

Prediction of adult height Almost 70% of height potential of a child is determined by genetics and 30% by environmental factors like nutrition, freedom from developmental defects, sound health, exercise, onset of puberty, and bone age.

(a) The rough adult height is approximately double the length of a boy at 2 years and a girl at 18 months.

(b) The calculation of mid-parental height is useful to evaluate the child's genetic endowment for linear growth. The determination is made by using the following formulae:

Boys = (Mother's height in cm) + (Father's height in cm) / 2 + 6.5 cm

Girls = (Mother's height in cm) + (Father's height in cm) / 2 – 6.5 cm

The projected target height by this method corresponds to within ±6 cm or ±2 SD. This represents the 3rd and 97th percentile for the child.

(c) Follow the curve method. The linear growth velocity of the child is recorded on the standard growth chart. The current height velocity curve of the child is extended up to 16 years in girls and 18 years in boys to predict the likely adult height of the child.

(d) Tanner's formulae

Adult height = Height at 2 years × 2

Adult height = Height at 3 years × 1.37

(e) Weech's formula

Adult height in inches:

Boys = 0.545 H_3 + 0.544 P + 14.84

Girls = 0.545 H_3 + 0.544 P + 10.09

wherein H_3 is height of the child at 3 years and P refers to mean height of parents. *This calculation is based on the assumption that height at 3 years is a good predictor of ultimate adult height.*

(f) Baby Height app is available for iOS devices to calculate the expected adult height of a child (Khamis Roche Height Predictor).

The weight and height charts and BMIs of Indian children of various ages are available at the site: http://iapindia.org/Revised–IAP–Growth–Charts–2015.php.

HEAD CIRCUMFERENCE

During fetal life, almost 70% of brain growth takes place. During infancy, 15% of brain growth occurs while the remaining 10% of brain growth takes place during pre-school years. If scalp edema or cranial molding is present, measurement of head circumference may be inaccurate until the third or fourth day of life. Head circumference is routinely recorded up to 5 years of age. The marasmic children are seen to have relatively large head for their body size because brain growth is minimally affected by malnutrition. During states of undernutrition of varying severity, weight (subcutaneous fat and muscles), linear growth (height) and brain growth are affected in that order. The occipitofrontal head circumference (OFC) should be measured with a narrow non-stretchable fiber-glass tape. The tape should encircle over the most prominent parts of occiput and supraorbital frontal areas with sufficient pressure to compress the hair and OFC recorded to the nearest 0.1 cm **(Figure 5.10)**. **Table 5.4** depicts the normal range of head circumference in under-five children. The head circumference growth velocity in under-5 children is shown in **Table 5.5**. The term macrocephaly refers to occipitofrontal circumference of more than 3 SD above the mean while microcephaly is diagnosed when OFC is more than 3 SD below the mean for age, sex, height and weight.

At birth, skull bones are separated by gaps or sutures and soft spots or fontanels to facilitate the growth of the brain. There are total of six fontanels, one anterior, one posterior and four lateral, two on each side of the skull (anterolateral and posterolateral). The lateral fontanels are usually closed at

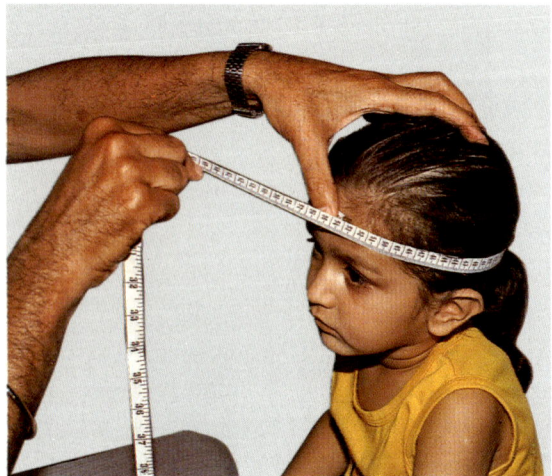

Figure 5.10 Method for recording head circumference. Use a non-stretchable fiber-glass tape and encircle the most prominent parts of occiput and supraorbital ridges.

TABLE 5.4 Head circumference (cm) in under-five children (10th–90th percentile)

Age	Head circumference
Birth (40 weeks)	32.0–35.5
1 month	34.0–37.5
2 months	36.0–39.5
3 months	38.0–41.5
6 months	40.0–43.5
9 months	42.0–45.0
1 year	43.5–46.5
1½ years	44.5–48.0
2 years	45.5–49.0
2½ years	46.5–50.0
3 years	46.8–50.3
3½ years	47.1–50.6
4 years	47.5–50.9
4½ years	47.8–51.2
5 years	48.1–51.5

TABLE 5.5 Head circumference growth velocity

First 3 months	2 cm/month
3 months–1 year	2 cm/3 months (1/3rd of initial velocity)
1–3 years	1 cm/6 months (1/12th of initial velocity)
3–5 years	1 cm/year (1/24th of initial velocity)

During first year, there is 12 cm increase in head circumference, while between 1 and 5 years age, only 5 cm gain occurs in head size. Adult head size varies between 53.0–58.5 cm in women and 56–61 cm in men.

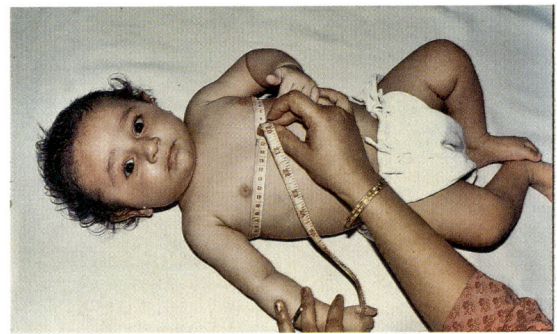

Figure 5.11 Measurement of chest circumference at the level of nipples.

birth while posterior fontanel closes by 3 months of age. The anterior fontanel usually closes by the age of 10–18 months.

Relationship between Head Size and Chest Circumference

At birth, head circumference is greater by up to 3 cm as compared to chest circumference. The head circumference is larger by more than 3 cm as compared to chest circumference at birth in preterms, small-for-dates and hydrocephalic infants. The chest circumference equals head circumference around 9 months to 1 year of age and subsequently chest grows more rapidly as compared to the brain. In preterm babies, chest circumference may exceed head circumference between 6 and 9 months of age. In malnourished children, chest size may be significantly smaller than the head circumference because growth of the brain is less affected by undernutrition. Therefore, there will be considerable delay before chest circumference overtakes head circumference. The chest circumference is measured at the level of nipples (Figure 5.11). Some workers recommend measurement of the chest circumference at the level of xiphisternal junction because the location of nipples may be variable.

AGE-INDEPENDENT CRITERIA FOR ASSESSMENT OF NUTRITIONAL STATUS

In developing countries, date of birth and hence accurate age of the child is often unknown thus invalidating above referred age-dependent parameters. The rough age may be deduced by using a local calender of events, seasons and festivals. In case the mother is totally ignorant about the age of the child, the following age-independent parameters can be utilized to assess the nutritional status of the child.

Mid-upper Arm Circumference

During 6 months to 5 years of age, the mid-upper arm circumference (MUAC) remains reasonably static between 15 and 17 cm among healthy children because fat of early infancy is gradually replaced by muscles. It is conventionally measured over the left upper arm. The child is asked to stand or sit with the arm hanging loose at the side. A point is marked over the lateral surface of the arm, midway between acromion (shoulder) and the olecranon (elbow) with arm bent at a right angle. Mid-upper arm circumference is measured with a fiber-glass or steel-tape at the midpoint between acromian and olecranon (**Figure 5.12A and B**). The tailor's tape is not accurate and should not be used. In children between 6 and 59 months of age, if the circumference of the upper arm is less than 11.5 cm, it is suggestive of severe malnutrition while MUAC between 11.5 and 13.5 cm is indicative of moderate malnutrition.

The UNICEF has developed four color-coded fiber-glass MUAC tapes for the benefit of paramedical workers to assess the nutritional status of children between 6 and 60 months. It circumvents the need to remember various cut-off limits of MUAC for classification and management of nutritional status of under-5 children.

- *Red color* MUAC <11.0 cm indicates severe acute malnutrition (SAM). The child should be immediately referred to a healthcare facility for treatment.
- *Orange color* MUAC between 11.0 and 12.5 cm indicates moderate acute malnutrition (MAM). The child should be immediately referred to healthcare facility for supplementation.
- *Yellow color* MUAC between 12.5 and 13.5 cm indicates that the child is at risk for acute malnutrition and should be counseled and followed up for growth promotion and monitoring (GPM).
- *Green color* MUAC >13.5 cm indicates that the child is well nourished.

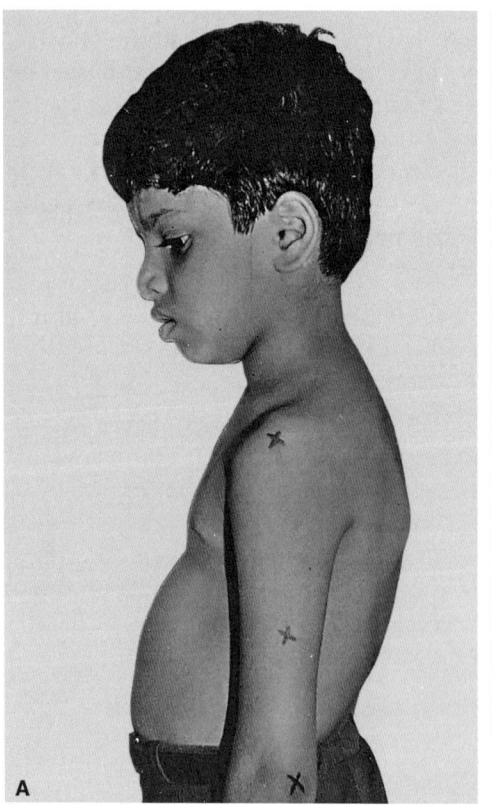
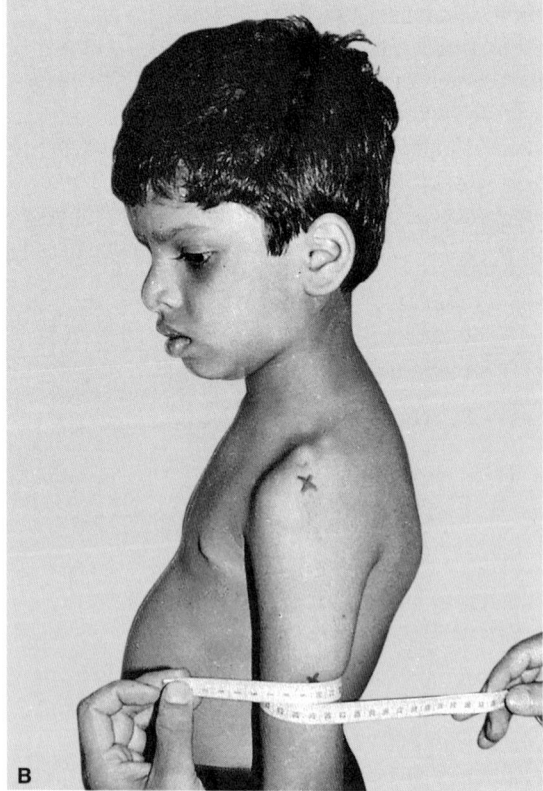

Figure 5.12A and B Method for recording mid-upper arm circumference. (A) Midpoint between acromion and olecranon is identified. (B) The circumference is measured with the help of a fiber-glass tape. The mid-upper arm circumference is recorded only in children between the ages of 6 months and 5 years.

Quac Stick

It is developed on the principle that acute starvation severely affects mid-upper arm circumference while height is unaffected. The child appears tall, thin and wasted. The Quac stick is a meter rod with two sets of markings. The expected height of the child against various sizes of mid-upper arm circumference of children between 1 and 5 years is inscribed on the rod. The malnourished child would be taller than the anticipated height derived from the mid-upper arm circumference (Table 5.6).

Thickness of Subcutaneous Fat

The subcutaneous fat thickness is measured with Herpenden or Lange caliper over the triceps, subscapular or suprailiac region (Figure 5.13). The skinfold measurements are taken on the right side of the body unless specified otherwise. The skinfold with subcutaneous fat is picked with left thumb and index finger, and caliper is applied beyond the pinch. Average of two readings is taken. On the basis of age, gender and skinfold thickness, it is possible to calculate percentage of body fat by various formulae. The fat-thickness is 10 mm or more among healthy children between 1 and 6 years of age. If it is less than 6 mm, it is indicative of moderate to severe degree of malnutrition. On the basis of skinfold thickness, age and gender of the patient, it is possible to calculate percentage of body fat. This method is cumbersome and mostly used in research protocols.

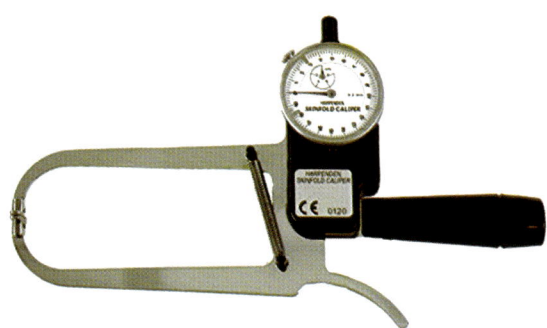

Figure 5.13 Herpenden skinfold caliper. It is a precision instrument used for measurement of skinfold thickness over the triceps and subscapular region with a resolution of ±0.2 mm

TABLE 5.6 Arm circumference for different heights in under-5 children

Mid-upper arm circumference (cm)	Height (cm)
16.50	133.00
16.00	129.00
15.50	125.00
15.00	121.00
14.75	118.00
14.50	116.00
14.25	113.50
14.00	110.00
13.75	106.50
13.50	103.50
13.25	97.50
13.00	90.00
12.75	80.00
12.50	70.00

Body Ratios

They are complicated and often unreliable.

Rao and Singh's weight-height index:

$$\frac{\text{Weight in kg}}{(\text{Height in cm})^2} \times 100.$$ The normal index is more than 0.15.

Kanawati and McLaren index (during 3 months to 4 years):

$$\frac{\text{Mid-upper arm circumference}}{\text{Head circumference}}$$

The normal ratio is more than 0.31 while a ratio of less than 0.25 suggests severe malnutrition.

Weight-for-Height

Weight-for-height is expressed as a percentage of the reference median weight expected on the basis of height of the patient and is calculated as follows:

$$\frac{\text{Weight of the patient (kg)}}{\text{Reference median weight against the actual height of the patient}} \times 100$$

The nutritional status can be expressed as follows on the basis of weight-for-height:

Weight-for-height*	Nutritional status
>90%	Normal
85–90%	Borderline malnutrition
75–84%	Moderate malnutrition
<75%	Severe malnutrition

*Reference standard NCHS or WHO data

Weight-for-Height and Height-for-age Classification

When malnutrition has been chronic, the child is "stunted", both his weight-for-age and height-for-age are low but his weight-for-height is usually normal. In acute malnutrition, however, the height-for-age is appropriate but child is "wasted" and underweight for his age. Based on the dynamics of malnutrition, there are various classifications of protein-energy malnutrition.

BODY MASS INDEX (BMI)

Body mass index is considered as a better criterion for the diagnosis of overweight and obesity because it expresses body weight in relation to height. It is calculated as weight in kg/(height in meters)^2. BMI can also be calculated by another mathematical formula, i.e. weight in pounds/(height in inches)^2 × 703. BMI-for-age percentile charts are available which can be used to diagnose obesity. A BMI-for-age of >85th percentile is suggestive of overweight and when it is more than 95th percentile for age and sex or when it is associated with triceps or subscapular skinfold thickness-for-age of >90th percentile, it is diagnostic of obesity. WHO has proposed a simplified classification of nutritional status on the basis of body mass index **(Table 5.7)**. In children aged 5–19 years, BMI percentile charts are available. BMI-for-age of >1 SD is classified as overweight, >2 SD as obese, <–2 SD as thin child and <–3 SD as severely thin.

BMI alone may not provide a reliable estimate of obesity among body builders and adolescents who have excessive lean body weight because of

TABLE 5.7 WHO classification of nutritional status on the basis of body mass index (BMI)

Classification	BMI
Underweight	<18.5
Normal weight	18.5–24.9
Overweight	25.0–29.9
Obesity grade I	30.0–34.9
Obesity grade II	35.0–39.9
Obesity grade III	≥40.0

BMI is calculated as kg/m^2 or lbs/(height in inches)^2 × 703

good muscle mass and heavy bones. Body volume index (BVI) is considered as a more reliable parameter of obesity, but it demands the availability of a special three-dimensional full body scanner to accurately assess both the quantum as well as the distribution of fat in the body. Body volume index provides computer-based data on BMI, waist circumference and waist-to-hip ratio. Waist circumference or waist-to-hip ratios alone can be used which are good correlates of increased risk for type 2 diabetes mellitus and cardiovascular disease. In general, Indians have greater amount of visceral and abdominal fat compared to the Western population. Waist circumference is measured just above the level of iliac crests. In adults, a waist-to-hip ratio of more than 0.9 in women and >1.0 in men is considered as abnormal. Various classifications of protein-energy malnutrition are summarized in Table 5.8.

Ponderal index (PI) is another parameter which is similar to BMI and is used for defining newborn babies with intrauterine growth retardation. Ponderal index is calculated by the formula: Body weight in grams/length (cm)^3 × 100. In malnourished small-for-dates babies (asymmetric IUGR), the ponderal index is less than 2.0 while it is usually more than 2.5 in term appropriate-for-gestation babies and hypoplastic SFD babies.

PROPORTIONAL TRUNK AND LIMB GROWTH

The mid-point of the body in the newborn is at umbilicus whereas in an adult the mid-point shifts

TABLE 5.8 Various classifications of protein-energy malnutrition (PEM)			
Classification	Criteria	Grading	Parameter
Gomez	% of median WFA	Mild (grade 1)	75–89% WFA
		Moderate (grade 2)	60–74% WFA
		Severe (grade 3)	<60% WFA
Waterlow	Z-scores (SD) below median WFH	Mild	80–90% WFH
		Moderate	70–80% WFH
		Severe	<70% WFH
WHO (wasting)	Z-scores (SD) below median WFH	Moderate	$-3\% \leq$ Z-score < -2
		Severe	$-3\% \leq$ Z-score < -3
WHO (stunting)	Z-scores (SD) below median HFA	Moderate	$-3\% \leq$ Z-score < -2
		Severe	$-3\% \leq$ Z-score < -3
Kanawati	MUAC divided by OFC of head	Mild	<0.31
		Moderate	<0.28
		Severe	<0.25
Cole	Z-scores of BMI-for-age	Grade 1	BMI-for-age Z-score < -1
		Grade 2	BMI-for-age Z-score < -2
		Grade 3	BMI-for-age Z-score < -3

Abbreviations: BMI, body mass index; HFA, height-for-age; MUAC, mid-upper arm circumference; OFC, occipitofrontal circumference; SD, standard deviation; WFA, weight-for-age, WFH, weight-for-height; WHO, World Health Organization. **Z-score** is a statistical expression of standard deviation (SD) and is calculated by the formula: Z-score = $(X-\mu)/\delta$; where x is the value of the parameter, μ is the population mean and δ is the standard deviation. Z-score of +2 or –2 means that the parameter of the subject is 2 standard deviations greater or lesser than the mean, respectively.

toward the symphysis pubis due to greater growth of limbs than trunk. The upper segment (vertex to upper edge of symphysis pubis) to lower segment (limb length, i.e. symphysis pubis to heels) ratio at birth is 1.8 to 1.0. There is gradual reduction in the ratio (due to rapid epiphyseal or limb growth) by 0.07–0.10 every year till ratio is around 1:0 to 1:0 at 10–12 years. Among healthy adults, the usual trunk to limb ratio is 1.0 to 1.1. In infants, upper segment (crown to symphysis pubis) can be measured by using infantometer as shown in Figure 5.14. The lower segment is obtained by subtracting the upper segment from total length. In older children, lower segment can be measured from symphysis pubis to the floor when child is standing and upper segment is deduced by subtracting lower segment from the height.

Infantile upper segment to lower segment ratio (trunk abnormally large or limbs abnormally small) is seen in achondroplasia (Figure 5.15), cretinism,

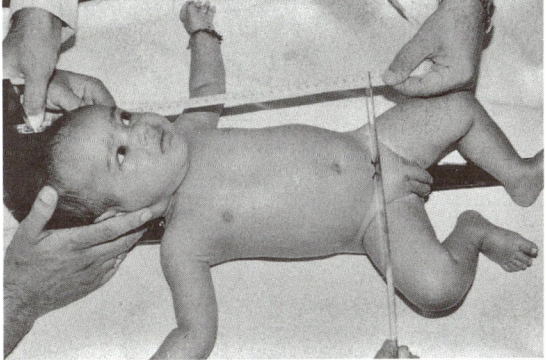

Figure 5.14 Method for recording upper segment in an infant with the help of an infantometer.

short-limbed dwarfism, sexual precocity, and bowed legs. Advanced upper segment-to-lower segment ratio (trunk abnormally short or limbs abnormally long) is seen in arachnodactyly, hypogonadism, eunuchoidism, Turner syndrome, Klinefelter syndrome, chondrodystrophy, and spinal deformities (rickets, Pott's spine).

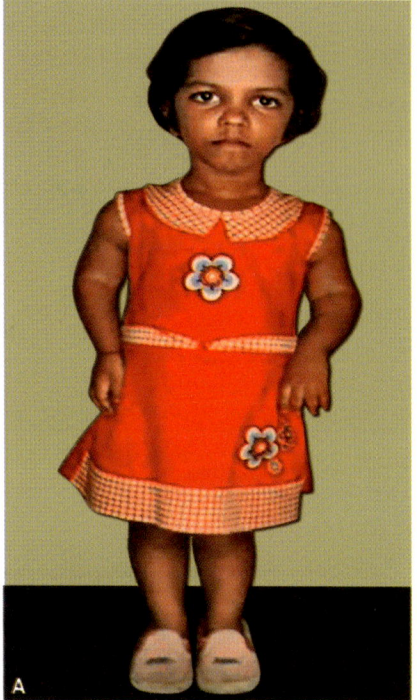
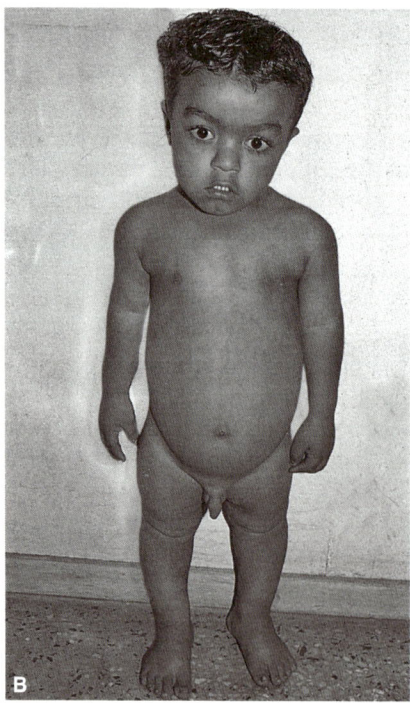

Figure 5.15A and B Achondroplasia. Upper segment is normal while limbs are short producing infantile upper to lower body segment ratio. The hands barely reach the thighs.

ARM SPAN

It is the distance between the tips of middle fingers of both hands when arms are outstretched at right angles to the body with palms facing forward. The arm span is measured across the back of the child. In under-5 children, span is 1 to 2 cm smaller than body length. During 10–12 years of age, span is equal to the height while in adults span is more than height by about 2 cm. Abnormally large span is seen in patients with arachnodactyly (Marfan syndrome), eunuchoidism, Klinefelter syndrome, and coarctation of aorta (due to relative over growth of upper extremities). Arm span is short as compared to height in patients with short-limbed dwarfism, cretinism and achondroplasia.

A complete list of anthropometric parameters is summarized in *Box 5.1*.

Box 5.1 Detailed list of anthropometric parameters
▪ Date of examination
▪ Date of birth, gestation and birth weight
▪ Corrected age or postconceptional age (up to 1 year in preemies between 30 and 36 weeks and 2 years in <30 weeks)
▪ Chronological age
▪ Weight (kg)
▪ Weight-for-age (%)
▪ Length/height (cm)
▪ Height-for-age (%)
▪ Weight-for-height/length (% and Z-score)
▪ Head circumference (cm) up to 5 years
▪ Chest circumference (cm) up to 1 year
▪ Mid-upper arm circumference (cm) 6 month–5 years (when date of birth is not known)
▪ Sitting height (cm)
▪ Upper segment–lower segment ratio
▪ Arm span (cm)
▪ Body mass index (kg/m^2)
▪ Waist circumference (cm)
▪ Waist-to-hip ratio
▪ Weight-to-height ratio
▪ Skinfold thickness (triceps or subscapular region)

OBESITY

It is true that protein-energy malnutrtion is a public health problem or a core health problem in children in developing countries. Nevertheless, over nutrition or obesity is being increasingly recognized in children belonging to affluent families having unhealthy dietary practices (intake of calorie-dense snacks and junk food) and sedentary lifestyle. Almost 25% of adolescent children attending private schools are obese. There is no satisfactory or standard definition for obesity in children. A weight-for-height of greater than 2 SD of NCHS or WHO data, > + 2 Z-scores or above 95th percentile is suggestive of obesity. The WHO expert committee recommends the use of body mass index-for-age. A BMI-for-age of >85th percentile is suggestive of overweight but when it is more than 95th percentile, it is diagnostic of adolescent obesity. BMI alone may not provide a reliable estimate of obesity among body builders and adolescents with good muscle mass and heavy bones. The constitutional or nutritional obesity should be differentiated from pathological or endocrinal obesity (Table 5.9). Pathological obesity during infancy is easy to diagnose and is usually due to endocrine causes or known syndromes (Figures 5.16 and 5.17). Apart from adverse psychological effects and orthopedic complications, obesity is a recognized risk factor for non-insulin-dependent type 2 diabetes mellitus, hypertension, coronary artery disease, osteoporosis and development of some cancers in adulthood.

Endogenous or pathological obesity is uncommon and occurs due to genetic and endocrine causes. The

TABLE 5.9 Differences between constitutional or familial obesity and pathological or endocrinal obesity

Feature	Constitutional or familial obesity	Pathological or endocrinal obesity
Family history	May be present	Usually absent
Eating behavior	Excessive intake of junk food, faulty eating habits, sedentary and lazy lifestyle	Eating may be normal or voracious, activity is affected after the onset of obesity
Distribution of fat	Generalized	Central obesity or "Buffalo hump" with greater deposition of fat over the face and cervicodorsal area
Height and bone age	Usually increased with advanced bone age	Usually decreased with retarded bone age
Blood pressure	Usually normal	May be raised
Endocrinal effects	May cause metabolic syndrome X and early onset of type 2 diabetes mellitus	Acne, hirsutism, acanthosis nigricans, amenorrhea or menstrual irregularity, and metabolic syndrome X
Hypogonadism	None but penis may be embedded in the pubic pad of fat	May be associated with several syndromes, such as Prader-Willi syndrome, Alstrom syndrome, GH deficiency, Laurence-Moon-Biedl syndrome, and hypothalamic disorders
CNS features	None	Excessive sleepiness, hydrocephalus with visual field defects (craniopharyngioma, pituitary tumor), papilledema or retinal degeneration, and mental retardation in association with certain syndromes (encephalitis, Prader-Willi syndrome, Vaquez syndrome, and Laurence-Moon-Biedl syndrome)

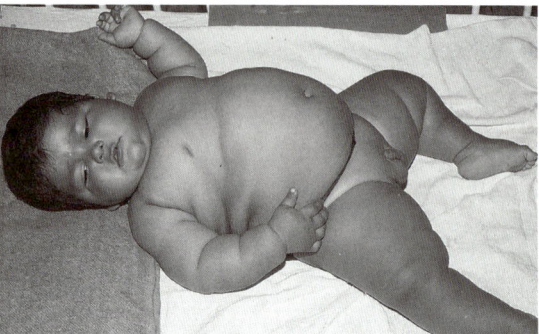

Figure 5.16 One and half-year-old boy with obesity, hypogonadism, and mental retardation due to Prader-Willi syndrome.

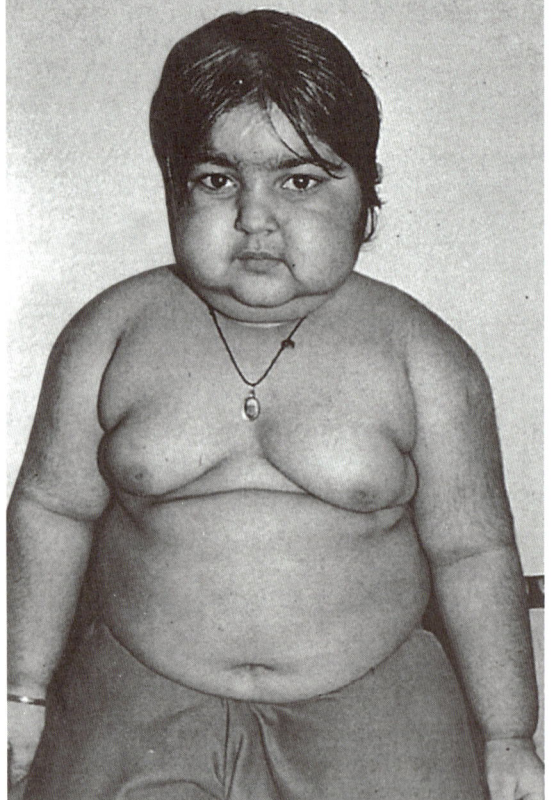

Figure 5.17 A 3-year-old girl with obesity due to Cushing syndrome as a result of carcinoma of adrenal cortex. Note moon-facies, double chin, hirsutism, buffalo-hump with enlarged overhanging breasts.

clinical features of pathological obesity due to various genetic and hormonal causes are listed in *Box 5.2*

> **Box 5.2 Causes and clinical features of endogenous obesity**
>
> **GENETIC CAUSES**
>
> - *Prader-Willi syndrome* Infantile obesity, marked hypotonia, short stature, and hypogonadotropic hypogonadism. Respiratory distress (Pickwikian syndrome) may develop due to deposition of fat in the interstitial tissue of lungs.
> - *Laurence-Moon-Biedl syndrome* Obesity, polydactyly or syndactyly, retinitis pigmentosa, renal anomalies, hypogonadism, and mental retardation.
>
> **HORMONAL CAUSES**
>
> - *Hypothyroidism* Excessive weight gain, constipation, coarse and dry skin, intolerance to cold, learning disability, deafness and goiter.
> - *Klinefelter syndrome* It is a form of hypogonadism in males due to 47XXY or XXY/XY mosaicism. It is characterized by delayed onset of puberty, obesity, gynecomastia and eunichoid body proportions (short trunk and long extremities). Penis and testes are smaller in size for the age with delayed development of secondary sex characters. There are varying grades of mental subnormality and learning disability.
> - *Polycystic ovary disease* (PCOD) Obesity during adolescence, hirsutism, acne, pigmentation over axillae and groin (acanthosis nigricans), delayed menarche, and type 2 diabetes mellitus or metabolic syndrome X.
> - *Cushing syndrome* Centripetal obesity, "buffalo-hump", hypertension, violaceous stria on abdomen, hirsutism, short stature and diminished glucose tolerance. The condition may occur because of excessive production of cortisol. It may occur due to prolonged or excessive intake of corticosteroids, ACTH-secreting pituitary micro-adenoma (Cushing disease), carcinoma or adenoma of adrenal cortex, other ACTH-producing tumors like carcinoids and lung cancer, bilateral hyperplasia of adrenal glands.
> - *Pseudohypoparathyroidism* Moon-shaped facies, depressed nasal bridge, stocky build, skeletal abnormalities (short metacarpals and metatarsals with index finger being longer than middle finger, curved radius, cubitus and genu valgus, coxa vara, exostosis), calcification of basal ganglia, cataracts, mental retardation, tetany with hypocalcemia, hyperphosphatemia and elevated PTH levels.
> - *Frohlich syndrome* Obesity, excessive appetite, short stature, sexual infantilism and visual abnormalities due to tumor in the hypothalamus.

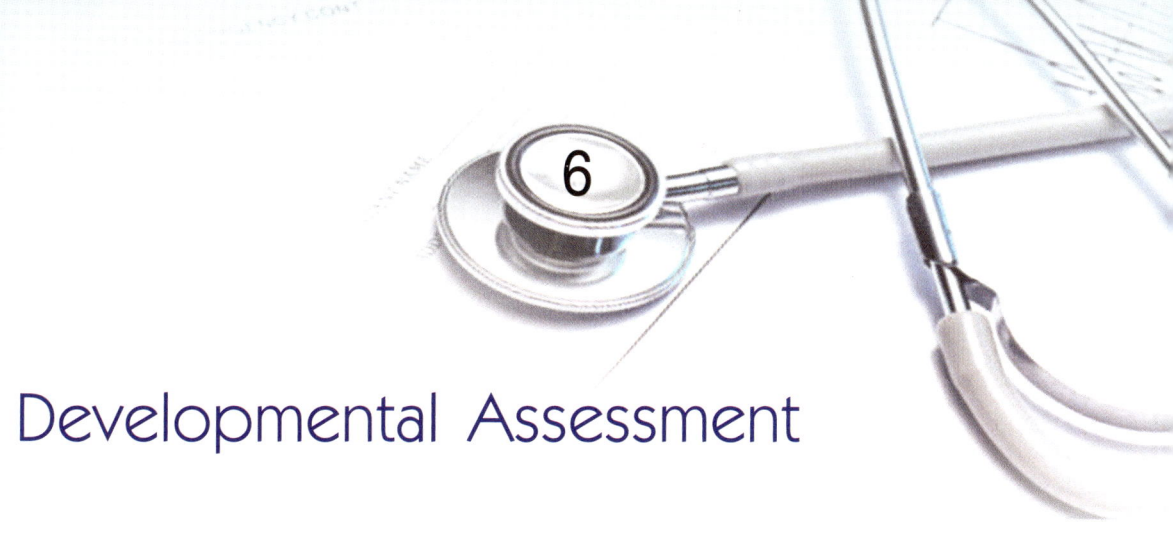

Developmental Assessment

Children, as opposed to adults, are characterized by a continuous process of physical growth and neuromotor development. The maturation of central nervous system is characterized by coordination of motor activity and as infants grow they respond to their environment in a purposeful manner with the help of special senses (touch, smell, taste, vision, acoustic and auditory inputs), integrity of labyrinthine, vestibular and musculoskeletal systems. Children achieve neuromotor milestones of development at predictable ages within a narrow range of a few weeks or months.

Development is dependent upon an interaction between innate genetic potential and environmental factors, like emotional security, love and attention, stimulating home environment, optimal nutrition, gender of the child, ethnic and cultural factors. When home conditions are unsatisfactory and children are reared in orphanages and foster homes, they are likely to have slower rate of neuromotor development because of lack of environmental stimulation. Neuromotor retardation may occur due to gestational immaturity, perinatal hypoxia, birth trauma, metabolic disorders (inborn errors of metabolism), hypoglycemia, kernicterus, intrauterine infections, postnatal CNS infections, hypothyroidism, developmental and chromosomal disorders.

PRINCIPLES AND CORRELATES OF DEVELOPMENT

1. It is the most distinctive attribute of children and is a continuous process from conception through adolescence.
2. Development is intimately related to the maturation of central nervous system.
3. The sequence of development is identical in all children but the rate of development varies from one child to another.
4. The generalized mass activity of early infancy is replaced by specific and subtle individual responses. It is a common observation that when shown a bright object, an infant shows wild excitement by moving the trunk, arms, legs and babbling while an older child merely smiles and reaches for the object.
5. The development proceeds in a cephalocaudal direction. The infant initially develops head control followed by ability to roll over and grasp, sitting, crawling, standing, and walking.
6. Certain primitive reflexes like grasp reflex and walking reflex must be lost before corresponding voluntary movements are acquired.
7. The development of language is early and advanced in girls as compared to boys.
8. Timing of dentition is unreliable for assessment of neuromotor development.
9. The child with an odd-looking face does not necessarily have associated mental subnormality.
10. The attributes, like creativity, future potentiality, various developmental quotients (intelligence, social, emotional, courage and spiritual), and mental superiority, cannot be predicted in an individual child by rate of development.

METHODS OF ASSESSMENT

A large number of methods have been standardized to assess the development of children. They demand the availability of skilled clinical psychologist and specialized kits for reliable assessment. Gessel development schedule evaluates gross motor, fine motor, social, adaptive behavior and language. Amiel-Tisson method of assessment pays special attention to muscle tone (active and passive), neurosensory responses (visual and acoustic) and neurobehavioral assessment. Vineland and Raval's Social Maturity Scale assesses the social and adaptive mental development. The other methods of neuromotor assessment include Bayley Scales of Infant Development (motor and mental), Brazelton Neonatal Behavior Scale, Vojta technique (postural reactions and central coordination) and Denver Developmental Screening Test (DDST) or Denver II and III. Among these, Bayley Scales of Infant Development (BSID) is most popular and widely practiced.

Bayley Scales of Infant and Toddler Development (Bayley III)

Bayley Scales of Infant and Toddler Development (Bayley III) is used to assess the development of children between 1 and 42 months. The scale is designed to test five major areas of development like cognitive, communication, motor (fine and gross), social-emotional and adaptive behavior. BSID scale is administered by early interventionists, sleep-language pathologists, occupational therapists, physical therapists, pediatric nurse practitioners and child psychologists. Depending upon the age and cooperation of the child, it may take 45 to 60 minutes to complete the assessment. The tool is useful to identify children with developmental delay and provides information to the practitioner for intervention planning. The involvement of the parents or caregivers is useful to facilitate testing and provide insight to them. It is a useful research tool.

Community Tools for Assessment of Development

In the community setting, health workers can be trained to screen development of children by using Baroda Development Screening Tests (BDST), Trivandrum Development Screening Chart (TDSC), and Woodside Screening System Test (WSST). The clinical adaptive test/clinical linguistic and auditory milestone scale (CAT/CLAMS) is a useful parental questionnaire to assess cognitive and language skills of under-3 children. Draw-a-man test (Good enough drawing test) is also a simple and a reliable tool of developmental assessment in pre-school children. Binet-Kamath (Stanford-Binet) and Wechsler Intelligence Scale for children are more sophisticated and can be used in some selected centers. The developmental quotient can be calculated as follows: DQ = developmental age/chronological age × 100. The quotient can be separately calculated for motor and mental or cognitive development (visual-motor and receptive and expressive language). The development is considered as slow or retarded, if developmental quotient is less than 70.

Basic Bedside Tools for Assessment of Development

The pediatric resident must acquire simple objects and instruments to undertake bedside assessment of development whenever indicated. These items include torch, dangling red ring of 6.5 cm diameter, red ball of 5.0 cm diameter, ten 2 to 5 cm sized colorful cubes, temple bell, rattle, cup with a handle, bunch of keys, pellets or beads, picture book, paper and crayons and percussion hammer.

Indications for Developmental Assessment

1. Follow-up of high-risk neonates discharged from NICU for early detection of cerebral palsy and/or mental retardation.
2. Complete evaluation of children with dysmorphism, developmental, chromosomal and neurological disorders.
3. To differentiate children with retardation in specific fields of development as opposed to those with global retardation.
4. Evaluation of children with learning disabilities.

DEVELOPMENTAL HISTORY

Accurate history of developmental milestones is often difficult to obtain due to poor observation and educational status of the mother. Early events in the life of child's development may be forgotten by the parents. The milestones should be asked in a chronological order in a simple and lucid manner. The social smile must be differentiated from spontaneous smile which even newborn babies may exhibit during sleep or fantasy. It is not enough to know when the child controlled his head or was able to sit. But it is equally important to know the quality of head control and whether the child could sit without support with a straight back or in a crouched posture.

It is important to ask the mother as to how the development of the index child compares with his siblings. She can recollect comparison more readily rather than precise ages for achieving various milestones. The mother should be asked whether the child interacts and plays with children of his age or likes the company of younger children or is self centered and is lost in his own world. At times, after having achieved certain milestones, the child may regress because of onset of a neurological disorder like seizures, autism, metabolic disorder, encephalopathy, etc. The efforts should be made to identify whether child is globally retarded or slow only in an individual or specific field, c.g. delayed speech in a deaf child, delayed walking in a child with protein-energy malnutrition or congenital dislocation of hips. The developmental progress of older children is best evaluated by consideration of school performance, proficiency in games, motor dexterity, social and emotional behavior.

DEVELOPMENTAL MILESTONES

Apart from assessing the developmental milestones, the resident should undertake a detailed neurological examination, evaluate the muscle tone (adductor angle, scarf maneuver, Landau reflex, parachute reaction, etc.) and special senses (vision and hearing). All high-risk infants must be subjected to detailed assessment of hearing and vision at the age of 3 to 6 months. Factors associated with deafness during infancy include prematurity, meningitis, craniofacial malformations, hypoxic–ischemic encephalopathy, congenital viral infections, kernicterus, prolonged use of aminoglycosides and furosemide, parental consanguinity and family history of deafness.

DEVELOPMENTAL ASSESSMENT

The child is placed in different postures and positions depending upon his chronological age and assessed for expected developmental responses as shown in Figures 6.1 to 6.19. *In preterm babies, corrected age (conceptional age calculated from expected date of delivery) should be used as the chronological age especially during first year of life.*

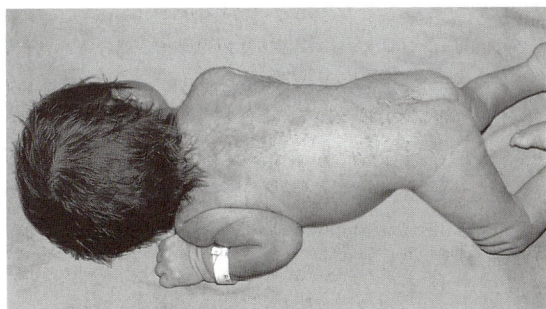

Figure 6.1 Prone position. Head is moved to one side and pelvis is raised in a newborn baby.

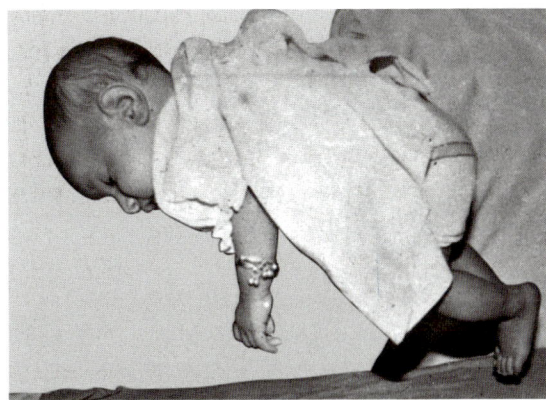

Figure 6.2 Head is momentarily lifted up on ventral suspension in a 4-week-old infant.

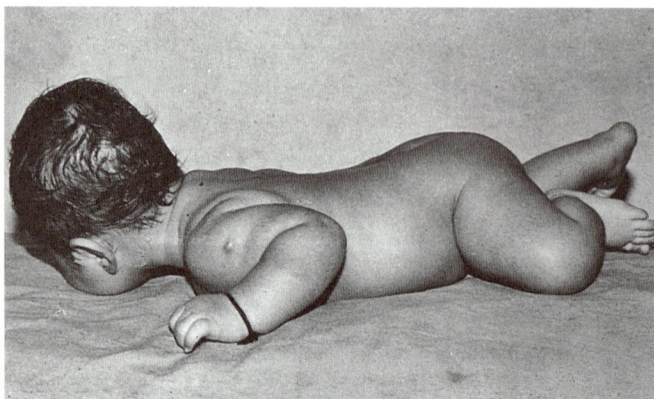

Figure 6.3 Prone position. The head is lifted off the couch momentarily around 6 weeks age.

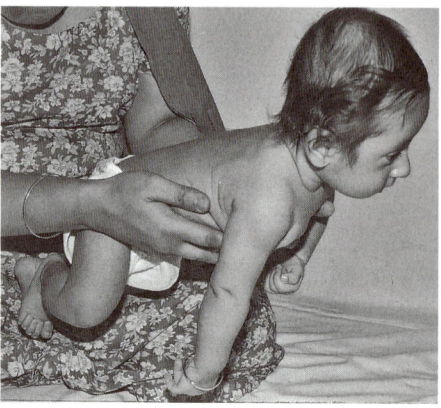

Figure 6.4 Ventral suspension. Head is lifted up beyond the plane of the body at 12 weeks.

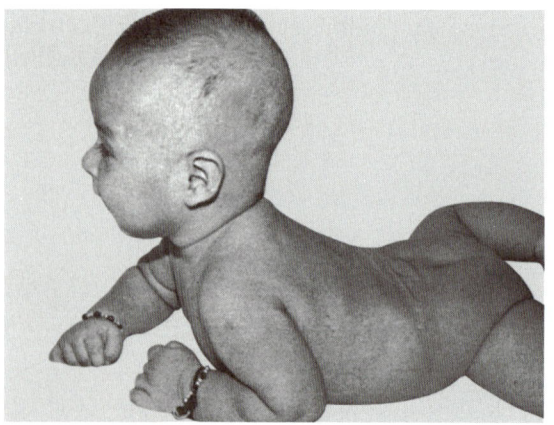

Figure 6.5 Prone position. Chest is maintained off the couch and body weight is supported on forearms during 16–20 weeks of age.

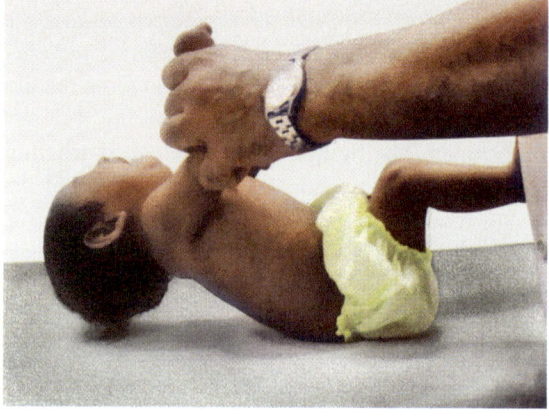

Figure 6.6 Traction response. Infant is being pulled from supine to sitting position by holding at forearms. There is complete head lag in a newborn baby.

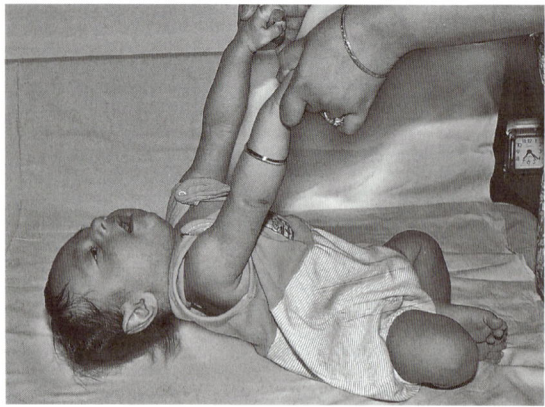

Figure 6.7 Traction response. Head is momentarily maintained in plane of the body around 6–8 weeks.

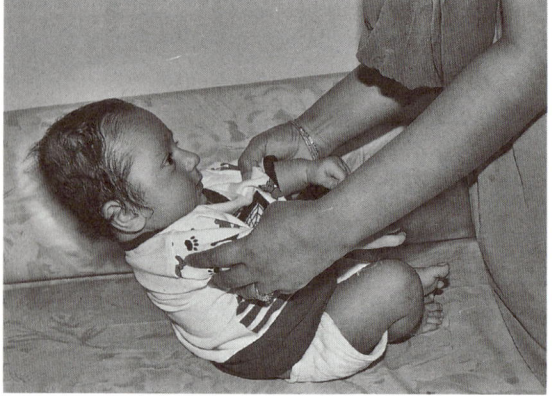

Figure 6.8 Traction response. There is no head lag at 12 weeks.

Developmental Assessment

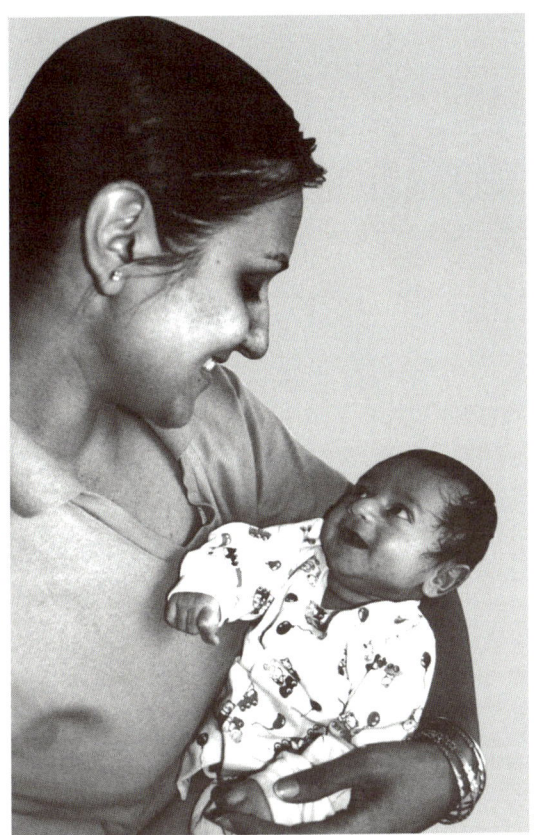

Figure 6.9 Baby is giving on interactive social smile at 6 weeks of age.

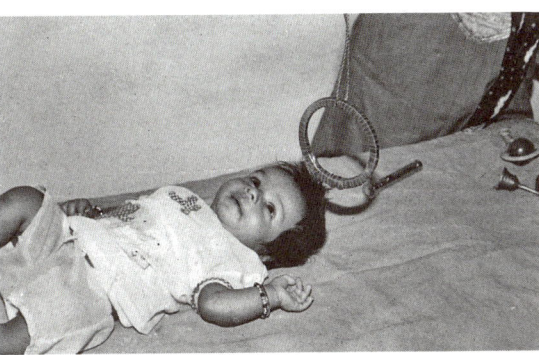

Figure 6.10 Infant follows a dangling red ring up to 180° at 12 weeks.

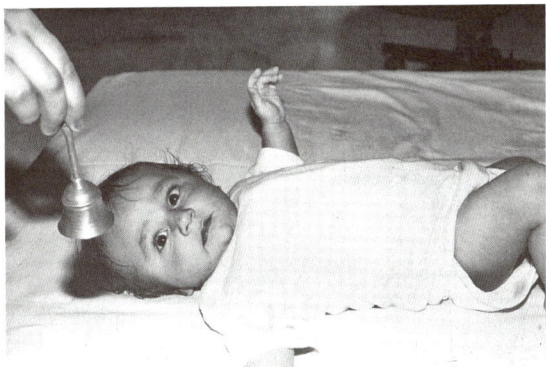

Figure 6.11 Infant turns towards the sound of bell around 16 weeks.

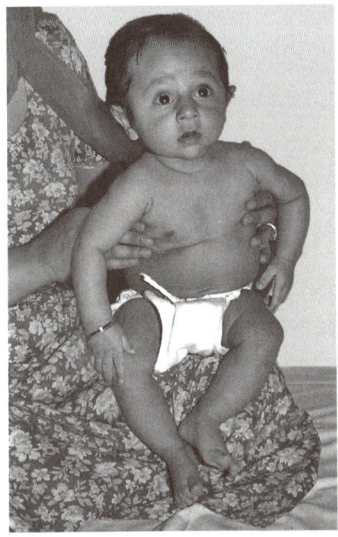

Figure 6.12 Steady head control at 4 months.

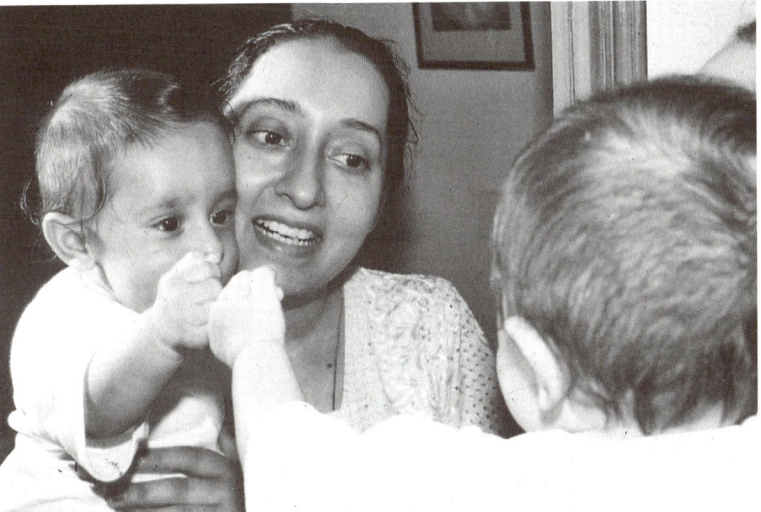

Figure 6.13 Plays and laughs at mirror around 4 months.

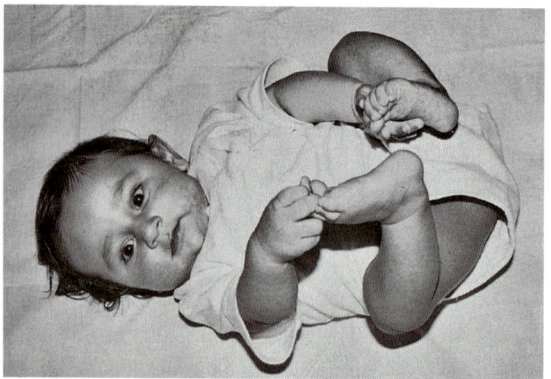

Figure 6.14 Holds feet and tries to put toes in the mouth at 16–20 weeks.

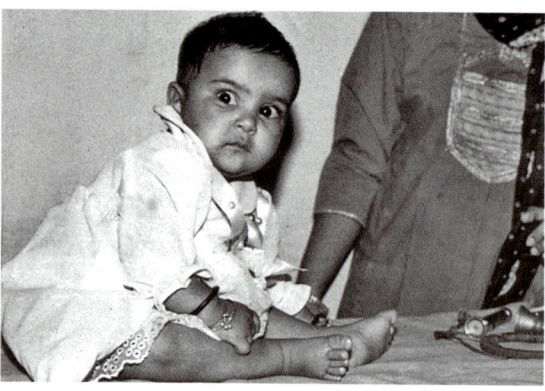

Figure 6.15 Sits with support of his hands around 4–5 months.

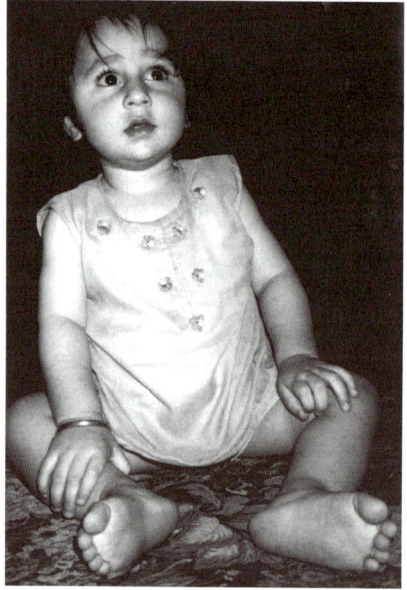

Figure 6.16 Sitting stable and independently with a straight back at 6 months.

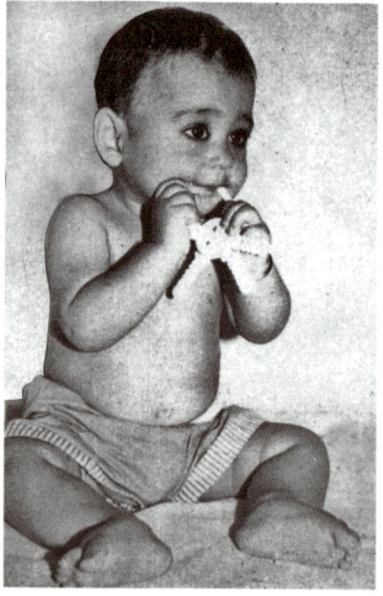

Figure 6.17 Holds a ring in both hands and puts it in the mouth around 5 to 6 months of age.

GROSS MOTOR DEVELOPMENT

The gross motor development is assessed by placing the infant in various postures and positions.

Ventral Suspension

The examiner suspends the infant in a prone position by supporting the abdomen of the baby on his palm. The extension of neck and flexion of the extremities are observed.

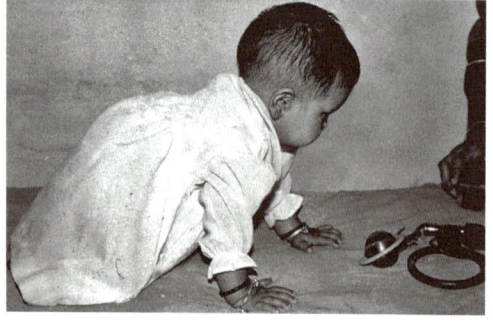

Figure 6.18 Crawls to retrieve toys around 8–10 months.

Developmental Assessment

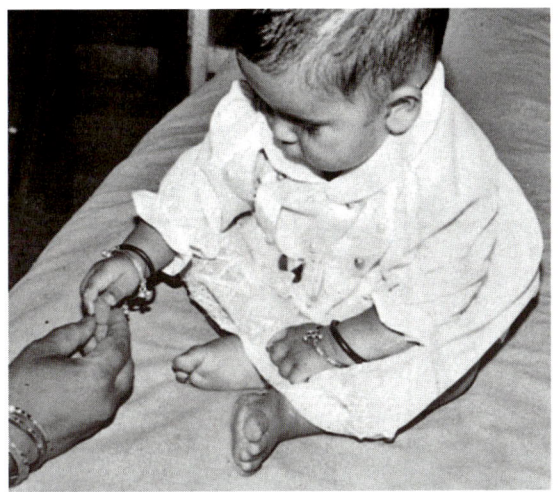

Figure 6.19 Pincer finger-thumb grasp to pick up a small object like a pellet or bead at 10 months of age.

Newborn — Head hangs completely and back is rounded.
4 weeks — Head momentarily lifted up, elbows flexed.
6 weeks — Head held momentarily in the same plane as rest of the body.
8 weeks — Head maintained in the same plane as rest of the body and momentarily lifted beyond the trunk.
12 weeks — Head maintained well beyond the plane of the rest of the body.

Prone Position

The infant is placed on the examination table in a prone position and watched for position of head, arms, pelvis and legs.

Newborn — Head is kept to one side, pelvis is raised, knees are drawn up under the abdomen.
4–6 weeks — Hips and knees are partially extended, can lift chin off the couch momentarily.
8 weeks — Head maintained in midline with chin lifted off the couch.
12 weeks — Pelvis is kept flat on couch with legs completely extended, chin is lifted off the couch.
16 weeks — Chest is maintained off the couch, arms are stretched out in full extension.
20 weeks — The body weight is supported on forearms.
24 weeks — Weight is supported on hands, and baby rolls from prone to supine. Indian babies first learn to roll from supine to prone because they are usually nursed in a supine position.

Supine Posture and Sitting

The infant is placed supine on the couch and pulled to sitting position by lifting at the forearms (traction response).

Newborn — Complete head lag.
4 weeks — Head maintained in plane of the body momentarily when baby is held in a sitting position, back is rounded. Chin may be lifted up momentarily.
12 weeks — Head held up when supported in a sitting position but it tends to wobble forwards.
16 weeks — When pulled up, there is slight head lag during the beginning and then head is flexed beyond the plane of the body. When held in sitting position and baby is swayed, the head wobbles.
20 weeks — No head lag, head is stable without wobbling and back is straight.
24 weeks — When about to be pulled up, lifts head off the couch in anticipation. Can sit supported in a pram or high chair.
28 weeks — Can sit on the floor with support of hands
32 weeks — Can sit momentarily on the floor without support.
36 weeks — Sits steadily without support and can lean forward and recover his balance.

40 weeks	Can sit up from supine position.
48 weeks	Can turn side ways and twist around to pick up an object.

Vertical Suspension, Standing and Walking

Newborn	Walking reflex during first 2 to 3 weeks.
8 weeks	Can hold head up for some time.
24 weeks	Puts almost all the weight of the body on the legs.
28 weeks	Bounces with pleasure.
36 weeks	Pulls self to stand, can stand with support.
44 weeks	Lifts one foot while standing.
48 weeks	Walks two hands held or on holding the furniture.
52 weeks (1 year)	Walks a few steps independently.
15 months	Creeps upstairs, can kneel without support.
18 months	Runs, can crawl up and down the stairs without help, pull a wheeled toy
2 years	Walks up and down the stairs with two feet on each step, walks backwards on imitation, picks up objects from the floor without falling, can kick a ball.
2½ years	Can walk tiptoes, jumps on both feet.
3 years	Goes upstairs with one foot on each step, jumps off the bottom step.
4 years	Comes down stairs with one foot on each step, can hop and skip on one foot.
5 years	Skips on both feet, can jump over low obstacles.

The salient gross motor milestones are summarized in Table 6.1.

Fine Motor, Visual-motor, Problem Solving and Social Responses (Manipulations)

Newborn	Grasp reflex is present.
4 weeks	Hands mostly closed.
8 weeks	Hands kept open more often

TABLE 6.1 Key gross motor milestones

4 months	Stable head control, rolls over, body weight supported on forearms in prone position
6 months	Sits with support with a round back
8 months	Sits without support with a straight back, can cruise and crawl (Figure 6.20)
10 months	Climbs from sitting position and stands with support
12 months	Stands without support (Figure 6.21)
15 months	Walks without support and creeps upstairs
18 months	Runs, throws a ball while standing, searches drawers
2 years	Jumps, can walk backwards, walks up and downstairs with two feet on each step, able to kick a ball (Figure 6.22)
3 years	Rides tricycle (Figure 6.23), goes upstair with one step on each stair
4 years	Hop and skip on one foot, comes downstairs with one step on each stair
5 years	Skips on both feet, can jump over low obstacles

12 weeks	Hands mostly open, grasp reflex disappears, plays with a rattle when it is placed in the hand.
16 weeks	Tries to reach objects but overshoots, hands come together during play.
20 weeks	Goes for objects and gets them usually with bidexterous approach, puts objects into mouth, plays with toes.
24 weeks	Drops one object when another is given, holds rattle, picks up a cube with crude palmar grasp.
28 weeks	Unidexterous approach to objects, transfers object from one hand to the other, feeds self with a biscuit, bangs object with each other or on table top, retains one cube when another is offered.

Developmental Assessment

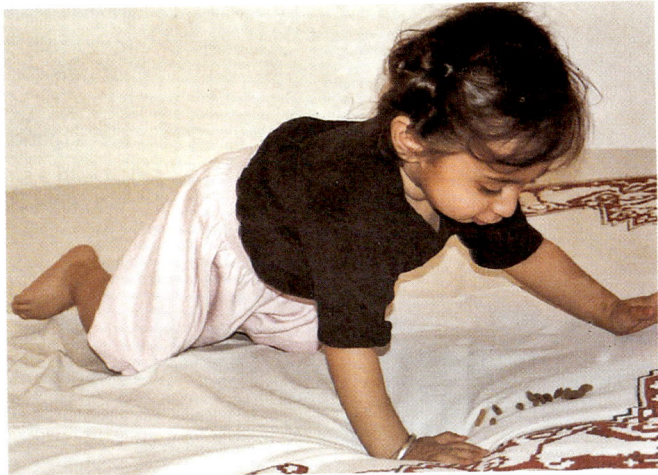
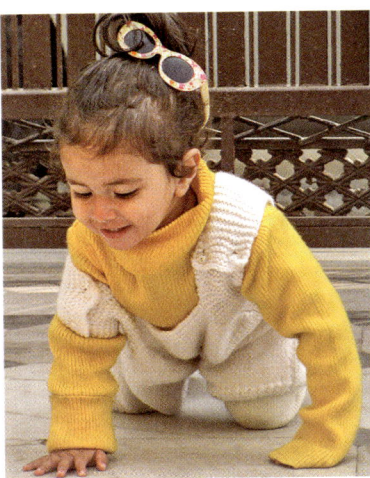

Figure 6.20 The crawling 8 months old toddlers.

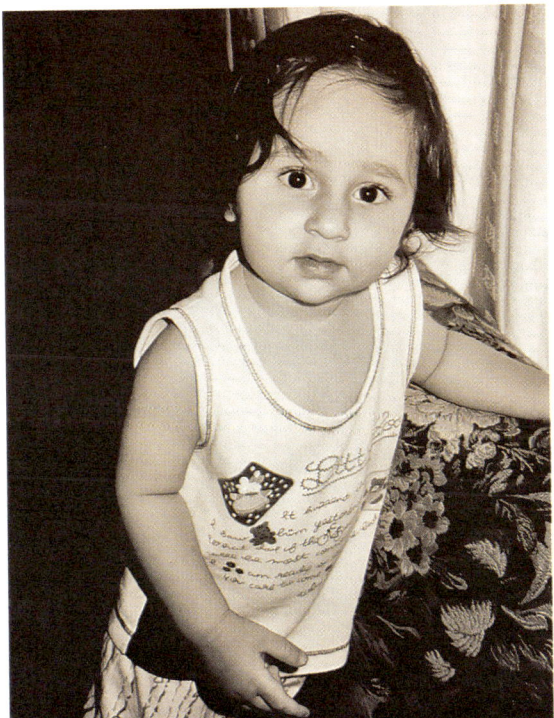

Figure 6.21 Standing with support at the age of 9 months.

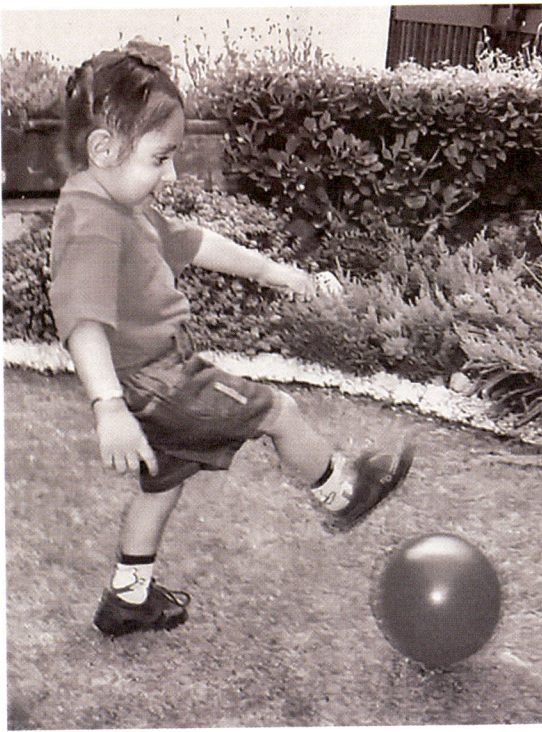

Figure 6.22 Able to kick a ball at 2½ years of age.

40 weeks	Pincer finger-thumb fine grasp to pick up a pellet or a bead.
1 year	Gives toy to examiner, uses mature pincer grasp, puts one object after another into the basket, mouthing is much reduced.
15 months	Self-feeds with a cup, builds tower of 2–3 cubes, holds two cubes in one hand, imitates scribbling.

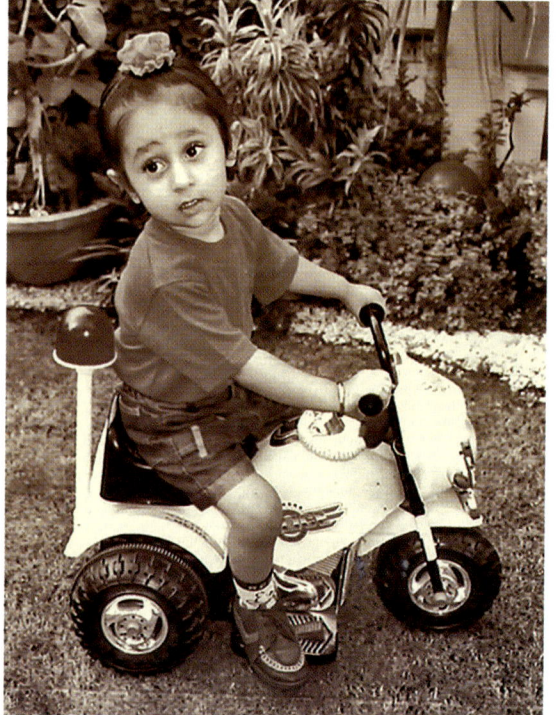

Figure 6.23 Rides tricycle at 3 years age.

18 months   Can self-feed with a spoon, makes a tower of 3–4 cubes, turns 2–3 pages of a book at a time.

2 years   Makes tower of 6–7 cubes, can turn pages one at a time, can turn door knob, puts on and takes off socks, shoes and pants.

2½ years   Can hold a pencil in hand to scribble lines.

3 years   Makes tower of 9–10 cubes, can dress and undress, can manage buttons, can draw a circle.

4 years   Copies a square and cross, makes a bridge with blocks, can dress self completely, can button the dress, catches a ball.

5 years   Copies a triangle, can tie shoe laces, can spread butter on the toast with a knife.

The salient fine motor milestones are shown in Table 6.2.

TABLE 6.2	The salient fine motor milestones
3 months	Hands mostly open, holds a rattle when placed in hand
4 months	Reaches out for objects with both hands (bidexterous)
6 months	Approaches objects with one hand, transfers rattle from one hand to the other hand
9 months	Immature or crude finger-thumb pincer grasp
1 year	Fine finger-thumb pincer grasp, mouthing is reduced
15 months	Self feeds with a cup, imitates scribbling, builds tower of 2–3 cubes
18 months	Can self-feed with a spoon, makes tower of 3–4 cubes, turns 2–3 pages of a book at a time
2 years	Can make a tower of 6–7 blocks, can turn one page at a time, can imitate vertical and circular strokes
3 years	Can make a tower of 9–10 cubes, can dress and undress, can draw a circle
4 years	Can make a bridge with blocks, can copy a square and cross, can unbutton and button
5 years	Can copy a triangle, can tie shoe laces

Social, Adaptive and Language Development

4 weeks   Watches mother intently when she speaks to him. Follows a dangling object up to 90°, quietens on sound of bell.

6 weeks   Gives an interactive or social smile which should be differentiated from a spontaneous smile which is present even in neonates, follows a moving object

8 weeks   Fixes and focusses gaze, eye-to-eye contact, vocalizes.

12 weeks   Hand regard, recognizes mother, can follow an object up to 180°, babbles when spoken to, squeals

Age	Milestones
16 weeks	with pleasure and gets excited on seeing a toy. Demonstrates excitement when feed is being prepared, laughs loud, turns head towards sound of bell/rattle.
20 weeks	Smiles at mirror image, imitates simple acts, dry during daytime if toilet trained, stranger anxiety.
24 weeks	No more hand regard, shows displeasure when toy is taken away, demonstrates likes and dislikes, when an object is dropped he looks for it searchingly.
28 weeks	Imitates actions and sounds, enjoys "peek-a-boo" and "pat-a-cake" games, responds to name, pats mirror image, says monosyllables, like ba, da, ma.
32 weeks	Imitates sounds, responds to 'No', produces disyllables, like ma-ma, ba-ba, da-da, etc.
40 weeks	Pulls clothes of mother to attract attention, waves bye-bye, repeats performance which is laughed at.
1 year	Gives toy to examiner, uses mature pincer grasp, interested in picture book, comes when called, imitates actions, shakes head for 'No', says 2–3 words other than ma-ma/pa-pa with meaning.
1½ year	Jargon speech, 10–15 words vocabulary, indicates the need for potty and when under garments are wet, knows 5 body parts.
2 years	Repeats what is said, uses the words 'I', 'me', 'you', asks for food, drink and tells need for toilet. Lisping and some stuttering is common, can use two-word sentences with vocabulary of 50–100 words.
3 years	Normal speech, with 3-word sentences with vocabulary of 250 words, attends to toilet needs except for wiping, can dress and undress, knows his name, age and gender.
4 years	Knows colors, develops right and left discrimination, can sing a song and recite a poem, asks questions, can tell a story, can cooperate to play in a group, goes to toilet alone.
5 years	Identifies 4 colors, asks meaning of words, plays competitive games, abides by rules, likes to help in household tasks.

TABLE 6.3 The salient social and adaptive milestones

Age	Milestone
2 months	Social and interactive smile
3 months	Hand regard, recognizes mother, anticipates feed, excited to see a toy
6 months	Stranger anxiety, pats mirror image, enjoys to play peek-a-boo and pat-a-cake games
9 months	Waves bye-bye, repeats performance when appreciated
12 months	Responds when name is called, imitates actions, shakes head for "No"
15 months	Jargon speech
18 months	Imitates various household tasks
2 years	Asks for food and drink and indicates needs for toilet
3 years	Knows his name, age and gender, and shares toys
4 years	Toilet trained, plays cooperatively in a group
5 years	Dresses and undresses, helps in household tasks

The key social and adaptive milestones and language milestones are summarized in Tables 6.3 and 6.4, respectively.

TARGET MILESTONES

The developmental milestones are achieved by healthy normal children within a narrow range of several weeks. The recommended corrected ages

TABLE 6.4 The salient language milestones	
1 month	Quietens or alerts to sound
3 months	Babbles and coos when spoken to
4 months	Laughs loud, turns towards the sound
6 months	Speaks monosyllables, like ba, da, pa, ma and ah-goo sounds
9 months	Utters disyllables, like mama, papa, dada
12 months	Speaks 2–3 words with meaning
18 months	Jargon speech with 7–10 words vocabulary
2 years	Can make 2–3 word sentences with a vocabulary of 50 words, can repeat what is said, use pronouns "I", "me", "you"
3 years	Can make 3-word sentences and has vocabulary of 250 words, normal speech, asks questions
4 years	Can tell a story, recite a poem or sing a song, inquisitive
5 years	Chatter box and asks meaning of words

Box 6.1 Red alerts for cerebral palsy

- Lack of social smile by 2 months.
- Absence of stable head control by 4 months.
- Inability to recognize the mother by 6 months.
- Inability to sit when pulled to sit by 6 months and lack of independent sitting without support by 8 months.
- Lack of creeping or crawling by 9 months.
- Inability to stand without support by one year.
- Inability to walk without support by 18 months.
- Lack of pincer or thumb-index finger grasp by the age of one year.
- Inability to play interactive games (peek-a-boo, pat-a-cake) by the age of one year.
- Absence of disyllabic babbling by the age of one year and failure to make meaningful sentences by 3 years of age.

(calculated from the expected date of delivery) for undertaking developmental assessement are 4 months, 8 months, 12 months and then every 6 months till 3 years of age. The children with red alerts should be subjected to a detailed developmental assessment by an experienced developmental psychologist *(Box 6.1)*. For assessment of hearing and vision refer to Chapters 14 and 15.

EARLY MARKERS OF CEREBRAL PALSY

The high-risk newborn babies should be followed up for early identification of neuromotor disability so that appropriate stimulation therapy can be initiated to enhance neuromotor development. Mother can be taught by the therapist to use simple culturally acceptable interactions to provide stimulation to the child. The child should be stimulated by music, bright-colored objects, lullabies and interactive overtures of the mother. It must be realized that mother is the best therapist and teacher for her infant. She should caress, touch, tease, talk, sing, tell stories and respond to child's pranks. The following clinical markers should be looked for to make an early diagnosis of cerebral palsy.

1. Episodes of inconsolable crying, chewing movements, lip smacking, excessive sensitivity to light and noise, spontaneous or excessive startle and Moro response.
2. Persistent neck tonic posture beyond 4 weeks of age.
3. Clenched fists with thumbs adducted and flexed across the palm beyond 8 weeks.
4. Paucity or absence of fidgety limb movements during first 6–12 weeks.
5. Abnormalities in tone (usually hypertonia but occasionally hypotonia) as assessed by scarf sign and various angles.
6. Persistence of automatic reflexes beyond 5–6 months (Moro reflex, grasp reflex, asymmetric tonic neck reflex).
7. Persistent asymmetry of posture, tone, movements and reflexes is abnormal.
8. Slow head growth.

Table 6.5 gives ages at appearance and disappearance of common primitive or automatic reflexes. Absence of parachute response and Landau reflex and persistence of automatic reflexes beyond the target ages are indicative of cerebral palsy.

Developmental Assessment

TABLE 6.5 Time table of primitive reflexes

Reflex	Age of appearance	Age of disappearance
Rooting	Birth	3 months
Moro	Birth	5–6 months
Palmar grasp	Birth	6 months
Tonic neck	Birth	9–10 months
Adductor spread of knee jerk	Birth	7–8 months
Landau	10 months	24 months
Parachute	8–9 months	Persists in normal children

ASSESSMENT OF MUSCLE TONE

Alterations in muscle tone especially hypertonia is common in cerebral palsy. Healthy term newborn babies have physiological hypertonia and there is gradual reduction of muscle tone during first year of life. Muscle tone should be assessed when baby is alert, wide awake, not hungry or crying. The infant should be placed in a supine position with head in the midline. The muscle tone is evaluated by (i) looking for abnormal posture of the limbs, (ii) palpation of muscles whether they are flabby or firm to feel, (iii) range of movements and resistance encountered at major joints and (iv) degree of flaility and range of movements on shaking various limbs. The range of movements at major joints is tested during infancy as follows:

Adductor angle Infant lies supine with legs extended and head in the midline. Both the hips are abducted maximally by holding at the knees with index finger resting over the front of thighs. The angle between the thighs is the adductor angle (Figure 6.24). The adductor angle is narrow and resistance is encountered during the procedure when infant is hypertonic. Asymmetry between the right and left leg should be noted.

Popliteal angle The infant lies supine on the cot. The hips are fully flexed onto the abdomen by holding at the knees. The legs are then extended by gentle pressure with examiner's hands placed behind the ankles and popliteal angle is measured.

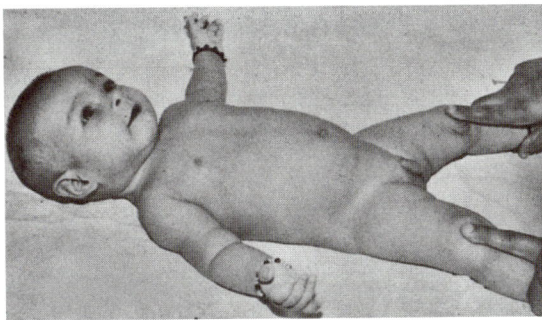

Figure 6.24 Adductor angle. Index fingers are aligned over the thighs to measure the angle.

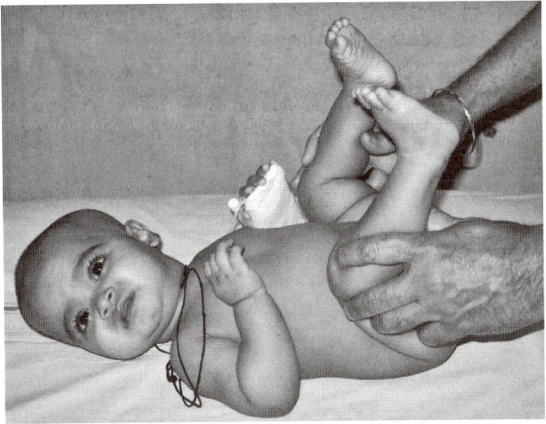

Figure 6.25 Popliteal angle. Assess angles on both the sides simultaneously and identify any differences in the tone on the two sides.

The resistance encountered to the maneuver is noted on both sides. The angle is measured separately on two sides (Figure 6.25).

Dorsiflexion angle of the foot The foot is passively dorsiflexed by applying gentle pressure with the thumb placed over the sole. Angle between dorsum of foot and front of leg is noted. During infancy, dorsiflexion angle at the ankle is 70° or less (Figure 6.26).

Heel-to-ear maneuver With the infant lying supine, the legs extended at the knees are held together and lifted as far backwards as possible towards the ears without lifting the pelvis from the table (Figure 6.27). Increased resistance on one side is suggestive of asymmetry of tone on the two sides.

Scarf sign The muscle tone in the upper limbs is tested by assessing the range of movements at the shoulders. The infant lies supine on the cot with head in the midline. The upper limb, flexed at the elbow, is pulled as far possible across the chest by holding at the hand and wrist. The position of the elbow in relation to midline of the body is noted (Figure 6.28). One limb is tested at a time followed by both the limbs together. The normal range of various angles during infancy is given in Table 6.6.

Transitory abnormalities in muscle tone (especially hypotonia) may be noted during first six months of life and they normalize by the age of one year.

Parachute response The child is held in a prone position by placing both hands around the lower chest. The child is suddenly lowered over a table top. There will be brisk extension and abduction of the upper limbs with extension of fingers as if to break the fall (Figure 6.29). It is a protective reflex and appears around 8 to 9 months of age. The reflex is absent in infants with spastic type of cerebral palsy.

Landau reflex The infant is suspended in a prone position by supporting the abdomen of the baby on the palm. The infant spontaneously extends the neck, trunk and legs after the age of 10 months. Forcible flexion of the neck is associated with flexion of hips and legs (Figure 6.30). The reflex is absent in floppy infants.

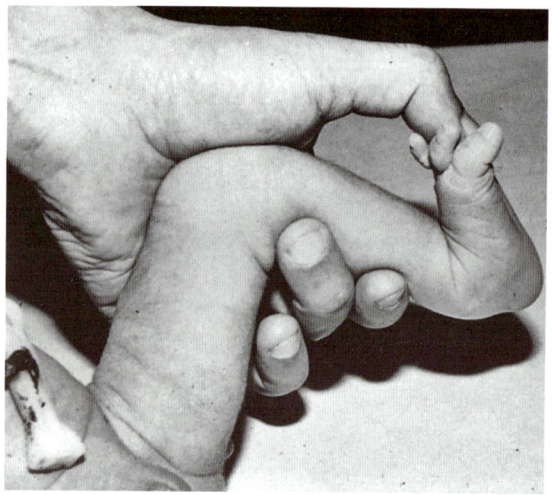

Figure 6.26 Dorsiflexion angle at the ankle.

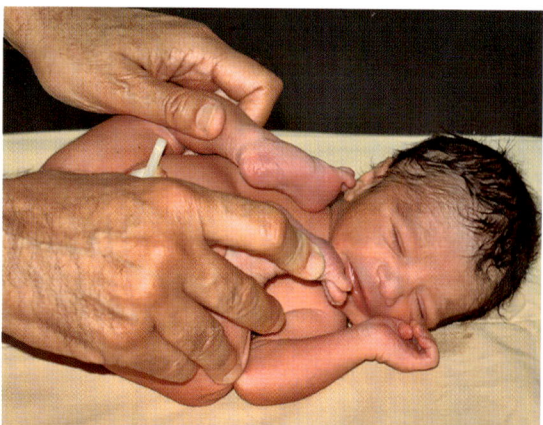

Figure 6.27 Heel-to-ear maneuver. The knees should be kept extended and trunk should not be lifted off the cot.

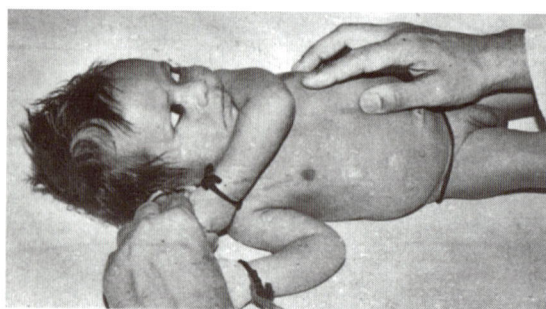

Figure 6.28 Method to assess the scarf sign. One arm at a time is held by the wrist and pulled across the chest towards the opposite shoulder. The position of elbow is noted against the plane of the trunk. The head should be kept in the midline while assessing tone in infants.

Developmental Assessment

TABLE 6.6 Normal range of angles during infancy

Age (months)	Adductor angle	Popliteal angle	Dorsiflexion angle of the foot	Scarf sign
0–3	40°–80°	80°–100°	60°–70°	Elbow does not cross the midline
4–6	70°–110°	90°–120°	60°–70°	Elbow crosses midline
7–9	110°–140°	110°–160°	60°–70°	Elbow goes beyond anterior axillary line
10–12	140°–160°	150°–170°	60°–70°	—

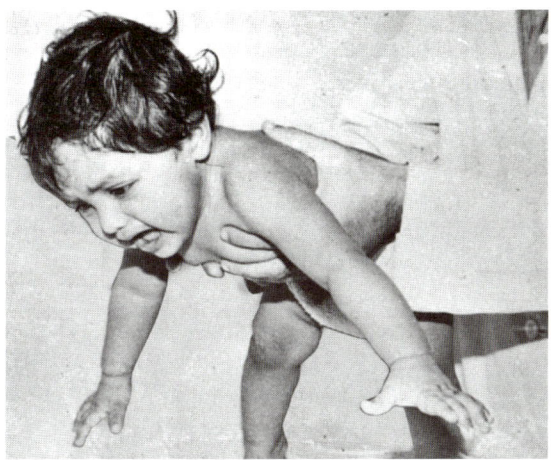

Figure 6.29 Parachute response. The response is normal in this child as he tries to ward off the fall by extension and abduction of upper limbs.

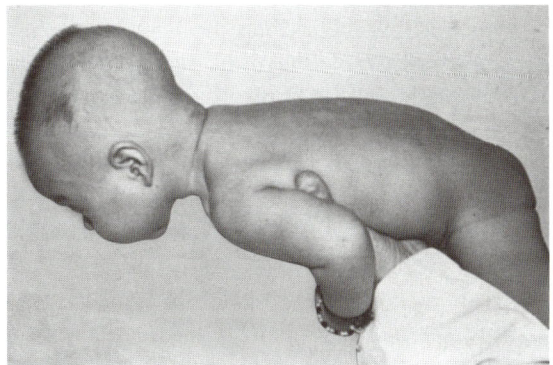

Figure 6.30 Landau response. On ventral suspension, infant extends the neck beyond the plane of the trunk with strong extension of lower limbs.

DEVELOPMENTAL SCREENING TOOLS

A number of parent-completed questionnaires are available for developmental screening like parent's evaluation of developmental status (PEDS) and ages and stages questionnaire (ASQ). A simplified Developmental Assessment Tool for *Anganwadis* (DATA) has been introduced for screening of toddlers between 18 and 36 months of age by the *Anganwadi* workers.

Sophisticated developmental testing instruments are time consuming and require the services of a trained developmental psychologist. They are useful for detection of borderline abnormalities as well as for research purposes. There is a need to develop reliable simple developmental charts which can be used by a busy clinician or basic health worker in the community. The ideal development screening tool should be reliable, simple, easy to administer, time-efficient, cost-effective and culturaly relevant.

Trivandrum Developmental Screening Chart (TDSC)

It is suitable for developmental screening of children below 2 years by a paramedical health worker. The range of each test item has been taken from the norms obtained on the Bayley Scales of Infant Development. It is based on 17 simple test items carefully chosen from among 67 motor items of Bayley Scales of Infant Development (Baroda norms). The left hand side of each horizontal dark line represents age at which 3% of children passed the item and the right edge represents the age at which 97% of the children passed the item in studies conducted at Trivandrum (Figure 6.31). A plastic ruler or a pencil is kept vertically at the level of chronological age of the child being tested. If the child fails to pass any item that lies to the left

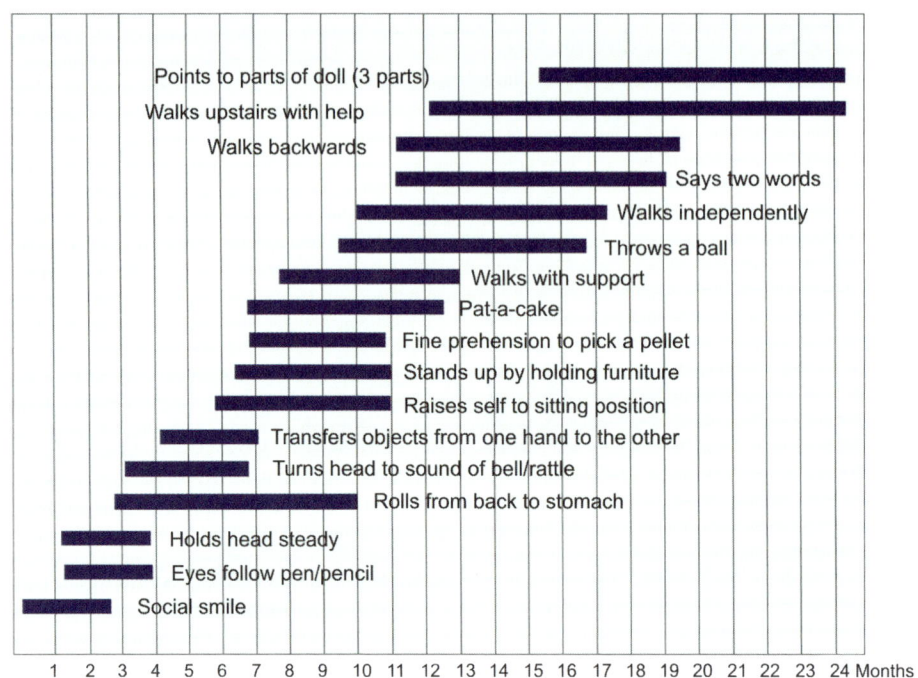

Figure 6.31 Trivandrum developmental screening chart.

side of the age marker, the child is considered to have developmental delay. It is simple to use and takes 5 to 7 minutes to administer. It is best suited to use in infants around one year of age because most of the test items are concentrated around that age period.

Baroda Development Screening Test (BDST)

To simplify the Bayley Scales of Infant Development, 22 motor items and 31 mental items, not requiring any standardized equipment have been retained. These items were grouped age-wise, one monthly intervals in the first 12 months and 3-monthly thereafter till 30 months. The 50% and 97% age placement of each item has been plotted on a graph and joined to have two smooth curves. The total number of the items passed by a child is plotted against his chronological age (or corrected age if preterm). When this point falls below 97th percentile curve, the child is considered to have developmental delay and is subjected to detailed assessment.

INTERPRETATION OF DEVELOPMENTAL FINDINGS

1. The developmental delay in two or more spheres (motor, adaptive, social, language, etc.) is called *global delay* and is suggestive of mental retardation. On the basis of global developmental status, the mental status or cognition can be clinically graded into dull normal, educable in an ordinary school, educable in a special school, trainable but not educable.

2. *Isolated delay* in development may occur in a single skill (DQ <70), e.g. isolated delay in walking due to congenital dislocation of hips, protein-energy malnutrition, rickets, neuromuscular disorder or delay in speech due to deaf-mutism.

3. *Deviancy* is defined as atypical development within a single stream when a milestone may be skipped or occur out of sequence, i.e. the child may crawl without sitting or walk before crawling. It may cause anxiety to parents but is of no significance.

4. *Dissociation* is defined as significant difference in the rate of development between two streams of skills. For example, there may be dissociation between motor and cognitive development in children with cerebral palsy (motor delay more than cognitive), mental retardation (cognition is delayed more than motor development) or motor milestones may be delayed without any significant adverse effects on cognition, i.e. benign congenital hypotonia, protein-energy malnutrition and rickets. In children with autism spectrum disorder, gross motor development is usually normal while language development and communication skills may be grossly delayed.

5. *Developmental regression* is diagnosed when a child loses previously acquired skills or milestones. The neuromotor regression may be sudden in onset or insidious and slowly progressive. The common causes of developmental regression include unrecognized head trauma, CNS infection, metabolic disorders, autism spectrum disorder, infantile myoclonus (hypsarrhythmia), degenerative disorders of central nervous system and post-vaccinal reactions (whole cell pertussis vaccine, sheep brain antirabies vaccine).

6. Apart from integrity of central nervous system, neuromotor unit and adequacy of nutrition, environmental stimulation through special senses (vision, hearing, touch, taste and smell) is essential for promotion of normal development. Lack of environmental stimulation and poor interaction between the child and working parents may adversely affect the process of development. Children in orphanages, divorced parents, parental discord or out-of-wedlock are likely to have delayed neuromotor development or behavior disorders.

7. Children with developmental disorders are at an increased risk to manifest behavior disorders. For example, temper tantrums, disruptive or introvert behavior may be a manifestation of language delay.

8. Children with *autism spectrum disorder* (ASD), which is pervasive development disorder, must be differentiated from children with mental retardation. The disorder is 4 times more common in boys than girls. Autistic children usually have normal development up to certain age and then regress especially in their social and communication skills. The manifestations are usually evident between 12 and 18 months of age. The autistic children do not like to be held or cuddled and they have no or only brief eye contact. They lack emotional warmth and social interaction. They may have stereotyped, compulsive and repetitive movements, like rocking, bouncing, head banging, swinging, spinning objects and flapping or twisting their hands and fingers. They are lost and engrossed in their own world. The child may not respond to his name when called.

   The child may be fascinated by visual stimuli like moving lights and fans. Other behavior abnormalities include toe walking, sniffing, licking or smelling objects. Speech may be absent or they may have a gibberish and repetitive (echolalia) language of their own. They may have intense liking or possessive behavior regarding some inanimate object and violently react to any change in their environment and daily routines. Some children may have a severe sleep problem. They may have associated macrocephaly, mental subnormality and seizure disorder. The Modified Checklist for Autism in Toddlers (M-CHAT-R™), a 23-item validated autism screen, is widely used to screen children between 16 and 30 months. Patients with fragile X syndrome, congenital rubella syndrome, tuberous sclerosis and Rett syndrome may have some autistic mannerisms. The salient or key features of autism spectrum disorders (ASD) are listed in *Box 6.2*.

9. Children with *attention deficit hyperactivity disorder* (ADHD) may have learning disability and school problems due to hyperactivity and poor attention span. The developmental

> **Box 6.2 Checklist for autism spectrum disorder**
>
> - No babbling by 12 months, no meaningful single word by 16 months, no two-word phrases by 24 months.
> - Speech may be absent, gibberish and repetitive (echolalia) language of their own.
> - Regression or loss of language or social skills at any age.
> - No gestures by finger pointing or saying bye-bye by one year.
> - No pretend playing or make-believe games.
> - Short attention span.
> - No eye contact.
> - Lack of response when his name is called from behind at one year of age.
> - Mostly self-occupied with no interest to make friends.
> - Repetitive behavior, like throwing of toys, rocking, flapping or twisting of hands, head banging, rocking, bouncing, swinging, spinning objects, asking repetitive questions, etc.
> - Resistance to change in an established routine or ritual.
> - Limited or lack of facial expression.
> - Limited gestures or non-verbal communications
> - They are likely to have the habit of toe-walking, sniffing, licking or smelling objects.
> - They have relative insensitivity to pain.
> - Head size may be large.

milestones are usually normal and some children may have exceptional congnitive abilities. They are unable to sit still and are perpetually "on the go". They are constantly on the move, fidget, squirm, aimlessly touch and poke their fingers into everything. They have trouble in completing their homework assignment, often forgeting and losing track of their personal belongings. They are unable to sit through a television program or listen to a story. They have short attention span with poor school performance. They have an impulsive behavior, blurting out answers before completion of questions and have trouble waiting for their turn. Their behavior becomes worse in crowded places and infront of guests. They demonstrate temper tantrums and crying episodes on minor pretexts. They are aggressive in their behavior and uncooperative with their classmates and have difficulty in cultivating friendship. They may have antisocial behavior, like disobedience, defiance, lack of discipline, destructiveness, fire setting and inflicting harm to others. They have associated language and learning disability due to distractibility and short attention span. They are likely to have sleep disorder and obsessive–compulsive disorder (OCD). The diagnosis of ADHD is facilitated by using Conners Parent Rating Scale-Revised: short form (CPRS-R:S), Conners Teachers Rating Scale-Revised: short form (CTRS-R:S), and Diagnostic and Statistical Manual-IV (DSM-IV).

10. Some children may have specific learning disabilities in the fields of reading (dyslexia), writing (dysgraphia), communication, or mathematical abilities (dyscalculia) despite having normal neuromotor development, normal cognition and social interactions. Dyslexia affects 1 in 10 individuals, many of whom remain undiagnosed and receive little or no intervention. It is a specific reading and writing disorder and does not reflect low intelligence. There are many bright and creative individuals with dyslexia who never learn to read, write, and/or spell at a level consistent with their intellectual ability.

THE CHILD WITH A LEARNING DISABILITY

The learning disability may be due to mental subnormality, visual, auditory or motor handicaps, emotional disturbances and lack of stimulation because of environmental disadvantages. There may be specific learning disability, like difficulty in understanding written or spoken language or child may have problems with attention span, listening, thinking, reading, speaking, writing, spelling and arithmetic due to perceptual handicaps, dyslexia and attention deficit hyperactivity disorder (ADHD). Due to learning disability and poor academic performance at school, the child may present with psychological or behavior problems including disruptive, aggressive, hyperactive, withdrawn, lazy, labile and immature behavior.

Assessment of children with learning problems is a multidisciplinary effort involving the pediatrician, ophthalmologist, audiologist and speech therapist, child psychologist, social worker and special educator or counsellor. Teacher's detailed report, parental perceptions and expectations and childs' own view of his problem should be sought. A detailed medical history should be taken regarding perinatal events, gestation, birth weight, Apgar score and neonatal course. History of any serious or significant medical illness should be sought. Family dynamics, parental discord and time spent by parents for interactions with the child should be assessed. A detailed physical and neurological examination must be done to identify any dysmorphism, abnormalities in shape and size of the head. The presence of soft neurological signs, like asymmetry of muscle tone, difficulty in standing on one foot, inability to perform rapid alternating movements, difficulty with right-left orientation, clumsiness, poor handwriting and graphesthesia, should be looked for.

The child should be specifically screened for visual acuity and hearing. A detailed psychological assessment is mandatory to assess cognition, perceptual deficit, communication and social abilities. A number of screening tests are available for diagnosis of autism spectrum disorder (ASD), dyslexia and attention deficit hyperactivity disorder (ADHD). Refer to Appendices XXXI, XXXII and XXXIII for screening of children for dyslexia, ASD and ADHD, respectively.

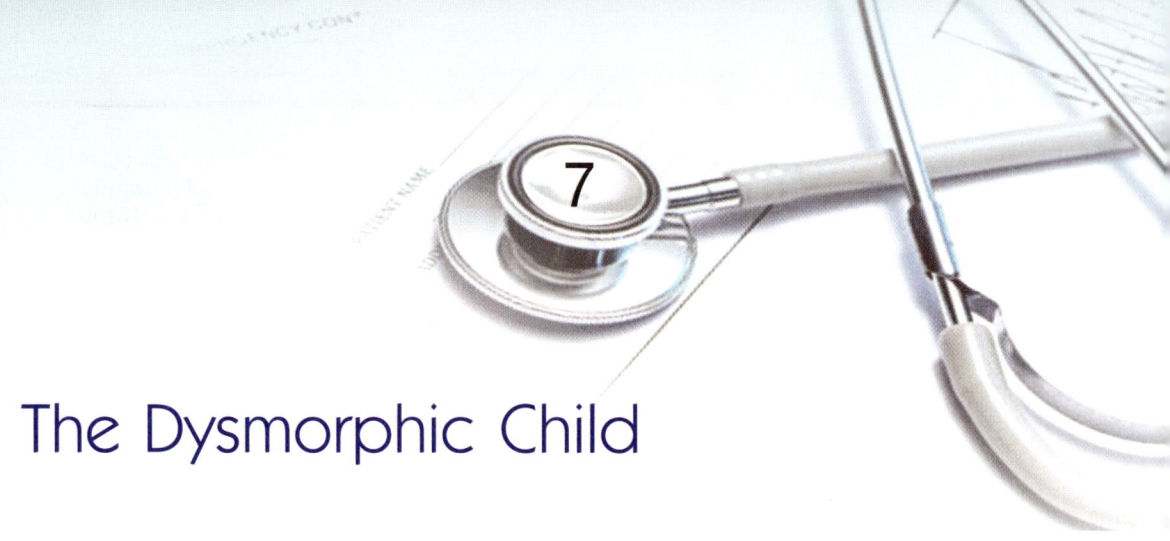

7

The Dysmorphic Child

Most developmental defects and chromosomal disorders are seen during childhood. A large number of childhood diseases can be diagnosed by identification of typical facies. By virtue of constant effort and practice, the pediatrician should sharpen his observational faculties to identify subtle abnormalities of head and face. Front, rear and profile views of face should be examined to identify facial dysmorphism. Look for size and alignment of eyes, distance between two eyes, shape of nasal tip and bridge, size of philtrum, size and position of ears, preauricular skin tags, size of chin and forehead (Figure 7.1). Look for congenital torticollis, short neck, webbing of neck, low hair line, spinal abnormalities, such as Klippel-Feil syndrome (fusion of the cervical vertebrae) and atlanto-

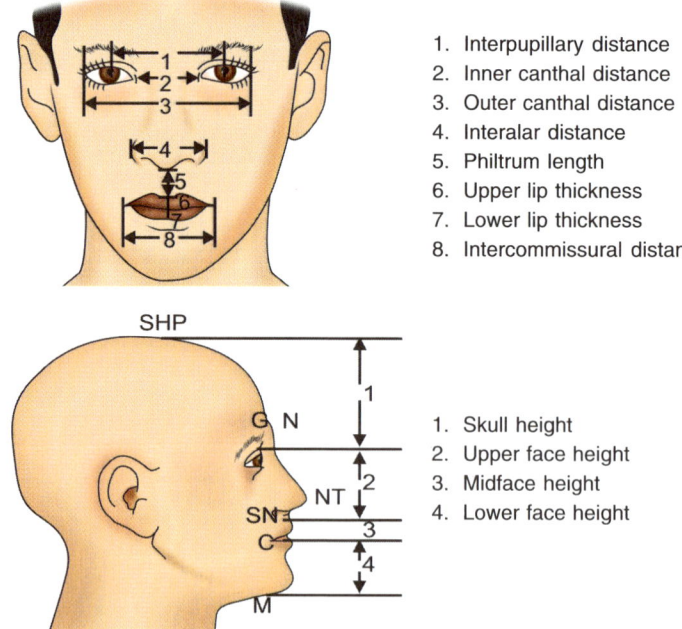

1. Interpupillary distance
2. Inner canthal distance
3. Outer canthal distance
4. Interalar distance
5. Philtrum length
6. Upper lip thickness
7. Lower lip thickness
8. Intercommissural distance

1. Skull height
2. Upper face height
3. Midface height
4. Lower face height

Figure 7.1 Guidelines for head and facial measurements for the diagnosis of facial dysmorphism.
Abbreviations: SHP, superior head point (vertex); G, glabella; N, nasion; NT, nose tip; SN, subnasion; C, cheilion; M, menton.

occipital assimilation. Data is available to make an objective assessment of dysmorphism in different ethnic groups and populations.

ABNORMAL SHAPE OF HEAD

The abnormalities in the shape and size of the head are common and easily visible. They may be isolated or associated with other anomalies as a part of syndrome. Abnormalities in the shape of scalp due to edema (caput succedaneum) or cephalohematoma are common at birth in vaginal born babies especially following prolonged labor or vacuum extraction. These abnormalities are transient and gradually resolve over a few hours or days. A number of physiological or pathological conditions may be associated with abnormalities in skull bones with odd-shaped skull and are listed in Table 7.1.

TABLE 7.1 Types of abnormal head shapes

- *Microcephaly.* Head circumference is less by more than 2 standard deviations below the mean for age and sex. Sutures and fontanels may be prematurely closed (craniosynostosis) or open (poor growth of brain).
- *Hydrocephalus.* Head circumference is more than 2 standard deviations above the mean for the age and sex. It is associated with rapid growth velocity of head, bossing of frontal and parietal bones, widely open and bulging anterior fontanel, visible and engorged veins over the forehead and sun setting sign due to paresis of upward gaze.
- *Dolichocephaly.* The head is elongated due to increase in anterior-posterior diameter of skull (premature fusion of sagittal suture, prematurely born baby). The skull may give an appearance of a boat (scaphocephaly).
- *Brachycephaly.* Flat head with reduced anterior-posterior diameter (Down syndrome, Carpenter syndrome).
- *Frontal bossing.* Prominent and overhanging forehead.
- *Caput quadratum or hot cross bun appearance of skull.* There is marked frontal and parietal bossing with depression in between the skull bones (rickets, beta thalassemia major)
- *Acrocephaly or oxycephaly or turricephaly.* Head is conical in shape with a pointed crown due to premature fusion of coronal suture (Crouzon disease, Apert syndrome)
- *Trignocephaly.* Forehead is pointed with prominent and elevated metopic suture due to its premature closure
- *Plagiocephaly.* Skull has bizarre or rhomboid shape with haphazard elevations and depressions in skull bones because of craniosynostosis of multiple sutures or it may be positional in premature babies
- *Flat occiput.* It is positional and commonly seen in premature babies
- *Prominent occiput.* The occiput is conical in infants with trisomy-18 and bulging and transilluminant in Dandy-Walker malformation.

Refer to Chapter 8 for causes of abnormal head shapes.

TYPICAL FACIES

In certain systemic disorders in children, the diagnosis can be suspected on the basis of characteristic facies. The typical facies are usually evident during the course of disease or when disease is well advanced. In genetic or chromosomal disorders, dysmorphism is evident at birth or early infancy.

Chronic hemolytic facies In beta thalassemia major, the increased erythropoiesis in the bone marrow results in the expansion of medullary cavity of various bones leading to development of typical facies. There is bossing of skull with flattened vertex giving an appearance of hot cross bun. The facial bones or malar eminences become prominent due to hypertrophy of maxilla. There is hypertelorism (expansion of lesser wing of sphenoid), epicanthic folds and depressed bridge of the nose. There is crowding of teeth with malocclusion and protrusion of teeth giving a "rodent look".

Cretinism The facial features are coarse with bloated cheeks, depressed nasal bridge, large protruding tongue and drooling of saliva. Anterior fontanel is large in size and cranial sutures are widely separated. The skin is usually dry, coarse, cold and mottled. Hair are coarse and brittle.

Mucopolysaccharidoses They belong to the group of lysosomal disorders and are characterized by coarse facial features, depressed or flat nose, thick lips, large tongue, clouded cornea and widely separated peg-like teeth (Figure 7.2). Additional features include short neck, pigeon-shaped chest, long extremities with stiff joints and hepatosplenomegaly.

Moon facies Moon-shaped facies are seen in children with cushingoid features due to prolonged corticosteroid therapy or Cushing syndrome. The face is rounded with prominent flushed or plethoric cheeks, double chin, hirsutism and acne. There is accumulation of fat over the upper back and supraclavicular region producing a typical buffalo-hump. In nephrotic syndrome, moon facies occur due to marked swelling of the face, puffiness and lid edema. During the course of corticosteroid therapy, cushingoid appearances supervene.

Hepatic facies In chronic liver disease and/or cirrhosis, facial features are characterized by icteric tinge, sallow or muddy complexion, pinched nose, sunken eyes, hollow temporal regions and cheeks.

Potter facies In infants with renal agenesis, there is oligohydramnios and the fetus is squashed *in utero*. Potter facies are characterized by small receding chin, low-set ears with folded helices, compressed nose, epicanthal folds, prominent skinfolds below the eyes and antimongoloid slant of the eyes.

Facial palsy In unilateral facial palsy, there is asymmetry of face with absence of nasolabial fold and inability to close the eye on the affected side (Figure 7.3).

Expressionless face Bilateral facial palsy either at the nuclear (bulbar palsy) or infranuclear level (bilateral facial nerve palsy) is characterized by expressionless or mask-like facies. The various conditions causing mask-like face include Mobius syndrome, Guillain-Barre syndrome, infantile botulism, Wilson disease, myotonic dystrophy, facioscapulohumeral muscular dystrophy and mental depression.

Risus sardonicus The infant with tetanus looks alert, the eyebrows are raised and angles of the mouth are drawn out due to spasm of facial muscles. The mouth may be kept slightly open due to downward pull because of spasm of the neck muscles. Trismus or reflex spasm of masseters is invoked when attempt is made to open the mouth. Apart from tetanus, other conditions that can produce features like risus sardonicus include dental abscess, peritonsillar infections, encephalitis or meningitis and intracranial hemorrhage.

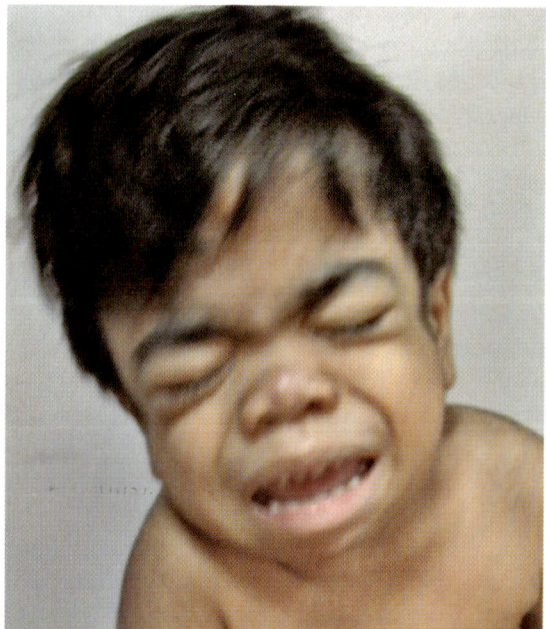

Figure 7.2 Note the coarse facial features, broad depressed nose, full pouting lips and thick eyebrows with peg-like teeth in a child with mucopolysaccharidosis.

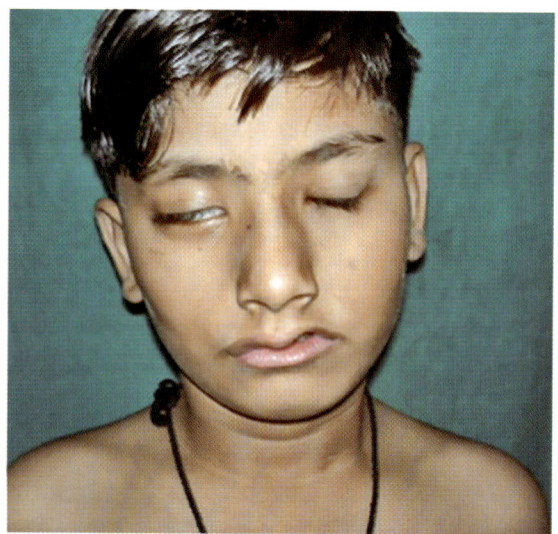

Figure 7.3 Partially recovered Bell's palsy on the right side. Note the inability to close the right eye.

THE DEVELOPMENTAL DEFECTS

The child with developmental defects or congenital structural anomalies is called a dysmorphic child. Dysmorphism is manifest during childhood and every pediatrician should be conversant with the clinical approach of such a child. The congenital structural anomalies may be classified as follows:

1. Structural or normal variants These are normal developmental or anatomical variations without any clinical or therapeutic implications. The examples include simian crease, clinodactyly (medial or lateral deviation of finger), camptodactyly (claw-like fingers), abnormal dermatoglyphics, wide anterior fontanel, wide forehead, sacral dimple, beaked or bulbous nose, etc. These variants may or may not be of any clinical relevance.

2. Minor anomalies They are true anomalies and are primarily of cosmetic concern. Isolated minor anomaly may be present in over 10% of normal newborn babies. Examples include pre-auricular skin tags, supernumerary nipple, various nevi and pigmentary disorders (Figure 7.4). Children with three or more minor anomalies are likely to have a dysmorphic syndrome.

3. Major anomalies The major developmental defects produce functional disability and may compromise normal life expectancy. Around 2 to 3% of newborn babies may have major anomalies. The anomaly may be detectable at birth or manifest any time during childhood.

4. Isolated versus multiple anomalies The majority of birth defects (almost two-thirds) are isolated involving a single organ or system. The common examples are cleft lip, cleft palate, congenital heart disease, etc. The cause of isolated major anomalies is usually multifactorial or polygenic. Less commonly, congenital anomalies may affect several organs or body systems producing multiple congenital defects. The common patterns of multiple structural anomalies include associations, sequences, field defects and syndromes.

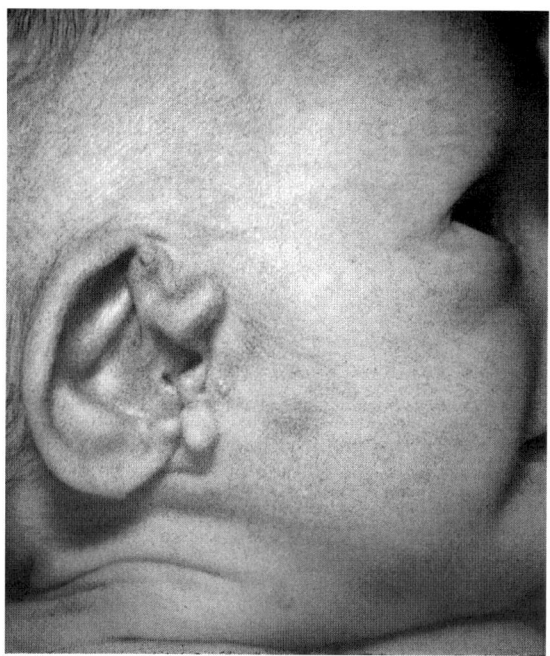

Figure 7.4 Preauricular skin tags in a child with Turner syndrome.

"*Association*" *defects* refer to non-random combination of anomalies wherein the individual components occur together more frequently than would be expected by chance. The clinical picture may vary from case-to-case but is consistent enough for recognition as a syndrome. For example, VACTERL association comprises of **v**ertebral anomalies, **a**nal atresia, **c**ardiac defects, **t**racheo-**e**sophageal fistula, **r**enal and **r**adial anomalies and **l**imb defects. The recognition of two or three cardinal features should prompt a search for other occult anomalies. CHARGE association is characterized by **c**oloboma of eye, **h**eart anomalies (tetralogy of Fallot, PDA, VSD, ASD), **a**tresia of choanae, **r**etardation (mental and physical), **g**enital hypoplasia (cryptorchidism and micropenis), **e**ar anomalies and deafness. VATER association is characterized by **v**ertebral (hemivertebrae or sacral deformity) or **v**ascular anomalies, **a**nal malformations, **t**racheoesophageal fistula, **r**adial or **r**enal defects. The recurrence risk of association anomalies is low and this information is useful for genetic counseling.

The "*sequence anomalies*" is a pattern of multiple congenital malformations that cannot be explained on developmental and embryologic basis and occur as a result of a cascade of seemingly unrelated consequences. The typical example of sequence anomaly is "Potter oligohydramnios" due to renal agenesis. Oligohydramnios due to renal agensis leads to intrauterine compression of fetus with limb deformities, flattened or compressed facial appearance and pulmonary hypoplasia which is usually the cause of death (Figure 7.5).

The "*field defects*" refer to constellation of anomalies of different body organs which differentiate during the same time of embryogenesis because of anatomical proximity. Some adverse uterine factors may interfere with the normal development of the structures differentiating during the critical phase of embryogenesis. They are often caused by an adverse vascular event and the recurrence risk is low. The examples include Poland anomaly and Moebius syndrome.

The "*syndrome*" is defined as a unique constellation of multiple anomalies that repeatedly occur in a consistent pattern. The presence of multiple dysmorphic features in a child is suggestive of a chromosomal defect. When there are two or more major anomalies affecting different body systems or one major and two minor congenital malformations, chromosomal disorder should be ruled out. In patients with multiple malformations, there are no confirmatory laboratory tests and diagnosis is based on identification of a typical pattern of anomalies.

At times, the constellation of anomalies in a patient may not conform to any recognized syndrome. A number of computerized dysmorphology databases are available to assist the clinician to make a reliable diagnosis of a child with multiple malformations. The popular computerized databases or software include LDDB (London dysmorphology database), LNDB (London neurogenetic database), POSSUM (Pictures of standard syndromes and unidentified malformations) and SYNDROC (syndromes of congenital

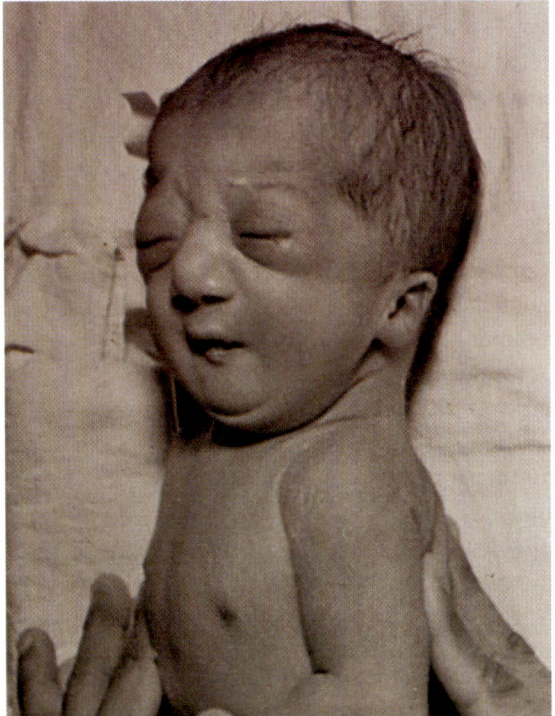

Figure 7.5 Potter facies due to oligohydramnios showing receding chin, low-set ears and prominent skinfolds below the eyes.

malformation database). These databases can be screened on a personal computer. If a database search does not suggest a definitive diagnosis, the combination of anomalies may be a new, hitherto, unreported syndrome. It is recommended to perform a prometaphase chromosomal analysis to rule out a rare chromosomal anomaly (usually interstitial deletions or translocations) as a cause of syndrome. Cytogenetic techniques like analysis of G-banded chromosomes, fluorescent *in situ* hybridization (FISH) and comparative genomic hybridization (CGH) are increasingly used. Chromosomal microarray analysis is useful to identify aneuploidies and unbalanced rearrangements of chromosomes.

Based on the nature of major anomalies present, the dysmorphic syndromes can be categorized into ten broad groups. The salient diagnostic features of common dysmorphic syndromes are discussed below.

1. Chromosomal Syndromes

Down syndrome (Trisomy 21) Brachycephaly, flat facies, hypertelorism with mongoloid slant (upwards and outwards) of eyes with epicanthal folds, excess skin over the nape of neck, open mouth with protruding tongue, low set small ears, Brushfield spots in iris, single transverse palmar crease or simian crease, small incurved little finger, clinodactyly, sandal gap in the toes, hypotonia, or hyperflexibility, and mental subnormality (Figures 7.6 and 7.7). The commonly associated congenital anomalies with Down syndrome include congenital heart defects (atrioventricular septal defect, atrial septal defect, ventricular septal defect, patent ductus arteriosus, coarctation of aorta and tetralogy of Fallot), digestive system anomalies (duodenal atresia, Hirschsprung disease, and tracheo-esophageal atresia), musculoskeletal anomalies (club feet, syndactyly, polydactyly, limb reduction), diaphragmatic hernia and cataracts.

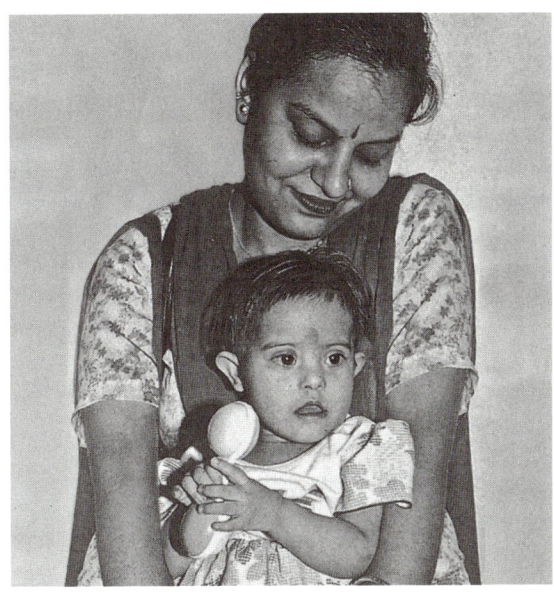

Figure 7.6 Down syndrome. Note hypertelorism, epicanthal folds, mongoloid slant of eyes, small hands and clinodactyly of little finger. The child had AV canal defect with congestive heart failure.

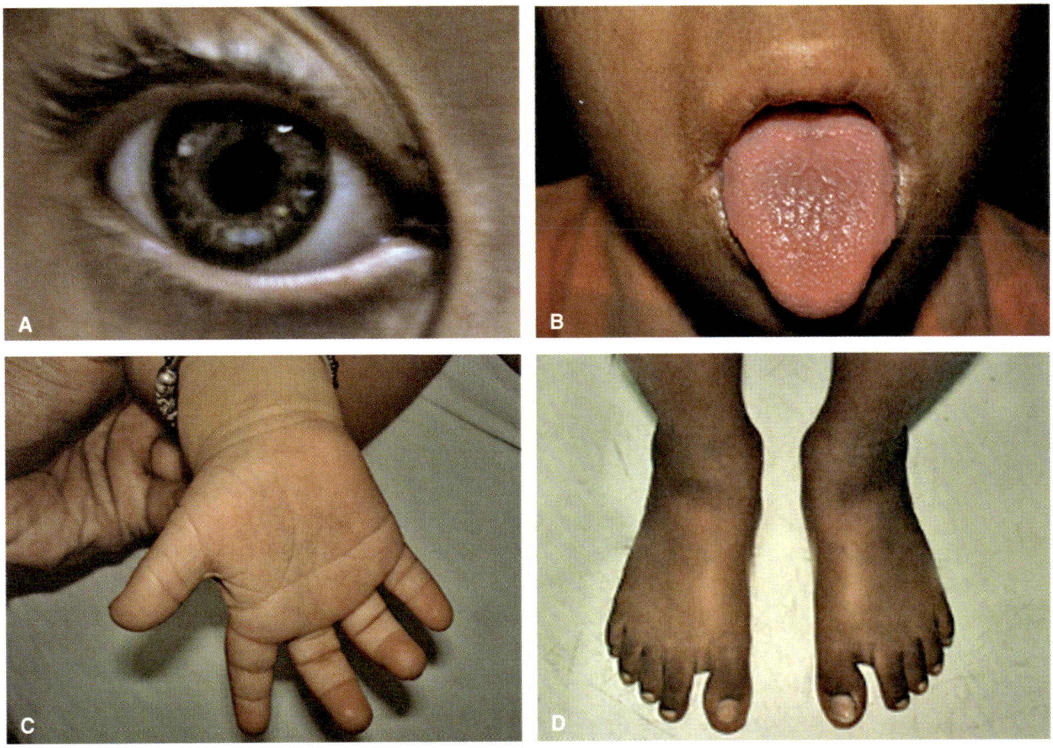

Figure 7.7A to D Spectrum of clinical findings in children with Down syndrome. (A) Brushfield spots in the iris, (B) large, thick, "scrotal" tongue, (C) Simian crease and (D) "Sandal gap" in the toes.

Edward syndrome (Trisomy 18) Intrauterine growth retardation, microcephaly with prominent occiput, low-set malformed ears, microphthalmia, clenched hands with index finger overlapping third finger and fifth finger overlapping fourth finger, short dorsiflexed big toe, short sternum, rocker bottom feet, inguinal or umbilical hernia, undescended testes, low-arch dermal ridge pattern, congenital heart defects (VSD, PDA, ASD), and severe neuromotor retardation (Figure 7.8 A and B).

Patau syndrome (Trisomy 13) Microcephaly with localized scalp defects (aplasia cutis congenita), holoprosencephaly (forebrain fails to develop into two hemispheres), cleft lip/palate or both, broad flat nose, hypotelorism, low-set ears, microphthalmia, coloboma of iris, postaxial polydactyly of hands and feet, inguinal hernia, undescended testes, omphalocele, congenital heart defects (VSD, ASD, PDA), and neuromotor retardation (Figure 7.9 A and B).

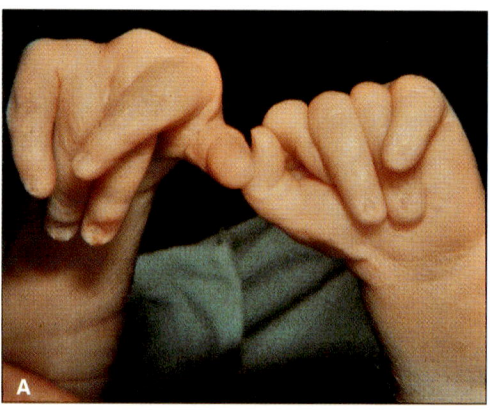

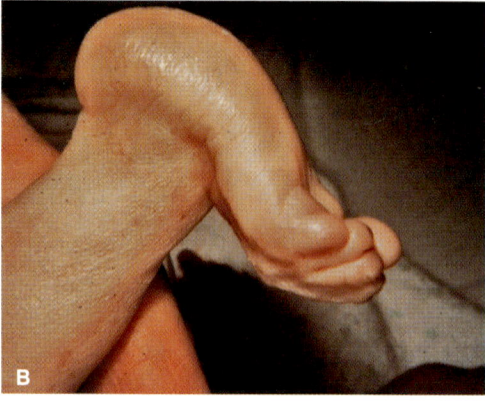

Figure 7.8A and B Edward syndrome. (A) Overlapping of fingers with hypoplastic nails. (B) Rocker-bottom feet.

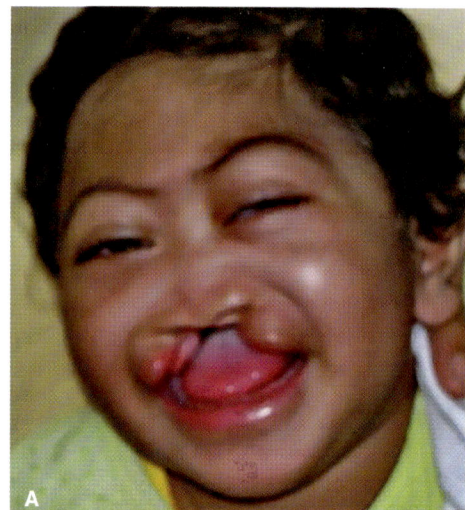

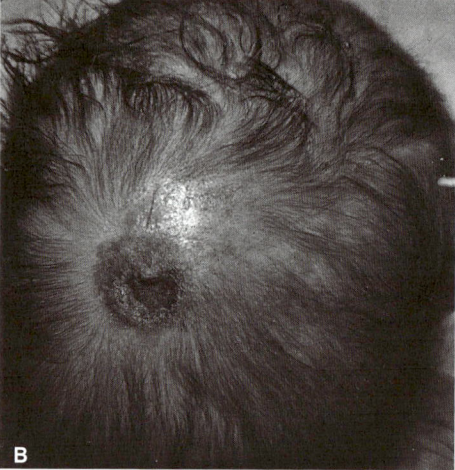

Figure 7.9A and B Patau syndrome. (A) Bilateral cleft lip and palate, broad flat nose and low-set ears. (B) There is localized punched-out defects in the scalp. It is usually associated with holoprosencephaly.

Cri-du-chat syndrome or Lejeune syndrome (5p deletion syndrome) Cat-like cry in infancy, round facies, microcephaly, hypertelorism, antimongoloid slant of eyes, epicanthal folds, hypertrichosis, single palmar crease, excessive drooling, failure to thrive, cardiac defects, neuromotor retardation.

Turner syndrome (Monosomy X or 45X) Short webbed neck, low posterior hairline, lymphedema of dorsa of hands and feet, cubitus valgus, shield-like chest with widely spaced nipples, short stature, primary amenorrhea. The associated findings include gonadal dysgenesis, renal anomalies, coarctation of aorta and deafness (Figures 7.10 A to C and 7.11). They are more likely to develop diabetes mellitus and hypothyroidism.

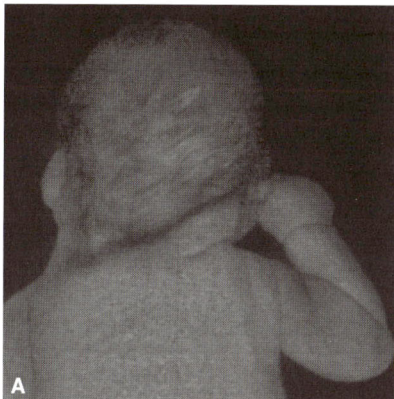
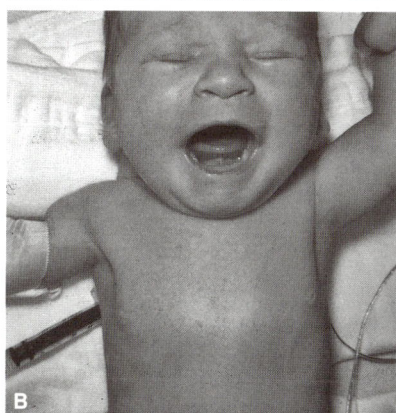
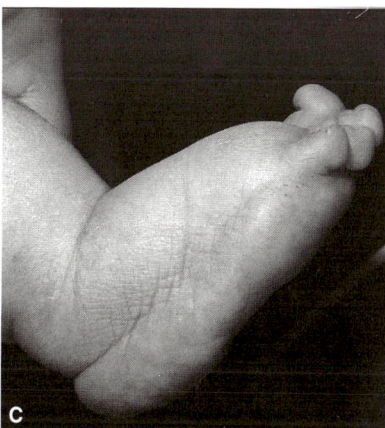

Figure 7.10A to C Turner syndrome in a neonate (A) Short webbed neck with lymphedema of dorsum of hand. (B) Shield-like chest with widely spaced nipples. (C) Lymphedema of dorsum of foot.

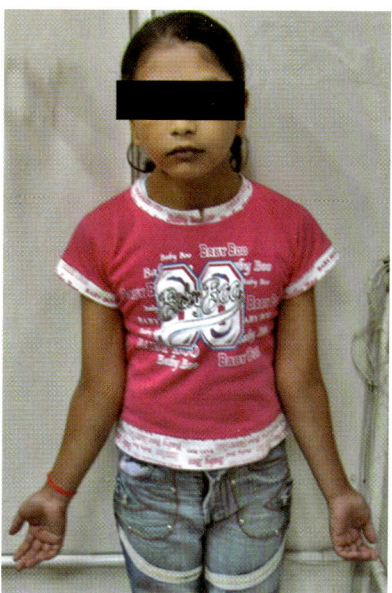

Figure 7.11 Turner syndrome. Note increased carrying angle at elbows in a 14-year-old short-statured girl without onset of menstrual periods.

2. Syndromes with Extremely Short Stature

Cornelia de Lange syndrome (CdLS) Microbrachycephaly, hirsutism, long curly eyelashes, thin downturned upper lip, long philtrum, bushy eyebrows with synophrys (eyebrows merge in the midline), micromelia, and mental retardation (Figure 7.12).

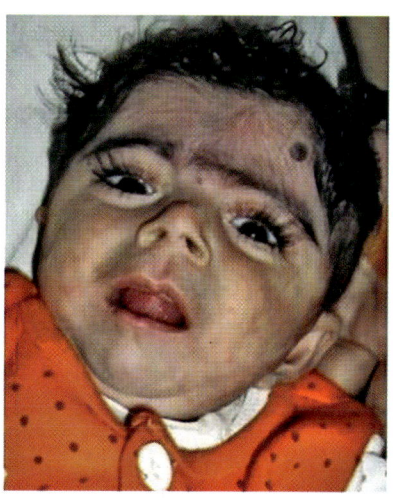

Figure 7.12 Cornelia de Lange syndrome. Hirsutism, long curly eyelashes, thin downturned upper lip and long philtrum.

Rubinstein-Taybi syndrome (RTS) Microcephaly, hypoplastic maxilla with narrow palate, low set ears, antimongoloid slant of palpebral fissures, beaked nose with nasal septum extending below the level of nares, hypertrichosis, broad thumbs and broad first toes (broad thumb-hallux syndrome), mental retardation, tendency to form keloids, lymphoma and leukemia (Figure 7.13 A to C). They are prone to develop complications during anesthesia especially administration of succinylcholine.

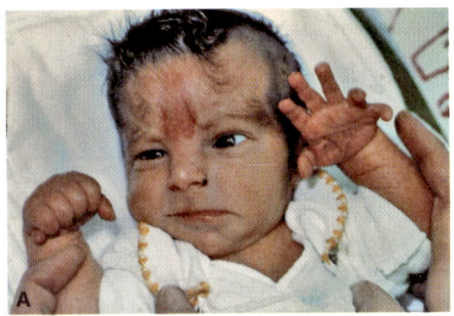
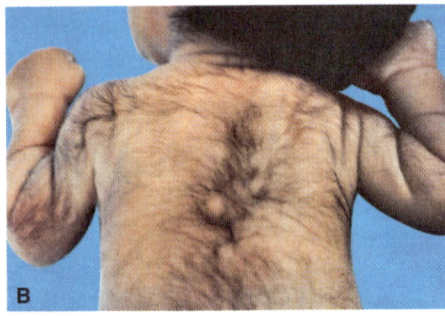
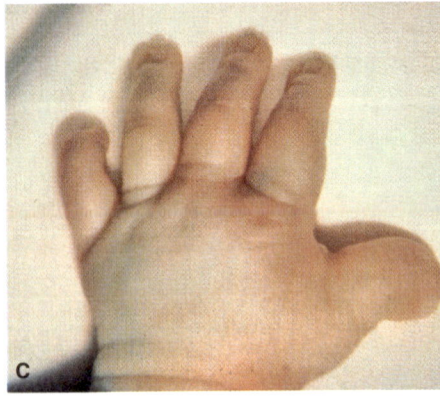

Figure 7.13A to C Rubinstein-Taybi syndrome. (A) Microcephaly, antimongoloid slant of eyes, strabismus, beaked nose with nasal septum extending beyond the level of nares. (B) Hypertrichosis over the back and (C) Broad thumb and fingers.

Russell–Silver syndrome (RSS) Triangular facies with down turning of corners of mouth, skeletal asymmetry (facial or limbs), clinodactyly, caféaulait spots, hypoglycemia, wide fontanels with delayed closure and dwarfism.

Seckel syndrome (bird-headed dwarf syndrome) Microcephaly, facial hypoplasia with small chin and prominent beak-like nose, prominent eyes, low-set malformed ears, and mental retardation (Figure 7.14).

Hallermann-Streiff syndrome Brachycephaly with frontal and parietal bossing, bird-like facies, hypotrichosis or sparse hair over scalp, eyebrows and eyelashes, bilateral microphthalmos with cataracts, small pinched nose, micrognathia with double chin, and dental abnormalities.

Laron syndrome Marked dwarfism (resistance or insensitivity to hGH), hypoglycemia, frontal bossing, saddle nose, "setting sun" sign, obesity, small genitalia, and high-pitched voice.

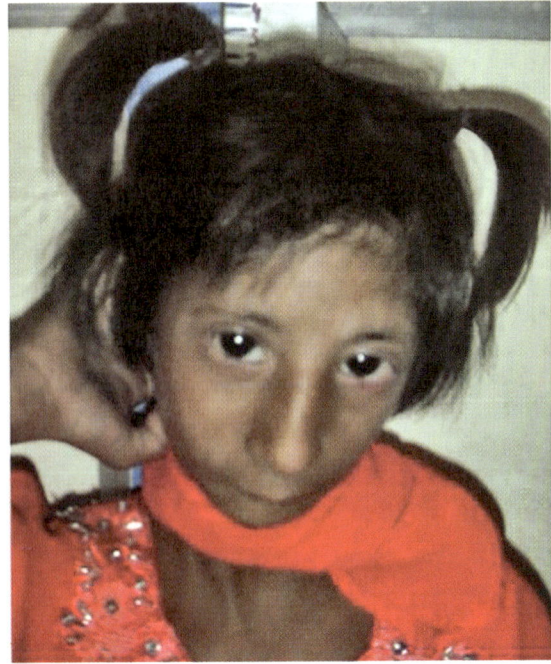

Figure 7.14 Seckel syndrome. Note small bird-like head and prominent beak-like nose.

3. Syndromes with Moderate Short Stature, Facial and/or Genital Defects

Rothmund-Thomson syndrome Photosensitivity, alopecia, cataracts, hypogonadism, and short stature.

Smith-Lemli-Opitz syndrome Ptosis, epicanthal folds, anteverted nostrils, low-set ears, micrognathia, syndactyly of second or third toes, hypospadias and cryptorchidism in males, failure to thrive, and mental retardation.

Laurence-Moon-Biedl syndrome Obesity, retinitis pigmentosa (night blindness), mental retardation, hypogenitalism, and polydactyly.

Williams syndrome Elfin facies, prominent forehead, long philtrum, anteverted or upturned nostrils, depressed nasal bridge, thick patulous upper lip with drooping lower lip, wide smile, hypertelorism, periorbital fullness, full cheeks, strabismus, blue eyes, hoarse voice, supravalvular aortic stenosis, peripheral pulmonary stenosis, friendly "cocktail party" mischievous personality, hypercalcemia during infancy, mental retardation with relative sparing of language, senile look due to wrinkling of skin and graying of hair (Figure 7.15).

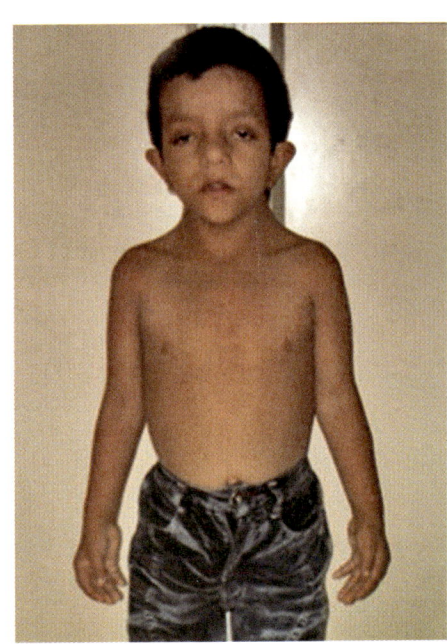

Figure 7.16 Noonan syndrome in a boy. Phenotype is similar to Turner syndrome. Note mild webbing of neck, widely placed downward slanting of eyes, low-set ears, shield-like chest with widely spaced nipples.

Noonan syndrome Turner-like phenotype, webbed-neck, hypertelorism with antimongoloid slant of eyes, broad forehead, ptosis, low-set posteriorly rotated or folded ears, pectum excavatum, carinatum or both, pulmonary valve stenosis or ASD, and cryptorchidism (Figure 7.16).

Aarskog syndrome Round face, small broad nose with anteverted nostrils, long philtrum with clinodactyly of 5th finger, "shawl scrotum" (scrotal skinfold encircles base of the phallus), and short stature.

4. Syndromes with Physical Over Growth and Associated Defects

Fragile X syndrome Long face, macrocephaly, prominent ears, large chin or prognathism, hyperextensible distal interphalangeal joints, postpubertal macro-orchidism, tall stature, mental subnormality, cluttered speech, hyperkinetic, autistic or aggressive behavior. It is the most common genetic cause of intellectual disability (Figure 7.17).

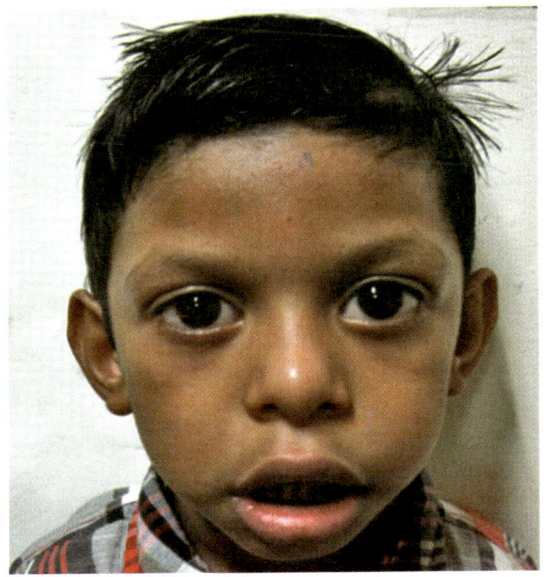

Figure 7.15 Williams syndrome. Prominent forehead and eyes, periorbital fullness, and thick patulous lips.

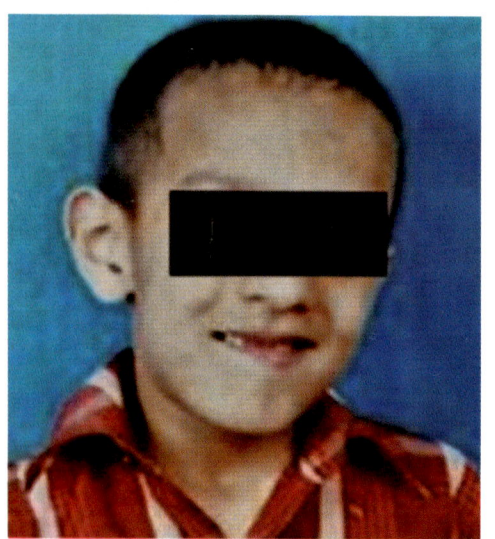

Figure 7.17 Fragile X syndrome. Note long face, large ears and prominent broad chin.

Sotos syndrome (cerebral gigantism) Large dolichocephalic head, coarse-looking facies, hypertelorism, antimongoloid slant of eyes, bossing of forehead, prominent chin (macrognathia), large hands and feet, overgrowth of all physical parameters, hypotonia, laxity of joints, advanced bone age, seizures, autistic features, mental retardation, and cardiac anomalies (Figure 7.18).

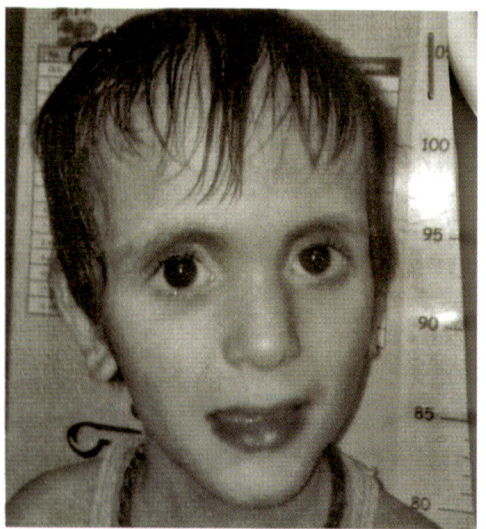

Figure 7.18 A 2-year-old boy with Sotos syndrome. Note long narrow face, frontal bossing, hypertelorism, and prominent chin.

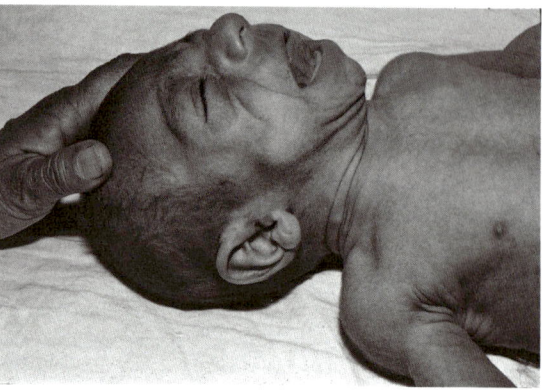

Figure 7.19 Beckwith-Wiedemann syndrome. Note macroglossia and classical clefts in the ear lobe. The infant had exomphalos and hypoglycemia.

Beckwith-Wiedemann syndrome The usual features include exomphalos, macroglossia, macrosomia, nevus flammeus over the forehead, prominent eyes, typical creases or clefts in ear lobes, visceromegaly, hypoglycemia, and hemihypertrophy (Figure 7.19). They are at increased risk to develop cancer.

Berardinelli lipodystrophy syndrome Muscular body habitus without subcutaneous fat, large hands and feet, acanthosis nigricans, phlebomegaly, hepatomegaly, and large phallus.

Marshall-Smith syndrome Large-for-dates, prominent forehead, upturned nose, blue sclerae, micrognathia, advanced physical and skeletal growth, and mental retardation.

Weaver-Smith syndrome Large baby at birth, macrocephaly, wide forehead, hypertelorism, antimongoloid slant of eyes, elongated philtrum, large ears, small chin, camptodactyly, broad thumbs, hypertonia with contractures.

5. Syndromes with Unusual CNS or Neuromuscular Findings and Associated Defects

Arthrogryposis multiplex congenita Multiple contractures of major joints, bilateral club feet, policeman-tip position of arms and hands, and decreased muscle mass.

Meckel-Gruber syndrome Occipital encephalocele, microcephaly, cleft lip/palate, abnormal genitalia, postaxial polydactyly, enlarged palpable kidneys due to multicystic dysplasia.

Sjögren-Larsson syndrome Ichthyosis, spastic diplegia, retinal degeneration, and mental retardation.

Ataxia-telangiectasia (Louis-Bar syndrome) Telangiectasia of bulbar conjunctiva, auricles and nasal bridge, progressive cerebellar ataxia, oculomotor apraxia, dysarthria, recurrent respiratory infections and sinusitis. They are at increased risk to develop lymphomas and leukemias.

Prader-Willi syndrome (PWS) Obesity because of excesive hunger, fish-like mouth, hypotonia, micromelia, short stature, almond-shaped palpebral fissures, hypogonadism in males, behavior problems and mental retardation (Figure 7.20).

Zellweger syndrome (cerebrohepatorenal syndrome) Long flat facies, high forehead, epicanthic folds, large fontanel, micrognathia, abnormal ears, hepatomegaly, hypomyelination of brain, hypotonia, hepatic and renal cysts.

Myotonic dystrophy syndrome Myopathic facies with atrophy of temporalis muscle, ptosis, cataracts (usually on slit-lamp examination), hypotonia during infancy and myotonia or lack of relaxation of muscles during childhood and testicular atrophy in pubertal boys.

6. Syndromes with Facial Dysmorphism as a Major Feature

Moebius syndrome Ptosis, bilateral 6th nerve palsy, bilateral facial nerve palsy with mask-like facies, and micrognathia.

Pierre Robin sequence (PRS) Micrognathia and retrognathia, glossoptosis with choking episodes, and U-shaped cleft of soft palate (Figure 7.21).

Frontonasal dysplasia sequence Broad-notched nasal tip or bifid nostrils with nasal tags, ocular hypertelorism or telecanthus, midline deficit of frontal bone with encephalocele.

Waardenburg syndrome Telecanthus or widely placed eyes, with nasal tags, outer displacement of inferior lacrimal puncti (telecanthus or dystopia canthorum), partial albinism or piebaldism (white forelock of hair), white patches of skin, heterochromia of iris, and sensorineural deafness. There is increased association with intestinal (Hirschsprung disease) and spinal defects.

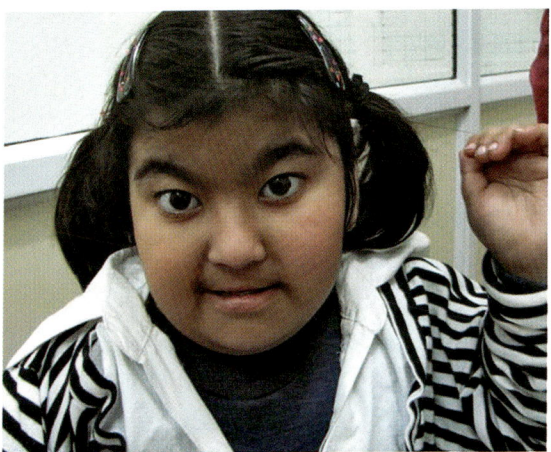

Figure 7.20 Prader-Willi syndrome. Obesity, almond-shaped eyes with mongoloid slant, thin upper lip, small hands with tapering fingers.

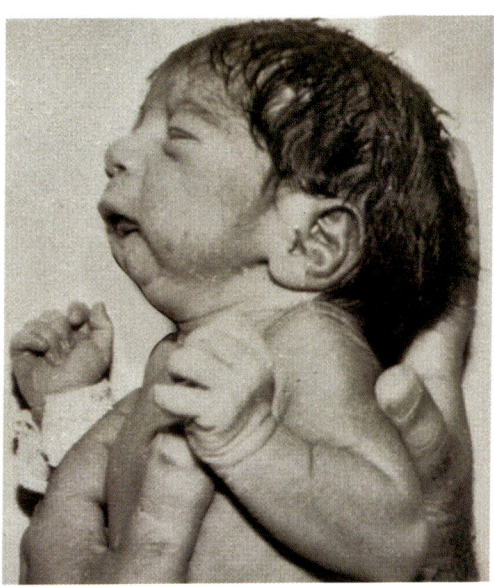

Figure 7.21 Typical appearances of micrognathia and retrognathia in an infant with Pierre Robin syndrome.

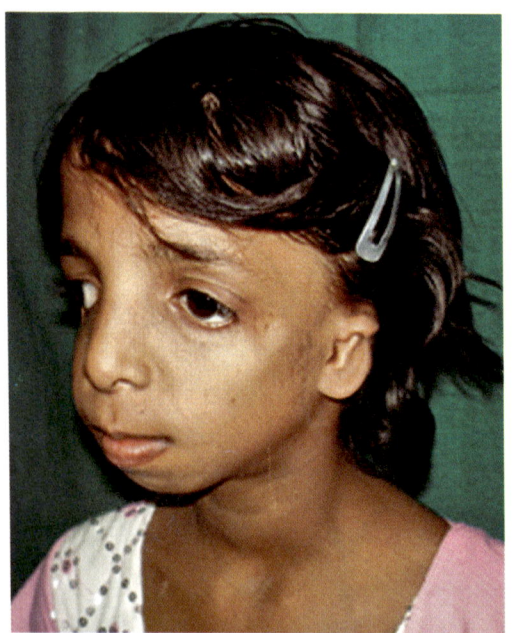

Figure 7.22 Treacher Collins syndrome. Note bilaterally symmetrical convex facial profile, prominent nose, antimongoloid slant of eyes, retrognathia, small and malformed rotated ears.

Treacher Collins syndrome (mandibulofacial dysostosis) Malar hypoplasia, antimongoloid slant of palpebral fissures, coloboma of lower eyelids, malformations of external ears, micrognathia and retrognathia (Figure 7.22).

Goldenhar syndrome Facial asymmetry, microtia (small, crumpled or complete absence of ears), preauricular skin tags, dermoid, lateral cleft-like extension of corner of the mouth, and cervical vertebral anomaly (Figure 7.23 A and B).

7. Syndromes with Facial and Limb Defects

Langer-Giedion syndrome (LGS) Prominent laterally protruding ears, large bulbous pear-shaped nose, sparse scalp hair, multiple bony exostoses, and cone-shaped epiphyses of phalanges. It is a rare autosomal genetic disorder.

Whistling face syndrome (Freeman-Sheldon syndrome) "Whistling face", small mouth with pursed lips, grooves over chin, contractures of small joints, and ulnar deviation of fingers.

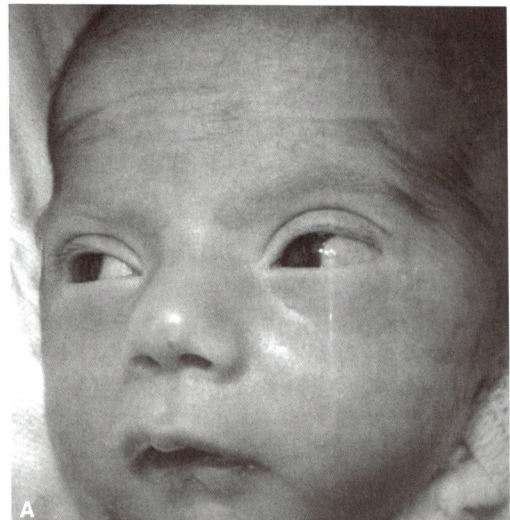

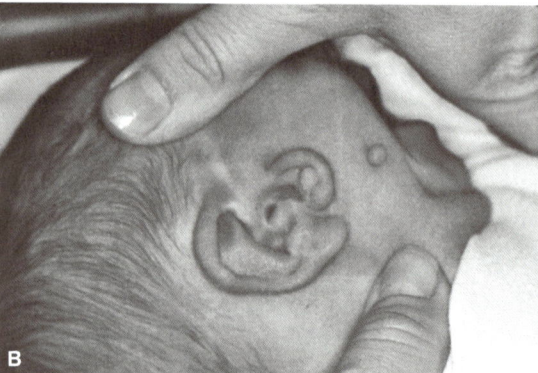

Figure 7.23A and B Goldenhar syndrome. (A) Facial asymmetry with lateral cleft-like extension of corners of the mouth. (B) Small, malformed ear with pre-auricular skin tag.

Coffin-Lowry syndrome Coarse facies, antimongoloid slant of palpebral fissures, bulbous nose, thick tapering fingers, drumstick appearance of distal phalanges, and severe mental retardation.

Coffin-Siris syndrome Coarse facies, sparse scalp hair, hypoplastic or absent fifth finger and toe nails, hypotonia, and mental retardation.

Pyknodysostosis Bossing of skull, large anterior fontanel, wide sutures, small mandible, parrot-like nose, blue sclerae, short-limbed dwarfism, osteopetrosis, dystrophic nails, widened drumstick appearance of fingers and toes, and increased tendency to fractures.

8. Syndromes with Limb Defects as a Major Feature

Poland syndrome Unilateral hypoplasia or absence of pactoralis major muscle with ipsilateral webbing of fingers or brachysyndactyly of hand and relatively shorter proximal segments of limbs (rhizomelic micromelia).

Escobar syndrome (multiple ptergyium syndrome) Ptosis, antimongoloid slant of pelpebral fissures, micrognathia, multiple pterygia or webbing of neck, axillae, antecubital, popliteal and intercrural areas, and rocker-bottom feet.

Holt-Oram syndrome (atrio-digital syndrome) Atrial septal defect with finger-like triphalangeal or absent thumb, complete or partial absence of radius and a number of associated anomalies. It is inherited as an autosomal dominant disorder.

Thrombocytopenia with absent radius syndrome (TAR syndrome) Thrombocytopenia with absence or hypoplasia of megakaryocytes in early infancy, bilateral absence or hypoplasia of radii (thumbs are usually present) and cardiac anomalies (ASD, tetralogy to Fallot).

Amniotic band disruption sequence Constriction rings or transverse amputation of digits or limbs, pseudosyndactyly of digits, unusual facial clefts not conforming to the usual anatomical embryonic planes of fusion (Figure 7.24).

9. Craniosynostoses Syndromes

Carpenter syndrome Brachycephaly, obesity, flat nasal bridge, lateral displacement of inner canthi, preaxial polydactyly of feet, partial syndactyly of hands and feet.

Apert syndrome Brachycephaly with high forehead (acrocephaly), midfacial hypoplasia, flat facies, antimongoloid slant of palpebral fissures, proptosis, syndactyly usually with complete fusion of 2nd, 3rd and 4th fingers (mitten hands), broad distal phalanx, thumb and hallux (Figure 7.25).

Crouzon syndrome Oxycephaly (pointed or conical vertex), maxillary hypoplasia, shallow orbits with ocular proptosis, strabismus, hypertelorism, and parrot-nose (Figure 7.26).

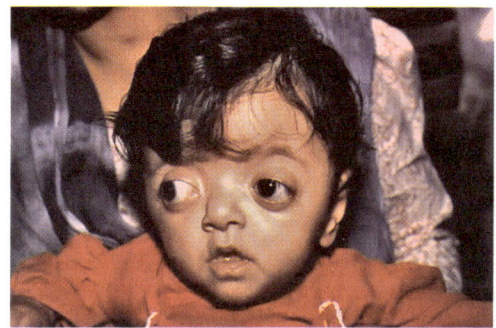

Figure 7.25 Apert syndrome. Proptosis, acrocephaly and midfacial hypoplasia. Infant also had mitten hands due to syndactyly.

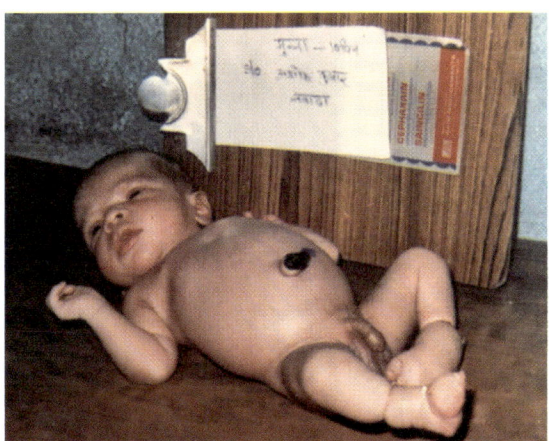

Figure 7.24 Constriction bands over the legs with pseudosyndactyly of toes.

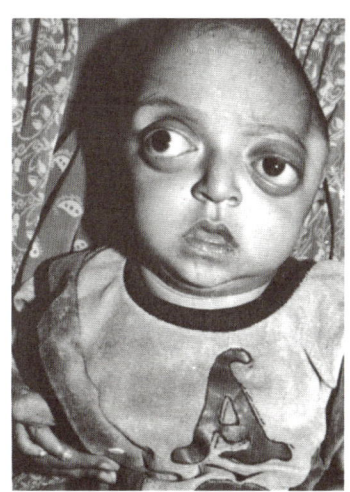

Figure 7.26 Crouzon syndrome. Note oxycephaly, ocular proptosis and maxillary hypoplasia.

10. Syndromes with Multiple Hamartomas

Sturge-Weber syndrome Phakomatoses with portwine hemangioma (nevus flammeus) involving facial area innervated by ophthalmic division of trigeminal nerve, ipsilateral meningeal hemangiomata with rail-track type of calcification, and ipsilateral choroid plexus hemangioma. Neurological manifestations include seizures, glaucoma, vascular headaches, hemiparesis and cognitive delay.

Incontinentia pigmenti (IP) It is a rare X-linked dominant genetic disorder which is characterized by irregular linear streaks and plaques of vesicles and verrucous patches which transform into pigmented skin lesions over trunk and extremities, alopecia, abnormal dentition, seizures, spasticity and mental retardation. The pigment is distributed in macular whorls, reticulated patches, flecks, splashes and linear streaks.

Tuberous sclerosis complex It is a multisystem genetic disorder with development of tubers or benign tumors in the skin and brain, and other vital organs like kidneys, heart, liver, eyes and lungs. Adenoma sebaceum on the face, ash-leaf macules, shagreen patches, retinal phakomas, pit-shaped defects in tooth enamel, phalangeal cysts, and renal angiomyolipomata. Neurological manifestations include seizures, low cognition, behavior and learning difficulties, pervasive development disorder, attention deficit hyperactivity disorder and obsessive compulsive disorder.

LEOPARD syndrome The mnemonic stands for **l**entigines, **e**lectrocardiographic conduction defects, **o**cular hypertelorism, **p**ulmonary stenosis, **a**bnormalities of genitalia, **r**etardation of growth and **d**eafness. It has features of Noonan syndrome with multiple lentigines.

Neurofibromatosis type 1 (Von Recklinghausen's disease) Multiple café au lait spots (>5 with a size of at least 5 mm), freckels in axillae and groins, multiple neurofibromata, and Lisch nodules (pigmented hamartomata of iris). Neurological features include seizures, learning disabilities, attention deficit, hyperactivity, autism spectrum disorder, speech difficulties, and macrocephaly. They are at an increased risk to develop hematologic malignancy.

Klippel-Trenaunay-Weber syndrome Asymmetric hypertrophy of a limb with phlebectasias and hemangiomata, port-wine stains, lymphangiomatous anomalies, syndactyly, polydactyly or macrodactyly, dislocated hips, kyphoscoliosis, and visceral hemangiomata.

Differential Diagnosis of Common Abnormal Physical Signs

FAILURE TO THRIVE

Most parents are worried about the growth of their children. Failure to thrive (FTT) is a common symptom for which children are brought for evaluation. It is defined as decelerated or arrested physical growth when height and weight measurements fall below the third or fifth percentile, or a downward trend in growth occurs across two major growth percentiles. It should not be confused with food fussiness of children of well-to-do parents when "*child is not eating or growing to the satisfaction of his parents.*" The diagnosis of FTT cannot be made on the basis of a single observation. It is characterized by failure to gain weight or weight loss is observed over a period of time. The diagnosis can be made reliably, if weight record of the child is maintained on a Road-to-Health card. In preterm babies, corrected age or post-conceptional age should be used for recording anthropometric measurements on Road-to-Health card during first one year of life. When growth curve runs along 25th percentile line without any downward trend, it indicates low genetic potential and not any disease process. The weight curve of the child with FTT shows a plateau or a downward trend so that it drops below two major percentile lines (Figure 8.1). The diagnosis of FTT can also be suspected, if the weight of the child is less than 3rd or 5th percentile on the WHO or National Center for Health Statistics (NCHS) weight-for-

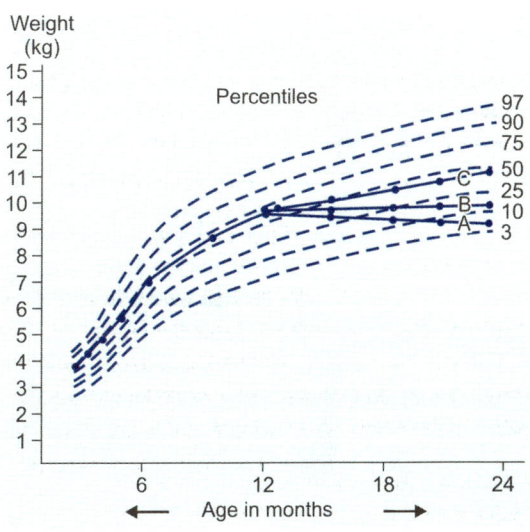

Figure 8.1 Failure to thrive. (A) Weight loss, (B) Slow weight gain, (C) Normal growth curve.

length/height charts. It is graded into mild, moderate and severe, when weight-for-age (% of median) is 75–90, 60–74 and <60%, respectively.

The child is diagnosed to be under weight when his weight is less than 2SD of the reference mean. Wasting is diagnosed when weight-for-height is less then 2SD of the reference mean value. A slowing in the rate of linear growth may take 6 months to manifest while slowing of weight gain or weight loss can be demonstrated during a short period of observation.

The size of the baby at birth depends upon the maternal health and adequacy of intrauterine environment rather than the genetic or constitutional factors. Children with poor genetic growth potential may grow normally during first 1–2 years of life. After the physiological adjustments, the child "finds his genetic growth curve" and then grows along a percentile line at a slow growth velocity (Figure 8.2). Some LBW infants with fetal developmental abnormalities (babies with symmetric IUGR) continue to follow the trend of intrauterine growth velocity after birth and grow as constitutionally light children (Figure 8.3). In these children, there is global retardation in all the growth parameters including body weight, head size and linear growth.

The causes of FTT may be psychosocial or organic. The majority of children with FTT in our country have nutritional or organic causes. The important causes of FTT are given in Table 8.1. The common psychosocial correlates of FTT include parental discord, lack of emotional support system, financial problems and substance abuse. There is history of irritability, sleep disturbances, excessive crying and temper tantrums. Infants with sensory deprivation are characterized by decreased vocalization, minimal smiling, abnormal posture,

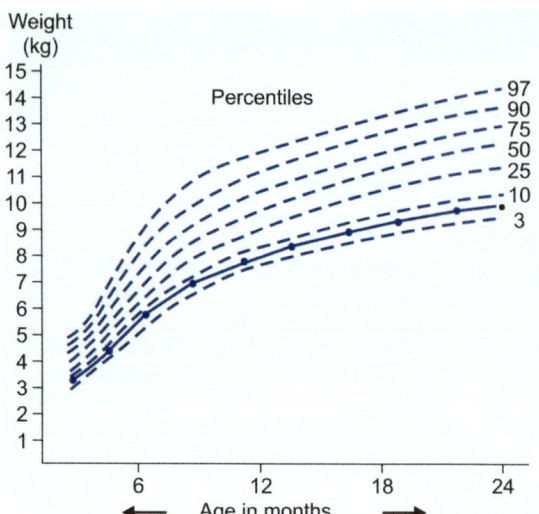

Figure 8.3 Low birth weight baby growing as a constitutionally slow growing child.

lack of cuddliness, head banging, rocking movements and rumination. In apparently healthy children, suboptimal physical growth and stunting may occur due to subclinical deficiencies of micronutrients (vitamins and trace minerals). Nutritional supplements containing micronutrients in these children can augment their growth by optimal expression of their genetic potential.

STUNTING OR SHORT STATURE

Stunting or short stature is diagnosed when height is less than –2SD or below 3rd percentile of mean height-for-age as per WHO growth reference standards. According to National Family Health Survey 2014–2015 (NFHS-4), about 37% under-5 children are stunted in India. *The prevalence of stunting should is taken as a poor social indicator for any nation just like the high infant mortality rate.* The height achieved at the age of 3 years is crucial because it is a good predictor of ultimate adult height. Dwarfism is diagnosed when height is less than –3SD below the mean height-for-age. Height velocity should be calculated over an observation period of 6 months. *In a school-going child, when height velocity is less than 5 cm per year, it indicates slow linear growth and a cause for concern.*

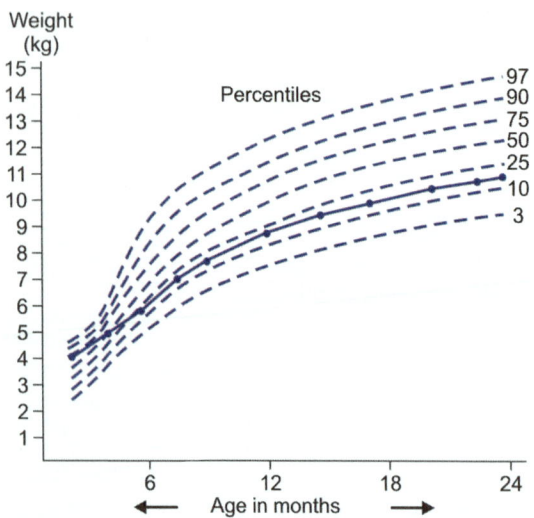

Figure 8.2 Normal neonate "finding his growth curve" during infancy.

A large number of conditions can adversely affect physical growth. Most conditions are associated with poor weight gain as well as subnormal linear growth. Nutritional disorders and systemic diseases are likely to have greater adverse effects on body weight than on linear growth and they are leading causes of failure to thrive. Stunting or dwarfism occurs more commonly due to endocrine disorders, skeletal dysplasias and dysmorphic syndromes because of chromosomal or genetic disorders (Table 8.2).

TABLE 8.1 Causes of failure to thrive

1. Psychosocial deprivation and child abuse

2. Prenatal events
Preterm and low birth weight babies (IUGR), intrauterine infections, fetal drug syndromes (alcohol, anticonvulsants), developmental defects, and congenital malformations

3. Faulty feeding practices
Failure of breastfeeding, excessive dilution of formula feeds, delayed and unsatisfactory weaning practices, and poor intake of micronutrients

4. Postnatal organic causes

Infections
Recurrent infections, tuberculosis, chronic malaria, kala-azar, and HIV infection

Gastrointestinal disorders
Recurrent or persistent diarrhea, celiac disease, protein losing enteropathy, inflammatory bowel disease, gastrointestinal allergy, giardiasis, gastroesophageal reflux, pyloric stenosis, aganglionic megacolon, worm infestations, and chronic liver dysfunction

Respiratory disorders
Bronchial asthma, recurrent chest infections, mucoviscidosis, tuberculosis, and bronchiectasis

Cardiovascular disorders
Congenital heart disease, acquired heart disease, and cardiac failure

Renal disorders
Recurrent urinary tract infections, renal tubular acidosis, and chronic renal dysfunction

Hepatic disorders
Chronic hepatitis, cirrhosis, and Wilson disease

Hemato-oncologic conditions
Nutritional anemia, beta thalassemia major, sickle cell anemia, and childhood malignancies

Neurologic disorders
Cerebral palsy, mental retardation, subdural hematoma, CNS tumors, diencephalic syndrome, and cranial irradiation

Immunologic conditions
Primary immune deficiency disorders, collagen vascular disorders and acquired immunodeficiency syndrome

Endocrine disorders
Diabetes mellitus, diabetes inspidus, cretinism hyperthyroidism, and pseudohypoparathyroidism

Genetic and chromosomal disorders

TABLE 8.2 Common causes of short stature

- **Psychosocial dwarfism** Parental discord, maternal depression or substance abuse, child neglect and abuse
- **Prenatal causes** Intrauterine growth restriction due to hypoplastic babies (developmental defects and intrauterine infections) and growth retarded babies with no catch up growth by 2 years of age
- **Nutritional dwarfism*** Faulty feeding practices and chronic systemic disorders, like celiac disease, mucoviscidosis, inflammatory bowel disease, chronic hepatic or renal disease, bronchial asthma, beta-thalassemia, and congenital heart disease
- **Endocrine disorders** Pituitary dwarf**, cretinism, diabetes mellitus, Prader-Willi syndrome, Cushing syndrome, corticosteroid therapy, and gonadal disorders (Turner syndrome, precocious puberty***)
- **Skeletal dysplasia** Achondroplasia, hypochondroplasia, short limb dwarfism, chondrodystrophies, osteogenesis imperfecta, diastrophic imperfecta, Ellis-van Creveld syndrome, X-linked hypophosphatemic rickets, vitamin D deficiency and vitamin D resistant rickets, and Pott's spine
- **Chromosomal and genetic disorders** Down syndrome, Turner syndrome, Noonan syndrome, and inborn errors of metabolism
- **Miscellaneous conditions** Familial short stature, constitutional delay in growth, and idiopathic short stature

* In nutritional disorders, body weight is more severely affected than height
** They have doll-like cherubic appearance with a single central maxillary incisor
*** In precocious sexual development, early linear growth is rapid with advanced bone age but ultimate adult stature is short due to early fusion of epiphyses

A detailed history should be taken to identify any psychosocial factors, faulty feeding practices and chronic systemic disorder. Anthropometric parameters should be recorded on a periodic basis on a Road-to-Health chart to identify the age of onset and severity of growth retardation. Height-for-age and height age (age calculated on the basis of actual height) should be recorded. The Target Height of the child should be recorded on the basis of mid-parental height as follows:

Boys: Father's height in cm + mother's height in cm divided by 2 + 6.5 cm

Girls: Father's height in cm + mother's height in cm divided by 2 – 6.5 cm

The child should be examined for any facial dysmorphism and skeletal dysplasia. Body proportions should be assessed to identify whether stunting is mainly affecting the trunk (hypogonadism, Turner syndrome, eunichoidism, chondrodystrophies, spinal deformities) or limbs (achondroplasia, short-limbed dwarfism, cretinism, sexual precocity, bowed legs). The distinctive clinical differences between constitutional growth delay (CGD) and familial short stature (FSS) should be identified (Table 8.3). Bone age should be checked by taking skiagram of left wrist and elbow in all children with stunting. Bone age may be retarded in children with hypopituitarism, hypothyroidism, Cushing syndrome, malnutrition, constitutional dwarfism with delayed adolescence, male hypogonadism and chronic systemic disease. *When bone age is less than the chronological age, it is possible to have catch-up linear growth.*

In constitutional growth delay, the onset of pubertal growth spurt is delayed but the ultimate adult height is normal. Sexual maturity rating should be assessed to diagnose sexual infantilism and precocious puberty because both can adversely affect the ultimate adult height. Precocious puberty is diagnosed in girls when breast development occurs before 8 years and menarche before 10 years of age. In boys, it is suspected when signs of puberty like facial hair and testicular enlargement occur before 9 years of age. Delayed puberty or sexual infantilism is suspected when there is no budding of breasts by 14 years or no menarche by 15 years in girls and absence of signs of puberty (facial hair and enlargement of testes) by 16 years in boys.

TABLE 8.3 Salient differences between constitutional growth delay and familial or genetic short stature

Feature	Constitutional growth delay	Familial or genetic short stature
Family history	Delayed puberty in one of the parents	One or both parents may have short stature
Sex	Mostly boys	Both sexes
Early growth	Growth is normal up to 1–2 years and then decelerates. The growth velocity remains slow without any spurt of growth during adolescence	Infant is normal at birth and after about one year the child identifies his genetic growth curve and grows slowly
Weight-for-height	Normal	Normal
Body proportions	Normal	Normal
Bone age	Retarded by 2 years against the chronological age but corresponds with the height age	Corresponds to the chronological age
Onset of puberty	Delayed*	Normal
Adult height	Normal	Short due to growth hormone receptor abnormality

*Puberty is considered as delayed in girls when there is no budding of breasts by 14 years or no menarche by 15 years and in boys with no signs of puberty by 16 years.

The term idiopathic short stature (ISS) is used to describe a child or adolescent with a height below −2SD of the mean height-for-age on the reference standard and in whom no cause has been identified on the basis of current diagnostic tools. Before assigning a label of ISS, it is important to exclude important causes of stunting, like celiac disease, Turner syndrome, hypopituitarism, cretinism, chronic inflammatory or systemic disease and renal tubular acidosis.

EXCESSIVELY TALL CHILD

As opposed to stunting, excessively tall stature is rare. It is suspected when height is more than +2SD (>97th percentile) of the mean height-for-age and the predicted adult height is >3SD above the mean, i.e. about 78 inches in males and 71 inches in females. Bone age should be checked and if it is less than the chronological age, there is greater likelihood of development of abnormally tall stature. The common conditions which are associated with excessively tall stature include familial or constitutional tall stature, exogenous obesity, Klinefelter syndrome (XXY), Marfan syndrome, fragile-X syndrome, precocious puberty, excess GH secretion, hyperthyroidism, and testicular feminization.

CYANOSIS

Cyanosis is characterized by bluish discoloration of skin and mucous membranes due to desaturation of arterial blood. It should be looked for in bright natural light. Cyanosis manifests clinically when level of deoxygenated hemoglobin exceeds 5 g/dL. Cyanosis is, therefore, unlikely to manifest in children with severe anemia. In contrast, infants with polycythemia become cyanosed at higher arterial oxygen tensions. Pulse oximetry is more reliable to assess oxygen saturation and cyanosis becomes evident only when arterial oxygen saturation (SaO_2) falls below 85%. The clinical manifestations of hypoxia include bradycardia, irritability, restlessness and excessive crying which is followed by lethargy and somnolence.

Cyanosis may be peripheral or central. *Peripheral cyanosis* occurs due to sluggish peripheral circulation as a consequence of exposure to cold, hypothermia, hypoglycemia, polycythemia, sepsis, shock and vasomotor changes. In peripheral cyanosis, bluish discoloration is limited to tip of the nose, nails and ear lobe. In newborn babies, peripheral or acrocyanosis usually manifests as circumoral grayness due to presence of prominent superficial venous plexuses in the region. In peripheral cyanosis, extremities are cold and arterial oxygen tension is normal but arterial oxygen saturation (SpO_2) as recorded by pulse oximetry is reduced.

Central cyanosis is characterized by blueness of mucous membranes, like lips, oral mucosa and tongue. When hypoxia or cyanosis is chronic, it is associated with elevation of hemoglobin and clubbing of nails of fingers and toes. In certain cardiac malformations, differential cyanosis may be seen. In coarctation of aorta with transposition of great arteries, hands and face may be blue while feet are pink. This can be reliably assessed by simultaneously recording SpO_2 on the right hand and left foot. On the other hand, in a patient with ductus arteriosus with reversal of shunt due to pulmonary hypertension or preductal coarctation of aorta, face and hands are pink while feet are blue. Cyanosis may occur because of cardiac, pulmonary, CNS, and metabolic conditions (Table 8.4).

The presence of cyanosis in the absence of respiratory difficulty is highly suggestive of cyanotic heart disease, methemoglobinemia, and polycythemia. The cyanosis due to right-to-left shunt becomes worse when the baby cries. The presence of severe respiratory difficulty with marked cyanosis is more common due to pulmonary rather than cardiac disorders. The respiratory cyanosis usually responds to oxygen administration or assisted ventilation.

In *hyperoxia test,* baseline ABG is checked preferably from the right radial artery when infant is receiving room air. The ABG is repeated after administration of 100% oxygen for 10 minutes. An arterial PaO_2 of <100 mmHg (failed hyperoxia test),

TABLE 8.4 Causes of central cyanosis
Cardiac causes
▪ *Cyanotic heart disease with decreased pulmonary blood flow.* Tetralogy of Fallot, tricuspid atresia, critical pulmonary stenosis or atresia, double outlet right ventricle with PS, and single ventricle with PS
▪ *Cyanotic heart disease with increased pulmonary blood flow.* Transposition of great arteries, and total anomalous pulmonary venous connection
▪ *Left ventricular outflow obstruction.* Severe aortic stenosis, hypoplastic left heart syndrome, and severe coarctation of aorta
▪ Persistent pulmonary hypertension of the newborn
▪ Acute cardiac failure due to any cause
Respiratory causes
▪ *Upper airway obstruction.* Congenital malformations, angioneurotic edema, epiglottitis, diphtheria, retropharyngeal abscess, foreign body, and macroglossia or glossoptosis
▪ *Respiratory failure.* Hyaline membrane disease, aspiration, congenital diaphragmatic hernia, pleural effusion, preumothorax, severe pneumonia, bronchiolitis, bronchial asthma, lobar collapse, cystic fibrosis, pulmonary hemorrhage, miliary tuberculosis, fibrosing alveolitis, interstitial pneumonitis, idiopathic pulmonary hemosiderosis, and pulmonary edema
CNS conditions
Cyanosis occurs due to apnea, hypoventilation or paralysis of respiratory muscles
Encephalitis, meningitis, status epilepticus, and intracranial hemorrhage
Paralysis of respiratory muscles: Paralytic poliomyelitis, Guillain-Barré syndrome, poisoning, and congenital myopathies
Metabolic causes
▪ Abnormal hemoglobins*, such as methemoglobinemia, sulfhemoglobinemia, and hemoglobin M
*The blood remains chocolate brown in color even when exposed to oxygen. Cyanosis cannot be corrected by oxygen administration

and/or rise in PaO_2 of less than 30 mmHg, in the absence of lung pathology, is virtually diagnostic of cyanotic CHD.

ANEMIA

Anemia or low hemoglobin is suspected on the basis of pallor of the skin (face, palms and soles), lower palpebral conjunctiva, dorsum of the tongue, lips, oral mucosa and nail bed. When anemia is severe (hemoglobin <5 g/dL), the pallor is marked and palmar creases become pale. You can compare the color of child's palm with yours, if you are not anemic! The skin of the face may appear pale in fair complexioned children and it should not be confused with pallor. Iron deficiency anemia may be associated with flat or spooning of nails (koilonychia) with longitudinal ridges but it is less common in children compared to adults. It is difficult to assess pallor in a severely jaundiced child. The extremities may become pale and cold in the absence of anemia in critically sick children with sepsis, shock, cardiac failure and generalized edema. The normal hemoglobin level varies widely in children with highest mean hemoglobin level of 16.5 g/dL at birth and the lowest level of 11.0 g/dL at 2 months of age due to physiological anemia. According to WHO, hemoglobin level below 11.0 g/dL in children between 6 months and 6 years and below 12 g/dL in older children is suggestive of anemia. The classification of anemia on the basis of associated clinical findings is shown in Table 8.5.

JAUNDICE

Jaundice manifests as yellowish discoloration of skin and mucous membranes because of accumulation of bilirubin in the blood. The jaundice should be looked for in natural daylight over the bulbar conjunctiva (yellow sclera), under surface of tongue, soft palate and skin especially over the face, palms and soles. Urine may be high colored and deep yellow when direct reacting or conjugated bilirubin is elevated. Anorexia is common when hepatic cellular dysfunction is present. The characteristic clinical features of jaundice due to various causes are listed in Table 8.6.

TABLE 8.5 Clinical classification of anemia

Anemia without any associated hematologic features
- Nutritional anemia (iron deficiency and megaloblastic)
- Thalassemia minor
- Celiac disease
- Red cell enzyme deficiencies
- Hypothyroidism
- Lead poisoning
- Chronic renal or hepatic disease
- Chronic blood loss
- Pure red cell aplasia

Anemia with petechiae but without any lymphadenopathy and hepatosplenomegaly
- Aplastic anemia
- Bleeding or coagulation disorder
- Immune thrombocytopenic purpura
- Disseminated intravascular coagulation

Anemia with hepatosplenomegaly but without any lymphadenopathy or petechiae
- *Hemolytic anemia*: Hemolytic disease of the newborn, G6PD deficiency, thalassemia major, sickle cell disease, hereditary spherocytosis, hemoglobinopathy, microangiopathic hemolytic anemia, burns, sepsis
- Chronic hepatitis with portal hypertension

Anemia with lymphadenopathy, hepatosplenomegaly and petechiae
- Leukemia
- Hodgkin's and non-Hodgkin's lymphoma
- Myeloproliferative disorders
- *Disseminated infections*: Infectious mononucleosis, miliary tuberculosis, and visceral leishmaniasis
- Neuroblastosis
- Storage disorders

EDEMA

Edema or swelling of subcutaneous tissues occurs due to accumulation of fluid in the interstitial spaces. Edema may occur due to fall in oncotic or osmotic pressure of plasma (fall in plasma protein especially albumin), rise in capillary hydrostatic pressure at the arteriolar end or passive venous congestion and capillary damage. Edema may be localized to certain parts of the body or generalized as manifested by puffiness, swelling of feet, legs and sacrum. Edema occurs more commonly over the periorbital region, scrotum, vulva, dorsum of hands and feet because of loose areolar tissue with reduced tissue tension. When edema is associated with collection of fluid in one or more serosal cavities, it is called generalized anasarca. Localized edema with signs of inflammation is a characteristic feature of infection or cellulitis. At times, edema may be limited to certain body organs, like airways (angioneurotic edema), brain, lungs or an isolated serosal cavity.

In newborn babies and infants, edema manifests as excessive weight gain, puffiness of face and swelling over the sacrum because they mostly lie in a supine position. Edema is assessed by looking for pitting after applying sustained pressure. It is best looked for over the medial malleolus, dorsum of feet and over the shins. A sustained pressure is applied with thumb or index finger for 5 seconds and the site is watched for visible or palpable depression. Edema due to accumulation of interstitial fluid pits on pressure and skin returns back to normal after some time. Abdominal wall edema is tested by pinching the skin and subcutaneous tissues with thumb and index finger or after sustained pressure with chest piece of stethoscope. Edema due to lymphatic obstruction feels firm and does not pit on pressure. It is associated with rough or coarse skin. The common causes of edema in children are listed in Table 8.7.

LYMPHADENOPATHY

Lymph nodes serve as protective sentinels to eliminate antigens or pathogens which are transported to them through the lymphatics. They are widely distributed throughout the body but are mostly concentrated over the neck, around the joints, axillae, groins, elbows (epitrochlear), knees, (popliteal), hilum of lungs, mesenteric and retroperitoneal sites. Lymph nodes (including tonsils and adenoids) are over reactive and readily enlarge in size in children to ward off infections through cell-mediated immune responses because young children lack specific humoral antibodies because of lack of previous exposure to pathogenic organisms.

TABLE 8.6 Clinical features of jaundice due to various causes

Characteristics	Hemolytic jaundice	Hepatocellular jaundice	Obstructive jaundice
Anorexia and nausea or vomiting	Absent	Common	May occur
Pain right hypochondrium	May occur when gallstones are present	Common	Very common
Fever	Uncommon	Common at onset	Hectic fever due to cholangitis at a later stage
Pruritus	Absent	May be present	Common with scratch marks on the skin
Anemia	Common	May occur during chronic stage	Absent
Skin color	Lemon yellow	Yellow	Greenish or orange yellow
Urine	Colorless when voided but may turn yellow on standing due to oxidation of urobilinogen to urobilin	Deep yellow	Mustard oil-colored
Stool	Yellow-colored	Usually yellow but may be clay-colored at some stage	White or clay-colored
Splenomegaly	Common	May be present	Occurs when portal hypertension supervenes
Hepatomegaly	Absent	Common in early stage but may disappear when cirrhosis supervenes	Invariable
Enlarged gallbladder	May be enlarged when gallstones are associated	Absent	May be palpable depending upon the cause and site of obstruction

Lymph nodes should be examined for their site, size, number, consistency, whether discrete or matted, free or attached to the underlying structures or overlying skin. Look for any softening with abscess or sinus formation and any evidences of acute inflammation, like pain, tenderness, redness and warmth. When lymph node enlargement is more than 1.0 cm (>1.5 cm in case of inguinal nodes) in size, it is considered as significant. In localized infections, regional group of lymph nodes are enlarged. When two or more lymph node groups are enlarged, it is designated as generalized lymphadenopathy. The common causes of lymphadenopathy are listed in Table 8.8.

DELAYED CLOSURE OF ANTERIOR FONTANEL

Anterior fontanel at birth varies in size between 2.0 ±1.0 cm and is slightly depressed relative to the frontal and parietal bones. It provides a useful acoustic window for imaging of brain by ultrasonography. The anterior fontanel normally closes between 10 and 18 months of age. Early closure of anterior fontanel should not be a cause for concern, if head growth is proceeding normally and there is no ridging of sutures. The presence of excessively large anterior fontanel and its delayed closure is a recognized clinical feature in several conditions listed in *Box 8.1*.

TABLE 8.7 Causes of edema

Newborn babies

Localized edema
- Edema on the presenting part
- Inflammatory edema
- Turner syndrome
- Milroy disease

Generalized edema
- Edema of prematurity
- Hydrops fetalis
  - Rh-isoimmunization
  - Non-immunologic causes
    - Severe anemia (homozygous alpha-thalassemia, twin-to-twin or fetomaternal hemorrhage, osteopetrosis)
    - Congenital malformations
    - Intrauterine infections
    - Miscellaneous conditions, like chorioangioma or hemangioendothelioma of placenta, arterio-venous anastomosis in the fetus or placenta, venous thromboses, fetal neuroblastosis, skeletal abnormalities

Older children

Hypoalbuminemia (decreased oncotic pressure)
- Protein-energy malnutrition, kwashiorkor
- Nephrotic syndrome
- Malabsorption syndrome
- Protein losing enteropathy
- Chronic hepatic and renal disease

Increased hydrostatic pressure
- Congestive heart failure
- Constrictive pericarditis
- Budd-Chiari syndrome
- Veno-occlusive disease
- Thrombophlebitis
- Superior vena caval obstruction
- Extrinsic pressure by a tumor mass

Sodium and water retention
- Congestive heart failure
- Acute glomerulonephritis
- Cirrhosis
- Chronic anemia
- Fluid and salt over load
- Corticosteroid therapy
- Premenstrual syndrome

Increased capillary permeability
- Allergic reaction: Urticaria, and angioneurotic edema
- Inflammatory reaction: Dengue fever, Rocky Mountain spotted fever

Lymphatic obstruction
- Turner syndrome
- Milroy disease
- Chylous ascites

TABLE 8.8 Common causes of lymphadenopathy

Infections

There may be regional lymph node enlargement or generalized lymphadenopathy

Bacterial: Non-specific cervical lymphadenitis due to oropharyngeal and scalp infections, tuberculosis (typical and atypical), BCG-adenitis, salmonella infection, brucellosis, tularemia, bubonic plague, cat-scratch disease, rat bite fever, *Yersinia enterocolitica*

Viral: Exanthematous illnesses (especially rubella), infectious mononucleosis, cytomegalovirus, and coxsackie virus

Fungal: Coccidioidomycosis, histoplasmosis, and candidemia

Spirochetal: Syphilis, leptospirosis, relapsing fever, and lyme disease

Parasitic: Toxoplasmosis, visceral leishmaniasis, and visceral larva migrans

Primary diseases of lymphoid or reticulo-endothelial tissues

There may be localized enlargement of lymph nodes or more commonly generalized lymphadenopathy with hepatosplenomegaly. The common conditions include leukemia, lymphosarcoma, Hodgkin disease, non-Hodgkin lymphoma, reticulum cell sarcoma, histiocytic lymphoma, Langerhans cell histiocytosis, non-endemic Burkitt lymphoma, rhabdomyosarcoma, neuroblastoma, carcinoma of the thyroid, and benign sinus histiocytosis

Immunologic or connective tissue disorders

Juvenile rheumatoid arthritis, systemic lupus erythematosus, serum sickness, and graft versus host disease (GVHD)

Immunodeficiency syndromes

Acquired immunodeficiency syndrome (AIDS), chronic granulomatous disease, combined immunodeficiency disorder, hyper-IGE syndrome, and hemophagocytic syndrome

Metabolic and storage disorders

Gaucher disease, Niemann-Pick disease, and cystinosis

Hematopoietic diseases

Thalassemia, sickle cell disease, and autoimmune hemolytic anemia

Miscellaneous disorders

Kawasaki disease (unilateral cervical lymph node enlargement), sarcoidosis, drug therapy with hydantoin and carbamazepine

> **Box 8.1 Causes of delayed closure of anterior fontanel**
>
> - Prematurity, intrauterine growth restriction and malnutrition
> - Hydrocephalus
> - Achondroplasia
> - Pituitary dwarf
> - Rickets
> - Apert syndrome
> - Cretinism
> - Trisomy 13 and 18
> - Down syndrome (trisomy-21)
> - Russell-Silver syndrome
> - Gorgoylism (mucopolysaccharidoses)
> - Hypophosphatasia
> - Congenital syphilis
> - Progeria
> - Thalassemia major
> - Hallermann-Streiff syndrome
> - Osteogenesis imperfecta
> - Pyknodysostosis
> - Cleidocranial dysostosis
> - Zellweger syndrome
> - Congenital rubella syndrome

> **Box 8.2 Causes of bulging of anterior fontanel**
>
> - Crying infant
> - Raised intracranial tension: Hydrocephalus, meningitis, encephalitis, subdural effusion, brain abscess, intracranial bleeding, shaken baby syndrome, tumor, sinus thrombosis, otitis media, and pseudotumor cerebri.
> - Hypoparathyroidism
> - Hypothyroidism
> - Congenital hypophosphatasia
> - Maple syrup urine disease
> - Urea cycle enzyme defects
> - Galactosemia
> - Tetracycline and fluoroquinolone therapy
> - Vitamin D-dependent rickets
> - Vitamin A poisoning
> - Nalidixic acid overdose
> - Corticosteroid therapy (following sudden cessation of prolonged therapy)
> - Lead poisoning
> - Roseola infantum

> **Box 8.3 Causes of craniotabes**
>
> - Rickets
> - Osteogenesis imperfecta
> - Marasmus
> - Lacunar skull and craniofenestria
> - Congenital syphilis
> - Hypervitaminosis A
> - Hydrocephalus
> - Thalassemia major
> - Mandibulofacial dysostosis (Treacher Collins syndrome)

BULGING OF ANTERIOR FONTANEL

The fontanel should be examined in a quiet child held in an upright position. The anterior fontanel is normally flat or slightly depressed relative to the frontal and parietal bones and is pulsatile. Bulging fontanel is a reliable sign of raised intracranial tension during infancy. The pulsations may disappear when fontanel becomes tense because of marked elevation of intracranial tension. The causes of bulging anterior fontanel are given in *Box 8.2*.

CRANIOTABES

Craniotabes refers to softened and parchment-like skull bones which can be indented like a ping-pong or table tennis ball. The cranial bones are soft, when pressure is applied they collapse and when the pressure is relieved, the bones snap back into place. The sign should be elicited away from the suture line. It is normally elicitable in preterm babies. The common causes of craniotabes are listed in *Box 8.3*.

BOSSING OF SKULL

The prominence of skull bones is called bossing. It may affect frontal, parietal or occipital bones though frontal bossing is most common. The important causes of bossing of skull are listed in *Box 8.4*.

HEAD NODDING OR BANGING

Nodding of head up and down or side-to-side and head banging or head rolling may be seen in some normal children. Nodding or bobbing of head is greater in the sitting than in the supine position. When head nodding is persistent or excessive, conditions listed in *Box 8.5* should be considered.

Box 8.4 Causes of bossing of skull

- Rickets
- Ectodermal dysplasia
- Thalassemia major
- Ehlers-Danlos syndrome
- Congenital syphilis
- Lowe's syndrome
- Achondroplasia
- Hallermann-Streiff syndrome
- Hurler syndrome (mucopolysaccharidoses)
- Generalized gangliosidosis type 1
- Crouzon syndrome
- Fragile X syndrome
- Pfeiffer syndrome
- Rubinstein–Taybi syndrome
- Russell-Silver syndrome
- Marfan syndrome
- Cleidocranial dysostosis
- 10 p deletion syndrome
- Pyknodysostosis

Box 8.5 Causes of head nodding

- Spasmus nutans (nystagmus, head bobbing and torticollis)
- Emotional deprivation
- Mental retardation
- Pelizaeus-Merzbacher disease (with poor head control and cog-wheel nystagmus)
- Ocular albinism
- Autism spectrum disorder
- Boredom and stress spectrum disorder
- Bobble-head doll syndrome (hydrocephalus due to lesion in the region of the third ventricle)

MACROCEPHALY

It is diagnosed when head circumference exceeds 2.5 cm of the mean-for-age or is above two standard deviations or above 97th centile of the mean-for-age, sex, height and weight of the child. The salient causes of large head are listed in *Box 8.6*. It may occur due to increase in the thickness of scalp, skull bones (cranial hyperostosis) and contents of the cranium (megaloencephaly and hydrocephalus).

Box 8.6 Causes of macrocephaly

- Familial macrocephaly (check head size of parents)
- Hydrocephalus. It is characterized by dilatation of ventricular system. The salient clinical features include large bulging anterior fontanel, separated sutures, bossing of frontal bones, engorged veins over the scalp and sun setting sign. Serial head circumference should be taken to identify whether it is progressive (active) or arrested hydrocephalus (Figure 8.4 A and B).
- Thick skull bones (achondroplasia, osteopetrosis, pyknodysostosis, craniometaphyseal dysplasia, oro-digito-facial dysostosis, rickets, osteogenesis imperfecta, hyperphosphatasia, leontiasis ossea).
- Cerebral gigantism (Sotos syndrome)
- Mucopolysaccharidoses
- Cerebral lipodosis (gangliosidosis)
- Metachromatic leukodystrophy
- Fragile X syndrome
- Porencephaly
- Subdural hematoma
- Hydrancephaly
- Dandy-Walker malformation
- Subdural effusion
- Intracranial tumor
- Sturge-Weber syndrome
- Neurofibromatosis type 1
- Tuberous sclerosis
- Weaver syndrome
- Glutaric aciduria type 1 (GA-1)
- Autism spectrum disorder
- Cowden disease
- Neurocardiofacial-cutaneous syndrome
- Intracranial hemorrhage

Hydrocephalus is caused by imbalance between CSF production and resorption that is of sufficient magnitude to result in net accumulation of fluid within the ventricular system. Non-communicating hydrocephalus may occur due to aqueductal stenosis, congenital malformation of the fourth ventricle, vascular malformation or a tumor. The causes of communicating hydrocephalus include intracranial hemorrhage, meningitis, cerebral venous or dural sinus thrombosis, and diffuse infiltration of the meninges by malignant cells.

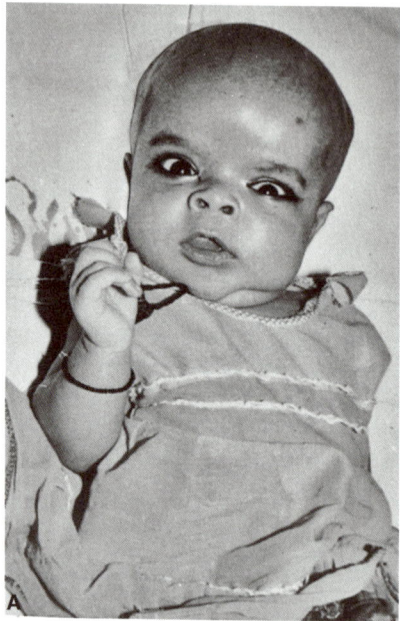

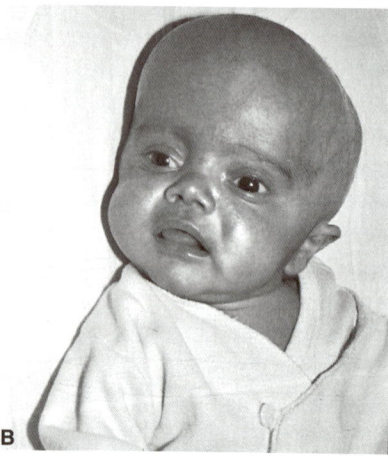

Figure 8.4A and B (A) Congenital hydrocephalus with marked frontal bossing. (B) Post-meningitic hydrocephalus.

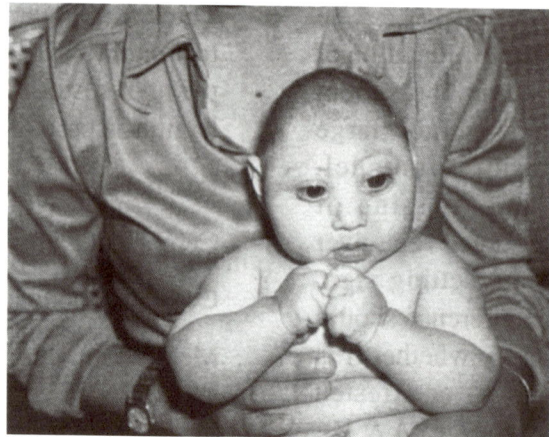

Figure 8.5 Primary familial microcephaly.

MICROCEPHALY

It is defined as head circumference below two standard deviations of the mean-for-age, sex, height and weight. It may be primary due to impaired growth of the brain or secondary because of premature fusion of sutures (Figure 8.5). It may be associated with seizures, mental subnormality and neuromotor disabilities. The common causes of microcephaly are listed in *Box 8.7*.

> **Box 8.7 Salient causes of microcephaly**
> - Familial primary microcephaly-5 (MCPH5)
> - X-linked microcephaly
> - Perinatal hypoxia and hypoglycemia
> - Low birth weight babies (premature and small-for-dates babies)
> - Cri-du-chat syndrome (5p-deletion)
> - Craniosynostosis (odd-shaped skull, prominence of sutures)
> - Trisomy-13, trisomy-18 and trisomy-21
> - Intrauterine infections (CMV, rubella, toxoplasmosis, syphilis, HIV, zika virus)
> - Cerebral dysgenesis
> - Cockayne's syndrome
> - Fetal alcohol, hydantoin, heroin or cocaine syndrome
> - Smith-Lemli-Opitz syndrome
> - Rothmund-Thomson syndrome
> - X-linked lissencephaly
> - Wolf-Hirschhorn syndrome (p-deletion)
> - Rett syndrome
> - Incontinentia pigmenti
> - 18 short-arm deletion (18p-) and long-arm deletion (18 q-) syndromes
> - Poland syndrome
> - Cornelia de Lange syndrome
> - Seckel syndrome
> - Holoprosencephaly
> - Inborn errors of metabolism
> - Radiation exposure

Differential Diagnosis of Common Abnormal Physical Signs

BLUE SCLERAE

The sclerae of infants and young children are usually grayish-blue in color and they become white as child grows. In infants, the sclera is thin so that underlying dark-colored structures are seen through the white of the eye. The conditions with distinctly blue sclerae are listed in *Box 8.8*.

Box 8.8 Causes of blue sclerae

- Physiological during early infancy
- Osteogenesis imperfecta
- Ehlers-Danlos syndrome
- Marfan syndrome
- Glaucoma
- Roberts syndrome
- Russell-Silver syndrome
- Marshall-Smith syndrome
- Hallermann-Streiff syndrome
- Pyknodysostoses
- Pseudoxanthoma elasticum
- Alkaptonuria
- High myopia

SUNSET EYE SIGN

The eyes are rolled downwards so that iris is completely covered by the lower eyelids and sclera is uncovered by the upper eyelids. It occurs due to involvement of center of upward gaze which is located in the pretectal area of brainstem. The sign is easily visible when infant is quickly lowered from sitting to supine position. The common causes of setting-sun sign are listed in *Box 8.9*.

Box 8.9 Causes of setting-sun sign of eyes

- Physiological. Transient and episodic "sun-setting" sign is common in preterm and some term infants
- Hydrocephalus (compression of brainstem due to dilatation of the third ventricle)
- Kernicterus
- Perinaud's syndrome (vertical gaze palsy)
- Laron dwarfism

HYPERTELORISM

Increased interpupillary distance between the two eyes is called hypertelorism (Figure 8.6). It occurs due to hypertrophy of the lesser wing of the sphenoid. In Waardenburg syndrome, the interpupillary distance is not increased but eyes look widely placed because both the inner canthi are displaced laterally. The important causes of hypertelorism are listed in *Box 8.10*.

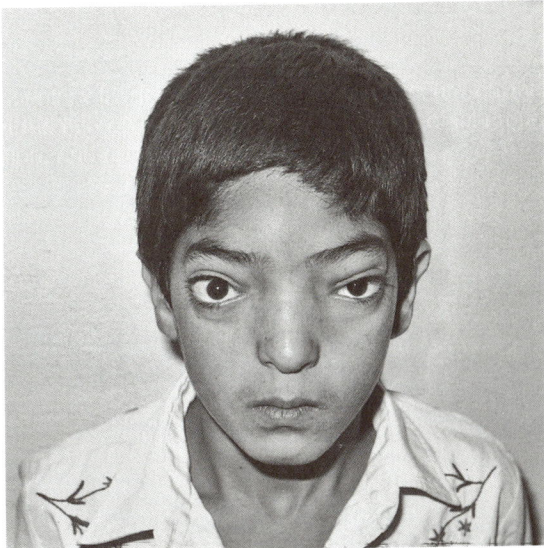

Figure 8.6 Hypertelorism with mongoloid slant of eyes.

Box 8.10 Causes of orbital hypertelorism

- Racial
- Cerebral gigantism (Sotos syndrome)
- Down syndrome
- Nevoid basal cell carcinoma
- Cretinism
- DiGeorge syndrome
- Chondrodystrophies
- Larsen syndrome
- Craniofacial dysostosis
- Multiple lentigines syndrome
- Thalassemia major
- Orofaciodigital dysostosis
- Ehlers-Danlos syndrome
- Apert syndrome

(contd.)

Box 8.10 Causes of orbital hypertelorism (contd.)

- Turner syndrome
- Coffin-Lowry syndrome
- LEOPARD* syndrome
- Waardenburg syndrome
- Crouzon disease
- Cri-du-chat syndrome
- Fetal hydrantoin syndrome
- Aarskog syndrome
- Whistling face syndrome
- Optiz syndrome
- Noonan syndrome
- Carpenter syndrome
- Rubinstein-Taybi syndrome
- 10q deletion syndrome

*Acronym for **L**entigenes, **E**lectrocardiographic conduction abnormalities, **O**cular hypertelorism, **P**rognathism and Pulmonary stenosis, **A**bnormalities of genitalia, **R**etardation of growth, **D**eafness

HYPOTELORISM

Decreased distance between the orbits is less common and is seen in conditions listed in *Box 8.11*.

Box 8.11 Causes of ocular hypotelorism

- Cyclops
- Fetal alcohol syndrome
- Metopic synostosis
- Patau syndrome (trisomy-13)
- Fragile-X syndrome
- Holoprosencephaly
- Ethmocephaly
- Cebocephaly
- Arrhinencephaly
- Prader-Willi syndrome
- Coffin-Siris syndrome
- Turner syndrome

PROPTOSIS

Proptosis or abnormal protrusion of eyeball(s) occurs due to a space occupying lesion in the orbit. It may be unilateral or bilateral. The term exophthalmos is used when proptosis occurs in association with Graves' disease. The sclera is visible above and below the cornea and lid lag is often present. Prominent eyes should not be confused with proptosis wherein the eyes bulge forwards. The severity of proptosis can be assessed with an exophthalmometer and CT scans of the orbits. The common causes of proptosis are listed in *Box 8.12*.

Box 8.12 Causes of proptosis

- Orbital cellulitis and abscess
- Retinoblastoma
- Thyrotoxicosis
- Anterior meningocele
- Hand-Schüller-Christian disease (Figure 8.7)
- Rhabdomyosarcoma (Figure 8.8)
- Optic glioma
- Orbital cellulitis and abscess
- Chloroma (acute myeloid leukemia)
- Crouzon disease
- Langerhans cell histiocytosis
- Polyostotic fibrous dysplasia
- Cavernous hemangioma or lymphangioma
- AV aneurysm
- Dermoid cyst
- Apert syndrome
- Cavernous sinus thrombosis
- Retro-orbital hemorrhage
- Basal skull fracture
- Pyknodysostosis
- Neuroblastoma
- Sickle cell disease
- Neurofibromatosis
- Visceral larva migrans
- Wegener's granulomatosis

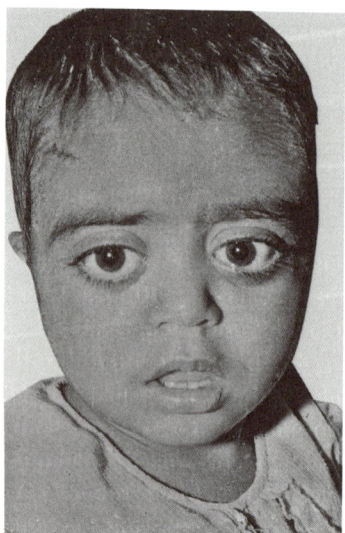

Figure 8.7 Hand-Schüller-Christian disease. Prominent eyes, seborrhea capitis, hepatosplenomegaly with diabetes insipidus.

Differential Diagnosis of Common Abnormal Physical Signs

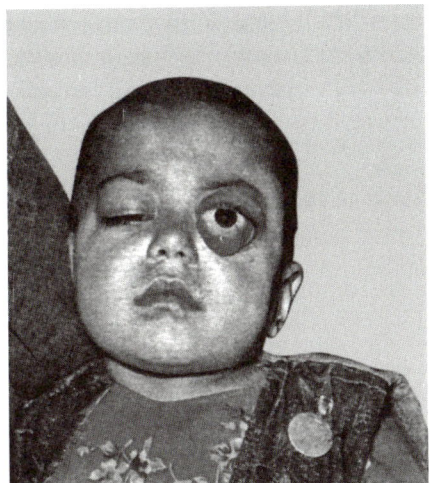

Figure 8.8 Proptosis of left eye due to rhabdomyosarcoma.

PTOSIS

Ptosis or drooping of upper eyelid may be congenital or acquired, unilateral or bilateral drooping of both eyelids. It may be present at birth or occur later in life. If congenital ptosis is not treated, it can lead to amblyopia (lazy eye). Rarely neurogenic ptosis may be associated with jaw-winking phenomenon, i.e. the droopy lid "flicks" open when child sucks on bottle or chews food. The common conditions which are associated with ptosis are listed in *Box 8.13*.

Box 8.13 Causes of ptosis

- Congenital unilateral/bilateral ptosis
- Aarskog syndrome
- Turner syndrome
- Oculomotor palsy (ptosis with mydriasis)
- Moebius syndrome
- Horner syndrome (ptosis, enophthalmos, miosis and lack of sweating)
- Intracranial tumor or hemorrhage
- Noonan syndrome
- Fetal alcohol syndrome
- Myasthenia gravis
- Whistling face syndrome
- Botulism
- Myotonic dystrophy
- Sticky eyes

CATARACT

The opacities in the lens are best seen through the +10 diopter lens of an ophthalmoscope at a distance of 10 inches from patient's eyes. The red reflex of the eye is replaced by white opacity. Cataract may be congenital or acquired, unilateral or bilateral, central or complete. If treatment is delayed beyond 2 months, the child develops "lazy" eye or ambylopia which leads to development of nystagmus, strabismus and inability to fix the gaze. A number of developmental disorders, genetic and chromosomal diseases and infections may be associated with cataracts *(Box 8.14)*.

Box 8.14 Causes of cataract

- Familial or idiopathic (developmental)
- Trauma to the eye
- Homocystinuria
- Rubella syndrome (Figure 8.9)
- Rothmund-Thomson syndrome
- Galactosemia
- Cortisone therapy
- Marfan syndrome
- Osteopetrosis
- Iridocyclitis
- Zellweger syndrome
- Conradi's disease
- Lowe's syndrome
- Ectodermal dysplasia syndrome
- Fabry disease
- Hallermann-Streiff syndrome
- Hypoparathyroidism
- Incontinentia pigmenti
- Progeria
- Refsum syndrome
- Alport syndrome
- Mannosidosis
- Intrauterine infections (toxoplasmosis, CMV, rubella, varicella, syphilis, herpes simplex)
- Mandibulofacial dysostoses
- Cockayne syndrome
- Trisomy 13, 18, and 21
- Smith-Lemli-Opitz syndrome
- Diabetes mellitus
- Turner syndrome
- Wilson disease

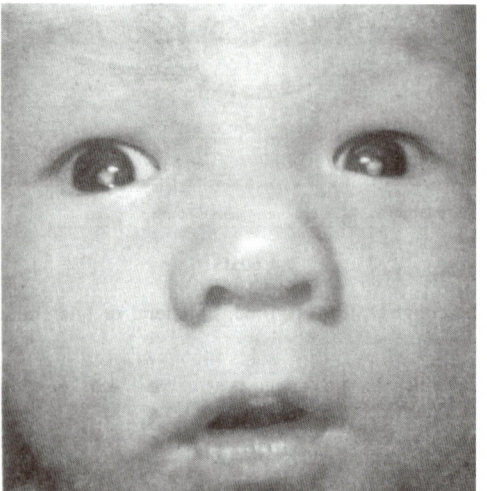

Figure 8.9 Cataract of both eyes due to congenital rubella syndrome.

WHITE REFLEX IN THE EYE (Cat's Eye)

When you shine a light through the pupil or look at the pupil through an ophthalmoscope, normally a red flare is seen. Absence of red reflex is a recognized feature of several conditions which demand urgent attention. The common causes of "white pupil" or leukocoria are shown in *Box 8.15*.

> **Box 8.15 Causes of white reflex**
> - Cataract
> - Retinoblastoma
> - Retrolental fibroplasia or retinopathy of prematurity
> - Pupillary membrane or persistent central hyaloid artery
> - Vitreous opacity
> - Eosinophilic granuloma (visceral larva migrans or toxocariasis)
> - Retinal detachment
> - Coats' disease
> - Choroidoretinal coloboma
> - Melanoma of ciliary body

DEPRESSED NASAL BRIDGE (Saddle Nose)

During vaginal delivery, most babies are born with a flat or misshapen nose which gets corrected within a few days. Flat nose is common in certain ethnic and racial groups. Depressed or flat nose may be associated with hypertelorism. The salient causes of flat nasal bridge are listed in *Box 8.16*.

> **Box 8.16 Causes of depressed nasal bridge**
> - Racial and ethnic feature
> - Osteopetrosis
> - Down syndrome
> - Cleidocranial dysostosis
> - Cretinism
> - Ectodermal dysplasia
> - Thalassemia major
> - Conradi syndrome
> - Congenital syphilis
> - Williams syndrome
> - Hurler syndrome
> - Smith-Lemli-Opitz syndrome
> - Chondrodystrophies
> - Fetal alcohol or hydantoin syndrome
> - Larson syndrome

SLANTING OF EYES

The face is normally symmetrical and both the eyes and palpebral fissures are aligned horizontally. A number of developmental defects and chromosomal disorders are associated with upward (mongoloid) or downward (antimongoloid) slanting of both the eyes (*Boxes 8.17 and 8.18*).

> **Box 8.17 Conditions with upward slanting of eyes (mongoloid slant)**
> - Racial
> - Down syndrome
> - Prader-Willi syndrome
> - Leri's pleonosteosis
> - Anhidrotic ectodermal dysplasia
> - Aarskog syndrome
> - Zellweger syndrome
> - 4p- 5p-syndrome
> - Conradi syndrome
> - Klinefelter syndrome
> - Hereditary spherocytosis

Box 8.18 Conditions with downward slanting of eyes (anti-mongoloid slant)

- Mandibulofacial dysostosis
- Whistling face syndrome
- Turner syndrome
- Alagille-Watson syndrome
- Trisomy 17 and 18
- Alport syndrome
- Cri-du-chat syndrome (5p-syndrome)
- Smith-Lemli-Opitz syndrome
- Apert syndrome
- Noonan syndrome
- Treacher Collins syndrome
- 10p depletion syndrome
- Weaver syndrome
- Sotos syndrome
- Launois-Bensaude syndrome

EPICANTHIC FOLDS

The folds of skin that project from the upper eyelids over the medial canthi of eyes are called epicanthic folds. They may be normally seen in some neonates during first 2 months of life *(Box 8.19)*.

Box 8.19 Common cause of epicanthic folds

- Racial or ethnic feature
- Down syndrome
- Turner syndrome
- Noonan syndrome
- Cri-du-chat syndrome (5p minus)
- Cornelia de Lange syndrome (CdLS)
- Smith-Lemli-Opitz syndrome

PUFFINESS OF EYELIDS AND PERIORBITAL TISSUES

Mild puffiness with dark circles under the eyes may be seen in children with recurrent respiratory infections, nasal allergy, chronic sinusitis or as a family trait. The important causes of puffiness are listed in *Box 8.20*.

ABNORMALITIES OF PHILTRUM

The midline depressed area or vertical groove between columella nasi (lower margin of nasal

Box 8.20 Causes of facial puffiness

- Familial
- Excessive crying
- Allergic rhinitis
- Chronic sinusitis
- Orbital trauma and cellulitis
- Conjunctivitis
- Mediastinal obstruction
- Insect bites
- Hypothyroidism (myxedema)
- Spasmodic cough
- Hypoproteinemia (nephritis, nephrotic syndrome, anemia, kwashiorkor, etc.)
- Ethmoid sinusitis
- Cavernous sinus thrombosis
- Angioneurotic edema or drug reaction (Figure 8.10)
- Chronic cor pulmonale
- Congestive heart failure
- Constrictive pericarditis
- Dermatomyositis (heliotrope color)
- Sickle cell veno-occlusive crisis

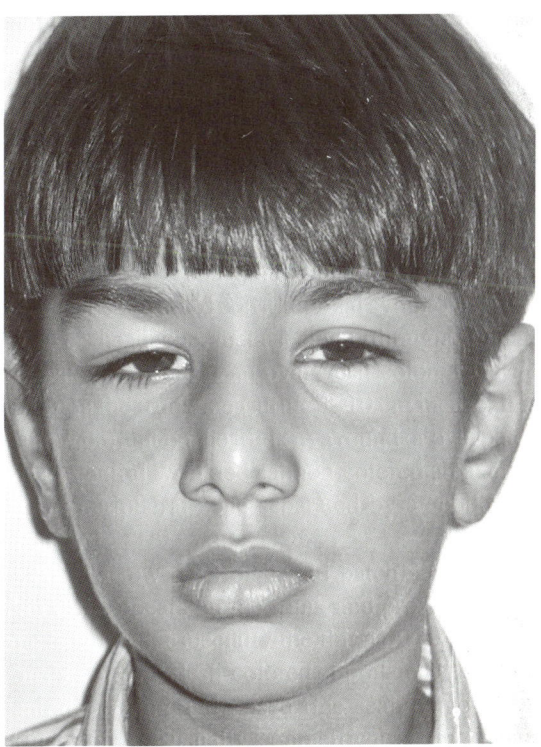

Figure 8.10 Puffiness and development of urticaria after intake of nimesulide.

septum) and the upper lip is called philtrum. Philtrum may be abnormally long in several developmental disorders listed in *Box 8.21*.

The philtrum may be abnormally short in children with DiGeorge syndrome, (CATCH-22 syndrome, 18q deletion syndrome), Martsolf syndrome and oral-facial-digital syndrome. The philtrum may be flat or smooth in children with fetal alcohol syndrome and Prader-Willi syndrome. The vertical groove in the philtrum is rather broad in children with autism spectrum disorder.

Box 8.21 Causes of long philtrum
▪ Hurler syndrome
▪ Robinow syndrome
▪ Fetal alcohol syndrome
▪ Facial femoral syndrome
▪ Fetal hydantoin and valproic acid syndrome (Figure 8.11)
▪ Aarskog syndrome
▪ Gangliosidosis
▪ Smith-Lemli-Opitz syndrome
▪ Wagler-Stickler syndrome
▪ Williams syndrome
▪ Weaver syndrome
▪ Ectodermal dysplasia
▪ Arthrogryposis multiplex congenita
▪ Coffin-Siris syndrome
▪ Cornelia de Lange syndrome

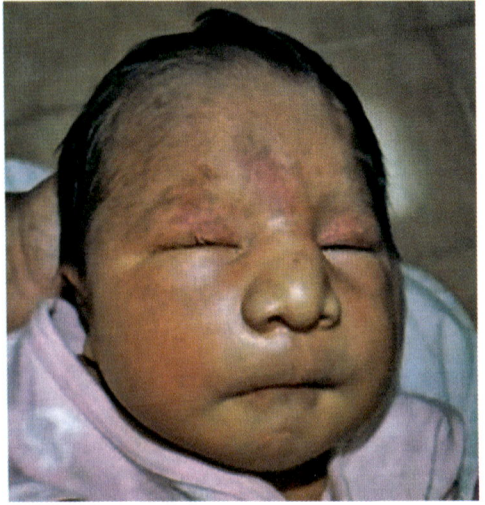

Figure 8.11 Note long philtrum and thin upper lip in an infant with fetal hydantoin syndrome.

LOW-SET EARS

The upper and lower borders of the pinna normally correspond to the level of eyebrows and base of the alae nasi, respectively. The horizontal interpalpebral line, when projected posteriorily, should bisect the ears into upper one-third and lower two-thirds. If the line passes above the ears or helix, it is suggestive of low-set ears. The common causes of low set ears are listed in *Box 8.22*. All newborns with external ear anomalies should be assessed for renal malformations and deafness.

Box 8.22 Causes of low-set ears
▪ Down syndrome
▪ Smith-Lemli-Opitz syndrome
▪ Renal agenesis (Potter facies)
▪ Treacher Collins syndrome
▪ Gargoylism
▪ Cri-du-chat syndrome
▪ Turner syndrome
▪ DiGeorge syndrome
▪ Noonan syndrome
▪ Edwards syndrome
▪ Patau syndrome
▪ Carpenter syndrome
▪ Trisomy 17–18, 13–15
▪ Apert syndrome
▪ Idiopathic hypercalcemia

MICROGNATHIA (Hypoplasia of Mandible)

Small chin giving an appearance of "bird facies" is a recognized feature of a number of developmental conditions and may be associated with posterior displacement of jaw or retrognathia. It may be associated with feeding and breathing difficulties. The salient causes of micrognathia are listed in *Box 8.23*.

HIGH-ARCHED PALATE

The hard palate is usually flat or slightly arched. The palate becomes dome-shaped or high-arched in children with mouth breathing, prolonged ventilation following orotracheal intubation and after surgical repair of cleft palate. Other causes of high-arched palate include Down syndrome,

> **Box 8.23 Causes of micrognathia**
>
> - Pierre-Robin syndrome (micrognathia, retrognathia, cleft palate and glossoptosis)
> - Treacher Collins syndrome
> - Cerebrocostomandibular syndrome (micrognathia, cleft palate, glossoptosis, multiple posterior rib gaps and cerebral maldevelopment)
> - Pyknodysostosis
> - Hallermann-Streiff syndrome
> - Cri-du-chat syndrome
> - Marfan syndrome
> - Seckel syndrome
> - Progeria
> - Turner syndrome
> - Arteriohepatic dysplasia (Alagille's syndrome)
> - Fetal alcohol syndrome
> - DiGeorge syndrome
> - Russell-Silver syndrome
> - Rubinstein-Taybi syndrome
> - Schwartz-Jampel syndrome
> - Smith-Lemli-Opitz syndrome
> - Wagner-Stickler syndrome
> - Trisomy 13 and 18
> - Weaver syndrome
> - Warkany syndrome
> - Juvenile rheumatoid arthritis

Marfan syndrome, Ehlers-Danlos syndrome, fragile-X syndrome, Friedreich ataxia, craniosynostosis and crowding of molars. It is usually asymptomatic but may cause difficulty in feeding, clarity of speech and obstructive sleep apnea.

BIG TONGUE (Macroglossia)

The tongue may be large and protrude out of the mouth in several conditions. The child with a long tongue may be able to protrude his tongue up to the chin or tip of the nose. The condition may be congenital or acquired. Rhythmic protrusion and retrusion of tongue (which is normal in size) is a feature of intracranial hemorrhage and cerebral edema in newborn babies, athetosis and Sydenham chorea. The common causes of macroglossia are listed in *Box 8.24*. It may be associated with difficulties in feeding, swallowing, speaking and sleeping (obstructive sleep apnea). In contrast, the

> **Box 8.24 Causes of macroglossia**
>
> - Cretinisim
> - Beckwith-Wiedemann syndrome
> - Down syndrome (tongue is normal but oral cavity is small)
> - Primary amyloidosis
> - Glycogen storage disease type 2 (Pompe disease)
> - Puppet-like syndrome of Angelman
> - New growth of tongue (lymphangioma, hemangioma, neurofibromatosis, rhabdomyoma)
> - Hurler syndrome
> - Klippel-Trenaunay-Weber syndrome
> - Lingual thyroid
> - Duchenne muscular dystrophy
> - Generalized gangliosidosis
> - Sandhoff disease

tongue may be small and atrophic (microglossia) in children with hypoglossal nerve palsy, multiple cranial nerve palsies (Moebius syndrome) and Werdnig-Hoffman disease.

GUM HYPERPLASIA

Hyperplasia of gums is most commonly due to poor orodental hygiene, mouth breathing and phenytoin therapy. It is more common in male children and adolescents. The common causes are listed in *Box 8.25*.

> **Box 8.25 Causes of hyperplasia of gums**
>
> - Poor oral hygiene (gingivitis)
> - Drug induced: Phenytoin, cyclosporin and calcium channel antagonists (nifedipine, amlodipine)
> - Xanthomatosis
> - Epulis
> - Hereditary gingival fibromatosis (HGF)
> - Neurofibromatosis 1 (von Recklinghausen's disease)
> - Scurvy
> - Diffuse fibromatosis
> - Acute myeloid leukemia
> - Hodgkin's lymphoma
> - Histiocytosis X
> - Hurler syndrome
> - Granulomatous diseases
> - Sweet's syndrome
> - Schinzel-Giedion syndrome

THRUSH

Oral thrush is caused by *Candida albicans*. It is characterized by white raised membranous patches that resemble milk curds and are located on the tongue, buccal mucosa, gums, lips and pharynx. The patches cannot be removed easily and when scraped, they leave behind mucosal lesions with oozing of blood. Except during newborn period, thrush does not occur in healthy individuals. Neonates may develop thrush, if mother is having vaginal candidiasis or candidal infection of the breast nipples or when infant is bottle fed. Prolonged use of broad-spectrum antibiotics may be associated with oral thrush. Recurrent or chronic oral and pharyngeal candidiasis is a recognized feature of acquired immunodeficiency syndrome (AIDS), severe combined immunodeficiency, T cell disorder, DiGeorge syndrome, biotinidase deficiency and autoimmune polyendocrine syndrome.

DELAYED DENTITION

Eruption of primary dentition usually starts around 6 to 8 months of age. In 1 in 200 births, a neonate may be born with one or two teeth. They may occur as an isolated anomaly or may be associated with cleft palate, Ellis-van Creveld syndrome, Hallermann-Streiff syndrome and pachyonychia congenita. The dentition may be delayed up to one year due to hereditary or constitutional factors. Dentition is considered as delayed, if there is no eruption of teeth by first birthday. Apart from constitutional delay (history of delayed dentition in siblings and parents), common causes of delayed dentition include nutritional or systemic disorders, chromosomal and genetic disorders associated with orofacial dysmorphism. The common causes of delayed dentition are listed in *Box 8.26*. The child should be evaluated by a dentist, if there is no primary dentition by 18 months or when secondary dentition is delayed beyond 8 years.

BROWNISH DISCOLORATION OF TEETH

Brownish discoloration of teeth may occur due to amelogenesis imperfecta because of malfunctioning

---

Box 8.26 Causes of delayed dentition

- Constitutional or hereditary delay
- Protein-energy malnutrition
- Chronic systemic disorder
- Rickets
- Down syndrome
- Endocrinal disorders like congenital hypothyroidism, hypopituitarism and hypoparathyroidism
- Amelogenesis imperfecta
- Apert syndrome
- Chondroectodermal dysplasia
- Osteogenesis imperfecta type 1
- Cleidocranial dysostosis
- Mucopolysaccharidosis
- Incontinentia pigmenti
- Progeria

---

of ameloblasts with poor formation of enamel or due to staining of teeth by drugs and endogenous metabolites (*Box 8.27*). Greenish-yellow staining of teeth may occur due to elevation of direct or conjugated bilirubin which is water-soluble.

Box 8.27 Causes of discolored teeth

- Poor orodental hygiene
- Iron medication
- Caries and fluorosis
- Erythrodontia (porphyria erythropoietica)
- Kernicterus
- Metabolic disorders like tyrosinemia and alpha 1-antitrypsin deficiency
- X-linked dominant hypophosphatemic rickets
- Tetracycline therapy
- Osteogenesis imperfecta

COSTOCHONDRAL BEADING

The common causes of costochondral beading include rickets, scurvy and chondrodystrophy. The beading is broad and dome-shaped in rickets while it is sharp like a bayonet because of posterior subluxation of sternum in cases of scurvy.

CLUBBING

Hippocrates was probably the first to document clubbing as a sign of disease. The exact mechanism of clubbing is unclear and is probably caused by hypervascularity and opening up of anastomotic channels in the nail bed. It appears to be due to production of a humoral substances which cause dilatation of blood vessels of the fingertips and endothelial proliferation. The clubbing can appear after about 6 weeks of the appearance of a predisposing factor. There are five clinical stages of clubbing.

Grade 1. Softening of nail bed with increased fluctuations.

Grade 2. Increase in the normal 160° angle between the nail bed and skinfold (Schamroth's window is obliterated).

Grade 3. Increased curvature and thickening of the nail producing parrot-beak appearance.

Grade 4. Drumstick appearance because of thickening of whole distal phalanx (Figure 8.12).

Grade 5. Hypertrophic osteoarthropathy. There is shiny or glossy change in the nails and adjacent skin with longitudinal striations. There may be thickening of periosteum and synovium of joints. It is commonly associated with lung cancer.

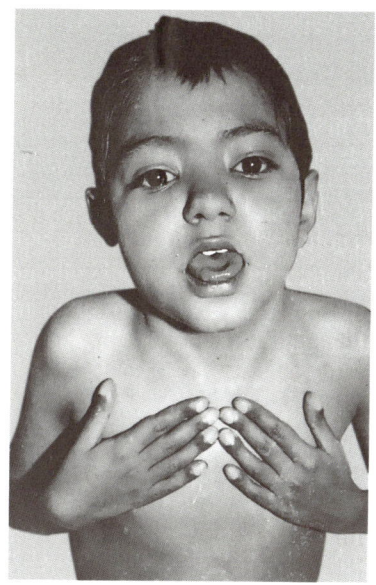

Figure 8.12 Clubbing in a child with tetralogy of Fallot.

Schamroth sign When dorsal surfaces of terminal phalanges of corresponding fingers are apposed, there is a diamond-shaped space at the base of nail bed. In clubbing, the diamond-shaped space is lost (Figure 8.13A and B).

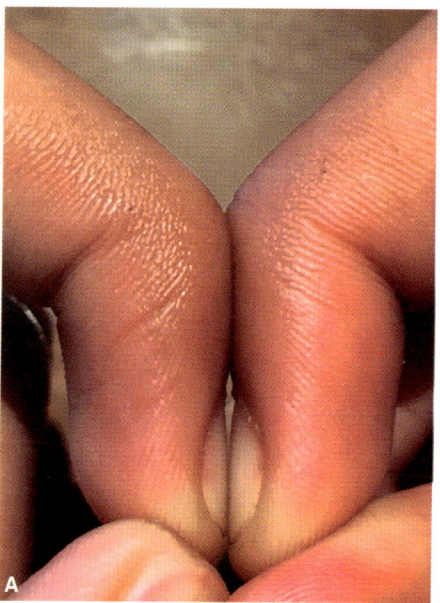
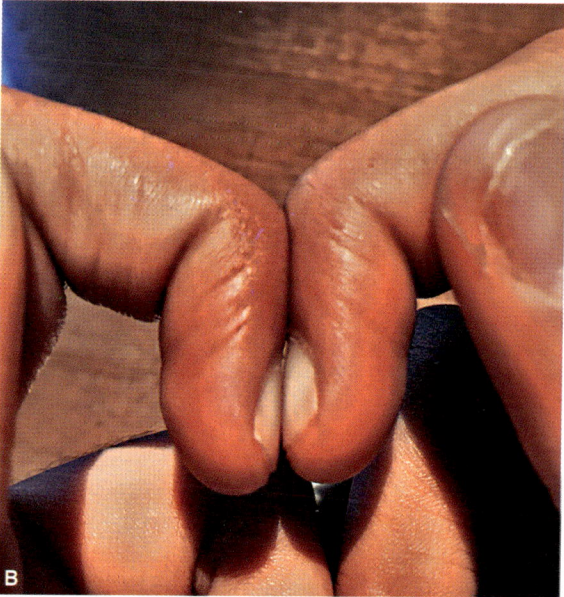

Figure 8.13A and B Schamroth sign: (A) The diamond-shaped space is seen normally at the base of nail beds when terminal phalanges of corresponding fingers are apposed. (B) The diamond-shaped space is lost in the presence of clubbing.

Examine the profile view of the distal phalanges. When clubbing is present, the vertical height at the base of nail will be greater than the height of distal interphalangeal joint. The angle between nail bed and adjacent skin or proximal nail fold (Lovibond angle) is normally less than 165°. In clubbing of the fingers, the Lovibond's angle is greater than 180°.

Clubbing occurs in association with a number of cardiopulmonary and abdominal conditions. The important causes of clubbing are listed in *Box 8.28*. Clubbing in association with pain over the wrists and ankles because of subperiosteal bone formation over distal diaphyses of the radius, ulna, tibia and fibula is called hypertrophic osteoarthropathy. It may occur due to mesothelioma, bronchiectasis and cirrhosis of liver.

Box 8.28 Causes of clubbing

- Familial or congenital
- Cyanotic heart disease (drumstick clubbing)
- Pulmonary suppuration (bronchiectasis, lung abscess, empyema, cystic fibrosis, lymphoid interstitial pneumonitis)
- Malabsorption syndrome
- Ulcerative colitis
- Polyposis of the colon
- Fibrocaseous pulmonary tuberculosis (parrot-beak type clubbing)
- Regional enteritis or Crohn's disease
- Subacute bacterial endocarditis
- Cirrhosis of liver
- Interstial lung disease
- Lung cancer
- Mesothelioma of pleura

Clubbing should be looked for in finger nails because toe nails may become curved due to tight shoes.

TRISMUS (Lockjaw)

There is inability or reduced ability to open the mouth. It may interfere with eating, speaking and maintaining proper oral hygiene. The condition is usually painful and may be associated with altered facial appearance. The common conditions causing lockjaw are listed in *Box 8.29*.

Box 8.29 Causes of lockjaw

- Tetanus
- Ankylosis of temporomandibular joint
- Syndrome of brainstem dysfunction
- Tumor of the jaw (rhabdomyosarcoma)
- Arthritis of temporomandibular joint
- Dislocation of temporomandibular joint
- Encephalitis
- Primary hypoparathyroidism (DiGeorge syndrome)
- Nasopharyngeal carcinoma
- Brain tumor
- Acute post-streptococcal polymyalgia
- Peritonsillar abscess
- Impacted third molar (pericoronitis)
- Odontogenic infection
- Acute parotitis
- Tetany
- Radiation fibrosis
- Teeth grinding
- Trauma to the jaw
- Strychnine poisoning
- Anesthetic-induced malignant hyperthermia
- Phenothiazines, metoclopramide, succinylcholine and tricyclic antidepressant toxicity
- Infantile Gaucher's disease
- Maple syrup urine disease
- Stress and hysteria

SHORT NECK

Webbing of neck (pterygium colli) gives an appearance of short neck due to presence of thick web of skin that extends from behind the ears to the outer end of the clavicles and the acromial process. A number of conditions are associated with short neck (*Box 8.30*).

NECK STIFFNESS AND OPISTHOTONOS

Neck stiffness is diagnosed when chin cannot be touched to the front of chest by flexion of the neck. In a struggling infant, the head should be suspended beyond the edge of the examination table to relax the neck. In infants below 3 months, severely malnourished and immunocompromised children, neck rigidity may not develop despite the presence of meningitis. Opisthotonos is characterized by

Box 8.30 Conditions associated with short neck

- Chondrodystrophy (Morquio's disease)
- Klippel-Feil deformity
- Down syndrome
- Platybasia
- Cretinism
- Turner syndrome
- Hurler syndrome
- Bilateral Sprengel's deformity
- Goldenhar syndrome
- Spondyloepiphyseal dysplasia congenita
- Noonan syndrome
- Rubinow syndrome
- Freeman-Sheldon syndrome
- Schwartz-Jampel syndrome
- Trisomy X syndrome

marked neck stiffness with extensor arching of the whole body. The causes of neck stiffness are listed in *Box 8.31*.

Box 8.31 Causes of neck stiffness

- Meningitis
- Kernicterus
- Meningismus*
- Acute poliomyelitis
- Tetanus
- Phenothiazine toxicity
- Vertebral anomalies
- Leukemic infiltrates in CNS
- Vertebral trauma
- Hypernatremia
- Caries cervical spine
- Toxic shock syndrome
- Retropharyngeal abscess
- Posterior fossa brain tumor with herniation
- Juvenile chronic arthritis
- Lyme disease
- Subarachnoid hemorrhage
- Calcification of cervical intervertebral disks
- Arnold-Chiari malformation
- Infantile Gaucher's disease (Figure 8.14)
- Leptospirosis
- Behcet syndrome
- Decerebrate rigidity
- Lesch-Nyhan syndrome

*Signs of meningeal irritation without any abnormalities in the CSF may be seen in children with pneumonia, pyelonephritis, salmonellosis, bacillary dysentery, leukemic infiltrates, etc.

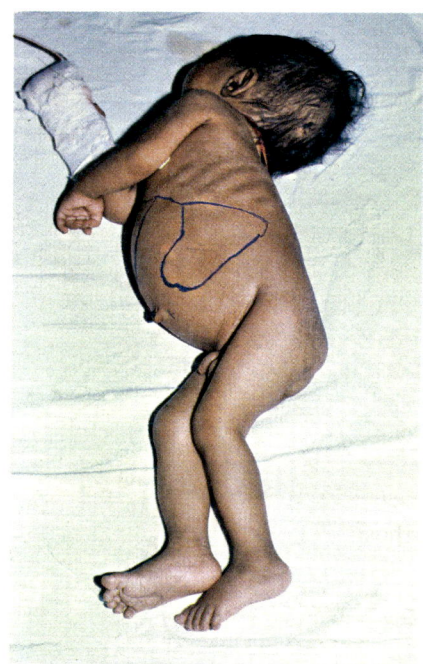

Figure 8.14 Infantile Gaucher's disease. There is marked neck retraction, hepatosplenomegaly and delayed neuromotor development

TORTICOLLIS (Wry Neck)

Torticollis is an asymmetric deformity of the neck and head characterized by lateral flexion or tilt of the head towards the involved side and rotation of the chin towards the opposite shoulder. In normal infants, the head can be turned so that chin can touch each shoulder and the ear can be made to touch the ipsilateral shoulder. Infants and children may tilt their head to avoid double vision. Sudden exposure to cold may lead to torticollis (*Box 8.32*).

Box 8.32 Causes of torticollis

- Sternocleidomastoid "tumor"
- Exposure to cold
- Viral infection
- Strabismus and diplopia (ocular torticollis)
- Klippel-Feil syndrome
- Acute oral infections and retropharyngeal abscess
- Trauma to head and neck
- Acute cervical adenitis
- Pott's disease of cervical spine

(contd.)

> **Box 8.32 Causes of torticollis (contd.)**
>
> - Torsion dystonia
> - Acute dystonic drug reaction
> - Athetoid cerebral palsy
> - Gastroesophageal reflux disease
> - Tumor of cervical spine (eosinophilic granuloma, osteoid osteoma)
> - Tonsillar herniation (astrocytoma of cerebellum)
> - Subluxation of the atlantoaxial joint
> - Down syndrome
> - Skeletal dysplasias
> - Juvenile chronic arthritis
> - Morquio's syndrome
> - Occipitalization and basilar impression of skull
> - Larsen syndrome
> - Pseudoachondroplasia
> - Congenital anomalies of the odontoid process
> - Benign paroxysmal torticollis due to faulty posture
> - Sandifer syndrome

ERYTHEMA NODOSUM

They are characterized by tender, painful, reddish-blue nodules which are typically located on the shins and rarely may spread to thighs and arms. They fade slowly over several weeks leaving behind bruised patches but they never ulcerate. It is a manifestation of hypersensitivity panniculitis because of a variety of inflammatory conditions. The common causes of erythema nodosum are listed in *Box 8.33*. In contrast, erythema induratum (Bazin disease) is a panniculitis of calves with formation of painful subcutaneous nodules over the calves and ankles which may ulcerate. They are more common in girls and are usually associated with cutaneous tuberculosis.

> **Box 8.33 Conditions associated with erythema nodosum**
>
> - Viral upper respiratory tract infections
> - Streptococcal infection
> - Tuberculosis
> - Hepatitis C and Epstein-Barr virus infection
> - Sarcoidosis
> - Behcet's disease
> - Leprosy
> - Systemic mycosis and histoplasmosis
> - Toxoplasmosis
> - Inflammatory bowel disease (Crohn's disease)
> - Systemic lupus erythematosus
> - Cat-scratch disease
> - *Yersinia enterocolitica* infection
> - Cancer, lymphoma, and histiocytosis
> - Sulfonamide and penicillin therapy
> - Alpha 1-antitrypsin deficiency
> - Idiopathic

MICROPENIS

It refers to a small penis. There is minimal growth of genitals during childhood followed by sudden spurt of growth during adolescence. The normal stretched dorsal length of penis in infants varies between 2.8 and 4.2 cm. Micropenis is diagnosed when stretched penile length is less than 1.9 cm or when stretched penile length is 2.5 standard deviation less than the mean-for-age without the presence of any other penile anomalies, such as hypospadias. The penis may be buried in the pubic fat in obese children. The length of stretched penis should be recorded from the pubic ramus to the tip of the glans penis (after retracting foreskin) over the dorsal side. The suprapubic pad of fat should be pressed inward as much as possible. A disposable 10 mL plastic syringe can be used to measure penile length. The needle-bearing end of the syring is cut and piston introduced through the cut end. The smooth flanged end of the syringe is firmly pressed against the pubis after enclosing penis into the barrel of the syringe. Gentle suction is applied to stretch the penis. Piston is aligned to the glans and length of penis is read with a scale. Micropenis is a recognized clinical feature of several syndromes (*Box 8.34*). It is usually caused by a defect anywhere along the hypothalamic-pituitary-gonadal axis, isolated growth hormone deficiency or part of a genetic syndrome.

ABNORMALITIES OF TESTICULAR SIZE

The volume of testes is best evaluated with the help of a Prader orchidometer or orchiometer which has testis-shaped plastic balls of different sizes strewn on a string. During preadolescence, the size of testes varies between 1.5 and 2.0 cm. The adult size of testes varies between 3.5 and 5.0 cm or an average volume of 20 mL (range 12–25 mL). The right testis is slightly larger in size while left testicle

> **Box 8.34 Syndromes associated with micropenis**
>
> - Hypogonadotropic hypogonadism (Kallmann syndrome, Prader-Willi syndrome, Ruds' syndrome, Alstrom syndrome, septo-optic dysplasia)
> - Hypopituitarism
> - Klinefelter syndrome
> - Fanconi's anemia
> - Carpenter syndrome (acrocephalopolysyndactyly type III)
> - Robinow syndrome
> - Williams syndrome
> - Hallermann-Streiff syndrome
> - Deletion of long arm of 18 chromosome
> - Noonan syndrome
> - X-linked hypogammaglobulinemia
> - Down syndrome
> - Cornelia de Lange syndrome
> - CHARGE association
> - Maternal intake of fertility drugs like diethylstilbestrol (DES)

usually hangs lower than the right. Failure of testicular enlargement by the age of 16 years is suggestive of delayed sexual maturation or hypogonadism.

Micro-orchidism. If testes are less than 1.0 cm in length or 12 mL in volume, it is suggestive of micro-orchidism. It is a recognized feature of following conditions:

- Rudimentary testes syndrome
- Klincfelter syndrome
- Laurence-Moon-Biedl syndrome
- Hypopituitarism
- Hypothalamic disorders
- Testicular atrophy due to mumps
- May be associated with various syndromes having micropenis.

Macro-orchidism. Testicular length that exceeds 2 cm or a volume of greater than 20 mL in preadolescent children or >30 mL in an adult is suggestive of macro-orchidism. It may occur in following conditions:

- Fragile-X syndrome (macro-orchidism occurs after puberty)
- Neurogenic or idiopathic sexual precocity
- Hypothyroidism

- FSH-secreting pituitary macroadenomas
- Testicular tumors (teratoma, interstitial cell tumor, and rhabdomyosarcoma)
- Aromatase deficiency

Sexual Infantilism and Delayed Puberty

The age of onset of puberty is variable but usually occurs between 10 and 12 years in girls and 12 and 14 years in boys. Puberty is considered as delayed, if there is no budding of breasts by 12 years in girls or there is lack of increase in the volume of testes by the age of 14 years in boys. The upper age limit for onset of menstruation is 15 years. Delayed puberty is more common in boys than girls. The most common cause of delayed puberty is constitutional delay in boys and Turner syndrome in girls. The common causes of delayed sexual maturation are listed in Table 8.9.

TABLE 8.9 Common causes of delayed sexual development

1. *Constitutional delay*
   The adolescent growth spurt may be delayed more often in boys than girls.
2. *Central causes (hypogonadotropic hypogonadism with low FSH and LH)*
   - Hypopituitarism
   - Hypothalamic disorders
   - Suprasellar cyst or tumor, trauma, irradiation, encephalitis, etc.
   - Kallmann syndrome (anosmia and color blindness provide useful clues)
   - Laurence-Moon-Biedl syndrome
   - Frohlich syndrome (adiposogenital dystrophy)
   - Prader-Willi syndrome
   - Vaquez syndrome
   - Septo-optic dysplasia
   - Alstrom syndrome
3. *Gonadal disorders (hypergonadotropic hypogonadism with elevated FSH and LH)*
   Boys
   - Congenital anorchia or testicular hypoplasia
   - Mumps or non-specific orchitis
   - Torsion of the spermatic cord
   - Trauma
   - Cryptorchidism with idiopathic fibrosis

(contd.)

TABLE 8.9 Common causes of delayed sexual development (*contd.*)

- Surgical or medical (chemotherapy) castration
- Klinefelter syndrome
- Weinstein syndrome

Girls
- Turner syndrome
- Gonadal dysgenesis
- Ovarian degeneration
- Gonadotropin resistant ovary syndrome
- Oophoritis

4. *Chronic systemic disorders*
   Hemoglobinopathies, end-stage renal disease, malabsorption, celiac disease, cystic fibrosis, chronic liver disease, inflammatory bowel disease, malignancy, severe obesity, severe zinc deficiency, and anorexia nervosa.
5. *Other endocrinal disorders*
   - Hypothyroidism
   - Diabetes mellitus
   - Hyperprolactinemia
   - Cushing syndrome
   - Congenital adrenal hyperplasia due to 17-alpha hydroxylase deficiency in girls.

CAFÉ AU LAIT MACULES (CALMs)

These are flat, sharply demarcated brown-colored (coffee with milk) macules on the skin. In children, up to 5 spots of less than 1.0 cm diameter are considered as normal. When the spots are large in size (>5 mm in preadolescents or >15 mm in adolescents) or excessive in number (>6), they serve as useful marker of diseases which are associated with café au lait spots (*Box 8.35*).

Box 8.35 Conditions associated with café au lait spots

- Familial multiple café au lait spots
- Neurofibromatosis type 1 (Figure 8.15)
- McCune-Albright syndrome (Figure 8.16)
- Gaucher disease
- Russell-Silver syndrome
- Ataxia-telangiectasia
- Marfan syndrome
- Bloom syndrome

(contd.)

Box 8.35 Conditions associated with café au lait spots (*contd.*)

- Tuberous sclerosis
- Chediak-Higashi syndrome
- Legius syndrome
- Hunter syndrome
- LEOPARD syndrome
- Noonan syndrome
- Pulmonary stenosis
- Watson syndrome
- Wiskott-Aldrich syndrome
- Fanconi anemia
- Basal cell nevus syndrome
- Turner syndrome
- Maffucci syndrome
- Jaffe–Campanacci syndrome
- Peutz–Jeghers syndrome
- Chronic myeloid leukemia
- Multiple lentigines
- Idiopathic

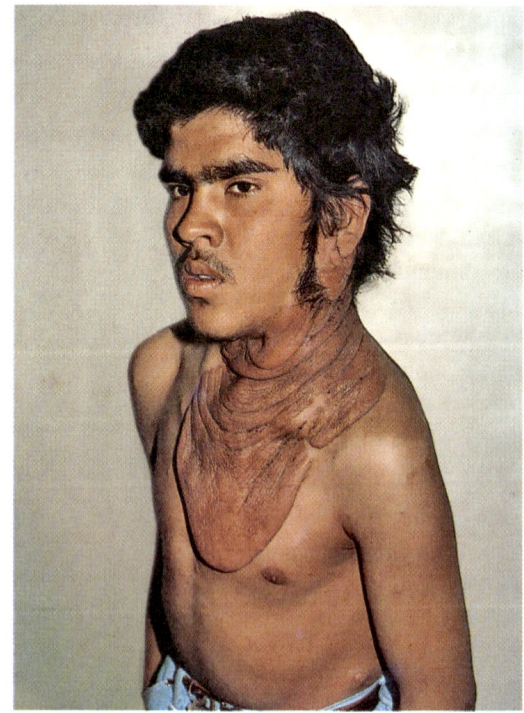

Figure 8.15 von Recklinghausen disease. Note the multilayered, overhanging plexiform mass of neurofibromatous tissue over the neck and chest in an adolescent boy.

Differential Diagnosis of Common Abnormal Physical Signs

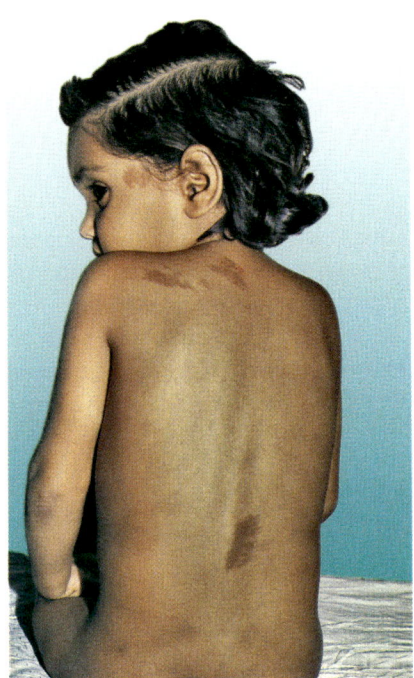

Figure 8.16 Café au lait macules in a girl with McCune-Albright syndrome. There was polyostotic fibrous dysplasia with polyendocrinopathy.

HEMIHYPERTROPHY

It is characterized by enlargement or hyperplasia of one-half of the body or hypertrophy may be limited to the face or one of the extremities. The condition is more common in girls and on the right side. These children should undergo regular monitoring of serum alpha-fetoprotein and abdominal ultrasound every 3 months until 5–7 years of age. The common causes and their correlates of hemihypertrophy are listed in *Box 8.36*.

PALMAR ERYTHEMA

There is marked erythema of the palms especially at the thenar and hypothenar eminences. Soles may or may not be affected. Erythema may occur due to elevation of estrogen level, inflammation, increased circulation, polycythemia, telangiectasia or increased vascularity due to release of nitric oxide. Palmar (and plantar) erythema may occur due to various physiological and pathological conditions (*Box 8.37*).

Box 8.36 Causes or conditions associated with hemihypertrophy

- Idiopathic
- Cutis marmorata telangiectatica congenita
- Beckwith-Wiedemann syndrome
- Russell-Silver syndrome
- Wilms tumor
- Klippel-Trenaunay-Weber syndrome
- Hepatocellular carcinoma
- Congenital arteriovenous fistula
- Neurofibromatosis
- Genitourinary abnormalities
- Proteus syndrome
- Skeletal dysostoses
- Hemi-3 syndrome
- Adrenocortical carcinoma
- Sotos syndrome

Box 8.37 Causes of palmar erythema

- Pregnancy
- Drugs like steroids, capecitabine, 5-fluorouracil and liposomal doxorubicin
- Chronic liver disease with or without portal hypertension
- Rheumatoid arthritis
- Kawasaki disease
- Infective disorders like scarlet fever, hand-foot-mouth disease, secondary syphilis and Rocky mountain spotted fever
- Chronic mercury poisoning (acrodynia)
- Thyrotoxicosis
- Polycythemia
- Deep telangiectasias
- Chronic hepatitis and cirrhosis
- Eczema
- Psoriasis
- Idiopathic

EPISTAXIS

Bleeding from the nose or epistaxis is common in children. It is usually benign and occurs during summer months because of excessive drying of nasal secretions and nose picking. The bleeding most commonly arises from Little's area (Kiesselbach's plexus) which is an anastomotic site for terminal arterioles. It is located over the nasal septum about 0.5 cm within the nostril and above the nasal floor. The common causes of epistaxis are listed in *Box 8.38*.

> **Box 8.38 Causes of epistaxis**
> - Bleeding from Little's area by picking or blowing the nose especially in dry weather
> - Chronic allergic or viral rhinitis
> - *Acute febrile illness*: Diphtheria, rheumatic fever, infectious mononucleosis, dengue fever and viral hemorrhagic fevers
> - *Bleeding diathesis*: Thrombocytopenia, hemophilia, von Willebrand disease
> - Prolonged instillation of nasal drops, insufflations and sprays
> - Nasal polyps
> - Septal deviation and spurs
> - Foreign body and nasal catheter
> - Nasal trauma and head injury with fracture of base of the skull
> - Hemangioma and hereditary telangiectasia (Osler-Weber-Rendu syndrome)
> - Tumors like juvenile angiofibroma, lymphoepithelioma and rhabdomyosarcoma of the nasopharynx. Capillary hemangioma and hamartoma may present as epistaxis
> - Drugs like steroids, antihistamines and nonsteroidal anti-inflammatory drugs (NSAIDs)
> - Chronic liver disease
> - Hypertension

DROOLING OF SALIVA

Saliva is produced to keep the oral mucosa wet and contains anti-infective agents and digestive enzyme ptyalin. It aids in swallowing, digestion and maintenance of oral hygiene. Drooling occurs either due to excessive production of saliva (sialorrhea) or inability to swallow the saliva as a result of oropharyngeal obstruction or neuromotor incoordination. Excessive drooling and choking during feeding in a newborn baby is suggestive of esophageal atresia. When atresia is suspected, attempt should be made to pass a Fr. 8 or 10 stiff rubber catheter into the esophagus. In esophageal atresia, it is not possible to pass the catheter into the stomach. Drooling with putting of fingers in the mouth is a physiological oral phase (mouthing)

of development and is often considered as a useful correlate of teething in infants. The dribbling of saliva through mouth may cause irritation and rash over the cheeks, neck or chest. Upper respiratory tract infection with nasal congestion is usually associated with drooling.

Persistent or excessive drooling is common in children with mental retardation, cerebral palsy, Bell's palsy, familial dysautonomia (Riley-Day syndrome), Rett syndrome, and pseudobulbar palsy (Wilson disease). Drooling of acute onset and short duration is seen in children with nose block, gingivostomatitis, tonsillitis, acute epiglottitis, diphtheria, peritonsillar or retropharyngeal abscess, foreign body, caustic ingestion, scorpion sting and organophosphate poisoning.

HALITOSIS

Halitosis or bad breath is uncommon in children compared to adults. It is a reliable index of orodental hygiene. Mouth breathing due to persistent nasal blockage is a leading cause of foul breath. The salient causes of halitosis are listed in *Box 8.39*.

> **Box 8.39 Common causes of halitosis**
> - Mouth breathing
> - Poor orodental hygiene
> - Caries teeth
> - Hypertrophy of adenoids or tonsils
> - Sinusitis
> - Nasal foreign body
> - Atrophic rhinitis
> - Vincent stomatitis or ulcerative gingivostomatitis
> - Prolonged febrile illness
> - Bronchiectasis and lung abscess

EXCESSIVE SWEATING

Excessive sweating or hyperhidrosis is a common complaint in children. It may be generalized or localized over the head, armpits, palms and soles. It is most commonly due to constitutional abnormality and is of no clinical significance although most parents are worried that it may cause

Box 8.40 Causes of excessive sweating

- Constitutional or idiopathic
- Hot and humid environment
- Lysis of fever
- Physical activity
- Hot and spicy food
- Hyperthyroidism
- Autonomic dysfunction
- Anxiety, nervousness and emotional stress
- Heart disease especially left-to-right shunt
- Shingles
- Spinal cord injury
- Pheochromocytoma
- Serotonin-secreting tumor of the gut (ganglio-neuroma or ganglioneuroblastoma), carcinoid tumor, non-Hodgkin's and Hodgkin's lymphoma
- Pulmonary tuberculosis (night sweating)
- Drugs like antidepressants, pilocarpine, propranolol, paracetamol
- Night terror
- Hypoglycemia
- Cystic fibrosis
- Fabry disease
- Shock (cold and clammy extremities)
- Substance abuse

TABLE 8.10 Causes of abnormal body odor*

Systemic diseases
- *Uremia*: Ammoniacal or fishy odor
- *Hepatic failure*: Mousy odor or fetor hepaticus
- *Diabetic ketosis*: Sweet and sickly smell of acetone

Suppurative conditions
Putrid smell in bronchiectasis and lung abscess

Inborn errors of metabolism
- *Maple syrup urine disease*: Maple syrup or burnt sugar smell
- *Hypermethioninemia and tyrosinemia*: Boiled cabbage or stale fish
- *Phenylketonuria*: Musty or mousy body odor
- *Isovaleric acidemia and glutaric acidemia type II*: Cheesy or sweaty feet
- *Cystinuria and homocystinuria*: Sulphurous smell
- *Multiple carboxylase deficiency*: Cat urine
- *Tyrosinemia, hypermethioninemia and trimethylaminuria*: Rotten fish

Poisonings and drugs
- Kerosene, alcohol, paraldehyde, insecticides or pesticides

*In a comatosed child, breath and urine should be smelled to identify any abnormal odor. Unusual odor is more readily smelt in a sample of frozen urine because organic compounds with different freezing points concentrate on the top. A filter paper soaked in urine can be smelled akin to evaluation of perfumes!

weakness. Increased perspiration is commonly seen in children with congestive heart failure, acute respiratory failure and narcotic withdrawal syndrome. Excessive sweating of palms along with nail biting is suggestive of anxiety. Teenagers with hyperhidrosis may develop anxiety, poor self-image, embarrassment, social withdrawal and emotional insecurity. The common causes of excessive sweating are listed in *Box 8.40*.

ABNORMAL BODY ODOR

Body odor depends upon a large number of factors including personal hygiene, odor of breath and smell of sweat, urine, feces or pheromones elaborated by the skin and use of medicated soaps and various cosmetics. Abnormal and specific odor may be observed in certain systemic disorders and inborn errors of metabolism (Table 8.10). However, among various special senses which are used for evaluation of a patient, the senses of smell and taste are least important.

XEROSTOMIA (Dry Oral Mucosa)

Reduced secretion of salivary glands with dryness of mouth and tongue may cause foul breath, tooth decay and poor digestion. The common causes include mouth breathing (nasal obstruction), severe dehydration, parotitis, calculus in one of the major salivary glands and psychological disorders like anxiety, stress and depression. Xerostomia is a recognized feature of Parkinson disease, human immunodeficiency virus (HIV) infection, cystic fibrosis, sarcoidosis and Sjögren syndrome. It may occur as a side effect of several medications namely caffeine, atropine, antihistamines, antidepressants, antipsychotics, sedatives, methyldopa, diuretics, chemotherapy agents and radiotherapy of head and neck.

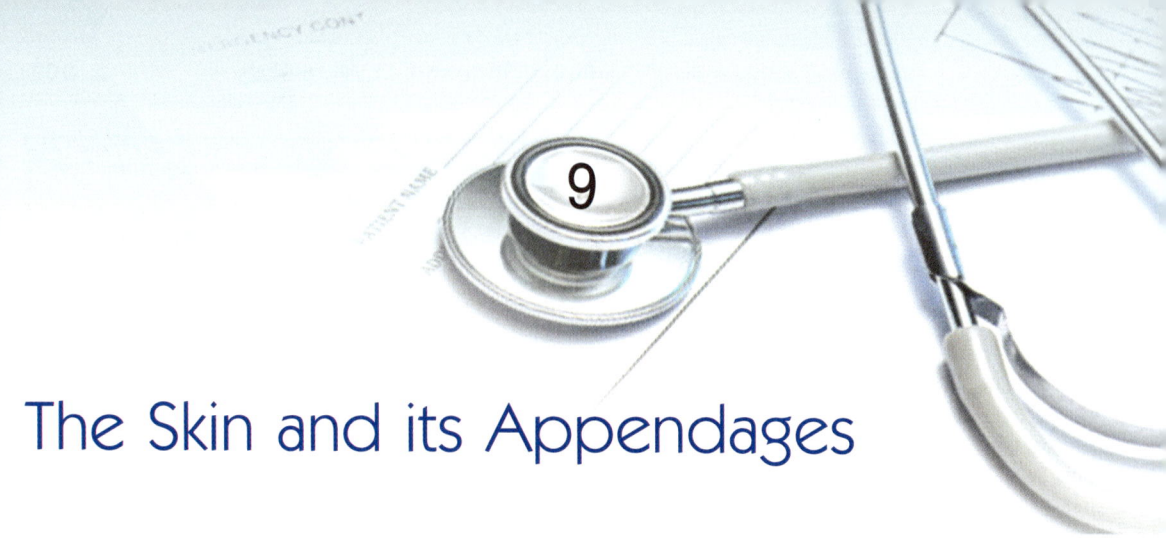

9
The Skin and its Appendages

Skin is the largest body organ providing protective covering to the underlying structures. It is thin and more delicate in children. Over 10% of children reporting to the primary care physician have a dermatologic disorder. Skin manifestations may occur due to a primary skin disorder or they may represent manifestations of an underlying systemic disorder. Most skin diseases are either transient and self-limiting or chronic and intractable. Rarely, skin condition may manifest as a life-threatening dermatological emergency, viz. drug reaction, Stevens-Johnson syndrome, toxic epidermal necrolysis (TEN), pemphigus, epidermolysis bullosa, erythroderma, and scalded skin syndrome (SSS). A number of viral exanthems are limited to children. A detailed examination of skin and its appendages is required when primary manifestations of a disease process are limited to the skin.

HISTORY

Apart from demographic details, enquiry should be made regarding the duration of skin lesions, involvement of initial site and their subsequent progression, evolution and distribution. The specific areas of the skin surface involved, whether predominantly over the extensor surfaces or flexor creases should be asked. Are skin lesions localized or generalized, symmetrical or asymmetrical, clustered or diffuse in distribution? The presence of itching, irritation and smarting sensation should be asked. Infants manifest itching by irritability and restlessness. The presence of associated constitutional symptoms like fever, malaise, joint pains, abdominal pain, evidences of inborn error of metabolism or any other systemic manifestations should be looked for. Skin manifestations may occur due to deficiency of essential nutrients and trace elements like vitamins, zinc and essential fatty acids.

History of drug intake and possibility of an adverse drug reaction should always be kept in mind. Administration of vaccines, sera, blood and blood components should be asked to exclude side effects of vaccines, serum sickness and host-versus-graft reaction. A detailed probing is required to elicit history of contact with an offending cosmetic agent, poison ivy or toxic plant, insects (mosquitoes, bed bugs, ants, honey bees, centipede, scorpion, etc.), and infested animals (fleas, visceral larva migrans, and cat-scratch disease). History of similar manifestations among household contacts is suggestive of an infective disorder like viral infection, pyoderma and scabies. Family history of eczema, atopic dermatitis, autoimmune disorder, vitiligo and psoriasis should be enquired. Exclude systemic manifestations by a detailed review of body systems. A detailed history of topical and systemic therapy taken should be recorded.

PHYSICAL EXAMINATION

Examination of skin must be conducted in a well-lighted room preferably with optimal sunlight. Magnifying glass with a built-in light should be used to study the morphology of skin lesions. A transparent spatula or glass slide is useful to view erythematous patch after applying pressure to assess whether it blanches or not (diascopy). It is desirable to completely undress the young child while older children can have a loose fitting gown. The presence of constitutional manifestations like fever, toxemia, anorexia and systemic symptoms demand a detailed physical examination. Vital signs should be checked in children with generalized skin disorder. All areas of skin including palms, soles, creases, scalp, mucocutaneous junctions like perioral and anogenital skin should be scrutinized. Because of ectodermal origin of both skin and CNS, many genetic or developmental defects of skin are associated with CNS malformations or hamartomas.

Spider nevi, palmar erythema, gynecomastia and xanthomas may be seen in patients with chronic liver disease with hepatocellular failure. Mucous membranes, hair, and nails are often involved in various skin disorders and should be examined in detail. The most important aspect of the physical examination of skin is the morphology of individual skin lesions. In addition to thorough inspection of skin, palpation of skin lesions may allow the examiner to appreciate subtle depression or elevation of skin lesions. A number of viral exanthems (Table 9.1) and acute bacterial infections (Table 9.2) can be diagnosed clinically by characteristic distribution and evolution of skin rash. The morphologic features of skin lesions should be carefully looked for and recorded on a human diagram for their extent and distribution.

TABLE 9.1 Characteristics of skin rash in common viral exanthems

Measles (rubeola, first disease)
Skin rash appears after 3–4 days of prodromal features of fever, coryza and conjunctival congestion. The fever shoots up on the day of onset of rash. Maculopapular or morbilliform confluent rash starts behind the ears and spreads to the forehead, face, neck, trunk and extremities (Figure 9.1). Koplik spots (grayish-white dots like grains of sand or sago with reddish areola, usually located over the buccal mucosa opposite lower molars) appear 24 hours before or 24–48 hours after the onset of rash are a characteristic early marker of measles. The rash starts to fade from the face on the third day and it disappears in the order of its appearance. When eruption fades, brownish copper discoloration of skin with powdery desquamation is seen for several days.

Rubella (German measles, third disease)
The rash appears after 1–2 days of mild prodrome of fever, cough and coryza. The exanthem begins on the face and extends over the body within a few hours as fine, light-pink discrete macules or scarlatiniform rash. Suboccipital and posterior auricular lymph nodes may be slightly enlarged and tender. The rash begins to fade after 2 to 4 days leaving behind fine desquamation. It is difficult to differentiate rubella from mild measles modified by prior immunity or immunization.

Chickenpox (varicella)
There is no prodrome except mild symptoms of upper respiratory catarrh for one to two days. Rash appears in crops over the trunk with simultaneous appearance of macules, papules, vesicles (like dew-drops or tear drops) which progress to develop pustules and crusts. Lesions spread to peripheral areas involving extremities and face (Figure 9.2). Pruritus is common. The crops of new lesions continue to appear over 4 to 5 days and exanthem lasts up to 8 to 14 days. Most lesions heal without scarring unless there is superadded bacterial infection. When all the lesions are crusted, the patient is no longer contagious.

Erythema infectiosum (fifth disease)
It is caused by parvovirus B19 and manifests as bright red confluent rash over the cheeks, malar prominences and nose giving an appearance of "slapped-face". Circumoral pallor may be present. Erythematous macules may spread over the lateral and extensor aspects of extremities, trunk and buttocks. During recovery, there is characteristic lace-like or reticular pattern due to central clearing of erythematous macules.

(contd.)

TABLE 9.1 Characteristics of skin rash in common viral exanthems (*contd.*)

Roseola infantum (exanthum subitum or sixth disease)
The onset is sudden with high grade fever at times with convulsions. Coryza is mild or absent. The fever falls by crisis after 3–4 days followed by onset of maculopapular skin eruption starting on the trunk and involving arms and neck. The rash is absent or minimal on the face or legs. The skin rash fades within 24 hours without any desquamation.

Dengue fever
Sudden onset of high grade continuous or saddle back or biphasic fever which comes down by lysis and profuse sweating. Fever is usually associated with headache, backache, pain in the eyes and vomiting. Transient maculopapular rash appears around the 3rd–4th day of fever, usually starts from trunk and spreads to arms and legs. There may be palmar and plantar erythema with marked itching and desquamation of the skin of palms and soles during recovery. Puffiness and swelling of dorsum of hands and feet may occur during the stage of marked capillary permeability with exudation of fluid into interstitial compartment and serosal cavities.

Herpes simplex (cold sores)
Herpes simplex 1 (HSV-1) produces cold sores or fever blisters, while HSV-2 causes most cases of genital herpes. There is variable fever for 2–7 days. Papulovesicular skin lesions start from the mucocutaneous junction and spread to lips, gingivae, palate, buccal mucosa and tongue. The skin lesions may be widespread in children with eczema (eczema herpeticum). Skin lesions may be associated with paronychia (herpetic whitlow) and keratitis.

Herpes zoster (shingles)
Grouped or clustered papulovesicular skin lesions are seen with background erythema over contiguous skin dermatome in the distribution of a peripheral or cranial nerve. The skin lesions do not cross the midline and last for 10–14 days. In adolescents, skin lesions may be associated with intense burning sensation or excruciating pain. The skin lesions may be widely disseminated in immunocompromised children. Varicella vaccine also provides protection against herpes zoster.

Hand-foot-and-mouth disease (HFMD)
It is usually caused by Coxsackie A16 and enterovirus 71. After an incubation period of 4 to 6 days, there is prodrome of low grade fever, anorexin and malaise for 12–36 hours. Initial symptoms include sore throat with oral ulcerations due to vesicles over the buccal mucosa and tongue. Fever is mild and precedes skin rash. Painful papulovesicular skin lesions appear over the palmoplantar surfaces of hands and feet, with erythematous papular skin lesions over the buttocks and thighs (Figure 9.3). The disease is self-limiting and resolves within 3–7 days.

Infectious mononucleosis (glandular fever or mono)
The causative agent is Epstein-Barr virus (EBV). There is a bright red morbilliform or scarlatiniform skin rash which is often precipitated by intake of ampicillin. The course is prolonged and there is associated generalized lymphadenopathy, herpangina (sore throat), mild jaundice, splenomegaly and extreme fatigue.

Enteroviruses
Coxsackie viruses A9 and B5 and echoviruses 4, 9 and 16 may produce maculopapular, morbilliform, urticarial or petechial skin rash. There are no characteristic or diagnostic clinical features.

Adenoviruses
Nonspecific maculopapular skin eruption is often associated with adenovirus infection.

The Skin and its Appendages

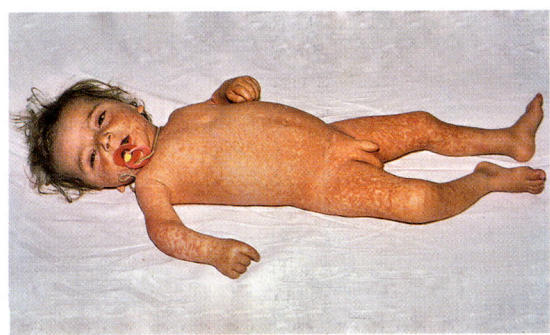

Figure 9.1 Generalized morbilliform rash due to measles in a one-year-old boy.

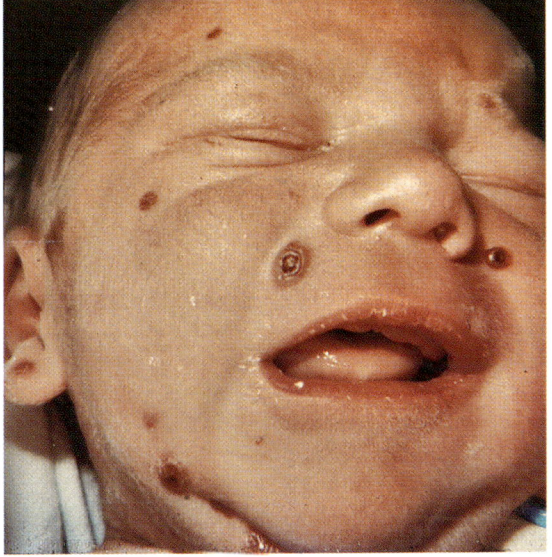

Figure 9.2 Typical lesions of chickenpox on the face of an infant with congenital varicella.

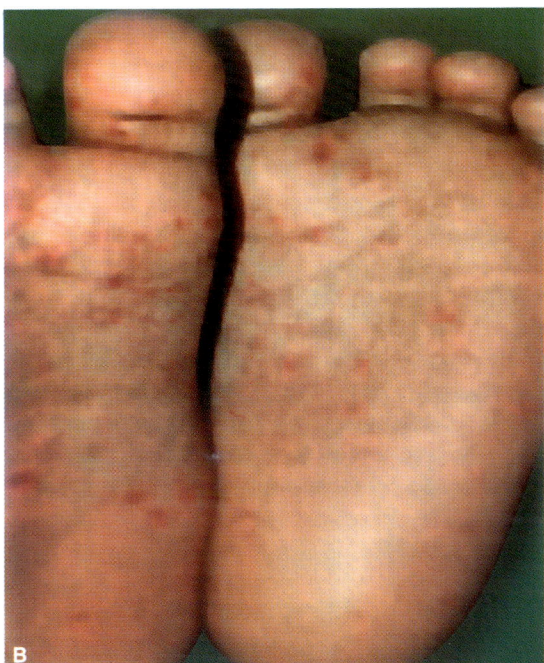

Figure 9.3A and B Papulovesicular skin lesions on the palms (A) and soles in a child (B) with hand-foot-and-mouth disease.

TABLE 9.2 Acute bacterial infections with a skin rash			
Disease	Organisms	Skin manifestations	Associated features
Anthrax (Black ulcer)	B. anthracis	Pruritic papule typically located on the face, enlarges to form an ulcer which is surrounded by vesicles and marked edema, heals by formation of eschar or black ulcer	Fever, headache and lymphadenopathy

(contd.)

TABLE 9.2 Acute bacterial infections with a skin rash (contd.)

Disease	Organisms	Skin manifestations	Associated features
Bacterial endocarditis	Streptococcus viridans, Streptococcus pneumoniae, Staphylococcus aureus, etc.	Osler nodes (tender pink nodules on finger tips or toe pads), Janeway lesions (painless erythematous or hemorrhagic macules over palms and soles), petechiae on skin and mucosa, splinter hemorrhages in the nail beds	Underlying heart disease with appearance of a new murmur, flame-shaped hemorrhages (Roth spots) in the fundus, and microscopic hematuria
Ecthyma gangrenosum	Pseudomonas aeruginosa and other Gram-negative rods	Indurated plaques evolve to form hemorrhagic bullae or pustules leading to sloughing and eschar formation. Mostly located in the axillae, groins and perianal region	Usually affects neutropenic children and newborn babies
Leptospirosis	Leptospira interrogans and Leptospira biflexa	Maculopapular skin eruption, conjunctivitis, and scleral hemorrhages in a few cases	Influenza-like illness with chills and headache, myalgias and aseptic meningitis in fulminant cases, jaundice and skin hemorrhages may occur (Weil's disease)
Meningococcemia	N. meningitidis	Extensive petechial and ecchymotic skin rash involving trunk and extremities, may evolve into gangrenous patches due to purpura fulminans	Hypotension, meningitis and disseminated intravascular coagulation
Rat-bite fever (RBF, Sodoku and Haverhill fever)	Streptobacillus moniliformis and Spirillum minus	Eschar at bite site, maculopapular violaceous or red-brown skin eruption over trunk, palms, soles, extremities specially over the joints with desquamation during recovery	Fever, myalgias, regional lymphadenopathy, arthritis and prolonged or recurrent fever
Rocky Mountain spotted fever	Rickettsia rickettsii	Rash begins on the wrists and ankles and spreads towards the trunk, may involve palms and soles and lesions may progress from blanchable macules to petechiae	Acute onset with high grade fever and chills, headache, myalgias and abdominal pain
Scarlet fever (second disease)	Group A Streptococcus haemolyticus	Diffuse blanchable erythema beginning on the face and spreading to trunk and extremities, circumoral pallor, "sandpaper" texture of skin, accentuation of linear streaks of erythema in skinfolds (Pastia's lines), "strawberry" tongue and desquamation during second week	Fever, pharyngitis and headache

(contd.)

TABLE 9.2 Acute bacterial infections with a skin rash (contd.)

Disease	Organisms	Skin manifestations	Associated features
Staphylococcal scalded skin syndrome (SSSS)	S. aureus Phage group II, mostly type 71	Diffuse tender erythema-like burns, often with bullae and marked desquamation (Figure 9.4). Nikolsky's sign is positive	Occurs in children below 2 years of age and neonates (Ritter's disease, pemphigus neonatorum)
Staphylococcal toxic shock syndrome (TSS)	S. aureus toxin 1 and enterotoxin B or C	Diffuse erythema starting from trunk and spreading to arms, legs, palms, mucosal surfaces and conjunctivae. Desquamation occurs after 7–10 days of illness	High fever, hypotension and multiorgan failure
Streptococcal toxic shock syndrome	Group A beta-hemolytic Streptococcus	Scarlatiniform rash with necrotizing fasciitis and pneumonia	Hypotension and multiorgan failure
Typhoid fever	Salmonella typhi	Transient blanchable erythematous macules and papules on the trunk (Rose spots)	Headache, diarrhea, splenomegaly, abdominal distension, and toxemia

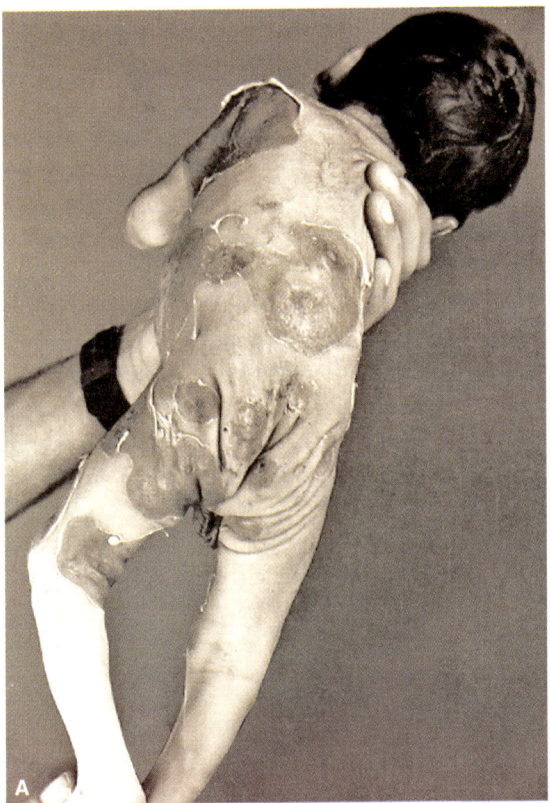 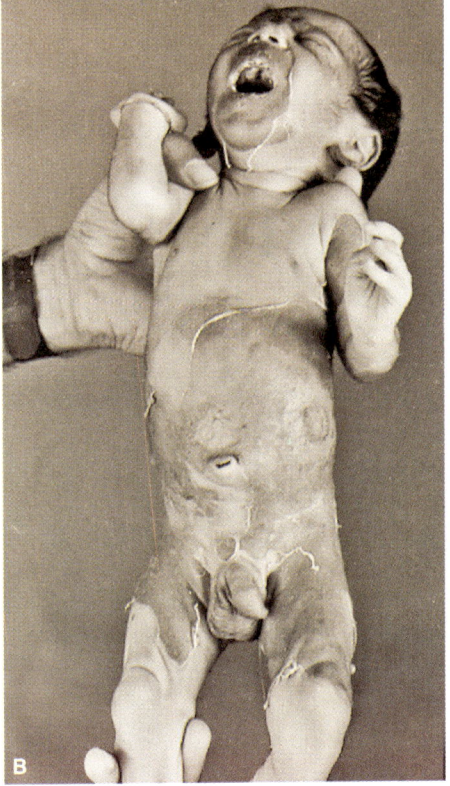

Figure 9.4 A and B Typical appearances of scalded skin syndrome due to staphylococcal infection.

PRIMARY SKIN LESIONS

Primary skin lesions provide the most vital clues for making a correct diagnosis. They are the most representative lesions of the disease process without any alteration by the patient by scratching, rubbing, secondary infection or therapy.

Macules They are flat, nonpalpable areas of color change of skin. Macules may be erythematous, hypopigmented or hyperpigmented. When a macule is larger than 1.0 cm, it is called a patch. They may be of any shape with well-defined regular or irregular borders. Examples include moles, lentigines, freckles, café au lait spots, vitiligo, Mongolian blue spot and port-wine stain.

Mole A pigmentary nevus is called a mole.

Freckles They are small, less than 0.5 cm, discrete brown macules that appear on the sun-exposed areas of skin. The condition is inherited as an autosomal dominant trait in light-skinned red-haired people. They are commonly seen on the face, back, chest, upper shoulders, sparing the mucous membranes.

Lentigines They are small, less than 0.5 cm, single or multiple brown to black, variegated or uniformly colored macules over the skin or mucosae. They are darker in color than freckles and are not affected by sunlight. They may be associated with LEOPARD (Lentigines, ECG conduction abnormalities, Ocular hypertelorism, Pulmonic stenosis, Abnormal genitalia, Retardation of growth, Deafness) syndrome, FACES (Facial features, Anorexia, Cachexia, Eyes and Skin lesions) syndrome, Sotos syndrome, LAMB (Lentigines, Atrial myxomas, Mucocutaneous myxomas and Blue nevi) syndrome, and Peutz-Jeghers syndrome.

Papules They are circumscribed raised skin lesions of less than 1.0 cm in diameter. They may be dome-shaped, flat-topped, conical, umblicated or verrucous. Examples include molluscum contagiosum, warts and miliaria rubra (prickly heat).

Papilloma It is a pedunculated lesion projecting from the skin.

Nodules Nodules are elevated skin lesions larger than 1.0 cm in diameter. They may be located in the epidermis, dermis or subcutaneous tissue. Examples include epidermoid cysts, fibromas and neurofibromas.

Tumors Tumors are large nodules, generally >2 cm in diameter. They may be benign or malignant and primary or metastatic.

Plaques They are well-circumscribed, broad-based discoid lesions of altered skin texture often formed by coalescence of a number of papules. The diameter or size of the lesions is greater than 1.0 cm. A plaque may be flat, elevated or depressed. A typical example is psoriasis.

Target lesion Annular patch or a plaque with central vesicle or pigmentation and a halo of erythema (erythema multiforme).

Wheals They are transient, raised, edematous skin lesions with irregular edges. The lesions are erythematous with a central pallor. Intense itching is usually present. They can be produced by dermatographism (Darier's sign and tache cerebrale), and are suggestive of urticaria, and insect bites.

Vesicles The elevated, fluid-containing skin lesions or blisters of <1.0 cm diameter are called vesicles. Examples include chickenpox, herpes simplex or zoster, and contact dermatitis.

Bullae When vesicles are larger than 1.0 cm diameter, they are called bullae. They may be intraepidermal or subepidermal. Examples include epidermolysis bullosa and staphylococcal scalded skin syndrome.

Cysts The circumscribed tumors containing semisolid or fluid contents are called cysts. The typical examples include epidermal cysts that occur after puberty on the face and upper back, dermoid cyst, sebaceous cyst, and branchial cyst.

Pustules The elevated well-circumscribed skin lesions containing purulent material or pus are called pustules. Unlike the transparent dew drop appearance of vesicles, the pustules may be turbid or opaque and white or yellow in color. Examples include folliculitis or pyoderma.

Callus Localized hyperplasia of horny layer on the palms or soles due to pressure.

Comedones These are characteristic skin lesions of acne due to dark horny keratin and sebaceous plugs which are distributed on the face and upper back. Open comedones or black heads are 2–5 mm flesh-colored papules with black centers. The closed comedones or white heads are 1–3 mm flesh-colored papules with a pinpoint opening.

Petechiae Pinhead-sized macules of extravasated blood. They cannot be blanched on pressure.

Purpura The leakage of blood in the skin is called purpura or ecchymosis. Unlike erythematous macules, purpura cannot be blanched by pressure with a finger or with a glass slide or a transparent plastic spatula (diascopy). Petechiae are small, pinpoint areas (<3 mm) of hemorrhages while ecchymoses are large areas of extravasation of blood in the skin (Figure 9.5). Ecchymotic skin patches may be flat or raised above the surface when there is associated vasculitis, viz. Henoch-Schönlein purpura and collagen vascular or connective tissue disorders (Figure 9.6).

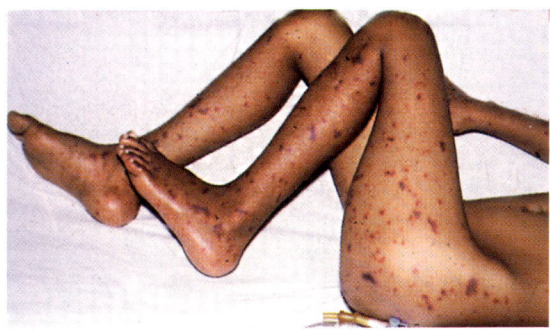

Figure 9.5 Typical irregular purpuric and gangrenous skin rash over the legs and buttocks in a child with fulminant meningococcemia.

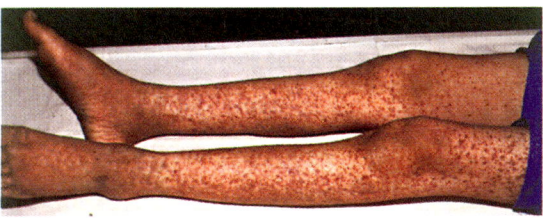

Figure 9.6 The characteristic purpuric skin rash which is slightly raised above the surface (due to vasculitis) gives a flea-bitten appearance in a patient with Henoch-Schönlein syndrome. The rash is distributed over the extensor surfaces of legs, buttocks and elbows. The condition is usually associated with arthralgias and pain abdomen.

Hematoma Swelling with or without fluctuation due to gross bleeding under the skin.

Telangiectasia Dilatation of superficial blood vessels which can be blanched by pressure.

Burrows They are linear, curved or serpentine elevations or tunnels in the superficial skin produced by the adult female mite as she travels through the stratum corneum. There is a black dot at the leading edge of the tunnel due to the lodgement of mite. Burrows are typically located in the interdigital areas of palms and soles.

The primary skin lesions enable classification into broad groups of skin disorders which is useful for consideration of differential diagnosis. The broad groups of primary skin lesions include maculopapular, papulosquamous, vesiculobullous, tumor-nodules, vascular reactions (urticaria, purpura), eczematous and pigmentary changes.

SECONDARY SKIN LESIONS

They are produced due to changes caused by scratching, touching, rubbing, secondary infection and because of local and systemic effects of medications.

Scales Desquamation or shedding of excess of normal and abnormal horny layer of stratum corneum.

Crusts They are formed by drying of blood, serum and any exudate overlying the diseased skin. They are often present in impetigo, in which they appear honey-colored and in weeping eczematous lesions.

Excoriations They develop as a result of linear loss of skin secondary to self-induced scratching and rubbing. Common examples include contact dermatitis, atopic dermatitis and insect bites.

Erosions There is partial loss of epidermis which heals without scarring.

Ulcers They occur due to deeper loss of the skin involving both epidermis and a variable depth of dermis or subcutaneous tissue. They may result from infection, vascular insufficiency or burns.

Eschar It is a necrotic skin lesion covered with a black crust.

Fissures They are linear clefts or cracks which are located deep in the epidermal layer in thickened or chronically inflamed skin.

Lichenification Thickening and hyperpigmentation of skin with exaggeration of skin markings due to chronic rubbing because of allergic or infective skin lesions is called lichenification.

Atrophy Atrophy of skin refers to loss or thinning of the epidermis or dermis. Epidermal atrophy is characterized by wrinkling of skin with telangiectases. In dermal or subcutaneous atrophy, the skin is depressed.

Sinus Tunnel within the dermis with an opening on the skin surface.

Eczematous skin lesions It refers to inflammatory skin lesions which have indistinct margins with erythema and vesiculation in the acute phase. Scaling, crusting and lichenification may be seen as the disorder progresses.

Striae Atrophic pink or white linear skin lesions over the abdomen and buttocks due to alterations in the connective tissue because of sudden changes in the girth as a result of obesity, pregnancy and ascites.

Hyperkeratosis It is a histologic term used to describe thickening of the stratum corneum. The presence of thick rough scales over skin lesions is a good clinical marker of hyperkeratosis.

Sclerosis Circumscribed or diffuse hardening of skin often due to fibrosis.

Scar Healing occurs by replacement with fibrous tissue. When formation of scar is excessive, it is called keloid.

MORPHOLOGY OF SKIN LESIONS

The configuration of skin lesions may provide useful diagnostic clues (Table 9.3). Linear lesions occur in a line and are characteristically seen in contact dermatitis and incontinentia pigmenti. Tache cerebrale is an erythematous raised linear streak that appears within 30 to 60 seconds after scratching with a fingernail or a sharp object (Darier's sign). It may be elicited in patients with encephalitis, meningitis and other acute CNS

TABLE 9.3 Differential diagnosis of skin lesions on the basis of their configuration

Nomenclature	Shape	Conditions
Nummular or discoid	Butterfly, round or coin-shaped	Lupus erythematosus, nummular eczema, and psoriasis
Circinate	Circular	Ringworm
Annular	Ring-shaped	Tinea corporis, and pityriasis rosea
Arcuate	Semicircular or curved	Erythema marginatum and granuloma annulare
Guttate	Like a drop of water or paint	Psoriasis
Gyrate or serpiginous	Wave-like or serpentine	Visceral larva migrans
Linear and along the lines of Blaschko*	Like a line	Contact dermatitis, incontinentia pigmenti, verrucous epidermal nevus, nevus achromicus, lichen planus, lupus erythomatosus, CHILD** syndrome
Grouped	Clustered	Herpes simplex
Dermatomal	Limited over a dermatome	Herpes zoster or shingles
Reticular	Net-like	Erythema infectiosum, cutis marmorata and livedo reticularis

*The lines of Blaschko refer to lines of normal development of embryonic cells in the skin. They are "V" shaped over the back, "S" shaped whorls over the chest and sides and "wavy" in shape over the scalp.
CHILD syndrome is an acronym for **Congenital **H**emidysplasia with **I**chthyosiform erythroderma and **L**imb **D**efects

inflammatory diseases. Annular or ring-shaped lesions are seen in children with ringworm (tinea corporis), pityriasis rosea and nummular eczema. Semicircular or arc-like (arciform) lesions are suggestive of erythema marginatum. The grouped lesions are called herpetiform lesions and are seen in herpetic infections. Reticulated eruptions give a net-like or interlacing pattern as seen in patients with erythema infectiosum and incontinentia pigmenti. A number of other descriptive terms are used that often connote a specific disease entity. For example, discoid (disk-shaped) usually refers to discoid lupus erythematosus, nummular (coin-shaped) is a type of eczema and guttate (drop-like) refers to a form of psoriasis. The lesions of lichen planus are slightly raised, flat-topped and have a violaceous hue. In polyarteritis nodosa, small aneurysms are strung like the beads of a rosary over the affected areas of the skin. The rosary sign is a useful diagnostic feature of vasculitis involving the small blood vessels.

DISTRIBUTION OF SKIN RASH

The distribution of skin lesions should be carefully examined and may provide useful diagnostic clues. When skin lesions are symmetrical in distribution, they are suggestive of endogenous causes while asymmetrical lesions may occur due to external factors. Flexor distribution of symmetrical skin lesions is suggestive of atopic dermatitis while extensor distribution is seen in psoriasis. Flexural distribution of rash occurs in a number of other conditions *(Box 9.1)*. In chickenpox and pityriasis rosea, skin lesions are centripetal (over the trunk) while in erythema multiforme and erythema nodosum, they are centrifugal (over the extremities) in distribution. In scabies, face is characteristically spared (except in infants) and lesions are mostly concentrated over the interdigital areas of palms and soles and genital region.

In Koebner phenomenon or isomorphic response, linear skin lesions appear at the sites of injury or self-scratching of healthy skin. The dermatological conditions which are associated with Koebner phenomenon are listed in *Box 9.2*.

Box 9.1 Flexural distribution of skin rash

- Atopic dermatitis
- Infantile seborrheic dermatitis
- Intertrigo
- Candidiasis
- Tinea cruris
- Ichthyosis
- Inverse psoriasis

Box 9.2 Skin conditions associated with Koebner phenomenon

- Psoriasis
- Vitiligo
- Molluscum contagiosum
- Lichen planus
- Lichen nitidus
- Warts
- Keratosis follicularis (Darier disease)
- Kaposi sarcoma
- Systemic lupus erythematosus
- Juvenile idiopathic arthritis
- Necrobiosis lipoidica
- Poison ivy

The presence of rash on the face may provide a diagnostic clue to the underlying collagen vascular disorder. Systemic lupus erythematosus is characterized by a typical sunlight-sensitive butterfly rash over the cheeks with marked erythema and papulovesicular lesions *(Figure 9.7)*. Heliotropic or lilac discoloration of the eyelids with periorbital edema is highly suggestive of dermatomyositis. In addition, there is scaly erythematous non-itching papules (Gottron papules) over the bony prominences, such as metacarpophalangeal, proximal interphalangeal joints, knees, elbows and medial malleoli. During recovery, the papules become atrophic and leave behind hypo- or hyperpigmented macules. Erythema of palms and soles with or without desquamation is a recognized feature of prolonged steroid therapy, rheumatoid arthritis, hepatocellular failure, scarlet fever, hand-foot-and-mouth disease, Kawasaki disease, and Rocky mountain spotted fever. Skin rash over the exposed parts of the body (face, extremities, hands

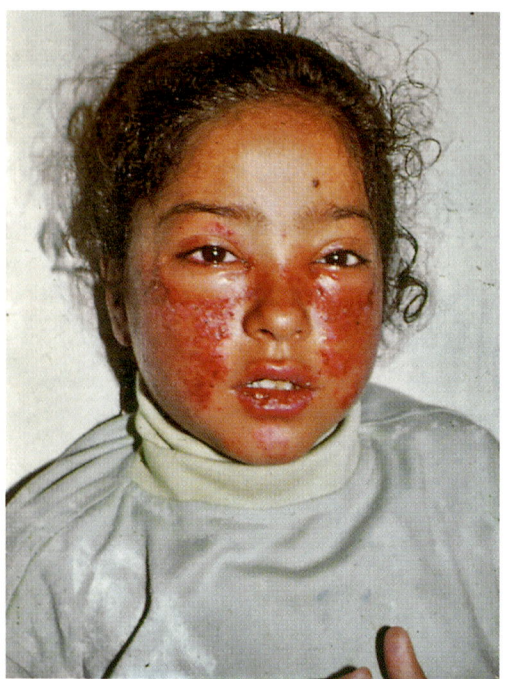

Figure 9.7 Typical erythematous "butterfly" rash involving malar areas and extending over the bridge of the nose in an adolescent girl with systemic lupus erythematosus. There is intense erythema with papulovesicular skin lesions having irregular margins.

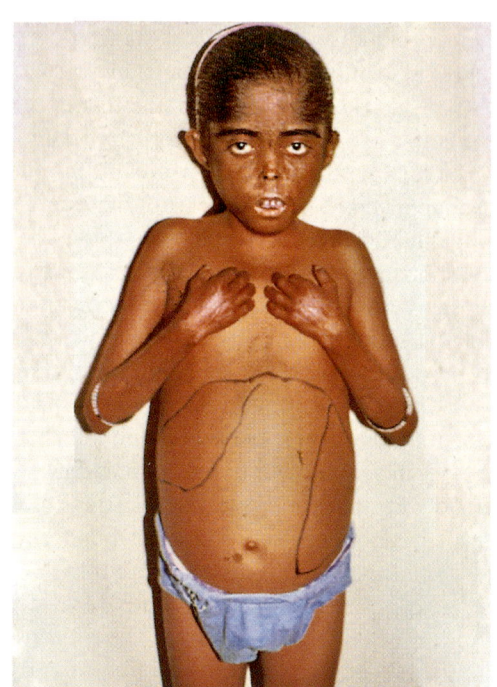

Figure 9.8 Photosensitive skin rash with pigmentation over the face and extremities with gross hepatosplenomegaly in a child with porphyria erythropoietica.

and feet) due to photosensitivity is a characteristic feature of a number of disorders (Table 9.4).

TABLE 9.4 Causes of photosensitivity skin rash

- Idiopathic polymorphous light eruptions (PMLEs)
- Pellagra
- Hartnup disease
- Porphyria erythropoietica (Figure 9.8)
- Drugs including phenothiazines, non-steroidal anti-inflammatory drugs, topical agents, cosmetics, etc.
- Phytophotodermatitis (Psoralen containing fruits and plants)
- Xeroderma pigmentosa
- Cockayne syndrome
- Bloom syndrome
- Rothmund–Thomson syndrome
- Primary skin diseases aggravated by sunlight (atopic dermatitis, acrodermatitis enteropathica, lichen planus, psoriasis, acne rosacea)

COLOR OF SKIN LESIONS

Macular erythematous skin lesions are most common. They occur due to viral exanthems as a result of dilatation of superficial cutaneous blood vessels. Erythema readily blanches on pressure. Purpuric skin lesions do not blanch on pressure and they undergo color changes from bright pink to bluish-pink, blue and dark brown over several days. Petechiae and ecchymoses may occur due to thrombocytopenia, vasculitis and life-threatening viral, bacterial and treponemal infections (Tables 9.1 and 9.2). The skin lesions may heal by desquamation and become lighter in color (hypopigmentation) after healing and recovery.

Depigmentation refers to total loss of pigment secondary to an autoimmune disorder (vitiligo) or due to hereditary disorders, like partial (piebaldism) and complete albinism. In leprosy, skin lesions may be depigmented or reddened with a slightly raised edge and they may be anesthetic to soft touch, pinprick or temperature. The café au lait spots should be differentiated from nevocellular nevus by irregular border and lighter color. Pigmentation of lips is a feature of Peutz-Jeghers syndrome which is characterized by multiple polyps of stomach or colon. Dark brown or black pigmentation of extremities at friction sites (knuckles) and buccal mucosa is a characteristic feature of Addison's disease. Carotenemia produces orange-yellowish discoloration of skin akin to jaundice but there is no discoloration of sclera. Livedo reticularis, a web-like pattern of reddish-blue discoloration mostly involving the legs, is seen in autoimmune vasculitis.

Special Examination and Signs

Magnifying hand lens with built-in light is useful to identify the morphology and configuration of skin lesions.

Diascopy A transparent spatula or a glass side is used to apply pressure over the erythematous skin lesions to look for blanching. Blanching occurs when there is vasodilation or telangiectasis (vascular nevus). When blood has leaked out of capillaries (purpura, ecchymosis), no blanching occurs. When a granulomatous skin nodule is examined with diascopy, brownish-yellow translucent "apple-jelly" appearance is suggestive of lupus vulgaris, granuloma annulare, sarcoidosis and tuberculosis.

Koebner phenomenon It refers to appearance of similar skin lesions along the line of injury or scratch. The examples include vitiligo, psoriasis, lichen planus, lichen nitidus, pityriasis rubra pilaris, keratosis follicularis (Darier disease) and molluscum contagiosum.

Dermatographism When skin is firmly stroked with a pointed object, wheal or urticarial response may occur in 50% of normal subjects. In mastocytosis or urticaria pigmentosa, mild stroking of skin with a finger nail or sharp object may lead to severe response resulting in formation of a blister (Darier sign).

Auspitz sign When thick white scales of psoriasis are gently scraped away from the surface of a plaque, tiny bleeding points are seen. The sign is highly suggestive but not diagnostic of psoriasis.

Nikolsky's sign In children with a blistering disorder, rubbing of skin with a finger or a rough rounded object like a pencil eraser may lead to peeling of skin in children with pemphigus and toxic epidermal necrolysis (scalded skin syndrome). The sign is not diagnostic or specific and may be seen in patients with erythema multiforme, epidermolysis bullosa, pemphigoid and variegate porphyria.

VASCULAR NEVI

Vascular birthmarks are hamartomas or benign tumor-like malformations composed of admixture of vascular components. They may be visible at birth or appear later in infancy. Almost 10–25% infants are likely to manifest vascular nevi by the end of first year. The vascular birthmarks are classified as flat (macular) nevi or elevated (papular, nodular or tumor-like). They may spontaneously regress (involuting type) and disappear during a few years or persist throughout life (non-involuting type).

Flat Vascular Nevi

Involuting Type

Salmon patches (nevus simplex) They are most common and found in almost 40% of neonates. They present as dusky pink blanching macules over the eyelids, glabella, forehead (angel kiss) and nape of the neck (stork bite). They invariably fade away during infancy, except nuchal erythemas which may persist much longer.

Spider nevus (nevus araneus) It is a small telangiectatic lesion consisting of a central arteriole from which superficial blood vessels radiate out. The radiating vessels collapse when central punctum is pressed.

Cutis marmorata telangiectasia congenita (congenital phlebectasia) It produces a mottled, marbled pattern of blue or dark-red erythema usually on an extremity. The skin overlying the lesions is depressed unlike livedo reticularis. It should be distinguished from symmetrical mottling of skin following exposure to cold which is a transient vasomotor phenomenon.

Non-Involuting Type

Port-wine stain (nevus flammeus) It presents as dark-red or purple-red macules on the face, neck or extremities with unilateral and segmental distribution. The presence of port-wine stain over the face affecting the skin innervated by the ophthalmic branch of trigeminal nerve may be associated with Sturge-Weber syndrome (ipsilateral glaucoma and leptomeningeal cerebral calcification due to meningeal angiomatosis). Nevus flammeus is a recognized component of Klippel-Trenaunay-Weber syndrome, Parkes Weber syndrome, hyperkeratotic capillary-venous malformation, Proteus syndrome, Rubinstein-Taybi syndrome, Beckwith-Wiedemann syndrome and trisomy-13.

Raised Vascular Nevi

Involuting Type

Hemangioma of infancy (strawberry nevus) The typical skin lesion is dark or bright red like a strawberry raised above the skin surface and compressible on pressure (Figure 9.9). They may be absent or small at birth and enlarge in size as the child grows. They may ulcerate, bleed or compromise the functioning of a vital organ. After one year, the involution starts from the center of the lesion which becomes pale and atrophic. When cavernous hemangiomas are multiple or deep seated, they may be associated with high ouput cardiac failure or disseminated intravascular coagulation (Kasabach-Merritt syndrome) because of trapping of platelets. The deepseated lesions should be differentiated from arteriovenous malformation which may be warm to touch and usually has a thrill or bruit and dignosis can be confirmed by Doppler sonography.

Non-Involuting Type

Cavernous hemangiomas (cavernous angioma) occur due to dilatation of deeply seated blood vessels. They appear pink and raised above the surface like a conglomeration of respberry structures because of the bubble-like caverns. They appear as a red-blue spongy mass of tissue filled with blood. They do not regress and may be complicated by bleeding, disfigurement and CNS manifestations.

Pyogenic granulomas and lymphangiomas are classified in this group but they are not truly vascular nevi. Lymphangioma produces skin-colored, ill-defined mass of lymphatics which hangs loosely, is compressible and transilluminant and feels like a bag of worms. They do not regress and are managed by laser therapy or surgical excision.

WARTS

Warts are caused by more than 200 types of human papillomaviruses (HPV). The virus enters the skin through breaks in the epithelium and cause hyperplasia of the squamous epithelium. The incubation period varies from 1 to 6 months, and the majority of lesions disappear spontaneously. Warts are well-circumscribed papules with an irregular, roughened, keratotic surface. Common warts or verruca vulgaris are skin-colored, rough, minimally scaly papules and nodules found on the exposed surfaces of the hands, face, arms and legs. Flat warts occur in clusters over the hands, arms

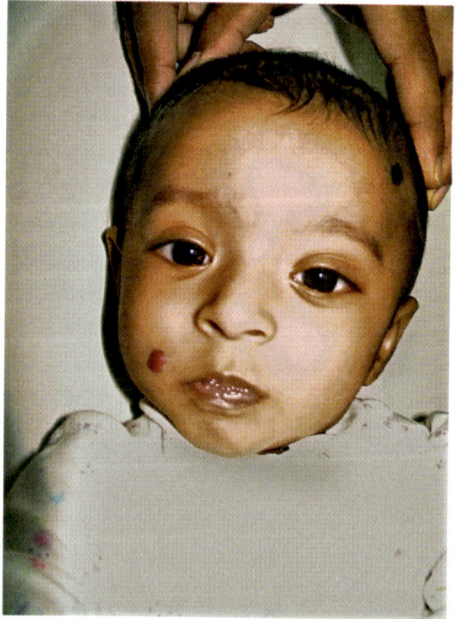

Figure 9.9 Strawberry nevus on the face of one-year-old infant.

and face. Periungual and plantar warts may be painful and occur due to inward-growing hyperkeratotic plaques and papules. Autoinoculation may occur along the lines of scratching (Koebner phenomenon). Anogenital warts occur in sexually active adolescents as a result of infection with HPV types 6 and 11. They are characterized by moist, fleshy, papillomatous lesions on the perianal mucosa (condylomata acuminata), labia, vaginal introitus, perineal raphe and on the shaft, carona and glans penis.

Molluscum Contagiosum

It is caused by a pox virus which is a large double-stranded DNA virus that replicates in the cytoplasm of host epithelial cells. The infection spreads by skin-to-skin contact, fomitis or autoinoculation. It is highly contagious with an incubation period of 2–8 weeks. The skin lesions are discrete, waxy, pearly-white or skin-colored, smooth, dome-shaped papules varying in size from 2–5 mm. They are characterized by central umbilication from which a plug of cheesy material can be expressed. The papules may occur anywhere on the body but the face, eyelids, neck, axillae and thighs are commonly affected. The lesions may develop along scratch marks (Koebner phenomenon). The lesions may be large in size or widespread in immuno-deficient children.

NEUROECTODERMAL DYSPLASIAS

Skin and central nervous system are both ectodermal in origin and presence of ectodermal dysplasias is a good marker of associated CNS abnormalities and seizures. Most of these diseases are inherited as autosomal recessive disorder except ataxia telangiectasia which is an autosomal dominant condition. Their clinical features are summarized in Table 9.5.

TABLE 9.5 Common neuroectodermal dysplasias

Conditions	Skin manifestations	CNS features	Investigations
Sturge-Weber syndrome	Unilateral nevus flammeus (port-wine stain) over upper face and eyelid	Vascular abnormality in the ipsilateral cortex with progressive tonic-clonic seizures on the opposite side, hemiparesis and mental retardation	CT scan of brain shows "railway track" type of calcification with atrophy of the underlying cortex
Tuberous sclerosis	Adenoma sebaceum (acne-like tiny nodules on the cheeks, nose and chin), shagreen patch (like orange peel), rough granulated skin of a shark or fibrous plaques on the lumbosacral region and hypopigmented skin macules like an ashleaf on the extremities and trunk (Figure 9.10). Other major features include subungual fibromas, cardiac rhabdomyoma, renal angiomyolipoma, multiple retinal hamartomas.	Intractable seizures starting as infantile spasms in infancy, mental retardation, behavior problems, noncancerous nodular growth in the kidneys, heart, lungs and eyes	MRI of brain shows typical subependymal calcification and multiple parenchymal tubers

(contd.)

TABLE 9.5 Common neuroectodermal dysplasias (contd.)

Conditions	Skin manifestations	CNS features	Investigations
Neurofibromatosis*	Café au lait spots of more than 5 mm size and more than 5 in number	Seizures with optic glioma and acoustic neuroma with Lisch nodules or hamartomas in the iris	CT scan shows high signal "unidentified bright objects" (UBOs) especially in the basal ganglia, and brainstem
von Hippel-Lindau disease	Cutaneous and visceral hemangiomas	Cerebellar hemangioblastomas and retinal angiomatosis, seizures, cerebellar signs and raised intracranial tension	CT scan of brain shows cystic cerebellar lesions
Ataxia telangiectasia	Telangiectasis of bulbar conjunctiva and skin (Figure 9.11)	Recurrent sinopulmonary infections and progressive disabling cerebellar ataxia with slurred or scanning dysarthric speech	CT scan shows cerebellar atrophy, serum IgA level is reduced and alpha-fetoprotein levels are raised
Epidermal nevus syndrome	Hyperpigmented verrucous epidermal nevi over unilateral side of upper arm, trunk, hip and lumbosacral area. There may be involvement of the skeleton, connective tissue, CNS, ocular, cardiac and genitourinary systems	Intractable seizures, paresis, developmental delay and mental retardation	Unilateral hemimegaloencephaly with multiple structural CNS abnormalities including defects of segmentation and migration
Incontinentia pigmenti (Bloch-Sulzberger syndrome)	It is a rare X-linked disorder due to mutation of IKBKG gene which encodes the NEMO protein. There is blistering skin rash along Blaschko's lines which heal as brown patches that fade with time. Other symptoms include pitted nails, hair loss, dental and visual abnormalities. The condition is seen more commonly in females because males die early	Seizures, cerebrovascular accidents, developmental delay, mental retardation, microcephaly and intellectual disability	Cerebral atrophy with formation of small cavities and loss of neurons in the cerebellum

*The other conditions which are associated with café au lait macules (CALMs) and neurofibromatosis include McCune-Albright syndrome, Bloom syndrome, Watson syndrome, Silver-Russell syndrome, ataxia telangiectasia, tuberous sclerosis and Gaucher disease.

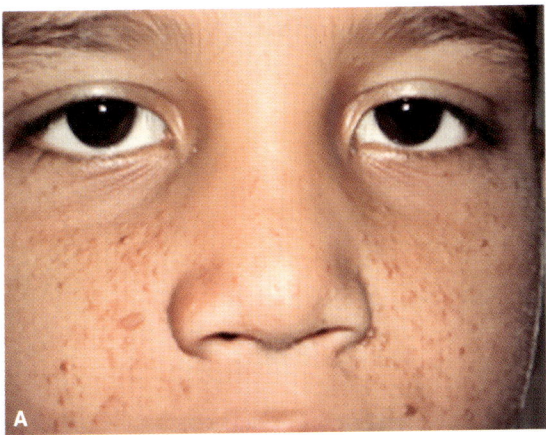
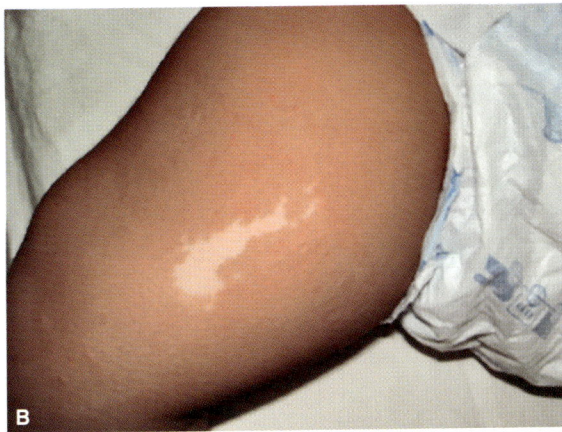

Figure 9.10A and B (A) Typical flesh-colored papulonodular skin lesions of adenoma sebaceum on the cheeks and nose. (B) Ash-leaf depigmented macule over the thigh. This patient had classic triad of tuberous sclerosis, i.e. adenoma sebaceum, intracranial calcification, and epilepsy.

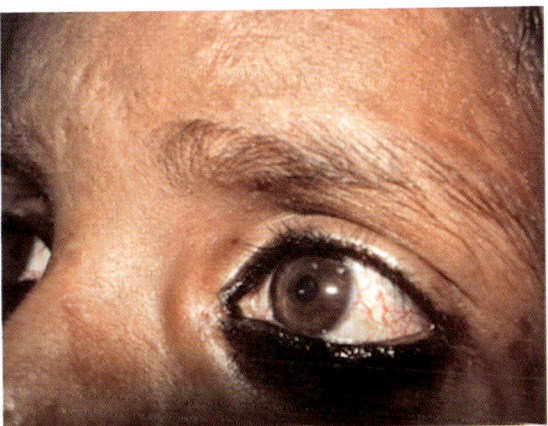

Figure 9.11 Characteristic telangiectasia over the bulbar conjunctiva in a child with ataxia telangiectasia.

APPENDAGES OF SKIN

Hair and nails provide protection to the skin and have common embryologic origin or background. Many developmental or acquired skin disorders may have associated abnormalities in the hair, nails, and teeth. Nails may be absent in nail-patella syndrome. *Splinter hemorrhages* under the nail bed may occur due to trauma, psoriasis, collagen vascular disorder, bacterial endocarditis and trichinosis. Several acquired disorders of skin are associated with abnormalities in the mucous membranes, hair and nails. Anhidrotic ectodermal dysplasia is characterized by hyperthermia (fever

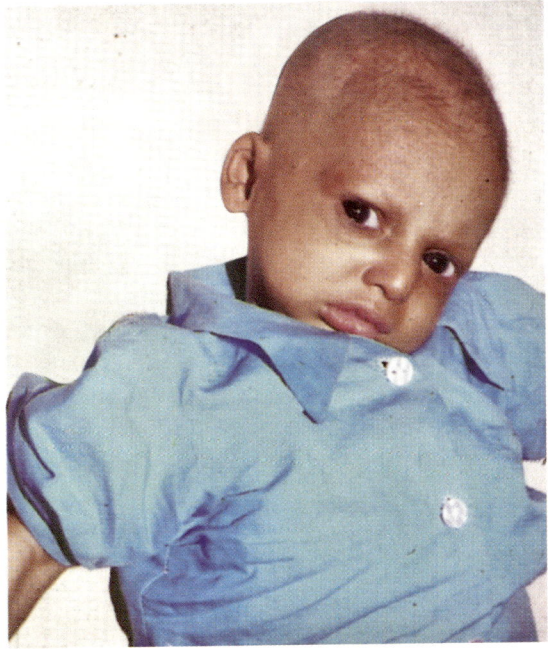

Figure 9.12 Alopecia, absence of eyebrows and eyelashes in an infant with anhidrotic ectodermal dysplasia.

due to rise of environmental temperature because of absence of sweat glands), alopecia, absence of eyebrows and eyelashes (Figure 9.12). Hypertrichosis or excessive generalized growth of body hair over the non-sexual areas of the body is seen in a number of systemic disorders (*Box 9.3*).

> **Box 9.3 Systemic conditions associated with hypertrichosis**
>
> - Familial or constitutional
> - Drugs like corticosteroids, phenytoin, cyclosporin, and minoxidil
> - Cushing syndrome
> - Chronic malnutrition or starvation
> - Porphyria cutanea tarda
> - Coffin-Siris syndrome
> - Cornelia de Lange syndrome
> - Treacher Collins syndrome (hair on the side of the face)

Hirsutism or androgen-related male-pattern of hair growth on the face and pubis in adolescent girls is most commonly idiopathic as a racial or constitutional trait due to end-organ hypersensitivity to androgens. The common causes of hirsutism are listed in *Box 9.4*. When there is androgen excess, libido is increased and menstrual cycles become irregular and scanty. The presence of regular menstrual cycles is a good evidence against significant androgen excess, suggesting that hirsutism is constitutional and not pathological.

Scalp should be examined for seborrhea, discoid lesions of tinea capitis and psoriasis, alopecia, pediculosis and depigmentation. The presence of an occasional grey scalp hair in a child is a cause for concern for some parents. It is of no clinical significance and is often ascribed to constitutional factors or chronic illness and nutritional disorder. The presence of white forelock or piebaldism may be associated with sensorineural deafness (Waardenburg syndrome) and Hirschsprung disease (Shah-Waardenburg syndrome.) Rarely, hair may show alternate bands of depigmentation producing typical flag sign in children with kwashiorkor. A number of systemic disorders are

> **Box 9.4 Common causes of hirsutism**
>
> - Racial or constitutional
> - Polycystic ovary disease (PCOD)
> - Late-onset congenital adrenal hyperplasia
> - Androgen-secreting ovarian or adrenal tumor (Cushing syndrome)
> - Acromegaly
> - Intake of androgens, progestogens and corticosteroids

> **Box 9.5 Causes of sparse, light-brown and brittle scalp hair**
>
> - Kwashiorkor
> - Cretinism
> - Chronic debilitating disease
> - Progeria
> - Ectodermal dysplasia
> - Hypervitaminosis A
> - Acrodynia
> - Adrenal insufficiency
> - Cartilage-hair hypoplasia syndrome
> - Langer-Giedion syndrome
> - Hallermann-Streiff syndrome
> - Trichotillomania (a ball of hair or trichobezoar due to swallowed hair may cause obstruction in the stomach)
> - Trichorrhexis nodosa ("paint-brush" hair)
> - Incontinentia pigmenti
> - Conradi disease
> - Congenital syphilis
> - Idiopathic hyperparathyroidism
> - Zinc deficiency
> - Copper deficiency
> - Acrodermatitis enteropathica
> - Biotinidase deficiency
> - Anorexia nervosa
> - Homocystinuria
> - Menke's syndrome (kinky hair disease)
> - Alopecia areata (no hair follicles with typical "exclamation mark" hair over the bald area)
> - Traction alopecia ("pony-tail" alopecia)
> - Tinea capitis
> - Coffin–Siris syndrome
> - Polyendocrine deficiency
> - Scarring alopecia (burns, severe infections, lichen planus, systemic lupus erythematosus, herpes zoster
> - Drug induced *(Figure 9.13)*

associated with sparse light-brown and brittle scalp hair *(Box 9.5)*. Many of these disorders are associated with a variety of skin manifestations.

Pitting of nails along with thickening, loss of lustre and subungual keratosis may occur in psoriasis, atopic dermatitis and onychomycosis. White spots or vertical lines in the nails (leukonychia) may be caused by trauma, nutritional deficiency and chronic debilitating disorders. Beau's lines are transverse ridges or grooves on the nails due to temporary interference in the formation of nail plate because of systemic illness, nutritional disorder, cytotoxic drugs or trauma.

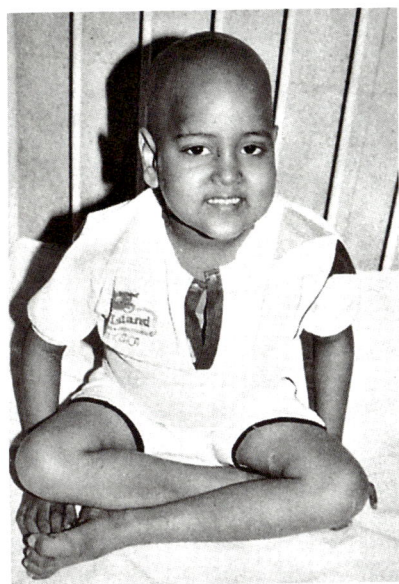

Figure 9.13 Alopecia due to cyclophosphamide therapy for Hodgkin disease.

Dystrophic nails is a recognized feature of epidermolysis bullosa, ectodermal dysplasia, chondroectodermal dysplasia and nail-patella syndrome. Dysplasia of nails is seen in infants with fetal alcohol and phenytoin syndromes. Tuberous sclerosis may have associated subungual and periungual fibromas arising from the groove of the nail beds of fingers and toes.

COMMON SKIN CONDITIONS

There are a number of relatively common and some unusual skin conditions which should be identified by the primary physician and pediatrician. Most dermatological conditions are diagnosed on the basis of morphology and distribution of skin lesions. The salient diagnostic clinical features of common skin disorders are given below. The list is merely representative and in no way exhaustive.

Acne Vulgaris

It is chronic inflammation of the pilosebaceous units due to excessive production of androgens during adolescence and puberty. The common predisposing factors include genetic predisposition, sex hormones, emotional stress and intake of certain drugs (corticosteroids, hydantoin, lithium). Seborrhea of the scalp and face due to excessive secretion of sebum may coexist. Microbial colonization (*Propionibacterium acnes*) and occlusion of pilosebaceous orifices with keratin plugs leads to perpetuation of lesions. The disorder is more severe in males, while it is more protracted in females. The sites of predilection of skin lesions include face, neck, upper arms, shoulders and back. A variety of skin lesions, like papules, nodules and cysts may occur. The characteristic skin lesions are open comedones, 2–5 mm flesh-colored papules with black plugs of keratin (black heads). The black tip of the comedone is not due to dirt but occurs because of oxidation of melanin. The closed comedones or white heads are 1–3 mm flesh-colored papules with pinpoint openings. The white heads out number black heads in a ratio of 10–20:1. Superadded bacterial infection and unnecessary squeezing of comedones or nodules may lead to formation of "ice-pick" scars which may be atrophic (pitted scars) or hypertrophic (keloids).

Scabies

It is a highly contagious disease caused by the bites of a mite *Sarcoptes scabiei var. hominis*. The incubation period is about 2–6 weeks. The symptoms may develop within 1–4 days in patients with reexposure and recurrence. The characteristic skin lesions include linear or S-shaped burrows with black dots at the leading edge mostly over the axillae, beltline, extremities especially flexor aspects of wrists, interdigital areas of palms and soles and genital region. Due to hypersensitivity reaction to the mites and their products, intensely pruritic papular or papular-vesicular rash develops over lower abdoman, buttocks, axillary folds and groins. The face is usually spared except in infants. There is intense and intractable itching especially at night. There is secondary excoriations, eczematous areas, pustules and crusting as a consequence of itching, rubbing and secondary infection. Itching may continue even after resolution of skin lesions because of hypersensitivity reaction of the mites. The disease is highly contagious and several family members are affected simultaneously.

Atopic Dermatitis

The distribution of skin rash in atopic dermatitis varies depending upon the age. In infancy, cheeks, wrists and extensor surfaces of the arms and legs typically develop papulovesicular, often weeping or wet lesions, which may develop fine scabs or lichenification (Figure 9.14). The scalp and postauricular areas are often affected while diaper area is usually spared. Secondary infection and traumatic lesions may develop due to scratching and rubbing. Primary herpes simplex infection may occur with crops of hemorrhagic vesiculopustular lesions limited to areas of pre-existing atopic dermatitis (eczema herpeticum). In older children, dry maculopapular lesions are mostly distributed over the flexor surfaces of extremities, neck, wrists and ankles. Xerosis and lichenfication commonly supervenes. In a number of disorders, skin rash is distributed over flexural surfaces. There may be personal or family history of atopy. Eosinophilia and elevation of serum IgE levels provide useful laboratory support to the diagnosis.

Wiskott-Aldrich syndrome (WAS) It is a rare X-linked disorder characterized by eczema, thrombocytopenia (reduced number as well as size of platelets), immune deficiency and bloody diarrhea. These infants are prone to develop auto-immune disorders.

Seborrheic Dermatitis

Seborrheic dermatitis is usually associated with seborrhea capitis (dandruff) and has predilection for infants and adolescents. The condition starts from scalp with greasy-yellowish scales and extends down the forehead to involve the eyebrows, nose and ears. Intertriginous areas and diaper area may be affected due to superadded candida infection. Loss of scalp hair and depigmented skin lesions are seen during the course of the disease. The clinical differentiation from atopic dermatitis may be difficult at times. Absence of eosinophilia and normal serum IgE levels support the diagnosis of seborrheic dermatitis.

Urticaria and Angioedema

There is sudden appearance of generalized wheals (edematous papules and plaques) which are intensely pruritic and may be associated with large edematous areas that involve the dermis and subcutaneous tissue (angioedema). The etiology is unknown in 80–90% cases and predisposing conditions include atopy, allergy to food or drugs, acute infection, physical stimuli (water, cold, sunlight, pressure) and emotional stress. Urticaria may be acute and recurrent (<6 weeks duration), which is usually IgE-mediated and associated with atopic background. Chronic urticaria is diagnosed when condition persists for more than 6 weeks, it is rarely IgE-dependent and often exacerbated by emotional stress. Angioedema is diagnosed when there is marked edema of the dermis involving the face (eyelids, lips, tongue), larynx or extremity.

Papular Urticaria

It is a common, intensely pruritic disorder caused by an allergic response to the bites of blood-sucking insects, especially dog and cat fleas, bed bugs and sometimes mosquitoes. The fresh lesions are papules with a central punctum on an erythematous

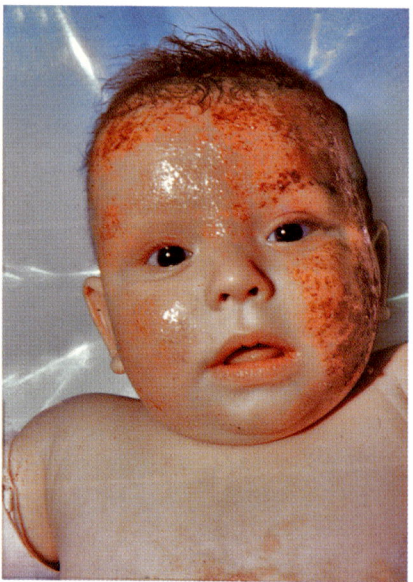

Figure 9.14 Infantile eczema. Papulovesicular weeping or wet lesions are classically distributed over the cheeks, wrists and extensor surfaces of arms and legs in infants with atopic dermatitis.

base mostly distributed over the exposed areas of skin. The lesions are markedly pruritic and frequently grouped or clustered. Most cases occur during summer and spring due to mosquito and flea bites. Excoriations and secondary infection may lead to hyperpigmentation in older lesions.

Nutritional Disorders

Acrodermatitis Enteropathica

It is a rare autosomal disorder of zinc transport due to defective gene which is mapped to 8q24. Breast milk contains compensatory zinc-binding ligand that facilitates absorption of zinc. The manifestations start after 1–2 weeks of weaning from breast-feeding. It is characterized by eczematous scaly skin rash which becomes vesicular, bullous, pustular or desquamative, involving peripheral or acral parts of the extremities, perioral and anogenital areas. Angular cheilitis (perleche) is a common early manifestation followed by paronychia. It is usually associated with intractable diarrhea, graying of hair, progressive alopecia and superadded infection with bacteria and *Candida albicans*. Acrodermatitis enteropathica is characterized by triad of acrodermatitis with special predilection for body orifices, diarrhea and alopecia. The condition should be differentiated from severe sehorrheic dermatitis, deficiency of essential fatty acids, niacin and biotin, and methylmalonic acidemia.

Zinc deficiency Skin manifestations are characteristically seen around the perioral, periorbital and perianal areas. Distal parts of limbs especially hands and feet also develop skin manifestations. The vesiculobullous skin lesions soon become dry, scaly and crusted with sharply demarcated borders. The vesicles rapidly rupture, revealing a moist, red base which subsequently dries and appears like a plaque. Diarrhea and alopecia are commonly associated. Affected infants are irritable, listless and fail to thrive.

Essential fatty acid deficiency It is characterized by generalized scaly dermatitis composed of thickened, erythematous, desquamating plaques. Alopecia, thrombocytopenia and failure to thrive are often associated.

Skin Lesions with Fine Scales

Pityriasis alba It is a common, asymptomatic skin condition of unknown etiology in young children between the ages of 6–12 years. It is considered as a mild form of atopic dermatitis. The lesions are more common in summer and following exposure to sunlight. The skin lesions are ill-defined hypopigmented round or oval patches with minimal fine lamellar or branny scales. The lesions, 1–3 in number, most commonly occur on the face but may be present on the neck, upper trunk and proximal parts of limbs.

Pityriasis or tinea versicolor It is characterized by appearance of asymptomatic ovoid or coin-shaped brown-colored or whitish macules over the neck, upper chest and back. The lesions have fine branny scales (pityriasis means "bran-like" scales) which can be easily scraped off with the edge of a glass slide. Pruritus is usually absent or minimal. Most cases occur after puberty during hot and humid summer months. KOH preparation may show characteristic round and elongated cells of *M. furfur*.

Pityriasis rosea It is a benign self-limited disorder of unknown etiology usually seen in adolescent children and young adults. There is some evidence that the disease may have a viral etiology because it is common in spring and autumn and one attack usually gives long-lasting immunity. The rash may be preceded by mild constitutional symptoms, such as fever, headache, malaise and arthralgia. In half the patients, there is an oval flesh-colored *herald patch* on the trunk measuring 1–10 cm in size. It is usually present on the trunk as a round or oval patch with a central wrinkled salmon-colored area and a darker peripheral zone separated by a "collarette of scales".

After a few days of herald patch, generalized skin rash appears on the trunk and proximal parts of extremities, especially the thighs. The eruption consists of oval flesh-colored or pink macules with central clearing and raised fine scaly edges. The skin lesions are usually symmetrical and their long axis follows lines of cleavage resulting in a pattern of christmas or fur tree on the back. Itching is minimal or absent. The disorder is often mistaken with tinea corporis and skin lesions at times are described as "lots of ringworms" by the young resident. The eruption continues to evolve for about 2 weeks and skin lesions usually persist for 4 to 8 weeks and at times for several months. Administration of oral erythromycin or doxycycline and exposure to UV light may hasten the recovery.

Fungal Infections (Dermatophytoses)

Tinea capitis There are no characteristic features. It often presents as a kerion with an inflammatory, boggy, pustular patch with localized alopecia of scalp. The typical scaly circular lesion with raised edges and central clearing that is seen in tinea corporis is uncommon in tinea capitis. There is formation of scales, eczematization, and scab formation. The condition should be differntiated from seborrheic dermatitis, pustular folliculitis and trichotillomania. The KOH preparation is not reliable in tinea capitis and diagnosis is best confirmed by fungal culture.

Tinea corporis It is characterized by annular erythematous ring lesions with active elevated margins and central clearing. The border is generally scaly, slightly elevated and often studded with microvesicles and tiny pustules. The lesions may be single or multiple. Tinea corporis should be differentiated from herald patch of pityriasis rosea, granuloma annulare and dry nummular eczema.

Candida infection Candida infection of skin has special predilection for moist areas like diaper area, neck, axillae, groin, perioral and perianal regions (Figure 9.15). It produces confluent bright-red erythema with maceration and fissuring. There are vesiculopustular lesions over the elevated edge or periphery of erythematous base as "satellite lesions". In candidiasis of diaper area, deep areas of inguinal folds are invariably affected. Oral thrush and paronychial candidal infection may coexist. There may be history of prolonged antibiotic therapy and poor response to conventional treatment of diaper rash. Examination of pustule contents by KOH preparation may reveal typical

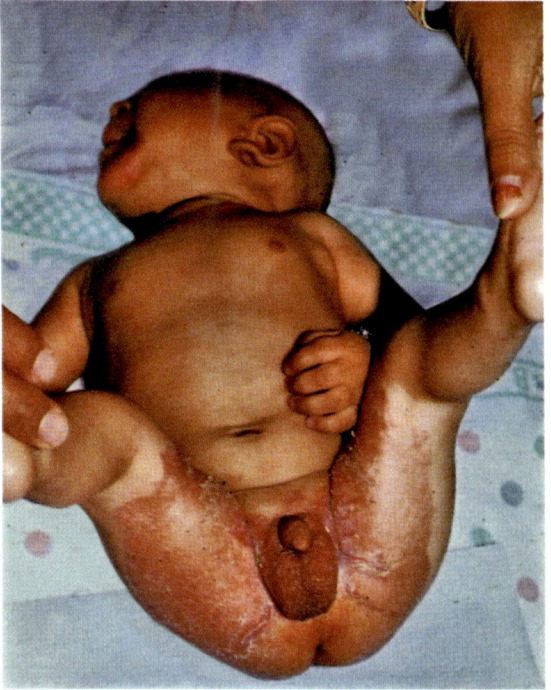

Figure 9.15 Scaly erythematous skin rash over the groins, perianal and perioral regions due to disseminated candida infection

budding yeasts and pseudohyphae of *Candida albicans*. Congenital cutaneous candidiasis is characterized at birth or within 12 hours of life by multiple erythematous macules or vesiculopustular lesions. After neonatal period, development of recurrent or persistent candidiasis should alert the pediatrician to look for an underlying cell-mediated immunodeficiency disorder, HIV infection, diabetes mellitus, hypoparathyroidism (DiGeorge syndrome), Addison's disease, biotinase deficiency and malignancy.

Miscellaneous Conditions

Miliaria (prickly heat or heat rash) It is an acute inflammatory eruption due to blockage or trapping of sweat in the eccrine sweat glands. The condition usually occurs in hot and humid weather. The rash is generalized with predilection for upper chest, neck, back and skin creases. The morphology of skin lesions depends on the depth of the obstruction of the sweat glands. In miliaria crystalline, ductal obstruction is in the uppermost epidermis with formation of minute, tense and transparent vesicles without any inflammation. In miliaria rubra, obstruction to sweat is deeper in the epidermis with formation of itchy erythematous papules with an intense "pins and needles" burning sensation. In miliaria profunda, there are deep-seated painful papules which are mostly limited to intertriginous areas. The lesions may become pustular with superadded bacterial infection (miliaria pustulosa).

Drug Eruptions

Adverse cutaneous drug eruptions are common and range from transient maculopapular skin rash to Stevens-Johnson syndrome or even fatal toxic epidermal necrolysis (TEN). The most common drug eruptions include maculopapular skin rash and fixed drug eruption. Drug eruptions may occur following any medication but are most common during administration of sulfonamides (co-trimoxazole), dapsone, antibiotics (especially penicillin and its derivatives), antiepileptics and antitubercular drugs.

The drug eruption is characterized by sudden appearance of skin rash during intake of drug(s) (Allopathic, Homeopathic, Ayurvedic, etc.), home remedies or topical agents. The skin rash is sudden or abrupt in onset, symmetrical in distribution (except in fixed drug eruption) and often pruritic. The morphology of the rash may be exanthematous (erythematous, macular, maculopapular), urticarial or vesicular. The skin eruption resolves on withdrawal of drug and would reappear when same or a similar drug is given again to the patient. In immune-mediated drug eruptions, there may be eosinophilia or elevation of IgE antibodies. *In any patient with sudden onset of skin eruption, adverse cutaneous drug reaction must be considered, if child is receiving medications.*

Fixed drug eruptions are uncommon in children but manifest with characteristic skin lesions which recur at fixed sites on re-exposure to the drug. There are single or multiple circular or oval erythematous macule(s) or plaque(s) with burning or tingling sensation. They are commonly located at the mucocutaneous junctions and leave behind coin-shaped slate-gray colored pigmentation on healing.

Phrynoderma (Toad Skin)

Phrynoderma is a type of follicular hyperkeratosis which is typically distributed over the extensor surfaces of elbows, knees, anterolateral thighs and buttocks. The morphology of skin lesions is variable and may range from filiform papules to small conical papules and at times large papules with horny puncta. Generalized xerosis with fine wrinkles and scales may be present. Phrynoderma is a classical manifestation of vitamin A deficiency but it may be associated with deficiencies of vitamin B complex, vitamin C, vitamin E and essential fatty acids. The condition should be differentiated from keratosis pilaris and Darier's disease.

Erythema Multiforme

It is characterized by erythematous lesions of pleomorphic morphology over the extremities. It is a distinctive acute hypersensitivity disorder, which is triggered by recurrent infection with herpes simplex virus (HSV). The lesions begin as erythematous macules and evolve into papules, vesicles, bullae, urticarial plaques or patches of confluent erythema. The pathognomonic lesions of erythema multiforme are iris or target-shaped lesions which have a dusky center, an inner pale ring and an erythematous outer border. The edges of lesions may vesiculate. In many cases, the initial crop of lesions may simulate urticaria but itching is minimal. The symmetric crops of skin lesions usually occur on extensor surfaces of arms and legs often involving palms and soles **(Figure 9.16)**. The constitutional symptoms are mild, consisting of low grade fever, malaise, and myalgia. The skin lesions may heal over 4–6 weeks with hypopigmentation or hyperpigmentation but without any scarring. When skin lesions are associated with involvement of two or more mucous membranes, the condition is called Stevens-Johnson syndrome **(Figure 9.17)**.

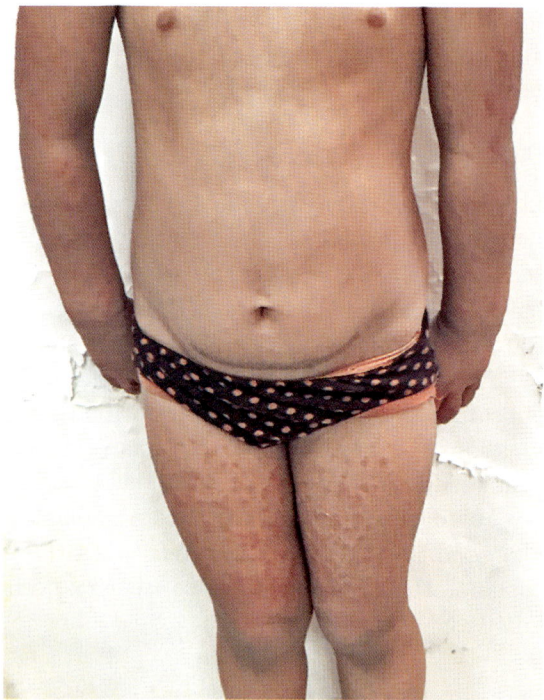

Figure 9.16 Polymorphous symmetrical target lesions widely distributed over the extremities in a 9-year-old girl.

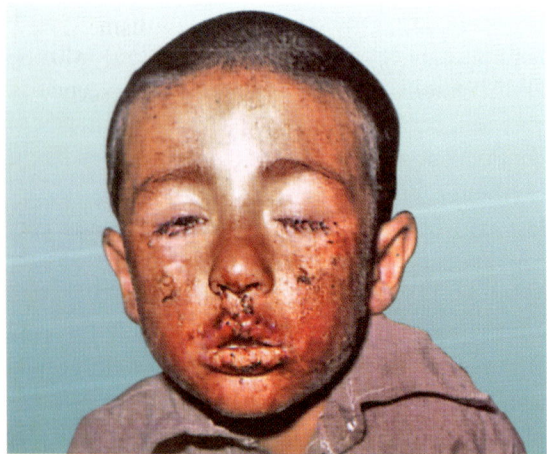

Figure 9.17 Stevens-Johnson syndrome due to intake of phenytoin. Erythema multiforme is associated with marked involvement of buccal mucosa, conjunctiva, perianal and urethral areas.

Lichen Planus (LP)

Lichen planus is a papulosquamous disorder characterized by pruritic, polygonal-shaped, flat-topped, shiny, violaceous papules and plaques. Examination with a hand lens may reveal a network of gray lines (Wickham's striae). The skin lesions have a special predilection for involvement of wrists, shins, lower back and genitalia. Involvement of scalp may lead to hair loss. Buccal mucosa is commonly involved leading to white net-like reticular eruption. There may be involvement of nails (dystrophy). Koebner's phenomenon may be present, i.e. the lesions may occur in areas of local injury, such as scratches. The etiology of LP is unknown but it may be immunologically mediated with genetic predisposition. Its course is variable but most patients have spontaneous remission within 6 months to 2 years. After resolution of primary lesions, there is a prolonged period of post-inflammatory hyperpigmentation. Topical steroids provide symptomatic relief.

Granuloma Annulare

It is an uncommon chronic skin disorder affecting school-going children and young adults. It is characterized by appearance of semilunar or arciform flesh-colored or pink smooth papules. The lesions coalesce to assume oval, round or ring shaped with central clearing. The size of lesions varies between 1 and 5 cm, single or multiple, may occur anywhere on the body but most commonly over the extremities. The skin lesions are smooth, without any scales or epidermal involvement. The lesions are asymptomatic and may take a few months to 2 years to resolve spontaneously. Absence of epidermal involvement, lack of scales, multiple lesions without itching differentiate granuloma annulare from tinea corporis.

Vitiligo

It is characterized by development of depigmented patches of skin due to dysfunction or destruction of melanocytes possibly because of an autoimmune mechanism. There is increased association with other autoimmune disorders, like thyroiditis, adrenal insufficiency, pernicious anemia, polyendocrinopathy and mucocutaneous candidiasis. Family history may be positive in one-third of patients. The distribution of lesions at the margins

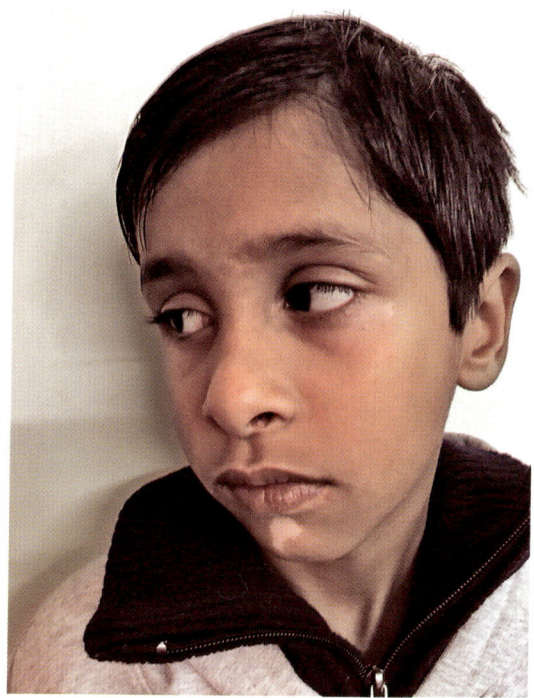

Figure 9.18 Classical milky-white skin lesions of vitiligo over the chin and angle of eye.

or adjacent to the eyes, nose, lips and genitals is characteristic of vitiligo (Figure 9.18). Skin lesions are usually oval in shape and form various geographic patterns with scalloped margins. In dark-skinned subjects, the patches assume milky-white or snow-white color. The distribution of skin lesion may be generalized and symmetrical or limited to a segment of the trunk or limb. The lesions are more likely to occur at the sites of repeated trauma (ankles, elbows, knees) or scratching (Koebner phenomenon). Depigmentation or graying of hair, choroid and retina (chorioretinitis) may be associated.

Psoriasis

It is a genetically determined, inflammatory and proliferative disorder of the skin because of unknown etiology. It is a chronic disorder characterized by appearance of sharply demarcated, dull-red or salmon-colored papules and plaques covered with silvery-white scales. When attempts are made to remove the scales, there is oozing of miniscule droplets of blood (Auspitz phenomenon). Skin lesions may occur at any site but are more common over the elbows, knees, intertriginous areas and scalp. The lesions over the palms and soles may become pustular. Rarely generalized erythrodermic psoriasis may be seen in infants. The skin lesions are aggravated by intake of certain drugs (oral corticosteroids, lithium, beta blockers, chloroquine, alcohol), exposure to sunlight, stress and obesity. There may be involvement of nails leading to pitting, subungual hyperkeratosis and yellowish-brown spots under the nail plate (oil-spots). Psoriatic arthropathy is uncommon in children.

Dermatitis Herpetiformis (DH)

It is a chronic autoimmune blistering disorder often associated with gluten intolerance. It has no association or relationship with herpes virus. There is symmetrical distribution of intensely pruritic urticarial papules and vesicles that are often excoriated by itching. Skin lesions are distributed over extensor surfaces (knees and elbows), back, buttocks and posterior scalp. Intake of wheat is known to exacerbate DH. There is an increased association with a number of autoimmune disorders including celiac disease, hypothyroidism, Type 1 diabetes mellitus, vitiligo and rheumatoid arthritis. Skin biopsy with direct immunofluorescence is diagnostic.

Graft-Versus-Host Disease (GVHD)

The acute form of GVHD manifests with maculopapular rash (which may progress to toxic epidermal necrolysis in a fulminant case) with diarrhea, tachypnea and hepatosplenomegaly. The chronic form of GVHD is characterized by hyperkeratotic skin rash, hepatosplenomegaly, hair loss, chronic diarrhea and wasting.

Toxic Epidermal Necrolysis (TEN)

It is characterized by loosening of large sheets of epidermis with formation of flaccid bullae. The bullae rupture leading to exposure of intensely pink, underlying epidermis or dermis which gives an appearance of scalded skin. Nikolsky sign is positive, i.e. epidermis can be readily peeled off by rubbing the skin at the normal sites. Other conditions with positive Nikolysky sign include pemphigus vulgaris and staphylococcal scalded skin syndrome.

TORCH Infections

Intrauterine infections may show manifestations of petechiae and ecchymoses over the trunk and extremities because of thrombocytopenia. "Blue berry muffin" spots are discrete, well-circumscribed skin lesions due to dermal erythropoiesis in severely affected infants with congenital CMV infection **(Figure 9.19)**.

Congenital Syphilis

It is a multiorgan disease, the clinical manifestations usually appear during third to eighth week of life and in all cases by third month of life. Early features include fever, malaise, snuffles (persistent nasal discharge) followed by development of fissures, cracks or linear scars (rhagades) especially at the angles of mouth and nose. The skin manifestations include features of secondary syphilis like scaly papules, plaques, bullae, desquamation of palms and soles, condylomata lata and mucous patches. There is generalized lymphadenopathy, hepatosplenomegaly, pseudoparalysis (pain due to osteochondritis or epiphysitis) with "saw tooth" metaphyses. The skull may look like "hot cross bun", with saddle nose deformity, multicuspid molars (mulberry molars) and notched central incisors (Hutchinson's teeth). The classical Hutchinson's triad includes Hutchinson's teeth (permanent upper central incisors are widely spaced, peg-shaped and notched), interstitial keratitis and eighth nerve deafness. Syphilitic chorioretinitis is characterized by "salt and pepper" changes in the fundus. There may be painless swelling of knee joints (Clutton's or Charcot's joints), saber tibiae, palatal perforation, neurosyphilis (tabes dorsalis, general paresis and localized gummata) and paroxysmal cold hemoglobinuria. Clutton's joints refer to symmetrical joint swelling (mostly knees) seen in patients with congenital syphilis. It is usually painless and occurs due to synovitis with joint effusions. In contrast, Charcot's joints refer to neuropathic osteoarthropathy because of progressive degeneration of weight-bearing joints (mostly ankles).

Cutaneous Tuberculosis

Mycobacterium tuberculosis can affect any organ of the body. The skin manifestations depend upon the immunity of the patient and route of inoculation. The diagnosis is confirmed by isolation of acid-fast bacilli and histopathology of skin lesions.

Lupus vulgaris It is characterized by a solitary well-demarcated reddish-brown plaque on head, neck and thighs. When lesion is pressed with a glass slide or transparent spatula (diascopy), pale yellow apple jelly nodules are visible. During recovery, center becomes atrophic and scarred with development of nodules.

Scrofuloderma The skin is involved by contiguous inoculation from tubercular lymph node(s) (usually cervical), bone (tibia) or joint (sternoclavicular). There is chronic discharging ulcer with non-healing undermined bluish edges.

Tuberculous verrucosa cutis It is a rare manifestation of cutaneous tuberculosis which is characterized by a solitary firm and warty plaque with a violaceous halo and central scarring.

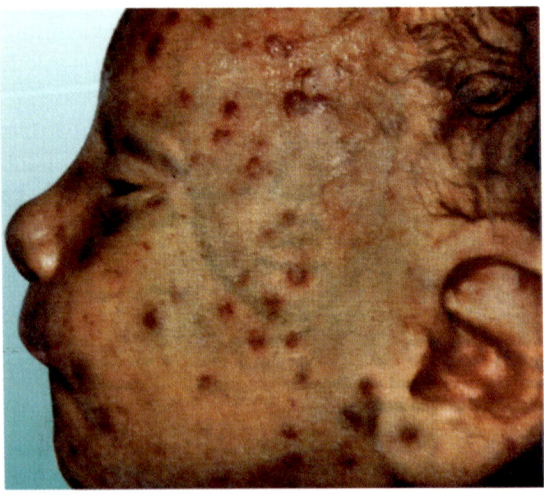

Figure 9.19 Classical "blue berry muffins" spots over the face due to dermal erythropoiesis in an infant with congenital CMV infection.

Tuberculosis cutis orificialis There are painful shallow ulcers with undermined bluish edges over the mucosa and skin adjoining the orifices in patients with advanced pulmonary, intestinal or urogenital tuberculosis.

Hansen's Disease

Hansen disease or leprosy is a chronic granulomatous disease affecting the skin and peripheral nerves. The disease has a long incubation period (usually >6 months) and is caused by *Mycobacterium leprae*. The infection is transmitted through aerosol spread from infected nasal secretions. Skin lesions consist of macules, plaques and nodules which are hypopigmented and erythematous with well-defined margins. There is atrophy of skin with loss of sweating and hair over the involved skin. The patches are characteristically hypoanesthetic or anesthetic due to involvement of peripheral nerves which become thickened and tender on palpation. Advanced cases develop sequelae, like trophic ulcers, deformities (saddle nose, claw hand and toes, foot drop) and ophthalmological complications. Demonstration of acid-fast bacilli from skin smear or biopsy material is diagnostic.

Scheme of Presentation

Systemic features None or there is irritability (due to itching), fever, toxemia, pallor, diarrhea, anorexia, developmental delay, involvement of joints, features suggestive of immunodeficiency disorder, autoimmune disorder, and hepatocellular failure.

Onset Acute (a few hours or 1 to 2 days), chronic (weeks or months), persistent, or there are remissions and relapses. Identify any aggravating triggers.

Distribution of skin lesions Site of skin lesions, localized or generalized, symmetrical or asymmetrical, over the exposed areas or covered areas, flexor or extensor surfaces, flexural areas or creases like neck, axillae, groins, sites of injury (Koebner phenomenon) hands and feet, external genitals and perianal areas. The distribution of skin lesions should be depicted on the front and back views of the human figure.

Morphology of skin lesions
Primary lesions Macules, papules, maculopapular, vesicles, bullae, pustules, wheals, skin patches or plaques, warts, comedones, adenoma sebaceum, ash-leaf macules, shagreen patches, café au lait spots, interdigital burrows, petechiae, purpura, ecchymoses.
Secondary lesions Excoriations or erosions due to scratching, scales, crusts, desquamation, fissures, lichenification, or atrophy, hyperkeratosis, scar or keloid.

Configuration and distribution of skin lesions Grouped or clustered, limited over a dermatome (shingles), coin-shaped or discoid, semicircular or arcuate, circular, annular or ring shaped, linear (Koebner phenomen or secondary to scratching), serpentine or gyrate, guttate like a splash of paint, reticular like a net (livedo reticularis).

Color of skin lesions Brown or skin colored, pale or hypopigmented, dark or hyperpigmented, erythematous, heliotropic, orange-yellow discoloration (jaundice, carotenemia).

Mucous membranes Spared or involved, nature and distribution of lesions over the mucosae of oral cavity, tongue and lips, anterior chamber of eyes, perivulvar, vaginal, urethral and anal areas.

Special signs When indicated look for features on diascopy, dermatographism or Koebner phenomenon, Darier's sign, Auspitz sign and Nikolsky's sign.

Appendages of Skin
Hair
Scalp Normal, brown colored, sparse, coarse and brittle hair, localized or generalized alopecia, tinea capitis, seborrhea, gray hair, white forelock or piebaldism.
Body Absence of eyebrows and eyelashes, lack of sweating or excessive sweating, hirsutism (facial hair in girls) and excessive body hair (hypertrichosis).

Nails Dystrophic or dysplastic nails, pitting of nails with white spots or vertical lines, Beau's lines, thickening of nails with loss of lustre, subungual keratosis or fibromas, koilonychia or clubbing of nails.

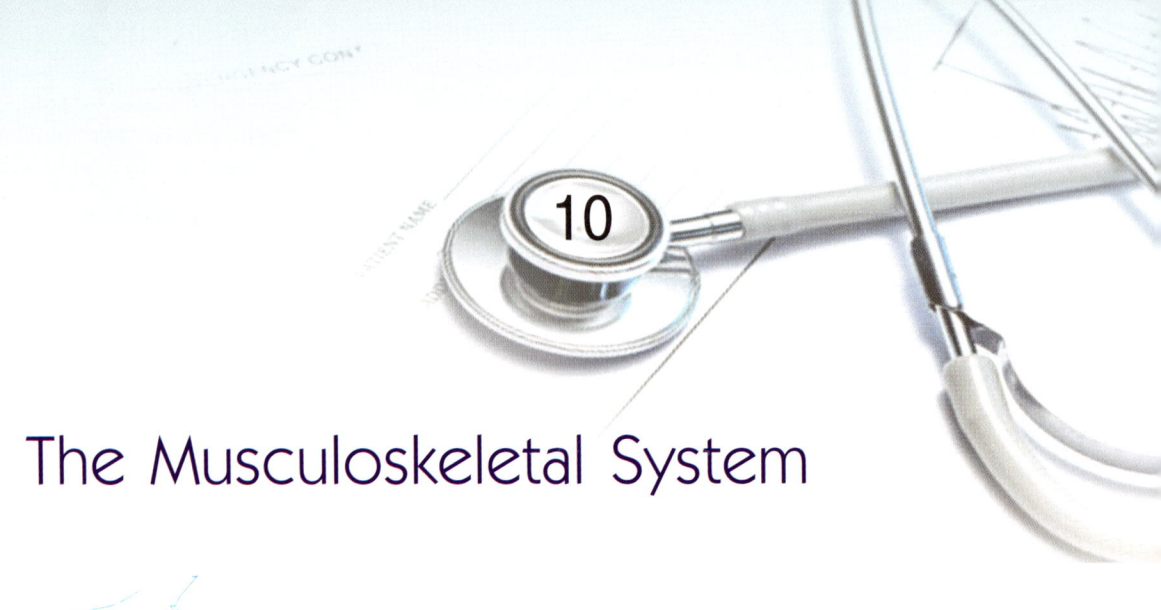

10

The Musculoskeletal System

HISTORY

The musculoskeletal system determines the body build, stature, posture and locomotion. The child should be watched for his gait and stance as he enters the examination chamber. Ask the presenting complaints in a chronological order with special emphasis on mode and type of onset, whether acute or insidious, and evolution of the disease process. Identify whether the symptoms are related to the muscles and other soft tissue structures or the underlying bones and joints by asking the child to point to the exact site and source of discomfort. The developmental, chromosomal and metabolic disorders of bones and muscles are extremely common and likely to have their onset at birth or early in life. Oligohydramnios may lead to postural defects due to *in utero* positioning. Trauma is a leading cause of locomotor disability and may be unrecognized or unreported as a consequence of child abuse. Post-infectious and autoimmune or connective tissue disorders are primarily limited to the muscles and joints but are recognized to involve several systems of the body including skin and integument.

Ask the details regarding history of discomfort, deformity, pain and disability. The degree of disability should be assessed by asking the child whether he can look after the "activities of daily living" (ADL), like toilet needs, bathing, dressing, eating, etc. independently or needs the help of the mother. At times, the pain in a joint may be referred from another joint or body organ, viz. pain in the knee or above patella may be referred from involvement of the hip joint, pain in the sacroiliac joint may be referred to the buttocks, shoulder pain may occur due to irritation of diaphragm by basal pneumonia or gallstones and pain of subluxation of the elbow is often referred to the wrist joint. Spinal pain due to involvement of intervertebral disks manifests as constriction or girdle pains over the chest or abdomen.

The distribution of the joints involved, whether the disease is predominantly affecting the large joints or small joints, and whether it is monoarticular, pauciarticular or oligoarticular (<5 joints) and polyarticular in nature should be recorded. A differentiation should be made between arthralgia (pain alone) and arthritis (pain with signs of inflammation). Monoarticular disease is usually suggestive of a sprain or injury, hemarthrosis, or pyogenic infection. Migratory or flitting and fleeting joint pains, i.e. involvement of 2–3 joints for 2–3 days and then moving on to involve other joints with partial relief to the previously affected joints, is a classical feature of rheumatic fever, but may also occur due to gonococcal arthritis, meningococcal arthritis, inflammatory bowel disease and acute leukemia. Early morning stiffness of joints is a recognized feature of acute inflammatory joint disease especially due to rheumatoid arthritis. Dactylitis, i.e. inflammatory spindle-shaped swellings of digits, may occur due to juvenile chronic arthritis, tuberculosis, acute lymphoblastic leukemia, congenital syphilis, sickle cell disease, chikungunya, and Reiter's disease. Diffuse swelling of dorsum of hands may occur due to periosteal reaction of the metacarpals as a manifestation of sickle cell disease, acute leukemia, tenosynovitis of flexor tendons and serum sickness.

When a toddler is pulled by traction, on holding at one or both the wrists or hands, subluxation of the radial head (Nursemaid's elbow) may occur. The child cries and keeps the elbow slightly flexed and hand pronated while supination is restricted and painful. The child is unable to lift the hand above the shoulder on the affected side. Preschool children commonly complain of pain in the legs especially in the evening or night. The condition is wrongly labeled as "growing pains" because discomfort actually occurs due to fatigue and tiredness in an overactive playful child. When body pains are present at multiple sites, and their are no constitutional symptoms, it is generally suggestive of a psychogenic disorder.

Localized pain in the bone may occur due to subperiosteal bleeding or periosteitis or green stick fracture because of trauma, infection, new growth or avascular necrosis due to sickle cell disease. Episodic intractable bone pains at multiple sites, especially at night, may occur in children with acute leukemia, metastases and metabolic bone disease. Back pain is uncommon in children but may occur due to viral fever, faulty posture, heavy school bag, sport injury, physical stress, spinal deformity, localized infection or tumor. Ask for associated constitutional symptoms like anorexia, sweating, fever, malaise, toxemia and weight loss. The family history may give clues to possible genetic disorders, such as congenital syndromes, muscular dystrophy and skeletal dysplasias.

GENERAL PHYSICAL EXAMINATION

Observe the gait and posture of the child as he enters the examination chamber. Assess nutritional status and look for any evidences of anemia and deficiencies of vitamins (especially vitamin C and vitamin D) and trace minerals. Eyes should be examined for blue sclerae as a marker of osteogenesis imperfecta. Conjunctivitis is commonly associated in patients with Reiter's syndrome, dry eyes in Sjögren syndrome and painful iritis in patients with ankylosing spondylitis. Subluxation of lens or ectopia lentis may be associated in patients with Marfan syndrome and homocystinuria. Iridocyclitis may occur in children with pauciarticular rheumatoid arthritis while chorioretinitis is a characteristic feature of TORCH infections. Look for any obvious swellings, deformities and functional limitations in the upper and lower extremities. Look for any abnormalities in the hands and feet, like polydactyly, and syndactyly. Camptodactyly or flexion deformity of little finger may occur in association with Down, Carpenter and Aarskog syndromes or as an isolated anomaly. Triphalangeal hand or bifid thumb is associated with Holt-Oram syndrome while broad thumb is a characteristic feature of Rubinstein-Taybi syndrome.

Temperature, pulse rate, respiration rate and blood pressure should be recorded. Hypertension is commonly associated in patients with connective tissue disorder. In children with systemic-onset rheumatoid arthritis, high grade spiking fever with evanescent salmon pink skin rash may precede joint involvement by several days or weeks. Lymph node enlargement in the draining areas of the disease sites and generalized lymphadenopathy should be looked for.

Skin should be examined for any evanescent macular rash, subcutaneous nodules, petechiae, erythema marginatum, café au lait spots and xanthomas. Painless, firm, nontender subcutaneous nodules due to rheumatic fever are characteristically seen over the pressure and friction sites, such as olecranon, extensor surfaces of forearms, shins and spine. Erythematous maculopapular rash in a shape of butterfly on the face is diagnostic of systemic lupus erythematosus. Non-bacterial arthritis, and mucosal lesions in the mouth and genital area are seen in adolescent children with Reiter's disease. Systemic examination, especially cardiovascular assessment is mandatory whenever a connective tissue disease or a metabolic disorder is strongly suspected. Slipped femoral epiphysis in an adolescent child may be associated with an endocrine disorder and obesity.

SPECIFIC EXAMINATION

A detailed head-to-toe examination should be conducted starting from vertex and gradually moving down to the face, jaw, neck, upper extremities, lower extremities, trunk and spine. The first aim of clinical assessment of the locomotor system is to determine whether the involvement is of the muscles, bones, joints or soft tissue structures, such as joint capsule, bursae, tendons and ligaments. A great tact and expertise is required for examination of a painful joint or extremity in children and it should be conducted in the end after completing the rest of physical examination. Observe the limb or joint for any swelling, redness and deformity. Active movements should be assessed before palpation and assessment of range of passive movements at various joints. The toddlers should be examined in the comfort of mother's lap while older children should be distracted by talking to them while examining the painful joint or limb and they should be handled with utmost gentleness and tact.

COMMON MUSCULOSKELETAL DEVELOPMENTAL DEFECTS

Musculoskeletal anomalies account for one-third of all anomalies in newborn babies. Apart from developmental or chromosomal defects, they may develop due to abnormal *in utero* posture or because of amniotic constriction bands.

Congenital talipes equinovarus (CTEV or club feet) There is adduction of forefoot, inversion of hindfoot and an equinus position (plantar flexion) of the heel. It is not possible to fully dorsiflex the foot by touching the dorsum of the foot with the shin. In isolated forefoot adduction (metatarsus adductus) and abduction (metatarsus varus), it is possible to dorsiflex the foot and correct the abnormality by passive stretching and physiotherapy. Club feet may be unilateral or bilateral and may be an isolated abnormality or a manifestation of caudal regression syndrome, meningocele, craniocarpotarsal dysplasia, Larson syndrome, diastrophic dwarfism and spinal tumor. Equinus position (plantar flexion) may develop due to tightness and shortening of the Achilles tendon because of cerebral palsy and in children with autism and pseudohypertrophic muscular dystrophy. Toe-walking is a characteristic feature in these children.

Talipes calcaneovalgus is less common and is characterized by eversion, abduction and dorsiflexion of the foot which is exactly reverse of CTEV. The toes point upward and arch of the foot is flat. It may be associated with dysplasia of hip and external rotation of tibia. It should be differentiated from congenital vertical talus or rocker-bottom foot in which foot is fixed in plantar flexion with reversed or convex arch of the foot.

Congenital dislocation or dysplasia of hip (CDH) is more common in first born, breech delivered female infants. It may be unilateral or bilateral and does not produce any visible abnormalities during newborn period. It is diagnosed by detailed physical examination by conducting Ortolani and Barlow tests (*see* Chapter 15). When early diagnosis is missed, it may produce asymmetry of inguinal or gluteal fold, relative shortening of femur on the affected side, limitation of hip abduction, delayed walking, limping or waddling gait (bilateral CDH). To test for apparent shortening of femur, both hips and knees are flexed and soles are placed flat on the table. Because of posterior dislocation of the hip, the knee on the affected side would be at a lower level than the normal side (Galeazzi sign).

Bowed legs (genu varum) During the first 2 years of life, there is physiologic bowing of tibia due to rotation at knees (Figure 10.1). The severity of bowed legs is assessed by measuring the distance between the knees when medial malleoli are closely aligned in a supine infant or standing child. In physiologic bowed legs, the distance between the knees is less than 5 cm. When tibial bowing is

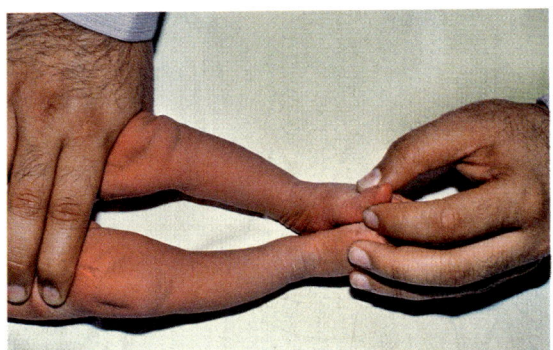

Figure 10.1 Bowed legs (genu varum). It is common and physiological during first 2 years of life. The distance between the knees is usually less than 5 cm when both ankles are closely opposed.

genuine or marked and persists beyond 2 years, exclude the possibilities of rickets, metaphyseal dysostosis, achondroplasia, neurofibromatosis, osteogenesis imperfecta, trauma, infection, tumor and osteochondrosis of the medial tibial condyle (Blount disease). Blount disease is characterized by tibia vara because of idiopathic growth disorder of medial aspect of the proximal tibial epiphysis leading to varus angulation and internal or medial rotation of tibia. It is usually bilateral but when unilateral it may cause leg-length discrepancy. Tibia vara is best diagnosed with an anteroposterior skiagram of both legs in a standing position. Blount disease is an autosomal recessive disorder and is characterized by beaking or nontender bony protuberance of proximal medial tibial metaphysis, fragmentation of medial tibial epiphysis and metaphyseal-diaphyseal angle of >11° (Figure 10.2).

Knock-knees (genu valgum) Physiologic bowing of legs is gradually replaced by knock-knees during 2–5 years of age. The severity of knock-knees is assessed by measuring the intermedial malleolar distance between the feet when child stands erect with knees barely touching each other (Figure 10.3). When severity of genu valgum is more than 5 cm (inter-feet distance) or it persists beyond 5 years, the possibilities of rickets, hypophosphatasia, Morquio disease, Hurler syndrome, and pes valgus should be excluded.

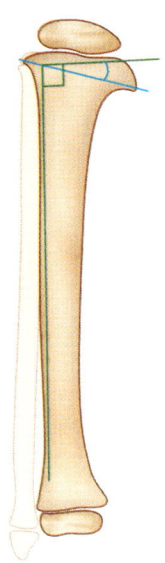

Figure 10.2 Diagrammatic depiction of metaphyseal–diaphyseal angle. A vertical line is drawn along the tibia, and a perpendicular (90°) line is created at the proximal tibial metaphysis. A second horizontal line is drawn along the slope of the metaphysis and the angle created with the perpendicular line is measured. In Blount disease, the metaphyseal–diaphyseal angle is usually greater than 11°.

Flat feet (pes planus) During first 2 to 3 years of life, arch of the feet is obliterated by the pad of fat producing physiological flat feet. When a child is asked to stand on tip toes, the arch of the foot is evident. Genuine flat feet are associated with pronation or eversion of forefoot and at times hallux valgus (adduction of big toe) and prominent medial malleolus. The children with flat feet have generalized relaxation of ligaments and their shoes wear off excessively on the medial side of the heel. When asked to walk with wet feet, a complete impression of the feet is left on the floor.

Pes cavus There is high longitudinal arch with excessive plantar curvature of the feet. It may be an isolated congenital abnormality or may occur as a manifestation or association of Friedreich ataxia, spina bifida, cauda equina lesion, metatarsus varus, diastematomyelia, peroneal muscular atrophy, Hurler syndrome and peripheral neuropathy (Charcot-Marie-Tooth disease or CMT). In CMT, there is foot drop, marked arching of foot, claw or

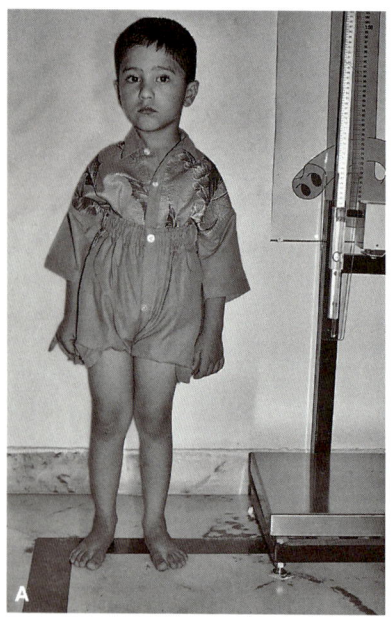 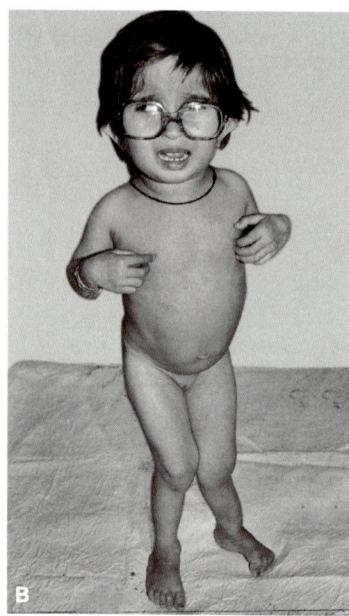 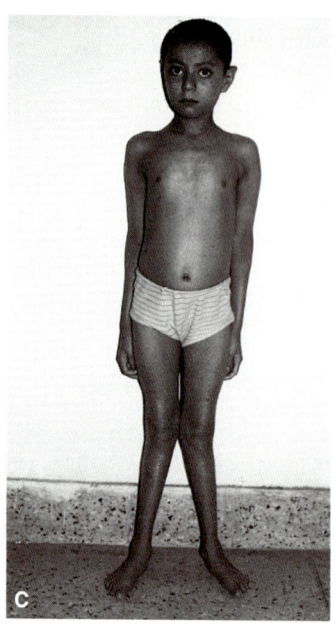

Figure 10.3A to C Knock knees (genu valgum). It is physiological during 2–5 years of age. (A) The distance between the medial malleoli at ankles is less than 5 cm when knees are touching each other. (B) Marked or pathological knock knees due to renal tubular dysfunction and (C) Marked knock knees without any identifiable cause.

hammer toes, peroneal muscular atrophy giving an appearance of "stork leg" or an "inverted champagne bottle."

Toeing-in (pigeon toes) Toeing-in is common in toddlers due to internal rotation of lower limbs. The child walks with knees slightly facing each other and toes pointing inwards like a pigeon. The abnormality is self-limiting and usually disappears by the age of 7–8 years. When toeing-in is marked and persists beyond 10 years of age, surgical correction may be considered.

Toe-walking Toe-walking is physiological during first one to two years of age. The child can stand on his heels without any difficulty and movements of ankles are normal. The habit disappears as the child learns to walk normally on his heels-to-toes. Persistent toe-walking occurs when tendo-Achilles is short and taut with inability to touch the dorsum of foot with the shin. Persistent toe-walking is a recognized feature of cerebral palsy, Duchenne muscular dystrophy and autism spectrum disorder.

Polydactyly Extra digits may occur in the hand or feet, either on the medial or preaxial side or the lateral side or postaxial. Polydactyly on the ulnar aspects (extra little fingers) of each hand is more common and may occur as an isolated anomaly or in association with chondroectodermal dysplasia (Ellis-van Creveld syndrome), Lawrence-Moon-Biedl syndrome, short-rib polydactyly, dwarfism, trisomy 13, and Meckel syndrome.

Syndactyly Fusion or webbing of the toes or fingers may be an isolated anomaly or may be associated with other anomalies especially premature fusion of the cranial sutures. Syndactylism is a recognized feature of Apert syndrome (mitten hand), Carpenter syndrome, Smith-Lemli-Opitz syndrome, oral-facial-digital syndrome, Poland syndrome and Pfeiffer syndrome (broad and deviated thumbs and big toes).

Trigger thumb or fingers Trigger thumb or flexion of thumb occurs due to idiopathic tightening of the underlying flexor pollicis longus tendon with inability to fully extend the interphalangeal joint of the thumb. A palpable nodule may be felt at the base of thumb. Trigger finger or isolated camptodactyly is uncommon and usually involves distal interphalangeal joint.

THE EXTREMITIES

Bony landmarks are used for measuring the length and girth of upper and lower limbs. Acromion of scapula, olecranon of ulna and lower end of radial condyle are reliable bony landmarks in the upper limbs. In the lower limbs, anterior superior iliac spine, upper and lower borders of patella and distal edge of medial malleolus are useful bony landmarks. Chest circumference is taken at the level of nipples or xiphoid cartilage while abdominal girth is measured at the level of umbilicus. Waist is measured just above the level of anterior-superior iliac crests.

Look for shortening, lengthening, hypertrophy and atrophy of limbs or their segments. Hemihypertrophy or hypertrophy of a limb or a localized segment of the limb may occur in cutis marmorata telangiectatica, Beckwith-Wiedemann syndrome, Russell-Silver syndrome, Klippel-Trenuanay-Weber syndrome, Wilms tumor, adrenocortical carcinoma, hepatocellular carcinoma, neurofibromatosis, congenital arteriovenous fistula, lymphangiectasia, and stimulation of epiphyseal growth following osteomyelitis or fracture near an epiphysis.

Shortening of an extremity may occur due to congenitally short femur or tibia, hypoplasia of femur (infant of a diabetic mother), congenital dislocation of the hip, slipped femoral capital epiphysis, coxa plana, poliomyelitis, hemiplegia, Ollier's disease and premature arrest of epiphyseal growth due to infection or trauma. In infantile cortical hyperostosis (Caffey disease) and vitamin A poisoning, there is a diffuse, painful and localized enlargement of mandibles, clavicles, ribs, scapulae and some long bones. Enlargement of ends of long bones or epiphyseal broadening may be seen in children with rickets, hypophosphatasia, chondrodystrophy, Morquio's disease and primary hyperparathyroidism. The ends of long bones may be enlarged and tender and there is associated clubbing of nails in patients with hypertrophic pulmonary osteoarthropathy.

In addition to enlargement of the wrists and ankles, rickets is characterized by frontal bossing, costochondral beading (rachitic rosary), pigeon-shaped (pectus carinatum) or funnel-shaped (pectus excavatum) chest, Harrison's sulcus, spinal deformities, bowing of legs or knock-knees and coxa vara (Figure 10.4). The skeletal manifestations of scurvy include subperiosteal hemorrhages in the long bones with marked irritability with pseudoparalysis of extremities with a frog-like posture and scorbutic rosary which is characterized by a bayonet-like angulation at the costochondral junction of ribs due to posterior dislocation of sternum.

Examine hands and feet for their size, shape, deformities and length of digits. A ganglion may develop over the wrist or ankle due to accumulation

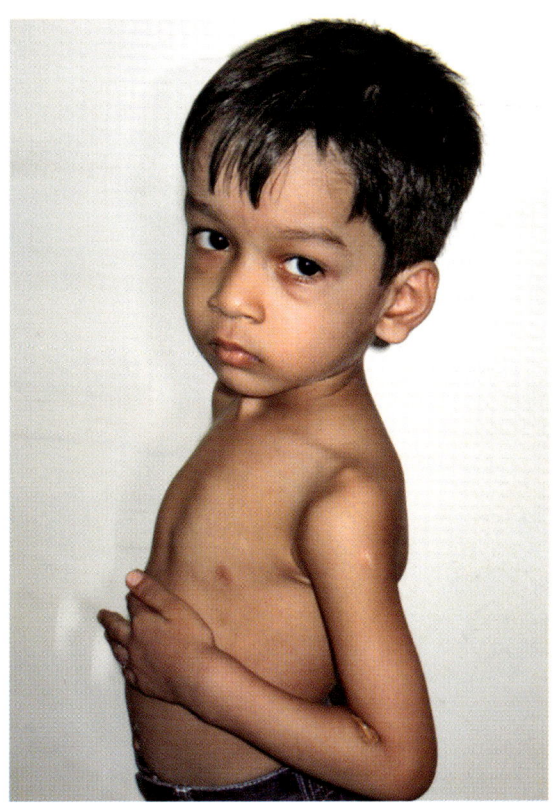

Figure 10.4 Pigeon-shaped chest with wide wrists in a child with rickets.

of synovial fluid or gelatin in the tendon sheath producing a painless and slippery or rubbery nodule. Long and thin extremities, hands, feet, fingers and toes are seen in patients with arachnodactyly (Marfan syndrome), homocystinuria, mucosal neuroma and Stickler syndrome. The Steinberg sign or "thumb sign", i.e. protrusion of the thumb beyond the palm when the hand is fisted, is a characteristic feature of Marfan syndrome (Figure 10.5). Small, short and stubby hands and digits may be seen in patients with Down syndrome, cretinism, Prader-Willi syndrome, Rubinstein-Taybi syndrome (short broad terminal phalanges of thumbs and great toes), and Pfeiffer syndrome (absence of middle phalanges). Distal hypoplasia of the digits and nails may be seen in fetal phenytoin and alcohol syndrome, chondroectodermal dysplasia and cleidocranial dysostosis. Turner syndrome should be considered in every short stature girl with delayed menarche especially if there is webbing of the neck or cubitus valgus, i.e. increased carrying angle of the arm. Look for anomalies of radial ray structures, i.e. thumb, radial metacarpal bones and radius. The common radial ray anomalies include underdevelopment or absence of the thumb, triphalangeal thumb, preaxial polydactyly and atrophy of radius. Absence or hypoplasia of the radius and thumb may be associated with thrombocytopenia (TAR syndrome), aplastic anemia (Fanconi anemia), and atrial septal defect (Holt-Oram syndrome).

THE BONES

It is difficult to examine the deep-seated bones (femur and fibula) as compared to the superficial bones like tibia and short bones of hands and feet. Bone pain is usually continuous (not related to movement of joint or posture), deep-seated and penetrating in character and usually disturbs sleep. Bone pains may occur without any physical findings in children with leukemia, metastases and metabolic bone disease. Exquisitely painful, tense and slightly warm swelling with erythema and tenderness may occur over one or more long bones due to vaso-occlusive bone involvement in patients with sickle cell anemia. Localized swelling of long bones may be caused by osteomyelitis, cyst or tumor. Osteomyelitis is associated with classical signs of inflammation such as redness (rubor), warmth (calor), pain and tenderness (dolor) and swelling (tumor). Osteochondritis at the distal ends of long bones may occur due to congenital syphilis, and other TORCH infections. Dactylitis is a recognized feature of syphilis, tuberculosis and chikungunya. Saber tibiae (anterior angulation or bowing of tibiae) may occur in children with congenital syphilis, neurofibromatosis, fetal malpositioning and congenital absence of fibula.

Fracture may occur because of trauma to healthy bones or spontaneously in diseased bones (pathological fractures). In children, trauma may be unrecognized and usually occurs during sport activities or may be unreported, if it is due to child abuse. Presence of multiple fractures at birth or early in life with deformed thin bones and blue sclerae is suggestive of osteogenesis imperfecta. When fracture occurs in a child with multiple café au lait spots, the possibility of fibrous dysplasia should be excluded. Due to presence of soft and

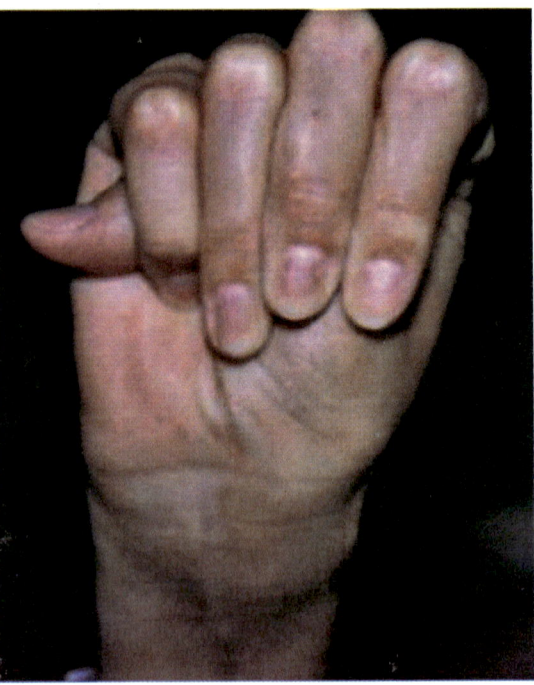

Figure 10.5 Thumb sign in an adolescent with Marfan syndrome

pliable bones, children may develop green-stick fracture without break in the continuity of bone. Fracture of clavicle and upper end of humerus or femur may occur due to difficult extraction of the baby during breech delivery.

The classical features of closed fracture include pain, tenderness, swelling, deformity of limb, bony crepitus (abnormal movement with a click at the site of fracture) and inability to use the limb. In Colle's fracture (fracture of distal end of radius), there is classical "dinner fork deformity" because of dorsal displacement and angulation, shortening and rotation of the wrist. In open or compound fracture, the soft tissues are damaged and broken bone ends may protrude out through the damaged skin. In a case of compound fracture, it is important to assess the blood supply, cutaneous sensations, and voluntary movements for any evidences of nerve injury distal to the site of fracture.

THE JOINTS

Hypermobility and hyperextensibility of joints is seen in a number of developmental disorders, like Ehlers-Danlos syndrome, Marfan syndrome, Stickler syndrome, homocystinuria, hyperlysinemia, osteogenesis imperfecta and primary hyperparathyroidism. Marked hyperextensibility of fingers and hands may be seen in children with cartilage-hair hypoplasia, cutis laxa and fragile-X syndrome.

Joint stiffness and limitation of joint mobility are seen in patients with arthritis, synovitis, osteomyelitis, fasciitis, contractures, dermatomyositis, scleroderma, muscular spasiticity and rigidity. A number of developmental and metabolic disorders like Morquio's disease, Hurler syndrome and arthrogryposis congenita multiplex, have generalized stiffness of joints. Recurrent hemarthrosis of weight-bearing joints (knees and ankles) due to hemophilia may lead to ankylosis, synovial thickening and atrophy of surrounding muscles (chronic arthropathy).

Subluxation and Dislocation

Developmental dysplasia or congenital dislocation of hip(s) must be ruled out by proper clinical examination in all newborn babies. Children with hyperextensible joints are more vulnerable to develop dislocation of various joints. Dislocation of multiple joints especially hip, knee and elbow is a recognized feature of Larsen syndrome. Some toddlers are vulnerable to develop recurrent episodes of subluxation of the elbow joint when they are pulled by holding them at their hands. Traumatic separation of an epiphysis may occur in newborn babies following a traumatic delivery. It occurs most commonly at the upper humeral epiphysis but may affect any joint causing localized swelling, pain and limitation of movements.

Arthritis and Arthralgias

The common causes of arthritis and arthralgias in children are listed in Table 10.1. Arthritis is characterized by local pain, swelling, redness, warmth, restricted and painful movements of joints, deformity and constitutional and systemic symptoms. Identify the site (whether large or small or both types of joints), and number of joints involved and whether involvement is symmetrical or asymmetrical in distribution. In superficial joints (especially knee joint), the presence of exudates or pus can be suspected on the basis of pitting edema, fluctuations and patellar tap. Neuropathic joint involvement is characterized by recurrent episodes of painless swelling of foot and ankle joints with loss of superficial and deep sensations (Charcot's or Clutton's joints). In certain children, cracking and creaking sounds may be heard during active and passive movements of certain joints especially metacarpophalangeal and knee joints but it is of no clinical significance.

Joint Movements

Both active and passive movements of the involved joints should be tested and compared with the normal side. Movements may be limited due to pain, muscle spasm and contractures rather than structural damage to the joints. The movements should be checked after placing the joint in the neutral position. The range of movements can be measured with the help of a transparent goniometer or protractor.

TABLE 10.1 Common causes of arthralgias and arthritis

1. **Arthralgias***
   Reactive or toxic arthritis, chronic active hepatitis, inflammatory bowel disease, toxic shock syndrome, transient synovitis, brucellosis, serum sickness, cystic fibrosis, immunodeficiency disorders, psychogenic pain and rheumatism
2. **Arthritis**
   - *Single joint*: Pyogenic or septic arthritis, tuberculous arthritis, and acute transient synovitis
   - *Migratory or flitting polyarthritis*: Rheumatic fever, gonococcal arthritis, meningococcal arthritis, inflammatory bowel disease, systemic lupus erythematosus, leukemia or non-Hodgkin lymphoma
   - *Multiple large joints*: Rheumatic fever, connective tissue disorder (juvenile rheumatoid arthritis, systemic lupus erythematosus, Kawasaki disease, polyarteritis nodosa), chikungunya, serum sickness, and Henoch-Schönlein purpura
   - *Multiple small joints of hands and feet (dactylitis)*: Juvenile rheumatoid arthritis, tubercular dactylitis, congenital syphilis, leukemia, sickle cell disease, and psoriatic arthropathy
3. **Traumatic arthritis**
   Hemarthrosis, ruptured cruciate ligament or torn medial and lateral meniscus of knee joint capsule
4. **Miscellaneous causes**
   Immunodeficiency disorders, disseminated lipogranulomatosis, sarcoidosis, Reiter syndrome, serum sickness, psoriatic arthropathy, sickle cell disease, and pulmonary hypertrophic osteoarthropathy

*Arthralgias are characterized by joint pains without any evidences of inflammatory signs.

The jaw Jaw movements are tested by opening and closing the mouth, protrusion and retraction of the jaw and side-to-side movements. The distance between the upper and lower incisor teeth on fully opening the mouth is a reliable measure of severity of ankylosis of temporomandibular joints.

The shoulder The neutral position is with arm to the side, elbow flexed to 90° with forearm pointing forwards. The scapula should be anchored between index finger and thumb while testing movements of the shoulder joint. Test the flexion, extension, abduction, rotation (both in abduction and neutral position) and elevation of the shoulder.

The elbow The neutral position is forearm in extension. Test the range of flexion, hyperextension, supination and pronation.

The wrist The neutral position is hand in line with the forearm and palm facing downward. Test for dorsiflexion and extension, palmar flexion, ulnar deviation and radial deviation.

The sacroiliac joints The sacroiliac joints are identified by two dimples on either side over the sacral region. There are no movements at the sacroiliac joints but their affection can be diagnosed by applying direct pressure over each sacroiliac joint, firm pressure over the sacrum and inward pressure at both the iliac bones. Pretzel test is useful to elicit tenderness of sacroiliac joints (Figure 10.6).

The hip The neutral position of hip is extension with patella pointing forwards. The pelvis should be stabilized with one hand while testing the movements of hip joint. Test hip flexion with knee bent, by doing abduction, adduction, rotation both in extension (prone position) and flexion. Hip extension is tested while patient is lying in the lateral position. Rotation of hip joints is best tested by asking the patient to lie in prone position with knees in flexion at 90° (Figures 10.7 to 10.9).

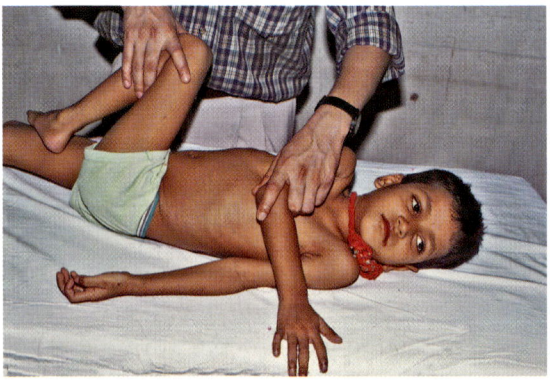

Figure 10.6 Pretzel test. The thigh on one side and shoulder on the opposite side are twisted to cross the midline. The sacroiliac joint on the side of twisted thigh gets stretched by this maneuver and minimal pain at the sacroiliac joint can be elicited.

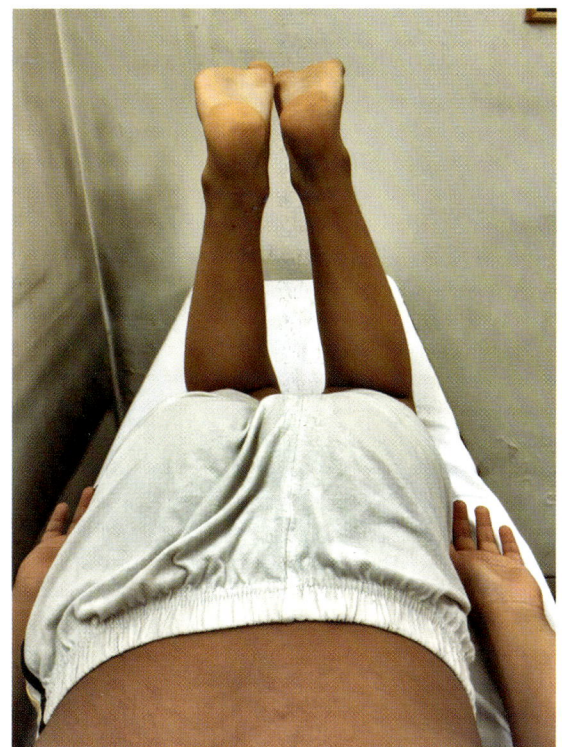

Figure 10.7 Patient is asked to lie prone with knees flexed at 90°. This is an ideal position to elicit ankle jerk and assess the movements at the ankles, knees and hip joints.

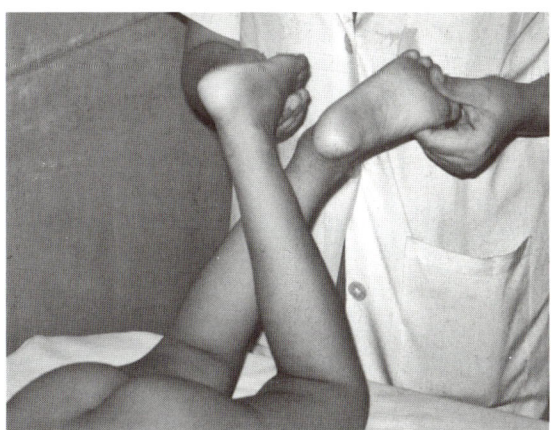

Figure 10.8 Movements at hip joints are best tested by asking the patient to lie in prone position with knees in flexion at 90°. The legs are adducted or crossed against each other to test internal rotation of hips.

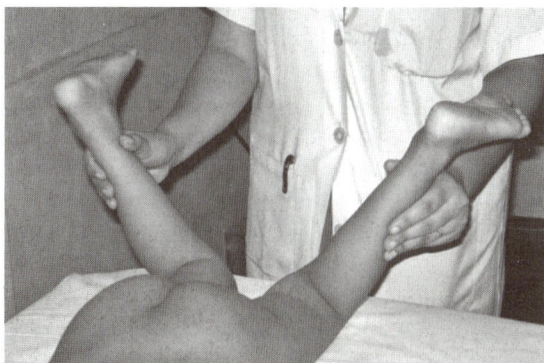

Figure 10.9 The legs are abducted to test external rotation of hip joints.

Patrick test or FABER (Flexion, Abduction, and External Rotation) test is performed to assess the involvement of hip joint and the sacroiliac joint. The child lies supine, the leg to be tested is flexed at the knee, the thigh is abducted and externally rotated by placing the ankle beyond the knee of the opposite leg. The flexed leg is pressed posteriorly by putting pressure over the inner side of the knee (Figure 10.10). If the pain is elicited

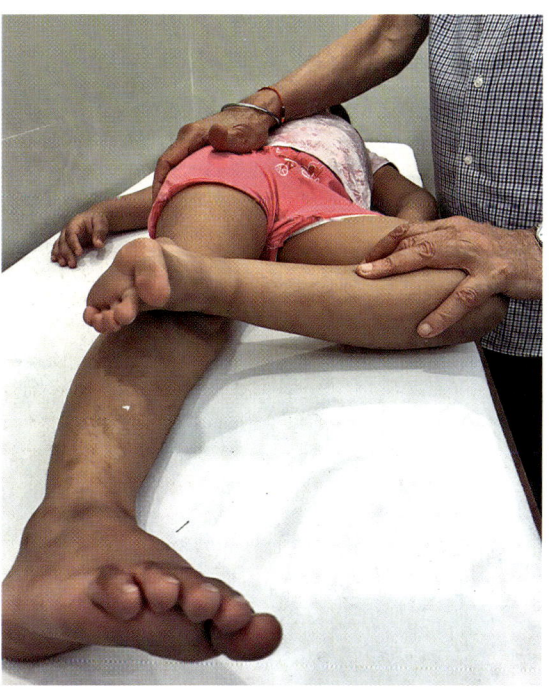

Figure 10.10 FABER test. See text for details.

on the ipsilateral side anteriorly, it is suggestive of hip joint disorder on the same side. When pain is elicited on the contralateral side posteriorly, it is suggestive of dysfunction of the sacroiliac joint.

Thomas test is useful to assess the hip joints. Both the hips are flexed so that the thighs touch the abdomen. One leg is kept flexed and child is asked to completely extend the other leg. Normally it is possible to completely extend the hip joint. Inability to completely extend the hip joint indicates the presence of hip flexion contracture and a positive Thomas test (Figure 10.11A and B).

Trendelenburg test is done for assessment of gluteus medius muscle and stability of hip joint. Observe the patient from behind and ask him to raise one leg. When one leg is lifted, the contralateral abductors try to stabilize the pelvis by raising the pelvis on the ipsilateral side. When hip joint is normal, the pelvis tilts upwards on the side with the leg raised. When hip joint is diseased or subluxated, the pelvis sags downwards when the leg is raised (Figure 10.12). Apart from weakness of gluteus medius muscle, Trendelenburg test is positive in patients with superior gluteal nerve palsy, herniation of lumbar disk, advanced degeneration of hip and Legg-Calvé-Perthes disease.

Lazarevic's test or straight leg raise sign is done in a patient with low back pain to diagnose herniated lumbar disk. The patient is asked to lie supine on a flat surface. The examiner lifts the patients' leg by keeping the knee in extension. The test becomes more specific when ankle is kept dorsiflexed and neck is flexed. The test is positive when patient experiences sciatic pain when lifted straight leg is at an angle between 30° and 70°.

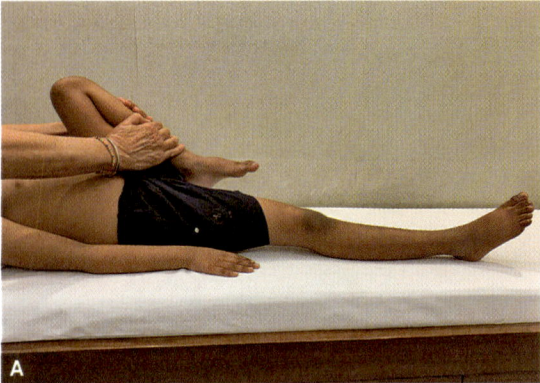
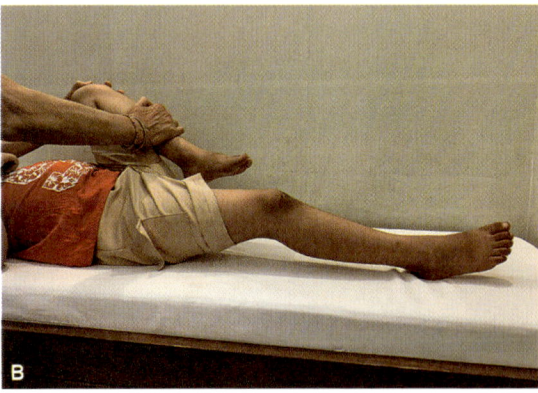

Figure 10.11A and B Thomas test: (A) In a normal child, complete extension of contralateral hip and knee joint is achieved. (B) The contralateral hip joint cannot be fully extended because of flexion contracture of hip joint. It is a characteristic feature of Legg-Calvé-Perthes disease.

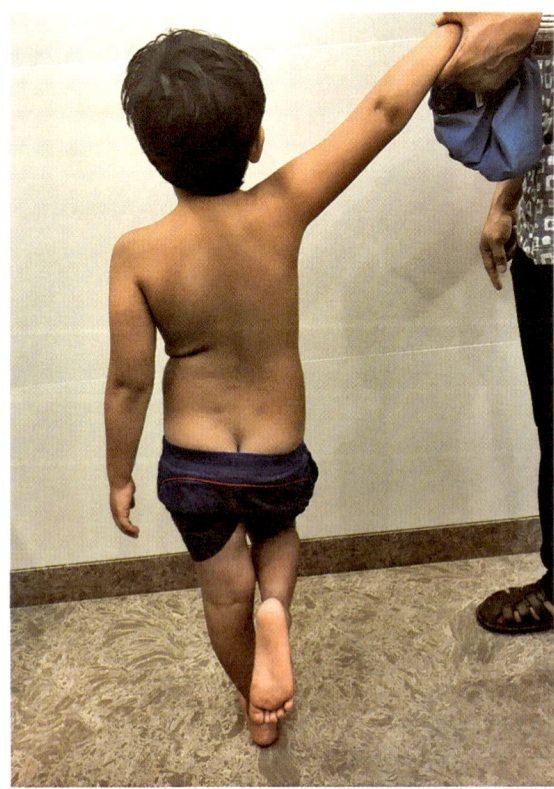

Figure 10.12 Trendelenburg test (*see* text for details).

The knee The neutral position is complete extension. Test flexion and extension movements of both knees. Check for hyperextension of knee joint (genu recurvatum). Patellar tap test is used to check for presence of effusion in the knee joint. Squeeze all the fluid from the suprapatellar space into the joint with your left hand and tap the patella with middle and index fingers of the right hand. If fluid is present, the patella will strike the deeper structures and bounce back.

The ankle The neutral position is with the outer border of the foot at an angle of 90° with the leg and midway between inversion and eversion. Test for dorsiflexion and plantar flexion with knee slightly flexed. Look for size and tone of calf muscles and tightness of tendo-Achilles.

The foot Test for eversion, inversion, forefoot abduction, adduction and flexion-extension of metatarsophalangeal and interphalangeal joints. Look for deformities, like hallux valgus or varus, toeing-in or out, claw toes, hammer toes (fixed flexion of terminal joints) and over-riding of toes.

The spine Examine the spine when child is standing and sitting in the erect position. The major landmarks for counting the vertebrae are the spinous process of C7 and the last rib which articulates with the 12th thoracic vertebra. There is physiological lordosis of cervical and lumbar regions with S-shaped curve of thoracolumbar spine. Look for kyphosis (diffuse posterior curvature) and gibbus (localized angular deformity) due to Pott's disease (spinal tuberculosis) and vertebral disk prolapse. Lateral curvature is termed as scoliosis and it is always associated with rotation of the bodies of vertebrae. *Adam's forward bend test* is useful to assess spinal deformity. The patient is asked to bend forward and viewed from behind which aggravates asymmetrical trunk rotation due to scoliosis.

When viewed from the side, one can more easily see subtle degrees of kyphosis (Figure 10.13A and B). *When scoliosis is caused by inequality of leg length, it disappears in a sitting position.* Examine cervical and thoracolumbar spine for various movements, like flexion, extension, rotation both sides and lateral bending towards right and left. All movements occur at the cervical spine while thoracic spine permits mainly rotation and

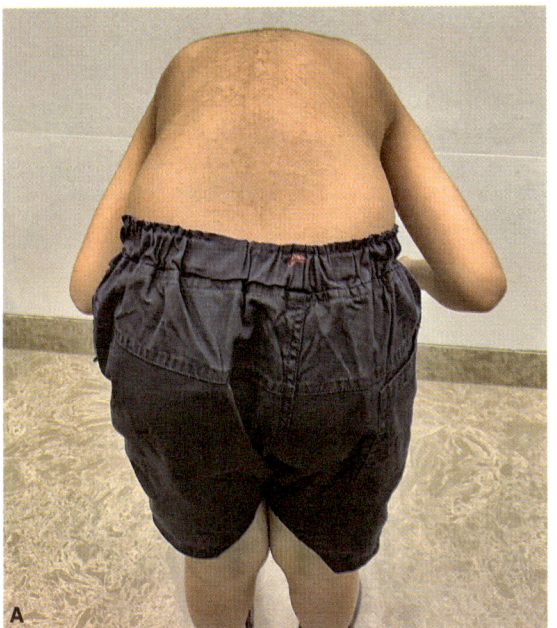
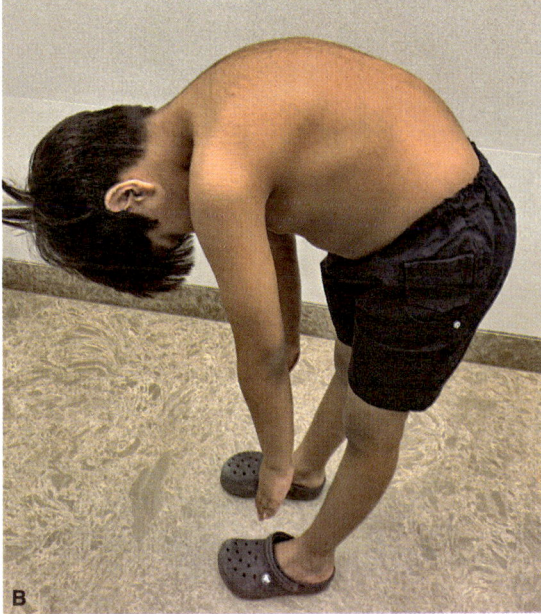

Figure 10.13A and B Adam's forward bend test. (A) The child is asked to bend forward and observed from behind for scoliosis; (B) Kyphosis is best seen when viewed from the side.

the lumbar spine can flex, extend and bend laterally. Assess the expansion of the chest which may be reduced due to ankylosing spondylitis even when there is no underlying lung disease. Pain and limitation of straight leg raising (SLR) and sensory loss over the sacral region are suggestive of prolapsed intervertebral disk. When limit of SLR is reached, passive dorsiflexion of foot further stretches the sciatic nerve causing severe pain. The lower back or sacral area should be examined for any pilonidal dimple, sinus, and hairy nevus.

THE MUSCLES

Look for muscle tone, power, localized atrophy or hypertrophy and whether involvement is symmetrical or asymmetrical. Enlargement or localized hypertrophy of muscles may be seen in patients with Duchenne muscular dystrophy, Becker muscular dystrophy, myotonia congenita, Schwartz-Jampel syndrome, chronic spinal muscular atrophy type 3 and amyloidosis. Rarely, generalized muscular hypertrophy is observed in patients with hypothyroidism (Kocher-Debre-Semelaigne syndrome) and glycogen storage disease associated with acid maltase deficiency. Generalized hypotonia and floppiness of muscles can occur in children due to a variety of causes (Table 10.2). Refer to Chapter 14 for testing muscle strength. The action of major muscles of the body and various maneuvers for their testing are summarized in Table 10.3. Muscle weakness may be minimal or severe, symmetrical or asymmetrical, limited to proximal (dermatomyositis) or distal (peripheral neuritis) muscles.

Body aches due to muscle pains are common during the course of viral infections and due to fatigue in pre-school children which are often labeled as "growing pains". Severe myalgias may occur during the course of leptospirosis, dengue fever, Rocky mountain spotted fever, toxic shock syndrome and plague. Staphylococcal infection may produce life-threatening suppurative fasciitis and myositis. Fibromyalgia in adolescents is characterized by chronic and persistent musculoskeletal aches and pains in at least 3 or more sites with fatigue and morning stiffness.

TABLE 10.2 Common causes of muscular hypotonia

- **Cerebral conditions** Atonic cerebral palsy, cerebral tumors and gliomas
- **Cerebellar** Cerebellar ataxia, Friedreich ataxia, cerebellar tumors, lesions of lateral hemispheres (neocerebellum)
- **Spinal causes** Spinal cord transection, spinal muscular atrophy, motor neuron disease, and transverse myelitis
- **Anterior horn cell disorders** Werdnig-Hoffmann disease, poliomyelitis, Guillain-Barré syndrome, and benign congenital hypotonia
- **Muscle disorders** Congenital myopathies
- **Hereditary connective tissue disorders** Ehlers-Danlos syndrome, and Marfan syndrome
- **Metabolic and genetic disorders** Glycogen storage disease, Zellweger cerebrohepatorenal syndrome, hypothyroidism, myopathic carnitine deficiency, periodic paralysis, 22q13 deletion syndrome (Phelan-McDermid syndrome), Aicardi syndrome, Canavan disease, CHARGE syndrome, Cohen syndrome, Costello syndrome, fragile X syndrome, myasthenia gravis, primary hypoparathyroidism, and Tay-Sachs disease
- **Miscellaneous causes** Protein-energy malnutrition, rickets, Down syndrome, Prader-Willi syndrome, Williams syndrome, Rett syndrome, and idiopathic hypercalcemia
- **Toxins** Infantile botulism and acrodynia

TABLE 10.3 Action of major muscles and their testing

Muscle	Testing
▪ Sternocleidomastoids	Flexion and rotation of neck
▪ Pectoralis major	Flexion of the arms at shoulders
▪ Latissimus dorsi	Extension of the arms at shoulders against resistance
▪ Trapezius	Shrugging of the shoulders
▪ Biceps	Flexing the elbow with palm facing upward
▪ Triceps	Extending the elbow with palm facing upward

(contd.)

Muscle	Testing
▪ Quadriceps	Extending the knee while sitting on the edge of a table
▪ Gluteus medius	Child is asked to lie on the side or lateral position and lift and abduct the upper leg at the hip. Keep the knee flexed to reduce the effect of iliotibial muscle
▪ Gluteus maximus	Patient lies prone with knees flexed to eliminate the effect of hamstrings. The child is asked to lift one thigh at a time off the table.
▪ Gastrocnemius and soleus	Plantar flexion of foot against resistance and ability to walk on toes

TABLE 10.3 Action of major muscles and their testing (*contd.*)

THE GAIT

Gait should be assessed with legs and feet fully exposed and without shoes or sandals. Observe the child as he enters your chamber. Ask the child to walk away from you, turn around at a given point and then walk back towards you. It is best to watch the gait of the child when he is not aware that his gait is being watched. The abnormality of gait due to disorders of central nervous system are listed in Chapter 14. Many children start walking on their toes but persistent toe-walking (equinus gait) is usually suggestive of spastic diplegia, spinal dysraphism, intraspinal and filum terminale tumors, pseudohypertrophic muscular dystrophy, shortening of tendo-Achilles and autism spectrum disorder. In-toeing and out-toeing gait due to torsional variations may occur but often resolves spontaneously. Medial or internal torsion of tibia is common during early infancy and is the most common cause of pigeon-toed or toeing-in gait. When the infant lies supine with knees extended, the lateral malleolus is normally 10°–15° posterior to the medial malleolus. Medial tibial torsion is diagnosed, if lateral malleolus is at the same plane or anterior to medial malleolus.

Transient synovitis of the hip joint ("observation hip") occurs in children below 10 years of age and is an important cause of fever of acute onset with pain in the hip or groin (sometimes referred to the knee) and limp. The lower extremity is held in flexion, external rotation and adduction. Internal rotation and abduction at hip joint are restricted. The limitation in abduction is best demonstrated by asking the patient to lie in a supine position with knees flexed and feet resting flat on the examination table. When the child is asked to let the knees fall apart while keeping feet together, the limited abduction on the involved side is evident. Internal rotation of the hip is tested by asking the child to lie in a prone position with knees flexed. A number of clinical conditions should be considered in the differential diagnosis of the transient synovitis, e.g. septic arthritis, Legg-Calvé-Perthes disease (avascular necrosis of femoral capital epiphysis), slipped femoral epiphysis, osteomyelitis, tuberculosis, osteoid osteoma and rheumatoid arthritis. Sudden alterations of gait and limping may occur from a variety of painful conditions involving muscles, joints, tendons and bones (Table 10.4). Identify whether limping is painless or associated with pain.

TABLE 10.4 Causes of limping in children

1. **Trauma** Sprain of ankle, splinter in the foot, traumatic periosteitis, contusions, tight fitting shoes, etc.
2. **Osteochondrosis** Involvement of femoral capital epiphysis, tibial tubercle, patella, metatarsal and tarsal bones
3. **Arthritis and osteomyelitis** Transient synovitis, slipped femoral episphysis, arthritis, bursitis and osteomyelitis involving joints of lower limbs
4. **Neoplastic diseases** Leukemia, sarcoma and metastasis from neuroblastoma
5. **Neurological disorders** Peripheral neuropathy, muscle weakness or paralysis, and spinal cord tumor.
6. **Miscellaneous conditions** Leg length inequalities, tight tendo-Achilles, inguinal or iliac lymphadenitis, muscular dystrophy, polymyositis, and conversion disorder or hysteria

	Scheme for Presentation
General physical examination	Nature and severity of physical disabilities, nutritional status and clinical evidences of vitamin C and vitamin D deficiency. Abnormalities of skull, facial dysmorphism and webbing of neck. Blue sclerae, ectopia lentis, iridocyclitis and chorioretinitis. Anemia, lymph node enlargement and hepatosplenomegaly. Temperature, pulse, respiration and blood pressure. Skin rash, subcutaneous nodules, petechiae, erythema marginatum, psoriasis, café au lait spots and xanthomas. Heart for any pericarditis or valvular involvement and evidences of congenital heart defects.
Specific examination	Head-to-toe examination starting with skull, face, neck, upper extremities, lower extremities, trunk and spine. Musculoskeletal developmental defects, like club feet, congenital dislocation of hips, bowed legs, knock knees, flat feet, pes cavus, toe-walking, pigeon-toes, compactodactyly or "trigger finger", triphalangeal, bifid or broad thumb, polydactyly and syndactyly of fingers and toes.
Extremities	Evidences for shortening, lengthening, hypertrophy and atrophy of limbs or their segments. Examine hands and feet for their size, shape, deformities and length of digits.
Bones	Localized or diffuse swelling, any warmth, redness, pain and tenderness. Identify any fractures, whether involving the healthy bones or diseased bones, nature of trauma (mild or severe) and whether isolated episode or multiple and recurrent.
Joints	Hypermobility or hyperextensibility of joints, any limitation of joint movements and stiffness of various joints. Arthralgias or arthritis, number and nature (large or small) of joints involved, symmetrical or asymmetrical. Look for any dislocation or traumatic separation of an epiphysis, active and passive movements of the involved joints, their range and restrictions, deformities and contracture of joints.
Spine	Lordosis, kyphosis, scoliosis or gibbus deformity, its exact location, whether painless or painful and tender. Spinal movements and their range and any limitation in flexion, extension, rotation and lateral bending.
Muscles	Muscle tone, power, localized atrophy or hypertrophy, swelling, inflammatory signs and tenderness. Degree of disability and whether child can independently look after the "activities of daily living" (ADL). Generalized hypotonia or floppiness, whether symmetrical or asymmetrical.
Gait	Sudden alterations of gait and limping, whether painful or painless and any abnormalities of gait during early life, such as toe-walking, in-toeing and out-toeing.

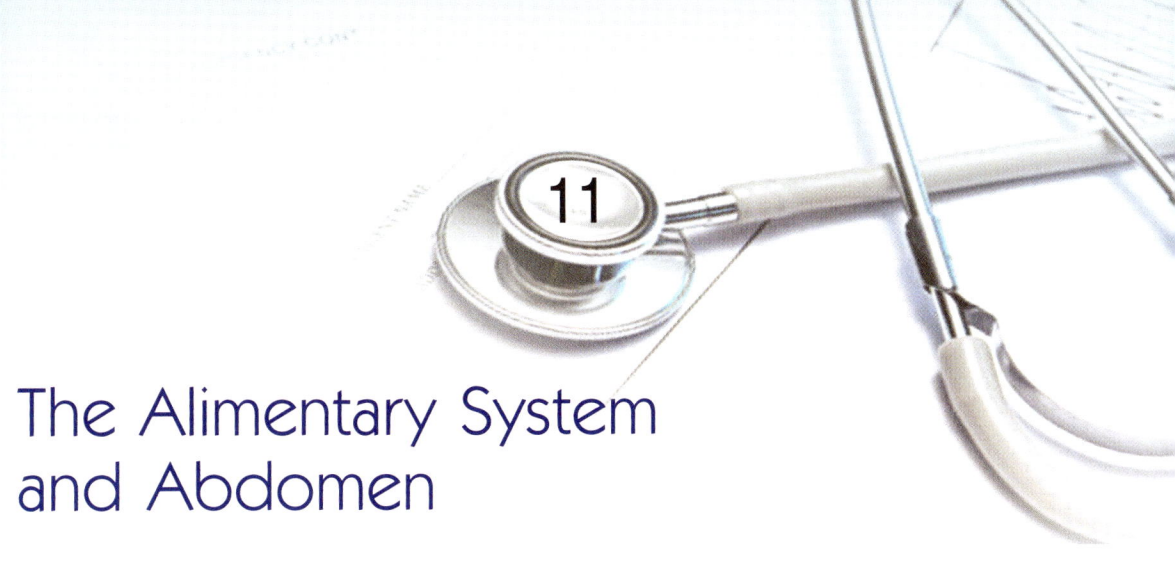

11

The Alimentary System and Abdomen

ANATOMY

The gastrointestinal tract extends from the mouth to the anus. It comprises of a long and curled stretch of 8 meters of hollow tubes for passage and processing of food and includes esophagus, stomach, pyloric antrum, duodenum, jejunum, ileum, cecum (appendix at the ileocecal junction), ascending colon, transverse colon, descending colon, sigmoid colon, rectum and anal canal. It serves the purpose of swallowing and propulsion of food with peristalsis and is conneted with intricate network of nerves and secretory glands which secrete ptyalin, amylase, lipase, colipase, proteolytic enzymes which help in the process of digestion and assimilation of food which is absorbed and metabolized in the liver. The partially digested and undigested food is propelled out as feces.

Apart from gastrointestinal tract, abdomen contains liver with gallbladder at its under surface in the right hypochondrium, spleen in the left hypochondrium, pancreas (with insulin-secreting islet cells) deep in the midline, two kidneys with adrenals, one in each lumbar region, with ureters which drain into the urinary bladder (Figure 11.1). The surface markings and location of non-alimentary viscera of abdomen is shown in Table 11.1. In females, uterus, fallopian tubes and ovaries are located in the pelvis while in males, the testes in the scrotal sacs and penis hang from the pubis. The left scrotal sac hangs slightly lower than the right. The peritoneum, a serous membrane, lines the abdominal cavity and provides a protective cover to many of the abdominal structures. Double folds of peritoneum around the stomach constitute the greater and lesser omentum. The mesentery, a fan-shaped fold of the peritoneum, covers most of the small intestines and anchors it to the posterior abdominal wall.

HISTORY

Obtain a lucid account of history of present illness in a chronological order without distorting the facts by asking too many direct or leading questions. Special attention should be paid to the onset (acute, subacute, insidious) and evolution (progressive, resolving, static) of the disease process and response to therapy. The common symptoms of gastrointestinal disorders include abdominal pain, vomiting, bowel disturbances (diarrhea, constipation), abdominal enlargement, jaundice, alteration in appetite (anorexia or excessive appetite) and failure to thrive (Box 11.1).

Fever may be a dominant feature in children with tuberculosis, malaria, kala-azar, viral hepatitis, cholangitis, amebic or pyogenic liver abscess, pyelophlebitis, cholecystitis, leptospirosis and malignant disorders. Septicemia due to Gram-negative microorganisms is common in children with chronic hepatic dysfunction because of by-passing of reticuloendothelial barrier of the liver by opening up of portosystemic channels.

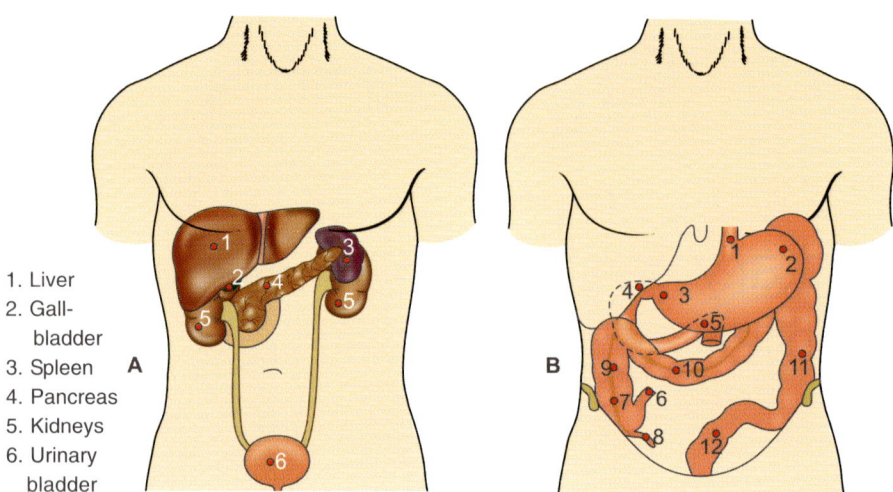

1. Liver
2. Gallbladder
3. Spleen
4. Pancreas
5. Kidneys
6. Urinary bladder

1. Esophagus
2. Stomach
3. Pyloric antrum
4. Duodenum
5. Duodenojejunal flexure
6. Terminal ileum
7. Cecum
8. Appendix
9. Ascending colon
10. Transverse colon
11. Descending colon
12. Sigmoid colon

Figure 11.1A and B (A) Surface markings of non-alimentary tract abdominal viscera. (B) Surface markings of the alimentary tract.

TABLE 11.1 The location and surface markings of non-alimentary abdominal viscera

Organ	Position
Liver	Upper border in the 5th intercostal space on full expiration and lower border about 2 cm below the costal margin in the midclavicular region on full inspiration
Spleen	Located against 9th, 10th and 11th ribs posterior to the mid-axillary line and tip may be normally palpable during first 3 months of life
Gallbladder	At the intersection of right vertical line (from mid-point of inguinal ligament) with the costal margin, i.e. tip of 9th costal cartilage
Pancreas	The body of pancreas lies at the level of L1, head lies below and to the right, and tail lies slightly above and to the left
Kidneys	Upper pole lies deep against 12th rib posteriorly in the lumbar region, the right kidney is 2–3 cm lower than the left and may be normally palpable in infants
Urinary bladder	When distended, it is palpable just above the symphysis pubis in the midline. It is an abdominal organ in infants

Box 11.1 Common symptoms of abdominal diseases

- Pain abdomen
- Nausea, dizziness and vomiting
- Dysphagia
- Dyspepsia, indigestion, heart burn, eructations, gastroesophageal "reflux"
- Constipation
- Diarrhea or malabsorption
- Anorexia or excessive appetite
- Flatulence and excessive wind
- Hiccups, burps or belchings
- Jaundice
- Abdominal distension
- GI bleeding: Hematemesis*, rectal bleeding, and melena
- Dysuria or difficulty in passing urine, frequency of micturition and red-colored urine
- Abdominal mass
- Weight loss or failure to thrive, malnutrition and anemia

*In epistaxis, the blood may be swallowed and vomited out

The potbelly contour of abdomen is normal in infants and should not be considered as an evidence of liver disease. The food fussiness and physiologic potbelly in preschool children is often attributed to liver dysfunction or "weak liver" by parents. Progressive abdominal distension may occur due to enlargement of abdominal viscera, ascites, tumor or gaseous distension.

Ask for history of jaundice at the onset of disease or in the past, whether jaundice is waxing and waning or is it progressively increasing in severity. A fluctuating pattern of jaundice is a characteristic feature of choledochal cyst, Dubin-Johnson syndrome, chronic active hepatitis, biliary calculi and cholestasis. Make sure that mother is not confusing pallor with jaundice by asking relevant questions. Information should be sought regarding the color of urine and stools. Urine is usually clear like water or high colored when concentrated due to dehydration or intake B complex vitamins. Urine may be dark yellow or green in obstructive, jaundice, tea-colored or smoky (microscopic hematuria), brown or red (excessive uric acid, hemoglobinuria), orange colored (intake of pyridium and rifampacin), black on exposure to air (alkaptonuria), blue or green (Hartnup disease, tryptophane gastrointestinal malabsorption intake of drugs like amitriptyline, indomethacin, propofol) or grossly blood stained due to hematuria. The passage of persistently clay-colored or acholic stools and generalized itching are highly suggestive of obstructive jaundice. History of intake of any hepatotoxic drugs or medicines from indigenous or alternative system should be enquired. The drugs which are known to be hepatotoxic include antitubercular agents, anticonvulsants, corticosteroids, androgens, sulfonamides, tetracyclines, macrolides, paracetamol and nimesulide. Ask for history of transfusion of blood products as a source of transmission of hepatitis B or C virus.

When abdominal pain is a dominant symptom, ask specific questions to identify its site (whether pointed with a finger or vaguely referred to by the whole hand), severity (mild or severe enough to make the child cry), nature (constant, boring, colicky), radiation, relieving and aggravating factors. Radiation of pain provides useful clinical guidelines (*Box 11.2*). Renal colic typically starts in the loin and radiates to the groin and sometimes towards genitalia and inner thigh. Midnight pain,

Box 11.2 Radiation of abdominal pain*

- Pain due to renal and ureteric colic radiates downward towards the groin, inner side of thighs and genitalia.
- Gallbladder pain usually radiates towards the tip of right scapula.
- Pain due to diaphragmatic inflammation (cholecystitis, basal pneumonia) may radiate to the top of one or both shoulders.
- Pancreatic pain is excruciating and boring in character and radiates towards the back.

*Radiation of pain occurs due to identical innervation of the affected organ and the sites where pain is radiated.

Box 11.3 Characteristic clinical features of acute appendicitis*

- The onset is with fever, vomiting, anorexia and epigastric pain which shifts to the right iliac fossa.
- Guarding and tenderness over the right iliac fossa or McBurney's point**.
- Rebound tenderness may be present, i.e. pain occurs when hand is released quickly after pressing the abdomen.
- Rovsing sign may be positive, i.e. pressure over the left iliac fossa is followed by pain in the right lower quadrant.
- Psoas sign may be positive, i.e. there is slight flexion of right hip due to irritation of psoas muscle.
- Obturator sign may be positive, i.e. flexion and internal rotation of right thigh causes abdominal pain.
- Ask the child to cough or jump. If there is no pain on coughing or jumping, acute appendicitis is unlikely.

*The features may be atypical, if appendix is located at an ectopic site. Constipation is common but diarrhea may occur with retrocecal or pelvic appendix.
**McBurnery point is located in the right lower abdomen at the junction of outer two-thirds and inner one-third of a line joining anterior superior iliac spine with umbilicus.

which awakens the child, is always pathological while morning pain may be a prank to miss the milk or school. Acute appendicitis is characterized by a combination symptoms and signs and should be ruled out (*Box 11.3*). Episodes of crying spells at night with arching of back, vomiting and poor feeding due to esophagitis are suggestive of gastroesophageal reflux disease. Peptic ulcer is characterized by epigastric pain which is aggravated by intake of NSAIDs, chillies and caffeinated drinks, and relieved by intake of food.

When a child complains of pain at multiple body sites, i.e. abdomen, chest, limbs, headache, etc. it is usually psychogenic or functional.

In adolescent girls, acute excruciating pain of sudden onset in lower abdomen or pelvic region may occur due to torsion of an ovarian cyst or acute pelvic inflammatory disease (PID). The latter condition may follow a sexual encounter and is characterized by abrupt onset of high grade fever and shaking chills in association with intense lower abdominal pain, nausea and vomiting.

Forceful or persistent vomiting in association with failure to thrive and bile-stained vomitus are invariably pathological. Ask duration, severity, frequency, nature of vomitus, aggravating and relieving factors, and associated features. Vomiting is a frequent complaint in viral hepatitis and liver dysfunction associated with intake of hepatotoxins and inborn errors of metabolism. Ask for history of gastrointestinal bleeding (hematemesis, dysentery, and bleeding per rectum or hematochezia) and any generalized bleeding tendency. Painless bleeding without much fecal matter is suggestive of rectal polyp. Anal itching may occur due to pinworms, chronic constipation, hemorrhoids, rectal prolapse, anal skin tags, perianal warts, and inflammatory bowel disease.

Most alimentary disorders are associated with anorexia. Excessive or voracious appetite may be seen in children harbouring ascaris, endocrine disorders (hypothalamic dysfunction, diabetes mellitus, hyperthyroidism), recovering from hepatic dysfunction or receiving corticosteroids. Ask discriminatory details regarding bowel disturbances. History suggestive of steatorrhea and evidences of deficiency of fat-soluble vitamins (A, D, E, K) should be sought. Failure to thrive and developmental retardation may occur as a consequence of chronic liver dysfunction, intra-uterine infections, and inborn errors of metabolism. Ask for any features suggestive of hepatic encephalopathy like changes in the mood or behavior irritability and sleep disturbances. They are followed by confusion, inarticulate speech, somnolence and stupor. The neurological features of Wilson disease are insidious in onset and include clumsiness, scholastic deterioration, behavior problems and dystonic movements. Family history of tuberculosis and history of a liver disorder in other siblings should be enquired.

GENERAL PHYSICAL EXAMINATION

Attitude or decubitus of the patient provides useful information. Children with peritonitis are motionless, while those with abdominal colic are restless. Pinched facies with sallow complexion are seen in cirrhosis. Dyspnea may occur due to massive ascites. Eyes should be examined for proptosis (chlorma, neuroblastoma), cataract, Kayser-Fleischer ring, macular degeneration, chorioretinitis, and signs of deficiency of vitamin A. Kayser-Fleischer rings are grayish-green or golden-brown colored rings located along the upper and lower borders of cornea due to deposition of copper in patients with Wilson disease, familial cholestatic syndrome and chronic active hepatitis. The finding may be visible to the naked eye or with the help of a magnifying glass or slit-lamp examination. When Wilson disease is suspected, look for CNS manifestations, like intention tremors, dysarthria, dystonia, behavior changes and deterioration in school performance. Aniridia or absence of iris is a recognized correlate of Wilms tumor, Rieger syndrome, neoplasms of adrenal cortex and liver. Enlargement of one-half of the body (hemihypertrophy) may be associated with Wilms tumor, Beckwith-Wiedemann syndrome, neurofibromatosis, visceral hemangiomas, hepatocellular carcinoma and adrenocortical carcinoma (**Figure 11.2**).

Record temperature, pulse, respiration, and blood pressure. Look for anemia, cyanosis (portal azygos shunt), jaundice and lymphadenopathy. Assessment of degree of pallor poses practical difficulties in a jaundiced child. Palpebral conjunctiva, dorsum of tongue, nails and skin of palm are reliable sites for clinical evaluation of anemia. In children, clinical jaundice is observed when serum bilirubin approaches 2 mg/dL while in a newborn baby, clinical jaundice does not manifest unless serum bilirubin is at least 4 mg/dL or more. Jaundice is evaluated by examining scleral

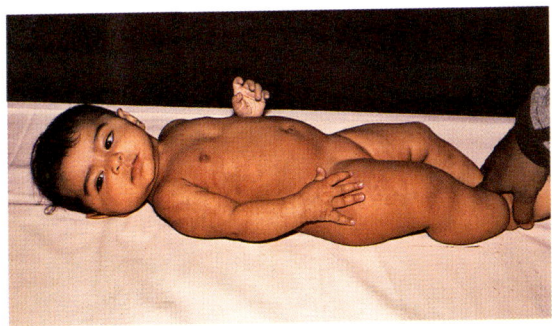

Figure 11.2 Hemihypertrophy on the right side in a child with Wilms tumor.

conjunctiva, under surface of tongue, buccal mucosa and skin in natural daylight. Muddy conjunctiva should not be mistaken with jaundice. In newborn babies, jaundice is best looked for by blanching the skin of the face around the nasolabial folds, root of the nose and cheeks. Jaundice is a characteristic feature of hepatocellular dysfunction, biliary obstruction or cholestasis. Jaundice is minimal or absent in patients with Reye syndrome and space occupying lesions of liver due to amebic and pyogenic liver abscess, hydatid cyst, primary benign or malignant neoplasms of liver.

Nutritional status It should be assessed by taking standard anthropometric measurements and by looking for evidences of protein-energy malnutrition and deficiencies of various micronutrients. A large number of gastrointestinal disorders are associated with nutritional disorders, e.g. chronic diarrhea, malabsorption syndrome, celiac disease, mucoviscidosis, inflammatory bowel disease, giardiasis, etc. Growth and neuromotor development are retarded in children with inborn errors of metabolism, intrauterine infections and chronic liver dysfunction.

Oral cavity Oral cavity is the portal of entry or window to the gastrointestinal tract and is likely to mirror and exhibit the inflammatory changes that take place in the gut. Look for thrush (monilial stomatitis), oral ulcers, membranous pharyngitis (streptococcal pharyngitis, diphtheria, infectious mononucleosis), herpangina, hypertrophied gums and macroglossia (glycogen storage disease, mucopolysaccharidosis, cretinism, Beckwith-Wiedemann syndrome, gangliosidosis and new growth of tongue). Recurrent episodes of oropharyngeal candidiasis is suggestive of cell-mediated immunodeficiency state including AIDS. Aphthous ulcers (acute herpetic gingivostomatitis) are small superficial painful ulcers with a white or yellow base with an erythematous halo of hyperemia. They are distributed over the gums, buccal mucosa, tongue and palate and cause difficulty in feeding. Stippled blue line over the edge of gums is suggestive of exposure to lead and may be associated with episodes of colicky abdominal pain, constipation and basophilic stippling. Diffuse hypertrophy of gums is common following phenytoin therapy, histiocytosis X, xanthomatosis, acute monocytic leukemia and Hurler syndrome while epulis is a localized swelling of gums due to trauma, granuloma or benign hyperplasia.

Pigmentation of lips and buccal mucosa is a recognized feature of Peutz-Jeghers syndrome which is associated with multiple polyps of stomach or colon. Bald and smooth tongue due to atrophy of papillae is suggestive of vitamin B_{12} deficiency, iron deficiency anemia, pellagra and celiac disease. "Strawberry tongue" is seen in patients with scarlet fever, bacterial toxic-shock syndrome and Kawasaki disease due to presence of white or bright-red enlarged papillae jutting against the bright-red surface of the tongue. Congenital fissuring of tongue or "scrotal tongue" is a common correlate of Down syndrome. Geographical tongue is characterized by constantly evolving and changing irregular red areas of desquamated epithelium and filiform papillae with a sharp whitish-yellow border giving an appearance of a map over the tongue. It is benign and of no pathological significance. Tongue-tie (ankyloglossia) is characterized by a short, thick and fibrous frenulum, inability to protrude the tongue and a midline notch at the tip of the tongue. Examine the floor of the mouth for any cysts. Ranula is seen as a bluish-white transluscent swelling due to formation of a mucocele because of ruptured salivary gland duct. Sublingual dermoid cyst, on the other hand, is an opaque sublingual swelling due to sequestration of epidermal tissue.

Skin and its appendages Skin should be examined for any petechiae, ecchymoses, scratch marks, angiomas, xanthomas, exanthem, seborrheic dermatitis and photosensitivity. Xanthomata over the extensor surfaces of extremities with xanthelasma in the eyelids may be seen in children with prolonged chalestatic jaundice due to biliary obstruction. Examine nails for clubbing (cirrhosis, ulcerative colitis, Crohn's disease, malabsorption syndrome, polyposis of colon) and leukonychia or white transverse lines in the nails (severe hypoalbuminemia due to nephrotic syndrome, Kwashiorkor, malabsorption due to celiac disease and protein losing enteropathy). Pedal edema, puffiness, ascites, and anasarca can occur because of hepatic and renal disorders and malabsorption.

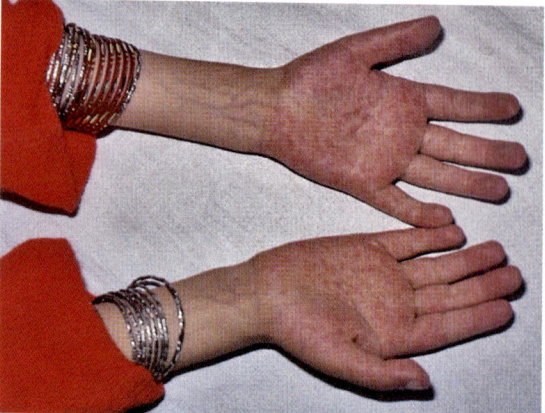

Figure 11.3 Palmar erythema due to hepatocellular failure.

Evidences of hepatocellular failure Jaundice, alterations in sensorium (behavior changes, irritability, sleep disturbances, drowsiness), fetor hepaticus (musty odor of breath due to mercaptans), "flapping tremors", palmar erythema, hyperreflexia, extensor plantars and spider nevi should be looked for (Figure 11.3). "Liver flap" or asterixis is demonstrated by asking the patient to extend both arms and try to maintain hands in a dorsiflexed position. There will be nonrhythmic jerky asymmetric flexion and extension movements of wrists and small joints of hands or drop of hands due to inability to maintain the dorsiflexed position (Figure 11.4). Rarely, gynecomastia and testicular atrophy may be seen in adolescent boys with chronic liver dysfunction because of accumulation of female sex hormones due to their reduced breakdown in the liver. In adolescent girls with chronic active hepatitis, there may be delayed puberty, menstrual irregularities, amenorrhea and acne.

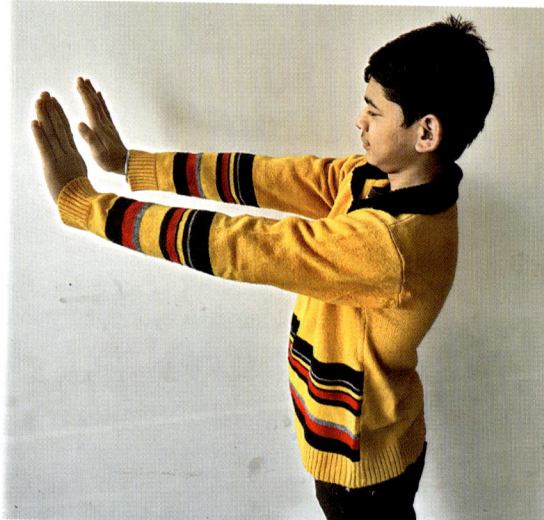

Figure 11.4 Method for elicitation of "flapping tremors". The patient is asked to extend both arms and try to maintain hands in a dorsiflexed position.

Acute kidney injury (AKI) Acute renal failure may occur due to hypovolemia (severe dehydration, blood loss, burns, diabetic ketoacidosis, septicemia), intrinsic renal damage (acute glomerulonephritis, hemolytic uremic syndrome, drugs and toxins) and obstructive anomalies of the renal system. Most cases of posterior urethral valves are diagnosed by prenatal ultrasonography showing evidences of hydroureteronephrosis, distended bladder and a thickened bladder wall. AKI is usually associated with reduced or absent urine output. At times urine output may be normal (non-oliguric AKI), especially when renal failure is caused by nephrotoxic drugs, birth asphyxia or sepsis.

Bony swellings and tenderness is an important sign of infiltrative disorders of bones especially acute leukemia. Skeletal deformities (mucopolysaccharidosis), evidences of osteochondritis (congenital infections especially syphilis), rickets (cystinosis and tyrosinosis) and pathological fractures (Gaucher's disease) should be looked for. Tumors of soft tissue (epidermoid cysts) and bones (osteomas) especially involving mandible may be associated with familial colorectal polyposis (Gardner syndrome).

Spine should be examined for Pott's disease. *Psoas sign* appears due to inflammation of psoas muscle due to appendicitis, iliac adenitis and perinephric abscess. It is characterized by slight flexion of thigh, limp and pain on sudden extension of hip joint. Flexion and internal rotation of thigh may cause abdominal pain (obturator sign).

EXAMINATION OF ABDOMEN

Clinical quadrants For clinical purposes, abdomen is divided into 9 quadrants, i.e. right hypochondrium, epigastrium, left hypochondrium, right lumbar (flank), umbilical, left lumbar (flank), right iliac fossa, hypogastrium or suprapubic region and left iliac fossa (Figure 11.5).

INSPECTION

Note the contour of abdomen, whether normal, bloated or bulging and depressed or concave. Look for any scar over the abdominal wall and ask for the nature of any surgical procedure done. Movements of all quadrants, fullness whether localized or generalized, position and shape of umbilicus (flushed or everted), discharge, inflammation, and nodule should be looked for. In ascites, there is enlargement of abdomen with fullness of flanks and umbilicus appears as a tranverse slit ("smiling face" sign). In obesity, umbilicus or belly button is invaginated to form a deep cleft. There may be umbilical granuloma or bright-red polyp in a newborn baby. Polyp may have a small opening discharging urine (persistent urachus or urachal cyst) or serosanguinous fluid or fecal matter through omphalomesenteric duct. Umbilical hernia consists of a symmetric protrusion of gut through the umbilical ring and manifests during early infancy. Paraumbilical hernias are more common and occur later in life. There is

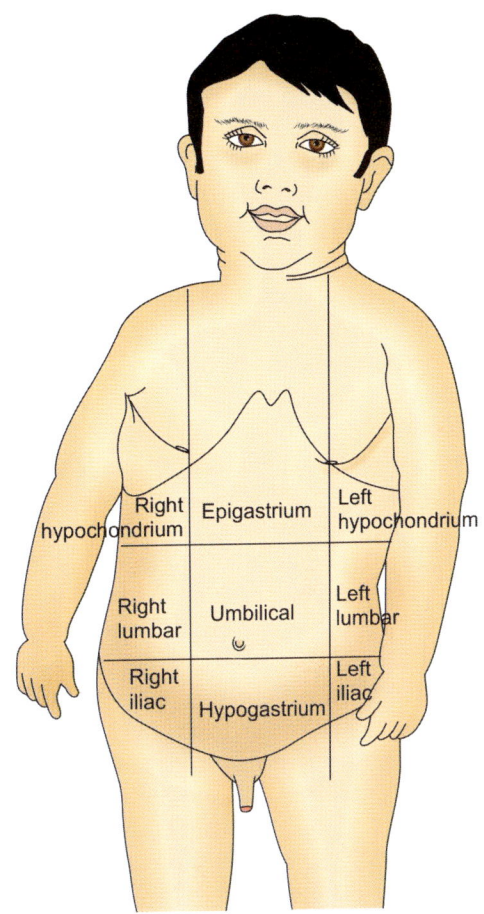

Figure 11.5 Clinical quadrants of abdomen. The vertical lines are projected upwards from mid-inguinal points. The upper horizontal line passes through the lower costal edges of the thorax. The lower horizontal line joins the two anterior superior iliac spines.

protrusion of gut through a gap above or below the umbilicus due to divarication of recti. Periumbilical ecchymosis (Cullen sign) and ecchymoses of one or both flanks (Grey-Turner sign) are suggestive of intra-abdominal hemorrhage due to pancreatitis and rupture of liver or spleen.

Look for any visible and engorged veins and assess direction of flow of blood. The direction of flow of blood is determined by placing both the index fingers at a point over the branchless segment of engorged vein. The vein is emptied by stripping one of the index fingers over it. One index finger at a time is taken off the vein to ascertain the direction of flow of blood. *The normal flow of blood is away from the umbilicus thus draining the blood from the umbilical veins into the portal system.* In portal hypertension, there are periumbilical engorged veins with exaggerated flow of blood away from umbilicus (caput medusae). In inferior vena caval obstruction, the engorged veins are at the flanks with flow of blood from below upwards while in superior vena caval obstruction, the engorged veins are above the umbilicus with flow of blood from above downwards. Apart from engorged veins, there may be edema of legs, buttocks and groins in children with inferior vena caval obstruction. Atrophic white or pink wrinkled striae may appear on the abdominal wall and buttocks due to rupture of elastic fibers because of sudden distension (due to ascites and obesity) and stretching of skin. Broad purple striae are characteristic of Cushing syndrome and prolonged steroid therapy.

Generalized distension and enlargement of the abdomen may occur due to fluid, gas, feces, fat or a mass. Abdomen is flat or scaphoid in an infant with diaphragmatic hernia. In obstructive uropathy, there is complete absence of muscles of abdominal wall giving a wrinkled appearance to the abdomen (prune-belly syndrome). Localized distension may occur around the umbilicus (small bowel obstruction, mesenteric cyst), hypochondriac regions (liver, spleen) or above the symphysis pubis (urinary bladder, uterus or ovary).

Site and direction of peristaltic waves should be looked for. Gastric peristaltic waves, passing across the upper abdomen from left to right, are classically seen in infants with pyloric stenosis. Distended coils of small bowel may be seen in the center of abdomen in a "ladder pattern" in children with subacute obstruction of small bowel.

PALPATION

The hands should be warm and nails should be trimmed for satisfactory abdominal examination. Divert child's attention by conversation during palpation. Infants are generally apprehensive and often cry and strain thus tensing the abdomen. It is best to examine an infant in the mother's lap. Breastfeeding is the best soother to elicit cooperation (Figure 11.6). Preschool children are

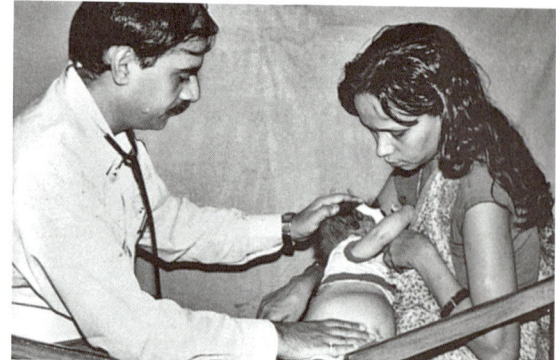

Figure 11.6 Infant is best examined in the mother's lap while she is breastfeeding.

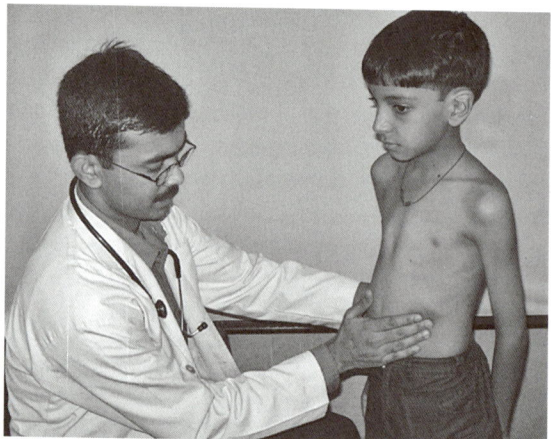

Figure 11.7 Examination of abdomen in a standing position in a preschool child.

best examined in a standing position (Figure 11.7). Older child can be asked to lie on the examination table, flex the hips and knees, relax and take deep breaths. Palpate the abdomen with flat of the hand with slight flexion of metacarpophalangeal joints rather than the tips of fingers. The site of abdomen where child localizes pain should be examined at the end after having palpated other areas of abdomen. During palpation, watch the child for any change in facial expression, wincing or screwing of eyes or forehead as an evidence of tenderness. It is unnecessary and unreliable to ask the child whether it hurts or not.

"Dipping technique" is used, if massive ascites is present. The viscera are explored by sudden but gentle dipping of fingers. At times satisfactory abdominal examination is possible only after paracentesis. Feel of abdomen may be normal, soft, doughy, tense and rigid. Tenderness may be localized, generalized and gurgling sounds may be palpable. Edema of abdominal wall is assessed by pinching the skin for 5 seconds (Figure 11.8) or by seeing the impression created by the diaphragm of stethoscope following auscultation.

When there is localized abdominal pain and tenderness, look for Carnett's sign. The child is asked to lie supine and raise both legs with extended knees or lift the head and shoulders in order to contract the muscles of abdominal wall. If the area or severity of tenderness increases with this maneuver, it indicates that the cause of pain is in the abdominal wall and not intra-abdominal.

Look for enlargement of liver (don't forget to identify the upper border and span of liver), spleen, kidneys, cecum and descending colon (Box 11.4). Liver is normally palpable up to 2 cm below the costal margin throughout childhood while spleen tip may be palpable in infants during first 3 months of age. In neonates, liver edge is palpable up to 3.5 cm below the right costal margin. The average liver span is 4–5 cm in newborns and 6–12 cm in children up to 12 years of age. The expected liver span in healthy Indian children between 1.0 month and 12 years is given in Table 11.2. The normal liver is soft and has a

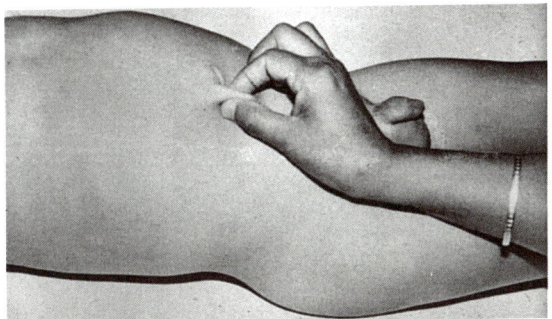

Figure 11.8 The skin of abdominal wall is pinched for a few seconds and released to look for pitting edema of abdominal wall.

Box 11.4 Key points for examination of liver and spleen

- Check for enlargement beyond the costal margin (cm)
- Edge: Round, sharp, well defined or ill defined, notch present or not
- Consistency: Soft, firm or hard
- Surface: Smooth, granular, nodular, or lobular
- Tenderness: Present or absent
- Upper border or level of dullness of liver and spleen (intercostal space)
- Span of liver and spleen by measuring it from upper border to the palpable margin (cm)

TABLE 11.2 Liver and spleen size or span in healthy Indian boys*

Age (years)	Liver span (cm)			Spleen span (cm)		
	Mean (SD)	3rd centile	97th centile	Mean (SD)	3rd centile	97th centile
1–3 mo	6.5 (1.23)	4.8	8.9	4.9 (1.44)	3.7	8.7
3–6 mo	7.1 (0.77)	5.9	8.9	5.4 (0.61)	4.4	6.6
6–12 mo	7.5 (0.88)	6.1	9.5	6.0 (0.86)	4.4	8.3
1–2 y	8.6 (0.85)	7.1	10.2	6.4 (1.01)	4.7	9.8
2–4 y	9.0 (1.34)	7.2	11.9	6.9 (1.01)	4.1	9.3
4–6 y	10.3 (1.27)	7.3	14.7	7.4 (0.99)	5.0	10.9
6–8 y	10.8 (0.94)	9.0	12.3	7.9 (0.94)	6.3	9.7
8–10 y	11.9 (1.08)	10.0	14.1	8.2 (1.02)	6.8	10.9
10–12 y	12.6 (1.2)	11.0	15.5	8.7 (1.84)	6.3	11.7

*There is no significant difference in the size of liver and spleen in boys and girls.
Source: Adapted from Dhingra B, Sharma S, Mishra D, et al. Normal values of liver and spleen size by ultrasonography in Indian children. Indian Pediatr 2010, 47:487–492.

rounded margin. Ascertain the consistency of liver and whether surface is smooth, granular or nodular. When margin of the liver is sharp and well defined, it is suggestive of firm or hard consistency of the organ. The liver may be pulsatile in children with tricuspid regurgitation. The presence of pitting edema or tenderness over the intercostal spaces overlying the hepatic region supports the possibility of underlying amebic or pyogenic abscess. Asymmetric or focal enlargement of liver with elevated upper level of hepatic dullness is seen in children with amebic or pyogenic liver abscess, hydatid cyst, focal nodular hyperplasia, benign neoplasms and primary or metastatic malignancy. Turn the child to right lateral position to feel the tip of just palpable spleen (Figure 11.9). Spleen becomes palpable when it enlarges to at least two to three times its size. The spleen enlarges downward and medially towards right iliac fossa.

The enlargement of liver and spleen is measured from the midcalvicular point over the costal margin to the lower most edge of the organ (Figure 11.10). The liver and spleen may become palpable due to downward displacement (without enlargement) because of contractual deformities of the thorax, hyperinflated lungs, basal pleural effusion, increased intrathoracic pressure, subphrenic abscess, or collection of air and relaxation of abdominal musculature because of gross hypotonia.

Kidneys should be palpated by bimanual technique (Figure 11.11). The lower pole of the right kidney may be normally palpable in some children. Renal angles, their fullness, tenderness and pitting edema should be looked for.

Look for any mass and assess whether it is intra-abdominal or in the wall of abdomen by *Rising test*. When a patient is asked to sit up from supine position, intra-abdominal mass becomes less prominent and difficult to palpate while a parietal

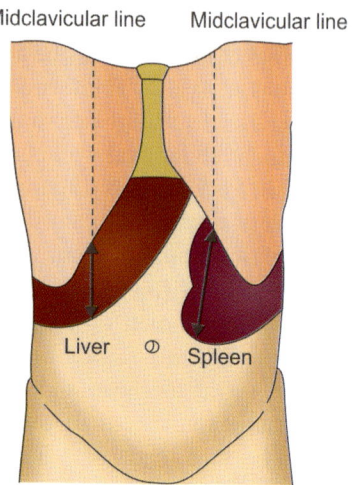

Figure 11.10 Landmarks for measuring hepatosplenomegaly. The maximum size of the organ is measured from midclavicular point over the costal margins up to the lower most margin of the organ with the help of a white plastic ruler.

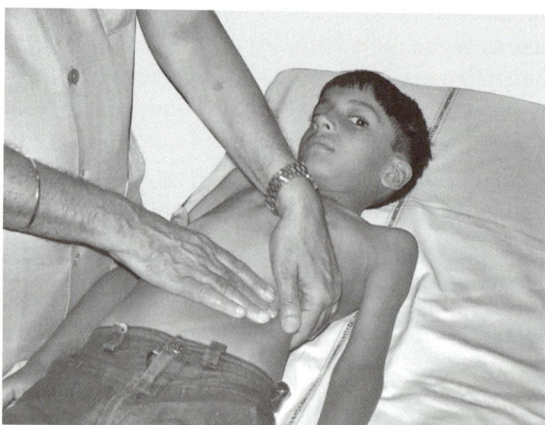

Figure 11.11 Bimanual palpation for kidneys. The hand over the loin lifts the kidney forwards which is explored by the other hand placed over the lumbar region.

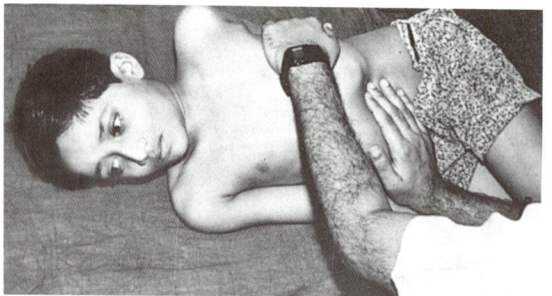

Figure 11.9 The child is turned to the right lateral position, left hand is placed over the lower part of the chest and upper abdomen and spleen tip is searched with the fingers of right hand by asking the patient to take relaxed deep breaths by inflating the abdomen with each inspiration.

mass becomes prominent and immobile. Divarication of recti is noted as a linear bulge between the recti muscles when a supine child is asked to sit up. Identify the site, size, shape, mobility of the mass with respiration and from side-to-side, bimanual palpability, does it cross the midline and whether it is pulsatile or not. Try to assess whether the upper and lower borders of the mass are distinctly felt or they are "lost" into the thorax (liver and spleen) or pelvis (bladder, uterus and ovary).

The main purpose of clinical examination of an abdominal mass is to assess the organ of origin and pathological nature of the mass. The consistency, margins, tenderness, percussion characteristics of the mass should be ascertained. The salient points for examining an abdominal mass are listed in *Box 11.5*. Nephroblastoma (Wilms tumor) and neuroblastoma are common intra-abdominal tumors in children and should be differentiated on clinical examination (Table 11.3). Special technique is used for palpation of pyloric tumor. While infant is being fed on the left breast, the pylorus is explored with fingers of left hand by palpating gently but deeply lateral to the edge of right rectus muscle in the epigastric region

> **Box 11.5 Salient points for examining an abdominal mass**
>
> - Is it parietal (located in the wall of abdomen) or intra-abdominal?
> - Location of the mass and its likely visceral origin
> - Size of the mass and whether it crosses the midline or not
> - Whether upper and lower borders of the mass can be reached?
> - Cystic or solid
> - Consistency: Soft, firm, or hard
> - Surface: Smooth, granular, nodular, lobular
> - Is mass pulsatile? Are pulsations transmitted or true expansile pulsations?
> - Is the mass tender or painless?
> - Mobility of the mass on breathing and side-to-side mobility
> - Ballotable and bimanually palpable or not
> - Percussion: Tympanitic, resonant, dull, with or without hydatid thrill
> - Auscultation: Look for any bruit or friction rub

(Figure 11.12). Pyloric mass, an olive-like firm swelling is located at a point 2 to 3 cm above and to the right of umbilicus. A mass of retroperitoneal origin is fixed while a mesenteric cyst or mass can be made to move freely from side-to-side. The

TABLE 11.3 Salient differences between Wilms tumor and neuroblastoma

Features	Wilms tumor	Neuroblastoma
Origin	Kidney	Adrenal gland or sympathetic neural pathway
Age	3–4 years	1–2 years
Constitutional symptoms	Uncommon like hematuria and elevation of blood pressure	Common like tenderness, irritability, wasting, "blueberry muffins" skin
Abdominal mass	Soft well-encapsulated smooth mass, mobile but does not cross the midline	Fixed and immobile and may cross the midline
Sites of metastasis	Liver and lungs	Skin, liver and bone marrow
Associations	WAGR (**W**ilms tumor, **a**niridia, **g**enital abnormalities, mental **r**etardation), hemihypertrophy and Beckwith–Wiedemann syndrome	Opsoclonus–myoclonus syndrome, Horner syndrome, "Raccoon eyes" or periorbital ecchymosis, neurofibromatosis
Catecholamine metabolites in urine	Normal	Elevation of vanillylmandelic acid (VMA) and homovanillic acid (HVA) levels
Ultrasound examination	Lobulated, smooth, well circumscribed mass arising from the kidney, rarely stippled calcification	Solid, irregular, nodular, heterogenous mass with curvilinear calcification

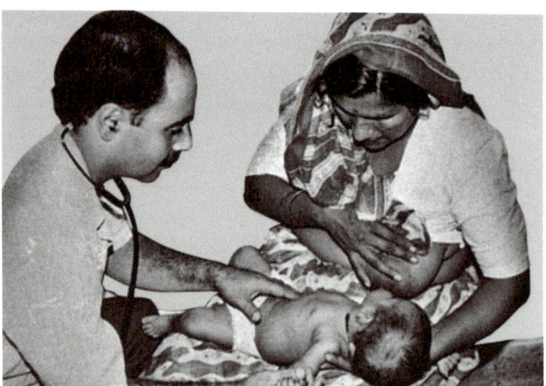

Figure 11.12 Method for examination of pyloric tumor. Refer to the text for details.

urinary bladder is an intra-abdominal organ in children and is easily palpable when full. Midline globular cystic mass over the suprapubic region is usually due to distended bladder. The swelling disappears after passage of urine. The common causes of distended bladder include postoperative state, posterior urethral valve, urethral stone, encephalopathy, neurogenic bladder due to meningomyelocele, paralytic poliomyelitis, transverse myelitis and Gullain-Barre syndrome. In children with constipation, hard fecal masses (which can be indented on pressure) are felt over the descending colon region in left iliac fossa.

The hernial sites should be examined for umbilical and inguinal hernia. Transillumination of swelling, whether parietal or intra-abdominal, is useful to differentiate between a cystic and solid mass. Examine external genitals for any abnormality.

PERCUSSION

Abdomen is tympanitic on percussion and it becomes excessively tympanitic or "resounding" in a child with intestinal obstruction or paralytic ileus. Look for shifting dullness, fluid thrill, puddle sign, and percuss over the mass. For eliciting shifting dullness, the patient is placed in a supine position. Percussion is performed from umbilicus towards one of the flanks (avoid the flank which is occupied by an enlarged viscus or mass) till dullness is elicited. The child is turned to the other side and held in lateral position to allow the fluid to gravitate towards the umbilicus. In this position, the nondependent flank will become resonant while percussion would be dull over the umbilicus and dependent flank, when there is free fluid in the abdomen.

Fluid wave or thrill appears later and is elicitable when ascites becomes moderate or massive. One hand is placed over the flank and sharp taps are given over the other flank with the index finger of dominant hand of the examiner. Distinct thrill due to movements of ascitic fluid shall be appreciated. To prevent transmission of tapping impulse to travel through the abdominal wall, assistant or patient is asked to firmly place hypothenar edge of his outstreched hand over the midline of abdomen (Figure 11.13). Massive ascites with non-pitting unilateral lymphedema of a limb is suggestive of chylous ascites (Figure 11.14). For the diagnosis of minimal ascites, the child is placed in knee-elbow position to ensure gravitation of fluid to mid-abdominal region. The chest piece of stethoscope is placed over the midabdomen and abdominal wall is gently tapped with index finger moving from one flank towards the centre till water puddle sound is audible when edge of the ascitic fluid pocket is tapped (Puddle sign).

Liver dullness, which is normally present between 6th rib and costal margin, may be

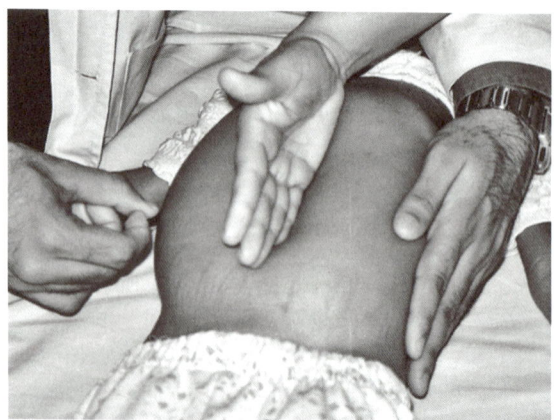

Figure 11.13 Method for elicitation of fluid thrill. One hand should be firmly placed over the midline of the abdomen to prevent transmission of tapping impulse to travel through the abdominal wall.

The Alimentary System and Abdomen

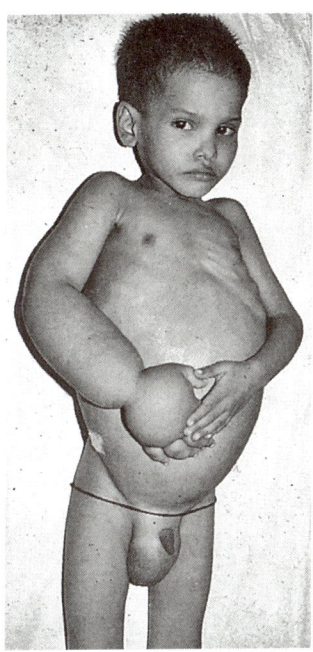

Figure 11.14 Chylous ascites with hydrocele and non-pitting lymphedema of right upper limb.

obliterated, if there is free gas in the peritoneal cavity. Splenic dullness extends from 9th to 11th ribs on the left side. Hydatid thrill should be looked for whenever there is gross isolated hepatomegaly or splenomegaly. When hydatid cyst is percussed, the displaced scolices and hydatid "sand" touch the pleximeter finger soon after the tap.

AUSCULTATION

Peristaltic sounds may be normal, decreased, absent or exaggerated. Exaggerated intestinal sounds or borborygmi are heard in children with intestinal obstruction and during an intestinal colic. In generalized peritonitis and state of paralytic ileus, the abdomen becomes silent. Friction sound over the enlarged liver and spleen is suggestive of perihepatitis and perisplenitis (infarction because of sickle cell anemia, abscess, leukemic infiltrates, infective endocarditis, following liver biopsy or splenic puncture). Bruit over the hepatic area suggests the possibility of hereditary hemorrhagic telangiectasia or hemangioendothelioma. Venous hum may be audible over the epigastric region in children in whom extensive portosystemic collateral circulation is established (Cruveilhier–Baumgarten syndrome). It is caused by a congenital patent umbilical vein draining into the portal vein. Bruit over the lumbar areas anteriorly on either side of midline should be looked for in children with hypertension. The abdomen should be firmly pressed backwards with the chest piece of stethoscope to identify the bruit due to renal artery stenosis. Succussion splash may be elicited by auscultating the stomach area while gently shaking the patient. A splashing sound like the noise made by hot water bottle partially filled with water and air is heard when stomach is distended with fluid.

GENITALS AND GROINS

Inguinal nodes are located in two chains, the horizontal chain below the inguinal ligament and a vertical chain along the line of saphenous vein. Look for enlarged lymph nodes in the inguinal region which are common and of no significance in children who walk bare feet. Inguinal lymph nodes may enlarge in association with generalized lymphadenopathy. Enlarged and exquisitely tender inguinal lymph nodes are seen in patients with bubonic plague due to *Yersinia pestis*. Look for any inguinoscrotal swelling due to hernia or hydocele. In hernia, the upper border of the swelling cannot be reached, swelling increases in size and has expansile impulse on crying or coughing and may reduce in size or disappear on lying down. Hernia is reducible by manipulation and it is opaque or gut is visible on transillumination unlike hydocele. Physiologic hydrocele may be present at birth and it usually disappears by 3 months of age. When inguinoscrotal swelling is not reducible, it is suggestive of hydrocele of the spermatic cord or an incarcerated inguinal hernia.

Male genitalia Look for tight prepuce or phimosis and balanitis (inflammation of glass) or meatitis and posthitis (inflammation of prepuce) which are important correlates of urinary tract infection. In uncircumcised boys, balanitis and posthitis are common due to entrapment of smegma within the foreskin. The foreskin is not retractable in children below 2 years of age but it causes no difficulty in voiding. Transient small epithelial pearls or inclusion cysts may be present on the distal portion of the prepuce in newborn babies. In adolescent boys, pearly white papules 1–3 mm size may be seen on the penile corona and should not be confused with venereal warts. Look for urethral opening which is normally located on the tip of the glans. In epispadias, urethral opening is located on the dorsal surface of penis while in hypospadias urethral meatus opens on the ventral surface of the penis. The opening may be located anywhere on the ventral surface of glans, shaft of the penis, penoscrotal region and perineum. When hypospadias is associated with ventral curvature of the penis, it is called chordee.

Look for cryptorchidism or ectopic testis and ambiguous genitals which may be missed by parents. The combinations of hypospadias and bilateral or unilateral cryptorchidism is highly suggestive of intersex unless proved otherwise. Retractile testis can be pulled down gently into the scrotum and should not be confused with undescended testis. The condition affects 1 in 200 male infants. The length of a gently stretched penis in a normal male infant varies between 2.8 and 4.2 cm (1.1–1.6 inches) with a circumference of 0.9–1.3 cm (0.35–0.5 inches). Micropenis is rare and diagnosed when penile length is less than 1.9 cm (0.75 inches) in infants. It is diagnosed when stretched penis is < –2.5 standard deviation of the mean in a child with normal internal and external male genitalia. It should not be confused with embedded penis in obese children. Enlargement of testis, with or without pain, may occur due to orchitis (mumps, coxsackie, rubella), epididymitis, leukemic infiltrates, Henoch-Schönlein purpura, Kawasaki disease, torsion of appendix of testis and tumor. Torsion of testis is characterized by sudden onset of severe pain, swelling of testis, tenderness and scrotal edema. The testis may assume horizontal lie and cremasteric reflex disappears. Elevation of testis does not provide any pain relief or pain may become worse. When appendix of testis undergoes torsion, a tender blue nodule is seen over the upper pole of the testicle (blue dot sign). Testicular torsion is a surgical emergency and must be relieved within 6 hours to salvage the testis. Acute epididymitis is characterized by swelling and pain over the back of testicle where coiled tubes of epididymis are located. Elevation of testis relieves pain due to epididymo-orchitis (Prehn's sign). Doppler ultrasound shows increased blood flow to the epididymis while blood flow is reduced in torsion of testis. Acute epididymitis usually occurs in adolescent boys due to sexually transmitted infection. The varicoceles due to varicosities of spermatic veins feel like a "bag of worms" in the scrotum. A painless swelling at the upper pole of testis may occur due to epididymitis or spermatocele. Priapism is a rare complication due to sludging of corpora cavernosa because of chronic myelogenous leukemia and sickle cell disease.

Assess the sexual maturity rate and stage. In precocious puberty, both testes and penis are large in size while in congenital adrenal hyperplasia (CAH), there is isolated enlargement of phallus.

Female genitalia The adolescent girl must be examined in the presence of a nurse or female attendant. Look for any vaginal discharge, redness, foreign body and hematocolpos due to labial adhesions or imperforate vagina. Vulvovaginitis may occur due to bacterial vaginosis, pinworm infestation, trichinosis, *Chlamydia trachomatis, Candida albicans*, herpes simplex, and trauma or sexual abuse. In adolescent girls, vulvar and inguinal irritation and pruritus may occur due to scabies and pubic lice. Look for specks of feces of parasitis on the underwear and careful examination of pubic area may show nits or adult lice (crabs) in children with poor personal hygiene. Look for ambiguous genitalia and clitoral enlargement or virilization, which is a characteristic feature of congenital adrenal hyperplasia (CAH). Clitoris has two paramedian frenulae (unlike penis which has a single frenulum) on its ventral surface and is covered with tissue on its superior aspect. Sarcoma botryoides is characterized by moist grape-like fleshy mass jutting out of vulva. It may be associated with multiple congenital anomalies. The sexual maturity rating should be assessed.

RECTAL EXAMINATION

Look for perianal excoriations, mucocutaneous lesions, skin tags, fissure, fistula, inflammation and diaper rash. Anal skin tags are common and are of no significance. They may occur due to chronic constipation or diarrhea, hemorrhoids, Crohn's disease or bowel inflammatory disease. Prolapse of a rectal polyp appears as a dark beefy-red mass compared to lighter pink mucosal appearance of rectal prolapse. The common causes of rectal prolapse in children include malnutrition, acute or persistent diarrhea, chronic constipation, intestinal parasites especially trichinosis, ulcerative colitis, cystic fibrosis, celiac disease, pertussis and Ehlers-Danlos syndrome. When there are rectal polyps, look for pigmentation of oral mucosa (Peutz-Jeghers syndrome). Anal fissure may occur due to severe constipation and is usually located at 6 o' clock position and is associated with a tear in the lining of anal canal. Digital examination is likely to be extremely painful and should not be attempted in such a patient.

Rectal examination is indicated in children suspected to have intestinal obstruction (Hrischsprung's disease, intussusception), mass extending into the pelvis, rectal bleeding and urethral stone. The child is made to lie in the left lateral position and the right thigh and right knee are flexed. The examination is conducted by using the smallest finger depending upon the age of the child. A well-lubricated little finger is used in newborn babies and infants, and index finger in an older child. Insert the finger slowly in a posterior or backward direction. The child should be asked to relax and take deep breaths. On withdrawing the finger after rectal examination, look at it for any staining with mucus, pus and blood. Microscopic examination of the material on the finger may show cellular exudates, ova of worms and protozoa such as Amoeba, Giardia and *Blantidium coli*. In Hirschsprung's disease, anal sphincter grips the finger and it is not possible to reach the feces due to presence of a narrow segment. But when finger is withdrawn, there is explosive passage of flatus and feces located in the distended rectum. In functional megacolon, anal canal is normal and finger enters the mass of firm feces. In anorectal stenosis, a ring or diaphragm is felt about 1.5–2.0 cm above the anal verge.

In meningomyelocele and spinal cord injury, anal sphincter may be lax and patulous. In distal or long-standing intussusception, a smooth rounded mass akin to uterine cervix may be palpable with staining of examiner's finger with blood.

CLINICAL CHARACTERISTICS OF COMMON ORGANOMEGALIES

Liver

The liver is normally palpable up to 2 cm below the right costal margin throughout childhood. It is normally soft in consistency and has a rounded margin. The pathological enlargement may occur upwards though it is generally downwards towards the right hypochondrium and umbilical regions. The margin is well defined and it moves freely with respiration. The fingers cannot be insinuated between the liver and costal margin. It is not bimanually palpable and is not mobile from side to side. The enlargement may affect any lobe of the liver but generally both the lobes are simultaneously enlarged. The left lobe of the liver may be more prominent in children with amebic abscess and portal hypertension. It is dull on percussion and dullness merges with subcostal hepatic dullness. The upper border of hapatic dullness must be identified on percussion to calculate liver span. Auscultate the liver to look for hepatic rub due to perihepatitis, liver abscess and leukemic infiltrates.

Significant isolated hepatomegaly with minimal or absence of splenomegaly is seen in children with cardiac failure, constrictive pericarditis, liver abscess, hydatid cyst, and glycogen storage disease (Figure 11.15), cirrhosis, primary or metastatic malignancy, mucopolysaccharidosis, veno-occlusive disease, Budd-Chiari syndrome, persistent hepatitis and tuberculosis.

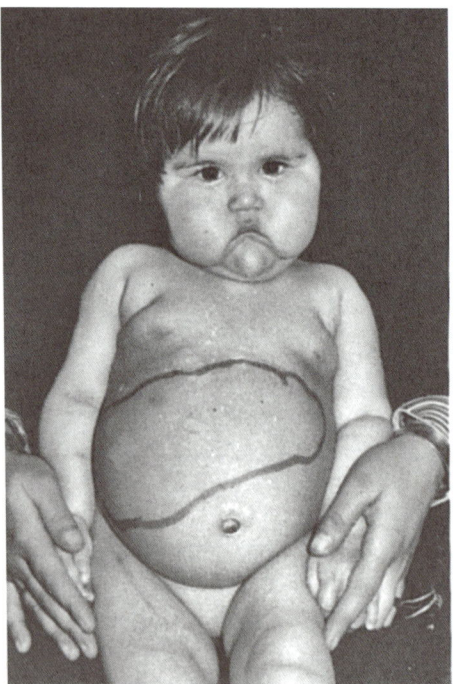

Figure 11.15 Glycogen storage disease. Note typical doll-like facies and massive hepatomegaly.

Gallbladder

The enlargement of gallbladder presents as a pear-shaped swelling which projects beneath the center of the undersurface of the liver. It is cystic in consistency and freely mobile from side-to-side. Murphy's sign may be positive in patients with acute cholecystitis. Maintain constant but gentle pressure over the gallbladder region and ask the patient to take a deep breath. The patient "catches his breath" due to pain when gallbladder touches the fingers. Choledochal cyst produces a cystic swelling at a site identical to gallbladder but swelling appears rather early in life and is fixed and non-mobile.

Spleen

The spleen has to enlarge by about two to three times before it becomes palpable. It enlarges downwards and medially towards the umbilicus. It moves freely with respiration. The margin is characterized by a notch. The finger cannot be insinuated between the spleen and the costal margin. Anteriorly it is dull on percussion while posteriorly it is resonant. It is not palpable bimanually. Auscultation may reveal spenic rub in a child with perisplenitis due to sickle cell disease.

Massive splenomegaly with minimal hepatomegaly is seen in children with portal hypertension, thalassemia major, chronic myeloid leukemia, myeloid metaplasia, chronic malaria, kala-azar, Gaucher's disease (Figure 11.16) and amyloidosis.

Kidneys

Either one or both the kidneys may be enlarged. The bean-shaped mass with rounded margins is located in the lumbar region. It does not move freely with respiration. It is located more posteriorly causing bulging of the renal angle. It is bimanually palpable and mobile from side-to-side. The kidney mass is resonant on percussion anteriorly but dull posteriorly. It does not cross the midline except when there is horseshoe kidney.

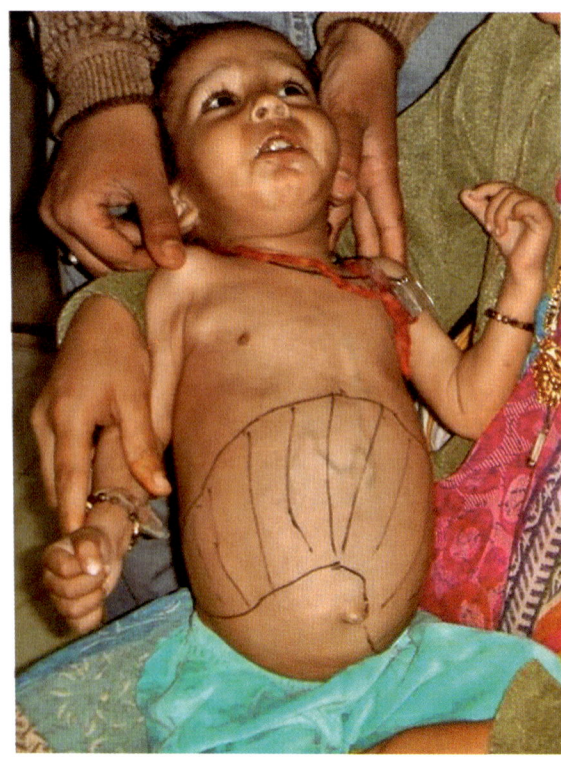

Figure 11.16 Massive hepatomegaly in an infant with Gaucher's disease.

Urinary Bladder

Bladder is an abdominal organ in infants. Distended urinary bladder produces a midline cystic swelling in the suprapubic region. The swelling is fixed and nonmobile with impaired percussion note. The swelling disappears after micturition or drainage of urine. In neonates with bladder neck obstruction, there may be three abdominal masses, one in each lumbar region due to enlarged kidneys and a distended urinary bladder in the midline over the hypogastrium.

\	Scheme for Presentation
General physical examination	Appearance, comfortable, sick, restless or immobile (peritonitis), nutritional status, growth and development, vital signs, anemia, cyanosis, jaundice, lymphadenopathy, evidences of vitamin A deficiency, proptosis, Kayser-Fleischer rings, aniridia, oral cavity and teeth, petechiae, ecchymoses, scratch marks, angiomas, spider nevi, xanthomas, clubbing, edema, ascites, bony tenderness, skeletal deformities, hemihypertrophy, and evidences of hepatocellular failure.
Inspection	Distension; localized or generalized, umbilicus, peristaltic waves, engorged veins, and spider nevi.
Palpation	Feel of abdomen, tenderness, edema of abdominal wall, flow of blood in the engorged veins, enlargement and characteristics of liver, spleen, kidneys and any other mass, renal angles and hernial sites.
Percussion	Shifting dullness, fluid thrill, percussion over various organomegalies and masses, upper border of liver, span of liver and spleen, and obliteration of hepatic dullness.
Auscultation	Peristaltic waves; normal, increased, decreased or absent, friction sound over the masses, bruit over the hepatic area and renal vessels.
Genitals and rectal examination	Perianal abnormalities, hernial sites, appearance and development of external genitals, hydrocele, developmental anomalies, epididymitis, orchitis, infiltration of testes and when indicated rectal examination.

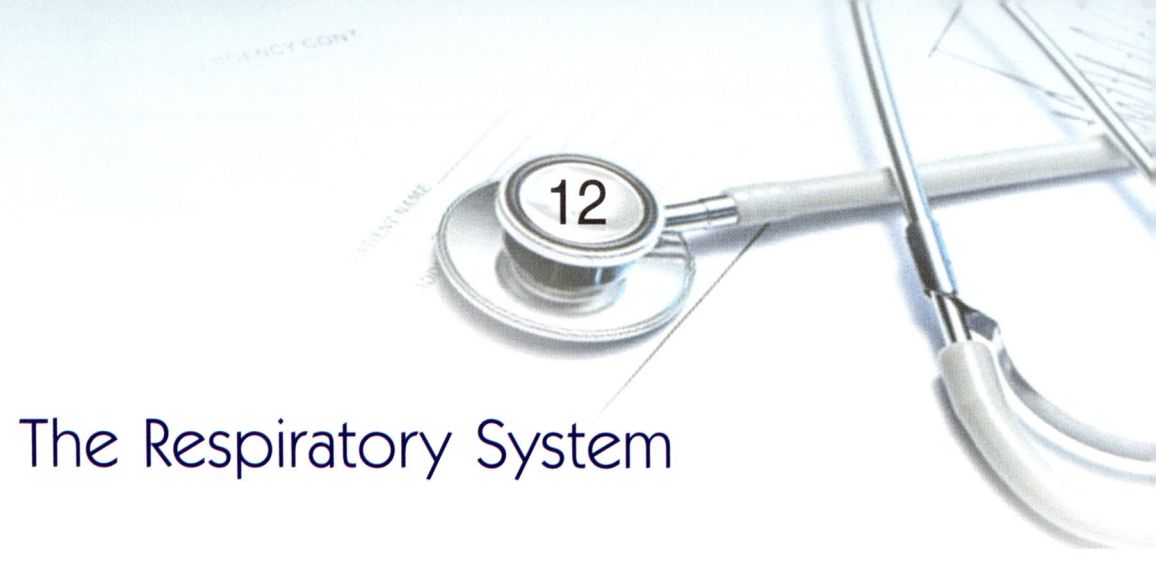

12

The Respiratory System

ANATOMY

The respiratory system consists of the upper airway (up to larynx) and the lower respiratory tract (trachea to alveoli). The upper airway starts from nose and mouth and includes oropharynx, nasopharynx, sinuses and larynx. The lower respiratory tract includes the trachea which bifurcates to provide bronchi, bronchioles and alveoli to both lungs. The right lung is bigger in size and has three lobes while left lung is smaller in size due to the presence of heart in the left hemithorax and has two lobes. The air passages are relatively narrow in children which predispose them to frequent development of croup, stridor, wheezing and atelectasis. The chest is relatively round with a larger anteroposterior diameter and chest wall is thinner in children.

The airways transport air along with oxygen to the alveoli during inspiration and eliminate carbon dioxide during expiration. The gas exchange takes place in the alveolar unit which consists of branching respiratory bronchioles with cluster of alveoli. Alveoli are tiny air sacs lined by flattened epithelial cells (type 1 pneumocytes) and are covered by a network of capillaries where gas exchange occurs. The lungs have two sources of blood supply, the bronchial arteries which arise from the aorta and supply oxygenated blood to the bronchial walls and the pulmonary arteries which circulate deoxygenated blood to the capillaries surrounding the alveoli.

Surface anatomy The bifurcation of trachea corresponds to angle of Louis or Ludwig anteriorly and 4th thoracic spine posteriorly. The angle of Louis is a transverse bony ridge at the junction of the the manubrium sterni with body of the manubrium. The ribs and intercostal spaces are best counted downwards from the angle of Louis which corresponds to the second costal cartilage. It also provides a cutoff for superior and inferior mediastinum. Lung fissures are a double-fold of visceral pleura that either completely or incompletely invaginates lung parenchyma to form the lung lobes.

Each lung has an oblique fissure separating the upper lobes from the lower lobes and the right lung has a horizontal fissure that separates the right upper lobe from the right middle lobe. There are accessory fissures which are not of any clinical relevance. A line drawn from 2nd thoracic spine to the 6th rib in the midclavicular line corresponds to the major interlobar fissure or upper border of lower lobe of the lung. The boundary between the upper and middle lobes is marked by a horizontal line drawn from sternum at the level of 4th costal cartilage to meet the major interlobar fissure line on the right side of chest. Mostly upper (middle also on the right side) and lower lobes are accessible to physical examination anteriorly and posteriorly respectively while all the lobes are accessible in the axillary area (Figure 12.1). The surface anatomy of bronchopulmonary segments of lungs both in front and back is shown in Figure 12.2 and Table 12.1.

The Respiratory System

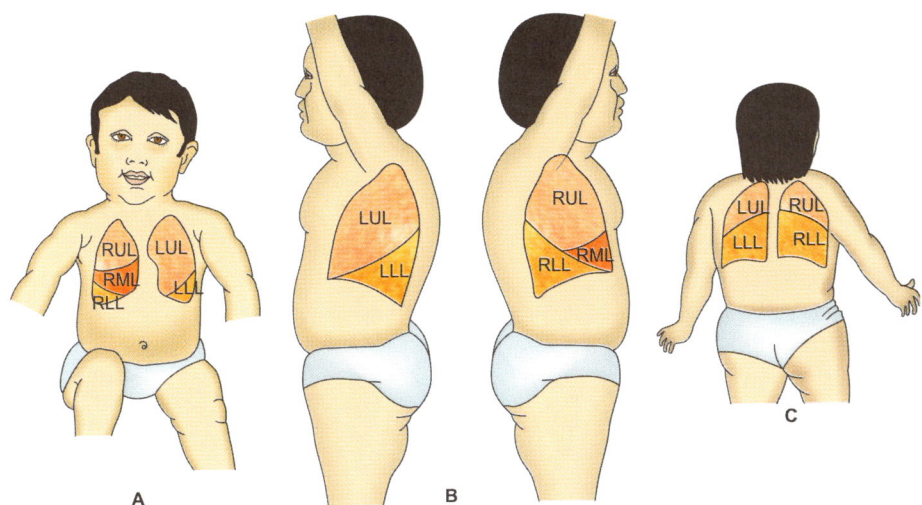

Figure 12.1A to C Surface anatomy of various lobes of the lungs on front (A), sides (B) and back (C). RUL, right upper lobe; RML, right middle lobe; RLL, right lower lobe; LUL, left upper lobe; LLL, left lower lobe.

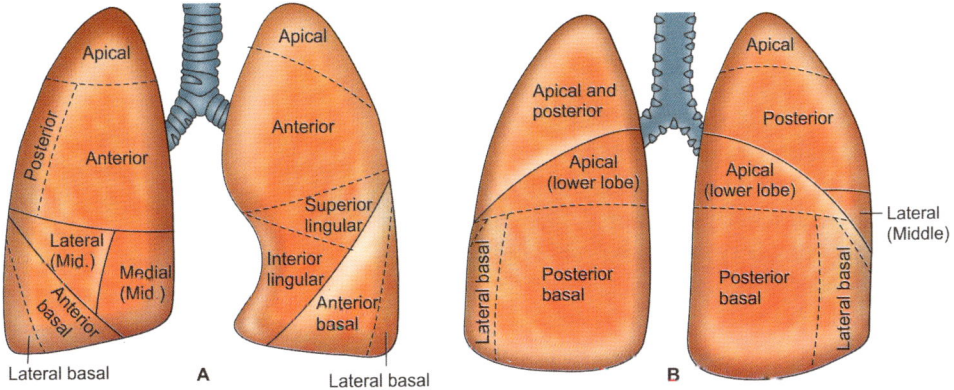

Figure 12.2A and B Bronchopulmonary segments of lungs as visualized from front (A) and back (B).

TABLE 12.1 Bronchopulmonary segments of lungs	
Right lung	*Left lung*
■ **Upper lobe** • Apical segment • Posterior segment • Anterior segment ■ **Middle lobe** • Lateral segment • Medial segment ■ **Lower lobe** • Superior segment • Medial basal segment • Anterior basal segment • Lateral basal segment • Posterior basal segment	■ **Upper lobe** • Apicoposterior segment • Anterior segment ■ **Lingula of upper lobe** • Superior lingular segment • Inferior lingular segment ■ **Lower lobe** • Superior segment • Anteromedial basal segment • Posterior basal segment • Lateral basal segment

HISTORY

Ask history of present illness with special emphasis on onset (sudden, acute, subacute, or insidious), evolution of the disease and response to therapy. The major symptoms of respiratory system disorder include fever, cough, coryza (viral URI or hay fever), sore throat, croup, stridor, chest pain and respiratory difficulty. Mouth breathing with snoring during sleep occurs due to oropharyngeal obstruction (adenoids). Rattling or wet sounds may be audible due to secretions in the oropharynx and upper airways. Rapid breathing with expiratory grunt (expiration through partially closed glottis to raise end expiratory pressure) is characteristically seen in infants with hyaline membrane disease and bronchopneumonia. Wheezing or predominantly expiratory whistling sounds are heard in children with obstruction or spasm of small airways. Inspiratory stridor is characteristically heard in children with obstruction in the larynx or trachea. The nature and characteristics of cough may provide useful diagnostic clues (Table 12.2).

Ask whether cough is mild or intractable, dry or associated with bubbling sounds in the throat or chest, diurnal or predominantly nocturnal. Cough aggravated by dust, acroallergens, smoke, physical activity (exercise-induced asthma), cold water bath, preservatives and synthetic colors in food, is suggestive of increased airway reactivity. Nocturnal and early morning cough is common due to asthmatic bronchitis, bronchial asthma, postnasal discharge, gastroesophageal reflux disease and left heart failure.

Gastroesophageal reflulx disease (GERD) in infants is characterized by frequent episodes of cough or wheeze, refusal of feeds, excessive crying at night with arching of trunk, frequent spitting of milk and palpable gurgling sounds on the back. Infants and young children cannot expectorate sputum and they often swallow it and may bring out the phlegm in the vomitus or pass it in the stools. Spasmodic hacking cough is suggestive of bronchospasm, tracheitis, pertussis, cystic fibrosis, foreign body and aspiration. In cough-variant asthma, there is intractable bouts of spasmodic cough without any significant wheezing. Cough is relatively an uncommon symptom in neonates and may occur due to aspiration and chlamydial infection. Inspiratory whoop following a bout of spasmodic cough is characteristic of pertussis but may occur in respiratory infections due to *B. parapertussis*, adenoviruses and chlamydiae. Cough with copious putrid expectoration is suggestive of bronchiectasis and pulmonary suppuration. There may be history suggestive of measles, pertussis and inhalation of foreign body at the onset of respiratory illness.

TABLE 12.2 Different types of cough and their interpretation

Nature of cough	Possible cause/s
▪ Dry hacking cough	Pharyngitis, tonsillitis, irritation of throat, and dry heated air
▪ Wet or productive or "chesty" spasmodic cough (worse at night or during sleep and early morning) followed by vomiting*	Bronchitis, bronchial asthma, gastroesophageal reflux (GER), bronchiectasis, foreign body, cystic fibrosis, congestive heart failure, and post-nasal drip
▪ Paroxysmal cough with a whoop and choking	Pertussis, chlamydial pneumonia, adenovirus infection, and cystic fibrosis
▪ Croupy, hoarse, low-pitched cough	Laryngitis and laryngeal edema
▪ Brassy or barking cough	Tracheitis, croup, mediastinal lymph nodes, and vascular ring
▪ Exercise-induced or cold-induced cough	Exercise and cold-induced asthma
▪ Cough-induced by feeding	Physiological, neuromotor disorder, laryngomalacia, bronchospasm, vascular ring, and gastroesophageal reflux disease
▪ Habit or psychogenic "throat clearing" or honking cough	Short low-amplitude brief bouts of honking cough, disappears during play or sleep

*Phlegm is passed in the vomitus which is followed by relief of cough

In children with *recurrent respiratory infections*, a detailed history should be taken to exclude inhalation of foreign body as evidenced by a sudden and dramatic episode of life-threatening choking, cough and cyanosis. Ask for history of abnormal sounds during inspiration (stridor) and expiratory grunting in pneumonia and wheezing in bronchiolitis and bronchial asthma. The triad of poor weight gain, steatorrhea and chronic cough since infancy is suggestive of cystic fibrosis. Sweat test (pilocarpine iontophoresis) is useful to confirm the diagnosis.

Psychogenic cough is characterized by short bouts of low-amplitude "throat clearing" cough which disappears in school, during play, and at night. The cough is worse during stress, unfamiliar circumstances and when child is being watched.

Stridor is a harsh, vibratory, high-pitched, shrill or crowing noise caused by obstructed air flow. The stridor may be inspiratory (upper airway obstruction), expiratory (lower airway obstruction below the level of larynx) or biphasic due to mid-tracheal or bronchial disorder. The additional features of respiratory obstruction include hoarseness, hypoxia, brassy cough, tachypnea and dyspnea with inspiratory retractions of chest and use of accessory muscles of respiration. The incidence of respiratory obstruction is relatively high in infants due to small size of larynx, presence of loose submucous connective tissue and rigid encirclement of the subglottic area by the cricoid cartilage. The common causes of stridor are listed in Table 12.3.

Epiglottitis or supraglottitis has become rare because of widespread vaccination against. *H. influenzae type b* (HIB). The condition usually occurs in children between 1 and 7 years with sudden onset of high grade fever, severe throat pain with dysphagia, drooling, dyspnea and anxiety. The child is markedly toxic and sits upright with neck extended and head held forward. Attempts to examine the throat in the outpatient department may lead to respiratory arrest. The affected child should be stabilized and escorted to the OT for intubation and management in the PICU. The lateral neck radiograph may show characteristic "thumbprint sign" due to swelling of aryepiglottic folds.

TABLE 12.3 Common causes of stridor

Infections
- *Viral*: Viral laryngitis, acute spasmodic laryngitis (croup), and acute laryngotracheal bronchitis.
- *Bacterial*: Diphtheritic laryngitis, acute epiglottitis, bacterial tracheitis, and retropharyngeal abscess (Quinsy).
- *Fungal*: Candidal laryngitis (AIDS).

Congenital malformations
- Laryngomalacia and tracheomalacia, laryngeal web or cyst, subglottic stenosis, vascular anomalies, Pierre-Robin syndrome, and macroglossia.
- *Laryngospasm*: Tetany, gastroesophageal reflux disease, acute infantile Gaucher disease.
- *Laryngeal edema*: Anaphylaxis (angioedema), trauma due to intubation and foreign body, ingestion of corrosives, and nephrotic syndrome.
- *Laryngeal paralysis*: Birth trauma, enlarged pulmonary conus with pulmonary hypertension, and Arnold-Chiari malformation.
- *Neoplasm*: Papilloma, hemangioma, fibrolipoma, mediastinal tumor or lymph nodes, goiter, and cystic hygroma

Croup is a viral condition of under-3 children that causes inflammation of upper airways (laryngotracheobronchitis). It is characterized by low grade fever, noisy breathing, hoarse cry, retractions and distinctive harsh "barking or brassy cough." Croup (inspiratory harsh crowing sound) due to spasmodic laryngitis usually occurs at night and during exposure to cold. The severity of croup can be assessed by a scoring system (Table 12.4).

Tachypnea and dyspnea are suggestive of acute lower respiratory tract infection, bronchospasm, atelectasis, and compression of lungs (pneumothorax, pleural effusion, mediastinal mass, diaphragmatic hernia). Retractions of chest are common and marked in children due to soft rib cage. Marked suprasternal retractions are seen in upper airway obstruction. The presence of cyanosis and feeding difficulty are suggestive of life-threatening respiratory disorder requiring immediate hospitalization. History of *recurrent episodes of cough with breathing difficulty* is suggestive of bronchial asthma, bronchiectasis, foreign body,

TABLE 12.4 Croup scoring system

Clinical parameter	Score			
	0	1	2	3
▪ Stridor	None	Mild	Moderate inspiratory	Severe both in inspiration and expiration, or no stridor with markedly decreased air entry
▪ Retractions	None	Mild	Moderate	Severe with marked use of accessory muscles
▪ Air entry on auscultation	Normal	Slightly decreased	Moderately decreased	Markedly decreased
▪ Color*	Normal	Normal (0 score)	Normal (1 score)	Dusky or cyanotic
▪ Level of consciousness	Normal	Restless when disturbed	Anxious and agitated even when not disturbed	Lethargic and depressed

*Pulse oximeter can be used as a reliable parameter of oxygenation.
The score of 2 or less indicates mild croup, 3–7 score is classified as moderate croup and score of 8 or more with marked chest wall indrawings is suggestive of severe croup.
Adapted from Westley CR, Cotton EK, Brooks JG. Nebulized racemic epinephrine by IPPB for the treatment of croup: a double-blind study. *Am J Dis Child* 1978, 132(5):484–487.

left-to-right shunt, cystic fibrosis, immunodeficiency state and gastroesophageal reflux. Ask for history of *dysphagia* which may be acute (acute pharyngitis or tonsillitis, diphtheria, acute epiglottitis, retropharyngeal abscess, etc.) or insidious in onset (mediastinal mass, vascular ring).

Hemoptysis is uncommon in children and may occur due to bronchiectasis, lung abscess, resolving lobar pneumonia, pulmonary hemosiderosis, pulmonary edema, mitral stenosis, tubercular cavity and bleeding disorder (*Box 12.1*). Unlike hematemesis, hemoptysis is preceded by a bout of cough, the blood is bright-red in color, and usually small in quantity (Table 12.5). Following epistaxis, the blood may be swallowed and spitted out with oral secretions. History of *chest pain* is uncommon and may occur due to pleurisy, pericarditis, pleurodynia, costochondritis, herpes zoster, trauma and coronary insufficiency (severe aortic stenosis or regurgitation, anomalous left coronary artery from pulmonary artery, Kawasaki disease). Ask whether pain is aggravated by breathing or not. Check for site of tenderness, whether over the ribs or intercostal spaces.

Box 12.1 Common causes of hemoptysis

- Bacterial pneumonia (rusty sputum)
- Fibrocaseous tuberculosis
- Bronchiectasis
- Lung abscess
- Pulmonary sequestration
- Pulmonary edema
- Foreign body
- Cystic fibrosis or mucoviscidosis
- Mitral stenosis, pulmonary hypertension or severe pulmonic stenosis
- Idiopathic pulmonary hemosiderosis
- Bleeding disorder

Family history of tuberculosis, bronchial asthma, and hay fever should be asked. Unsatisfactory living conditions, over crowding, environmental pollution, parental smoking and smoky *chulla* at home, are associated with increased incidence of respiratory tract infections and episodes of bronchospasm. History of contact and allergy to pet animals and exotic birds (pigeons, parrots, macaws, budgerigars, parakeets) may predispose to development of rhinitis, bronchial asthma and psittacosis.

TABLE 12.5 Differences between hemoptysis and hematemesis

Hemoptysis	Hematemesis
- It is preceded by cough	- Epistaxis (vomiting of swallowed blood), nausea and vomiting may precede it
- Amount of blood is small	- Amount of blood may be copious
- Blood-stained sputum is mixed with air (frothy) and it is bright-red in color	- Blood is often altered in color and may be dark red or brown
- Symptoms suggestive of cardiovascular or respiratory disease	- Symptoms suggestive of gastrointestinal or hepatic disorder
- Bronchoscopy is confirmatory	- Gastroscopy is confirmatory

Allergic manifestations may occur due to exposure to certain foods, artificial colors and preservatives. Exposure to strong perfumes or deodorants and smoke of *havan* and incense may aggravate reactive airway disease. The vaccination status of the child should be enquired. It provides useful guidelines to assess the likely cause of respiratory disorder and make a correct diagnosis.

GENERAL PHYSICAL EXAMINATION

Assess whether the child is comfortable, tachypneic or dyspneic. Look for any scars on the chest wall due to prior surgical procedure. While recording history, note whether accessory muscles of respiration and alae nasi are working or not. In order to improve the patency of airway in acute epiglottitis, the child sits with his mouth open and drooling, tongue protruding and head bent forward with neck slightly flexed. The child with pleural effusion is more comfortable on splinting the chest by lying on the side of effusion. Inspiratory dyspnea occurs due to obstruction of upper airways while expiratory dyspnea is seen in children with obstructive lung disease. State of consciousness, build and nutrition, and putrid odor from the mouth should be noted. Audible sounds during breathing, e.g. stridor, croup, hissing, grunting, stertorous, pharyngeal snores and wheezing may be heard. Stridor is a harsh, vibratory, high-pitched crowing sound due to inspiratory obstruction to the air flow. Grunting occurs when infant makes expiratory efforts through a partially closed glottis to increase end expiratory pressure to prevent collapse of alveoli during expiration. Nature of cough whether intermittent, spasmodic, whoopy, metallic, bubbly, etc. should be recorded. Note the character of voice or cry.

Temperature, pulse rate and its ratio to respiration (normal ratio being 4 to 1) should be noted. Respiration rate per minute, type of breathing rhythm (normal, reversed, Cheyne-Stokes, Biot's breathing), character (normal, inspiratory distress, expiratory distress), depth (normal, shallow, deep or Kussmaul's breathing) and suprasternal, intercostal, subcostal recessions and movements of alae nasi should be looked for. WHO cut offs for fast breathing in under-5 children are given in *Box 12.2*. Normal rhythm of breathing is characterized by inspiration – expiration – pause. Reversed rhythm, i.e. expiratory grunt – inspiration – pause is seen in children with acute lower respiratory infection.

Deep sighing breathing or Kussmaul breathing occurs in response to metabolic acidosis due to severe diarrhea and dehydration, diabetic ketoacidosis, acute renal failure, lactic acidosis, inborn error of metabolism, salicylate and methanol poisoning. Cheyne-Stokes breathing is characterized by temporary cessation of breathing (apnea) followed by respiratory efforts which gradually increase in magnitude to a maximum and then gradually diminish until apnea occurs once again. It occurs due to depression of respiratory center because of hypoxia, encephalitis or meningitis, increased intracranial pressure, uremia and congestive heart failure. Biot's breathing occurs in

Box 12.2 WHO cut offs for fast breathing in under-5 children

Age	Breaths/min
Birth–2 months	60 or more
2–12 months	50 or more
1–5 years	40 or more

children with raised intracranial pressure and is characterized by episodes of apnea followed by 4–5 irregular breaths (irregular nonrhythmic). Anemia, cyanosis, jaundice and lymphadenopathy should be looked for.

ENT check up is essential to rule out upper respiratory tract infection, otitis media and sinusitis. Examine oral cavity and throat for any acute or chronic infection and nose for any discharge, polyp. and deflected septum. Itching of nose (and eyes), upward rubbing of the nose with open palm (allergic salute), horizontal crease over nasal bridge, dark circles and allergic "shiners" over lower eyelids may be associated with allergic rhinitis (hay fever). Infraorbital folds of skin below the lower eyelids (Dennie–Morgan folds) are highly suggestive of allergic rhinitis. They occur due to continuous spasm of Muller eyelid muscles because of associated allergic conjunctivitis.

The sphenoid sinuses are present at birth while ethmoid and maxillary sinuses are of clinical importance during early childhood. The frontal sinuses usually appear after 10 years of age. Acute sinusitis is characterized by sudden onset of fever, nasal congestion, persistent nasal discharge, throbbing pain around the eyes which become worse on bending forward. There is swelling and tenderness over the location of sinuses. In a severe case of frontal sinusitis, exquisitely tender, doughy midline frontal swelling (Pott's puffy tumor) may occur due to formation of subperiorbital abscess. Chronic sinusitis is associated with nasal obstruction with persistent mucopurulent nasal discharge, slight puffiness of eyelids and dark circles under the eyes. The important causes of chronic sinusitis include cleft palate, nasal allergy, Kartagener's or immotile cilia syndrome, ataxia telangiectasia, Hurler's syndrome, cystic fibrosis, choanal atresia and immunodeficiency disorders.

Look for clubbing of nails and osteoarthropathy (clubbing with pain in the wrists and ankles). The common pulmonary causes of clubbing include bronchiectasis, lung abscess, empyema, recurrent or chronic pneumonia due to foreign body, fibrocaseous pulmonary tuberculosis, cystic fibrosis, interstitial lung disease, pulmonary alveolar proteinosis and neoplasms. The presence of severely engorged non-pulsatile jugular veins are suggestive of mediastinal mass and may be associated with facial plethora, "brassy" cough, hoarseness, stridor or dysphagia. Erythema nodosum and phlyctenular conjunctivitis may be associated with tuberculosis. Look for scar of BCG vaccination over the left shoulder. Subconjunctival hemorrhage, facial puffiness, suffusion of eyes and subcutaneous emphysema may occur in children with pertussis.

Assessment of Respiratory Distress

The severity of respiratory distress is assessed by following criteria:
 (i) Mental status: Alertness, irritability, drowsiness or stuporose
 (ii) Severity of tachypnea, dyspnea and use of accessory muscles of breathing
 (iii) Color: Blue (cyanosis) or pale (shock)
 (iv) Pulsus paradoxus and its severity (>20 mm Hg difference in blood pressure during end of inspiration and expiration)
 (v) Arterial oxygen saturation <85% on pulse oximeter
 (vi) Peak expiratory flow rate of less than 80% of the predicted or actual average of the patient.

Peak Expiratory Flow Rate (PEFR)

Children above the age of 5 years can be taught to use peak flowmeter to recognize an impending attack of wheezing. The marker of the mini-flow meter is slided to zero. The child is asked to stand up and take a deep breath. The mouthpiece of the flow meter is then taken in the mouth and lips are tightly closed over it. The child is asked to exhale out with a maximal effort and force. The procedure is repeated 3 times and the highest reading is recorded. The child can be asked to record his PEFR twice a day (Figure 12.3). It is a useful home device for early identification of an attack of bronchial asthma and its severity. Depending upon the actual PEFR of the child, three categories are identified.

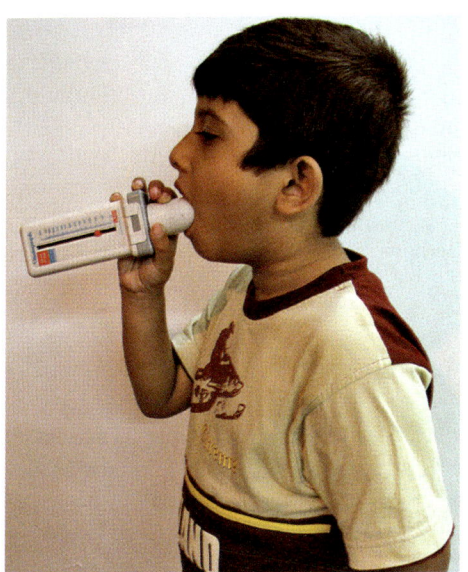

Figure 12.3 The technique for using a mini peak flow meter. See text for details.

Green zone Peak expiratory flow rate within 80% of the predicted average (Patient's known highest PEFR when well) indicates that patient is doing well on current medications (or without medications).

Yellow zone Peak expiratory flow rate between 50 and 80% of the predicted or actual average PEFR of the patient is indicative of a mild attack and need for stepping up the inhalation therapy on ambulatory basis.

Red zone Peak expiratory flow rate of less than 50% of predicted or actual average indicates moderate to severe attack of bronchial asthma. The child should be immediately referred to the hospital for further management.

Single Breath Count (SBC)

The single breath counting is done by asking the child to take a maximal inspiration and count at a normal speaking rate of 2 numbers per second. It is a useful bedside screening test to monitor respiratory adequacy of the patient. The best of three readings is documented. The child with a count of less than 20 per breath is considered as "breathless" with a risk of impending respiratory failure.

Acute Respiratory Failure

It is characterized by impending respiratory failure, apprehension, anxiety, restlessness, worsening of tachypnea, dyspnea, chest retractions and cyanosis. The air entry to the lungs may be severely compromised due to upper airway obstruction or marked bronchospasm with minimal or absent breath sounds on auscultation. The breathing may become slow, shallow and gasping or irregular due to CNS depression and neuromuscular disease or terminally when respiratory muscles become exhausted due to overwork. Pulse oximetry may show arterial oxygen saturation of <85% and PaO_2 of <60 mm Hg in an FiO_2 of >0.6 (in the absence of cyanotic heart disease) or $PaCO_2$ of >50 mm Hg (hypercarbia) and arterial pH <7.35.

EXAMINATION OF CHEST

The ready availability of roentgenographic examination and advances in imaging technology have rusted the art of clinical examination of chest. Anatomical areas for purposes of clinical examination of chest are as follows:

Front Supraclavicular, infraclavicular, mammary and inframammary areas.

Side Superior, middle and inferior axillary areas.

Back Suprascapular, interscapular, and infrascapular areas.

INSPECTION

The exposed chest should be inspected by standing at the head or foot side of the patient with eyes at the level of chest. The child, however, is best examined while sitting comfortably on a stool or standing with arms hanging limply by the sides.

Position of the patient The child with cardiac failure is orthopneic and prefers to sit upright or in a semireclining position. In asthmatic bronchitis, or attack of bronchial asthma, child is more comfortable while sitting and leaning forward. In a case of pleural effusion, hemothorax or lung abscess, the patient prefers to lie towards the side of pathology to splint the chest.

Shape of chest It is nearly circular or cylinderical in infants. The shape may be normal, barrel-shaped or emphysematous, pigeon chest or pectus carinatum (rickets, chondrodystrophy, spondyloepiphyseal dysplasia congenita, Noonan syndrome, Schwartz-Jampel syndrome, asphyxiating thoracic dystrophy, bronchial asthma), and funnel-shaped chest or pectus excavatum (rickets, absent pectoralis muscle, Marfan syndrome, mucosal neuroma syndrome). Agenesis or hypoplasia of the pectoralis major may be associated with hypoplasia or absence of the breast and nipple (Poland syndrome). Harrison's sulcus (rickets, upper airway obstruction), kyphosis, levo- or dextro-scoliosis of spine should be looked for. Costochondral beading (rickety rosary) may be the sole evidence of early rickets. In every child with a chest deformity, the spinal deformity must be excluded.

Symmetry of chest Note whether chest is bilaterally symmetrical or not. Note the distance of medial borders of scapulae from midline on both the sides which is useful to assess any asymmetry of the chest. Drooping of one shoulder may occur in patients with fibrocaseous tuberculosis. Look for localized bulge (whether costal or intercostal bulge) or retraction (collapse or fibrosis). There is bulging of intercostal spaces in cases of pleural effusion or empyema. When empyema points through an intercostal space as a cystic swelling, it is reducible and cough impulse is present, it is called empyema necessitans. The bony cage of chest may show localized bulge due to long-standing cardiomegaly, intrathoracic mass lesion, deformities of ribs and spine.

Movements of chest The breathing is mostly abdominal or abdominothoracic in infants. When the diaphragm is paralyzed, the upper part of abdomen may be drawn in (instead of being forced out) with each inspiration. In paralysis of intercostal muscles, there is very little expansion of chest with abnormal expansion of abdomen with each inspiration. The range of movements, respiratory lag on the affected side and indrawing of suprasternal, intercostal and subcostal spaces should be looked for. Marked suprasternal recessions are suggestive of narrowing or obstruction of upper airways due to laryngeal diphtheria, acute laryngotracheobronchitis, acute epiglottitis, laryngeal or tracheal foreign body, and angioneurotic edema.

The position of trachea and apex beat should be localized. The trachea is examined with child in supine position or sitting with slight flexion of neck. Place the index finger into the suprasternal notch, and gently push it backwards. Normally, the finger should touch the trachea in the midline. If trachea is deviated, the finger will slide into the tracheosternomastoid space (Figure 12.4A and B).

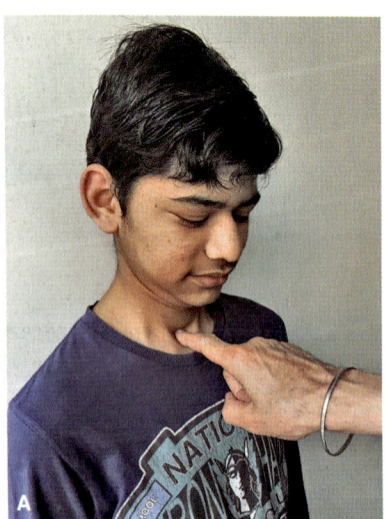 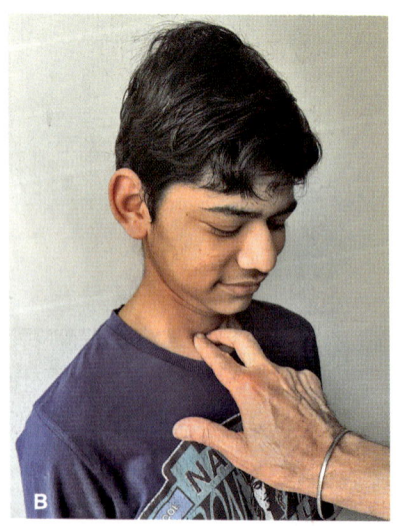

Figure 12.4A and B (A) In a child with slight flexion of neck, index finger is inserted in the midline of suprasternal notch. It will touch midline of trachea, if it is central in location. (B) Index and middle finger can be inserted into tracheosternomastoid space to assess whether trachea is displaced or central.

In a child with marked tracheal displacement, the clavicular head of the sternomastoid muscle is pushed forward as a visible bulge on the displaced side (sternomastoid or trail sign). In normal children, trachea may be slightly deviated to the right. Trachea may be pulled (towards the diseased side) due to collapse, fibrosis and thickened pleura. It may be pushed (towards the normal side) by pleural effusion, pneumothorax and a mass lesion. Scoliosis may cause tracheal deviation and should be excluded.

PALPATION

The findings of inspection should be confirmed. Look for any tender areas, crepitus (subcutaneous emphysema, fracture rib) and assess any differences of movements on two sides of chest. Feel for any abnormal vibrations, e.g. rhonchi, friction rub, coarse crackles and characteristic spongy feeling of subcutaneous emphysema (Figure 12.5). Vocal or tactile fremitus is looked for by comparing tactile transmission of spoken words (like one, two, three) or cry in infants, over identical areas on two sides of the chest. Hypothenar eminence or ulnar aspect of the hand should be used to look for vocal fremitus. It may

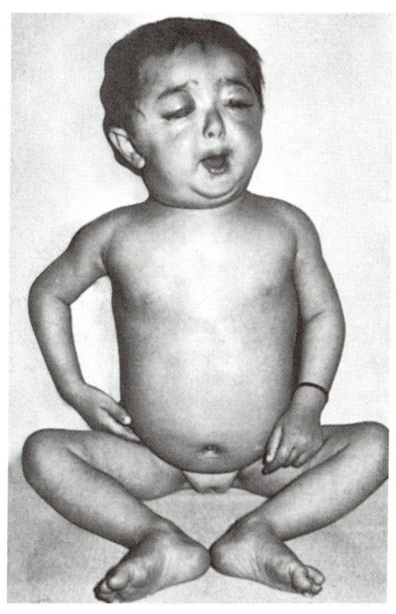

Figure 12.5 Massive subcutaneous emphysema following bouts of spasmodic cough in a child with pertussis.

be normal and equal on two sides or decreased/increased over a particular area. It has the same significance as vocal resonance but is unreliable in children. Assess the expansion of chest on two sides (Figures 12.6A and B and 12.7A and B).

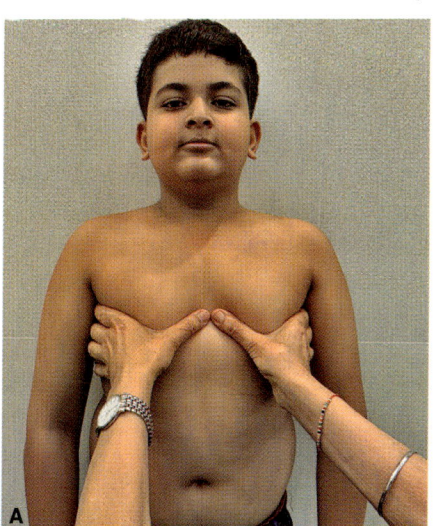
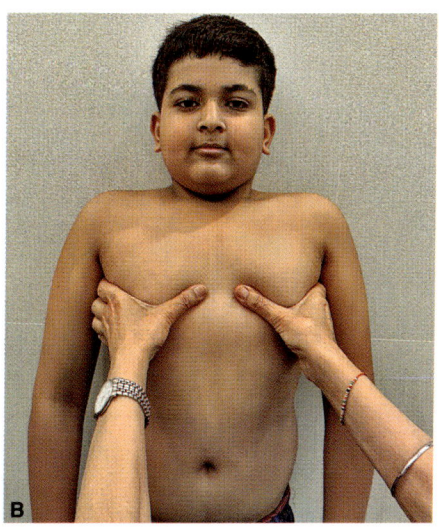

Figure 12.6A and B Assessment of chest expansion on the front. (A) Hands firmly grasp the chest and thumbs just touch each other in the midline over the lower sterum. (B) Child is asked to take a deep inspiration and distance between two thumbs is observed. The distance between two thumbs after deep inspiration is suggestive of adequacy of lung expansion.

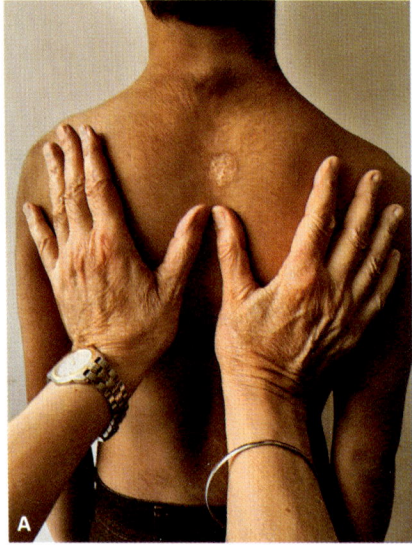 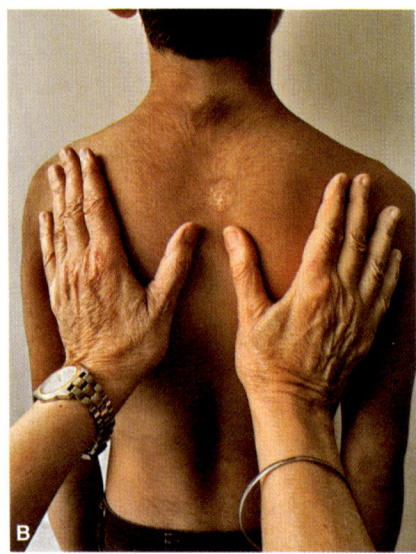

Figure 12.7A and B Assessment of chest expansion on the back. (A) Hands are firmly placed over the sides of the chest and thumbs are opposed in the midline over the spine. (B) Child is asked to take a deep inspiration and the movements of thumbs are observed. The distance between two thumbs on deep inspiration is suggestive of adequacy of lung expansion.

When pneumothorax is suspected in a newborn baby and infant, transillumination of the chest can be done with a fiberoptic cold light source in a dark room. The hemithorax will glow with light, if there is pneumothorax and decompression can be done without delay.

PERCUSSION

"We must not explore the chest by percussing our ideas into it. We must rather give our attention to listening to what comes out."

Friedrich Muller

The pleximeter finger (middle finger of the non-dominant hand) should be placed in firm contact with the chest while rest of the fingers should be lifted off the chest because they may dampen the resonance. The pleximeter finger should be held parallel to the margin of the organ to be outlined. It is kept parallel to the ribs except for eliciting mediastinal dullness when the pleximeter finger is kept vertical and percussed from lateral to the medial side. *The pleximeter finger should move from resonant towards the possible dull area.* The tap should be 'free' and gentle and is best done with the middle finger (plexor) of the dominant hand by striking the middle phalanx of the pleximeter finger (Figure 12.8). If organ or tissue to be percussed is superficial, it is advised to do light percussion. For example, direct (without pleximeter) light percussion over the clavicles is done to assess the apices of the lungs (Figure 12.9).

The strokes should be of uniform force and executed by movements at the relaxed wrist. The plexor finger must be withdrawn immediately after the stroke. The intensity and quality of the sound produced and 'feeling' of resistance imparted to the pleximeter finger should be observed. The identical areas of chest on two sides should be compared simultaneously. The chest may be normally or equally resonant on two sides, there may be unilateral or bilateral hyper-resonance (pneumothorax, emphysema), tympanitic note (large cavity, pneumothorax, diaphragmatic hernia). The percussion note may be impaired (consolidation, collapse, fibrosis), dull (consolidation, pleural thickening) or stony dull (pleural effusion or empyema). Rising dullness (higher level of dullness in the axilla as compared to front and back) and

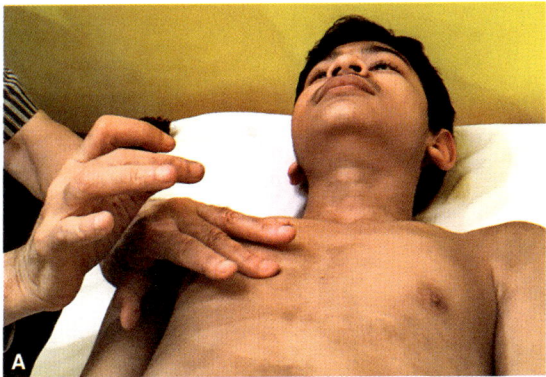

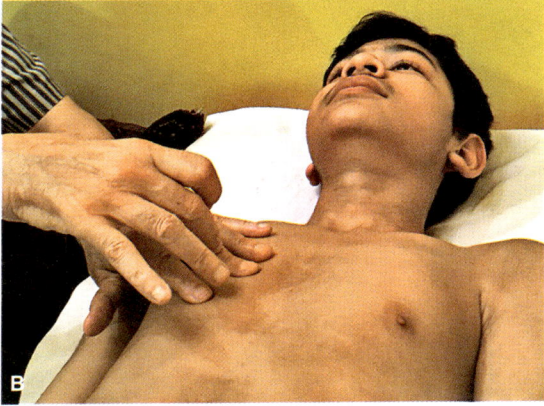

Figure 12.8A and B (A) The middle finger (pleximeter) of left hand is placed firmly on the chest while keeping it parallel to the ribs. The other fingers should preferably be lifted off the chest. (B) The middle phalanx of pleximeter finger is tapped gently by middle finger of the right or plexor hand by producing a free movement at the relaxed wrist joint. The plexor finger should be withdrawn immediately after the tap.

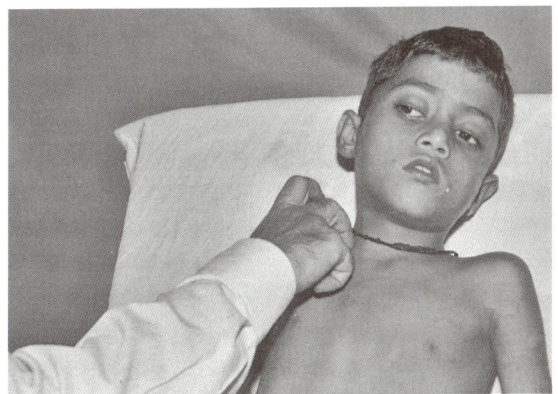

Figure 12.9 Direct percussion over the middle of the clavicle to assess the apices of lungs.

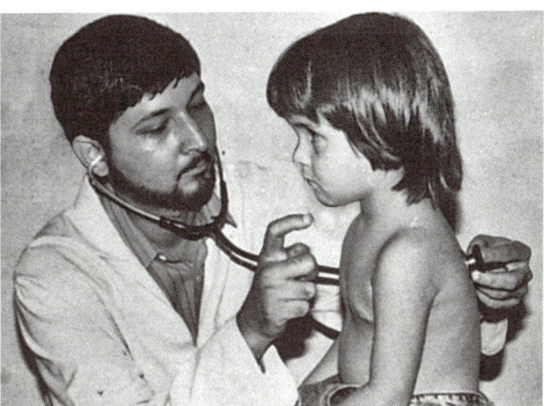

Figure 12.10 Method for auscultatory percussion. Refer to text for details.

shifting dullness (the level of dullness is more on lying down than on sitting up) should be looked for when pleural effusion is suspected.

Auscultatory percussion It is more reliable and informative than the conventional percussion and can pick up small lesions up to 3 cm in diameter especially hilar or mediastinal lymph nodes, pulmonary infiltrates, atelectasis and patches of pneumonia. The patient sits up with arms resting on his thighs. The examiner stands or sits on either side of the patient. The examiner percusses over the manubrium sterni by tapping lightly with the middle or index finger of dominant hand while listening with the diaphragm piece of stethoscope applied snugly by the other hand over the posterior chest wall (Figure 12.10). It must be ensured that percussion is applied with equal intensity over the same area of the manubrium while stethoscope explores both lung fields by comparing the intensity and quality of percussion note on the corresponding anatomical areas from upper border of the chest to the base. In the end, paravertebral areas are auscultated to detect possible mediastinal and hilar masses.

AUSCULTATION

The infants and young children are best auscultated while mother or father supports the child against the security of their shoulders (Figure 12.11). Infants are usually uncooperative and may cry which may actually facilitate auscultation. Children

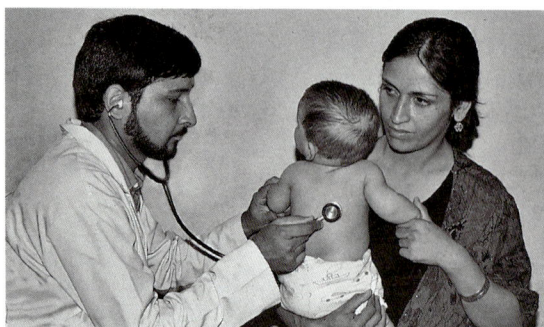

Figure 12.11 Method for auscultation of chest in an infant.

above 2 years can be asked to take deep breaths during auscultation. During auscultation, the identical areas of the chest on two sides are compared.

Character of Breath Sounds

Vesicular The normal breath sounds produced in the alveoli are called vesicular. The inspiration is loud, high-pitched and long, there is no pause after the inspiration, expiration is low in intensity and short in duration and is followed by a pause (Figure 12.12). In children, the normal breath sounds are peurile or harsh vesicular with slightly prolonged expiration (bronchovesicular).

Bronchial The inspiration is low in intensity, and is followed by a pause while expiration is harsh, blowing, guttural, high-pitched, loud and prolonged. The duration of inspiration and expiration is almost identical. The sounds have definite tubular quality. It may be normally heard over the neck and thoracic spine up to 4th thoracic vertebra (trachea). The bronchial breathing may be of the following types:

(a) High-pitched or tubular (consolidation)
(b) Medium-pitched (consolidation, small cavity or atelectasis with a patent bronchus).
(c) Low-pitched or cavernous (large cavity)
(d) Amphoric (bronchopleural fistula). It is low-pitched bronchial breathing with metallic overtones.

Intensity of breath sounds It may be normal, decreased or absent on one or both sides.

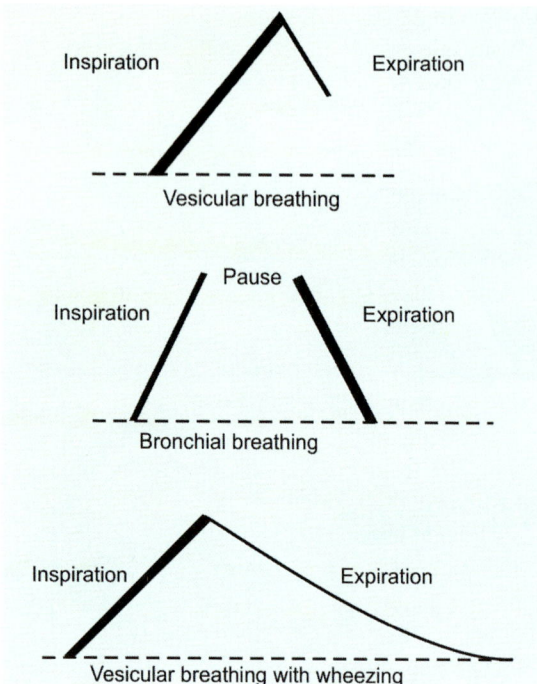

Figure 12.12 Diagrammatic representation of various types of breath sounds. Refer to text for details.

Vocal resonance It is similar to tactile fremitus but is evaluated by auscultation and is thus more reliable. Both the intensity and quality of sound transmitted through the chest-piece of the stethoscope are assessed when child is asked to repeat some words (1–2–3 or ma–ma) or cries. The intensity of vocal resonance may be equal and normal on two sides, absent or decreased (pleural effusion, pleural thickening, pneumothorax, emphysema, atelectasis) or increased (consolidation, cavity, infarction, atelectasis with patent bronchus). *Bronchophony* refers to increased vocal resonance when it is so loud that it appears as if the sound is being produced in the earpieces of stethoscope (consolidation, cavity). The audible vocal resonance, when child is asked to whisper certain words, is called *whispering pectoriloquy* and is indicative of markedly increased vocal resonance (bronchopleural fistula). The nasal twang or "bleating of a goat" quality of vocal resonance is called *egophony* and is audible at the upper level of pleural effusion due to partially collapsed underlying lung. It is produced by selective transmission of high frequency components of breath sounds.

Adventitious Sounds

The adventitious sounds may arise from the pleura or lungs. Extrapulmonary adventitious or abnormal sounds may be heard due to shivering or rigors, rubbing of chest-piece over the hairy skin or clothes and crepitus produced in the region of broken rib(s).

Wheezes or rhonchi (an increasingly absolete term) These are dry musical sounds produced due to narrowing of air passages. The expiration is prolonged in an attempt to expel the inspired air through the narrow air passages. They are monophonic in character when there is a localized obstruction of a bronchus (foreign body, lymph node) or polyphonic when there is generalized airway obstruction (asthma and bronchitis). The common causes of wheezing are listed in *Box 12.3*. They are classified on the basis of their pitch and site of origin.

(a) High-pitched or sibilant rhonchi are produced in the bronchioles. They are audible during the end of inspiration or beginning of expiration and are better appreciated by placing the chestpiece in front of infant's mouth and nose (acute bronchiolitis).

(b) Medium-pitched rhonchi are produced in medium-sized bronchi.

(c) Low-pitched or sonorous rhonchi are produced in large bronchi. They are heard throughout both the phases of breathing and are often audible even without a stethoscope.

(d) When airway obstruction becomes extreme, the movements of airflow becomes minimal with disappearance of breath sounds (silent chest) and rhonchi but worsening of condition of the patient with impending respiratory failure.

Crackles They are short, explosive bubbling or wet sounds produced by passage of air through the exudates collected in the alveoli, bronchioles, bronchi or trachea. The fine crackles are produced by sudden opening of previously closed small airways or alveoli. The older terms, like crepitations and rales, are no longer used. The nature and origin of crackles is given below:

(a) Fine crackles produce a sound like rustling of paper and are audible during the late phase of inspiration (bronchopneumonia, bronchiolitis and congestive heart failure).

(b) Medium-pitched crackles are heard in patients with bronchitis and resolving pneumonia and pulmonary edema.

(c) Low-pitched or coarse crackles are audible throughout both the phases of respiration and are loud in intensity (bronchiectasis).

The crackles must be differentiated from pharyngeal sounds or stertorous breathing and rattling sounds. The pharyngeal sounds disappear after suction or by asking the patient to cough and are better heard by auscultation by keeping the chest piece of stethoscope infront of the mouth and front of upper neck. In small infants, adventitious sounds from one side of the chest may be transmitted to the opposite side.

Pleural friction rub It is produced when inflamed parietal and visceral pleurae rub against each other.

Box 12.3 Common causes of wheezing

- Reactive airway disease due to asthmatic bronchitis
- Acute bronchiolitis or viral pneumonia
- Aspiration pneumonia or aspiration of a foreign body*
- Gastroesophageal reflux disease (GERD)
- Cystic fibrosis or mucoviscidosis
- Extra bronchial pressure due to enlarged mediastinal nodes*, endobronchial tuberculosis, tumor, cystic adenomatoid malformation
- Vascular ring*
- Lobar emphysema*
- Isolated tracheoesophageal fistula
- Visceral larva migrans and Loeffler's syndrome
- Allergic bronchopulmonary aspergillosis (ABPA)
- Ciliary dyskinesia syndromes
- Cow's milk hypersensitivity (Heiner syndrome)
- Interstitial pneumonitides
- Cardiac failure or large left-to-right shunt
- Bronchopulmonary dysplasia
- Drug-induced: β-blockers, opioids, NSAIDs
- Conversion reaction

*In these conditions, wheezing is usually unilateral.

It is unaltered by cough (unlike crackles), is more localized, and augmented by snug contact of chestpiece of stethoscope to the chest wall. It is heard during the identical phases of inspiration and expiration and has a peculiar superficial grating, creaking and leathery character. It increases in intensity when chestpiece of stethoscope is pressed against chest wall. If the pleura adjacent to the pericardium is inflamed, a pleuropericardial rub may also be heard. It disappears when two leaves of pleura are separated by further accumulation of exudates. At times pleural rub may be palpable with the palm. There may be localized chest pain.

The cardiovascular system should be examined for any evidences of chronic cor pulmonale and loud second heart sound because of pulmonary hypertension.

SPECIAL SIGNS

Hippocratic succussion or succussion splash Whenever pleural effusion is suspected, splash should be elicited to rule out hydropneumothorax. The chestpiece is placed at the upper border of dullness and child is suddenly shaken to elicit splash of fluid.

Coin test (Bell tympany) A coin is placed over the front of chest and tapped with another coin while chestpiece is placed at an identical spot on the back. A loud bell-like tinkle is audible in patients with pneumothorax.

Friction test The chestpiece is placed on the center of the chest and friction is produced on either side of chest wall with a wooden spatula or finger nail. The conduction of the sound is distinctly better when chest is scratched on the side having pneumothorax.

Ewart's sign The bronchial breathing and bronchophony may be audible over the left lower interscapular area in a patient with pericardial effusion due to compression of left main bronchus leading to collapse.

d'Espine sign The presence of bronchial breathing and increased vocal resonance in the midline over the back below the level of 4th thoracic vertebra in a patient with a mediastinal mass.

Mediastinal crunch (Hamman's sign) In children with mediastinal emphysema, especially when associated with left-sided pneumothorax, systolic crunching sounds may be heard on auscultation over left sternal border from third to fifth interspaces. Mediastinal air leaks may be associated with crepitus over the supraclavicular region without any subcutaneous emphysema of chest wall.

DIAGNOSTIC FEATURES OF COMMON RESPIRATORY DISORDERS

The salient physical signs of common diseases of lungs in children are shown in Table 12.6.

Lobar Pneumonia (Consolidation)

Sudden onset of fever, cough, chest pain, dyspnea and rusty sputum are characteristic symptoms. Trachea is central. The chest movements may be slightly impaired on the affected side, percussion note is dull, tubular bronchial breathing with crackles, and increased vocal fremitus and vocal resonance are classical signs of consolidation. Pleural friction rub, overlying the site of consolidation, may be heard at times.

Pleural Effusion or Empyema

There is history of chest pain, breathing difficulty, fever and cough. Onset may be sudden but is generally insidious. The patient prefers to lie on the affected side, to splint the chest. Trachea and heart are displaced towards the opposite side. The chest may be bulging (especially intercostal spaces) on the affected side with reduced movements. There is stony dullness, rising dullness and sometimes shifting dullness on the affected side. Breath sounds are vesicular, diminished or absent without any adventitious sounds. Tactile fremitus and vocal resonance are reduced.

Atelectasis or Collapse of Lung

History of inhalation of foreign body, aspiration and recurrent chest infections should arouse the suspicion of atelectasis. Trachea and heart are pulled towards the side of atelectasis due to increased negative pleural pressure. Intercostal

TABLE 12.6 Salient physical signs in common diseases of lungs

Signs	Consolidation	Collapse	Fibrosis	Pleural effusion	Pneumothorax	Emphysema
Chest wall	Normal	No or minimal retraction	Significant chest wall retraction with impaired movements of chest	Bulging of intercostal spaces with reduced chest movements at the base	Diffuse asymmetric inflation of hemithorax with reduced chest movements on the affected side	Barrel-shaped symmetrical chest with poor expansion of chest
Mediastinal shift	None	Same side	Same side	Opposite side	Opposite side	None
Vocal fremitus	Increased	Normal or decreased	Decreased	Grossly diminished	Diminished	Diminished
Percussion note	Dull	Impaired	Impaired	Stony dull with rising or shifting dullness	Tympanitic	Hyperresonant with loss of liver and cardiac dullness
Breath sounds	Bronchial	Absent or bronchial*	Diminished or bronchial*	Diminished or absent, may be bronchial at upper border of effusion	Amphoric (if there is a bronchopleural fistula) or diminished	Diminished with prolonged expiration
Vocal resonance	Bronchophony or whispering pectoriloquy	Diminished or bronchophony*	Diminished or bronchophony*	Diminished or absent with egophony at the upper border of effusion	Diminished	Diminished
Adventitious sounds	Fine crackles	None	Coarse crackles	Friction rub in early stages and above the level of effusion	Metallic crackles, succussion splash, if there is hydro-pneumothorax	Expiratory wheezes

*In children with collapse or fibrosis, bronchial breathing is heard, if bronchus is patent. At times, more than one condition coexist, giving cumulative clinical signs of the underlying disorder.

spaces may be narrowed on the affected side. Percussion note is impaired. Breath sounds are reduced in intensity, vesicular or distant bronchial, if connecting bronchus is patent. Vocal fremitus and vocal resonance are reduced or increased depending upon the patency of connecting bronchus. The opposite lung may show compensatory emphysema.

Fibrosis of Lung

Thickened pleura, chronic infection with fibrosis, mucoviscidosis and idiopathic insterstitial fibrosis produce chronic respiratory insufficieny with dyspnea, cyanosis and clubbing. If unilateral or localized, chest is retracted and moves less on inspiration. Mediastinum is pulled towards the affected side. Percussion note is impaired. Breath sounds are vesicular and reduced in intensity. Crackles are commonly present. Associated consolidation or collapse may produce additional clinical findings. Evidences of chronic cor pulmonale may be seen in long-standing cases. It is characterized by pulmonary arterial hypertension, right ventricular enlargement and hypertrophy, and right heart failure.

Pneumothorax

Sudden chest pain, dyspnea and cyanosis herald the onset of pneumothorax. Subcutaneous emphysema may be evident over the neck and upper chest. Trachea and heart are pushed towards the opposite side. The affected side shows hyperinflation and reduced movements on breathing. Percussion note is hyperresonant, or tympanitic. Breath sounds are vesicular and reduced in intensity, tactile fremitus and vocal resonance are reduced. When there is bronchopleural fistula, amphoric bronchial breathing with whispering pectoriloquy is audible. Coin test and friction test may be positive.

	Scheme for Presentation
General physical examination	Comfortable, tachypneic or dyspneic, whether alae nasi and accessory muscles of respiration are working or not, audible sounds during breathing (grunt, stridor, croup, wheezing, etc.), state of nutrition, growth and development, and level of consciousness. Temperature, pulse, respiration (rate, type, character, depth, abnormal sounds, recessions, etc.), and blood pressure. Anemia, cyanosis, jaundice, lymphadenopathy, BCG scar, engorgement of neck veins, detailed ENT check-up, clubbing, osteoarthropathy, position of trachea and apex beat, evidences of chronic cor pulmonale.
Inspection	Describe findings in accordance with the standard format of clinical areas of chest on front, sides and back. Shape of chest on front, sides and back. The presence of localized bulge (costal or intercostal spaces) or retraction, deformities (exclude spinal deformity), movements of chest on breathing, and expansion of chest.
Palpation	Check position of trachea (including sternomastoid sign) and apex beat. Assess the movements of chest on two sides, tenderness, crepitus (clavicular or rib fracture, subcutaneous emphysema), wheezes, crackles, friction rub and tactile fremitus on two sides.
Percussion	Describe the character (resonant, tympanitic) and intensity (hyperresonant, normal, impaired, dull, stony dull) of percussion note over identical sites on two sides, and rising or shifting dullness on change of position.
Auscultation	Describe the character (vesicular, harsh-vesicular, bronchial, amphoric) and intensity (normal, increased, decreased, absent) of breath sounds, adventitious sounds and their character (crackles, wheezes, pleural friction rub), vocal resonance (normal, decreased, increased, bronchophony, whispering pectoriloquy and egophony) and various diagnostic clinical signs whenever indicated, such as Hippocratic succussion, coin test, friction test, Ewart's sign, d'Espine sign, Hamman's sign, etc.

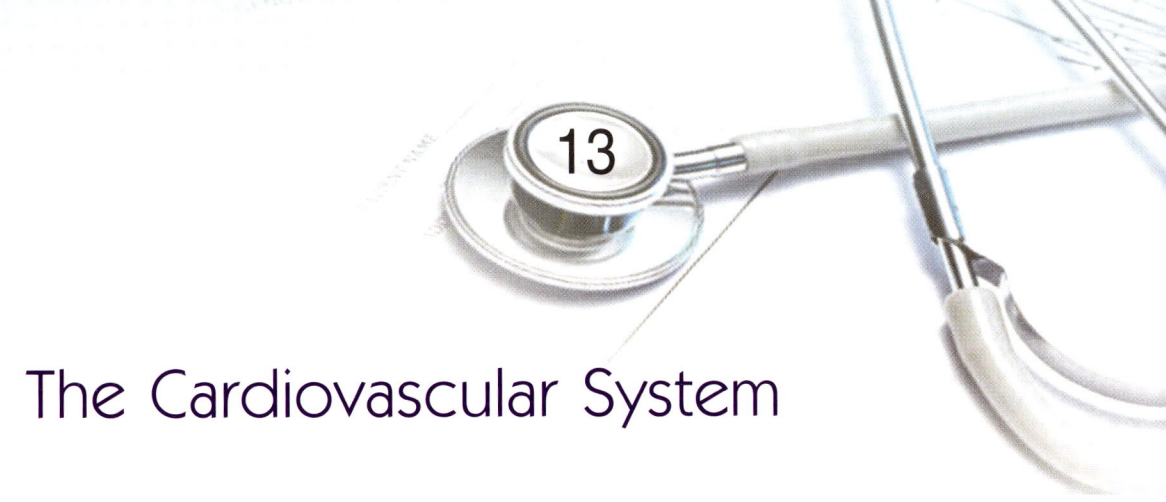

13

The Cardiovascular System

ANATOMY

The heart is located in the middle and left side of hemithorax. It comprises of two muscular pumps working in series, covered in a serous sac (pericardium) which allows free movements with each heart beat and respiration. The right heart (right atrium and ventricle) pumps blood returning from systemic veins (inferior and superior venae cavae) into the pulmonary circulation at a relatively low pressure. The left heart (left atrium and ventricle) receives oxygenated blood from the lungs and pumps it throughout the body through aorta and systemic arteries at a relatively higher pressures. The heart muscle (myocardium) is thicker in the ventricles than the atria and in the left heart than the right heart in order to generate higher pressures. However, in term newborn babies, there is physiologic right ventricular preponderance. Cardiac silhouette as seen on a PA skiagram of the chest is illustrated in Figure 13.1.

The atrioventricular valves (tricuspid on the right side and mitral on the left) separate the atria from the ventricles. They are attached to the papillary muscles in the myocardium of the ventricles by chordae tendineae which prevent them from prolapsing into the atria when the ventricle contracts. The pulmonary valve on the right side of the heart and the aortic valve on the left, separate the ventricles from the pulmonary and systemic arterial systems, respectively. Each of these valves has three cusps and are called

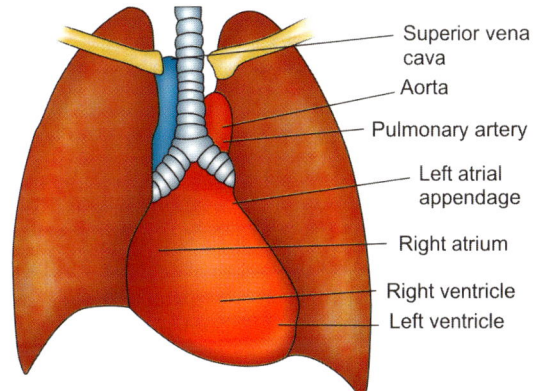

Figure 13.1 The cardiac silhouette in the antero-posterior position.

semilunar valves because they are half-moon-shaped. Cardiac contractions are coordinated by a specialized neural mechanism. The cells in the sinoatrial node act as a cardiac pacemaker. The further spread of cardiac impulse ensures that atrial contraction is completed before ventricular contraction (systole) begins. At the end of systole, the atrioventricular valves open, allowing blood to flow from the atria to refill the ventricles (diastole).

HISTORY

Ask for presenting symptoms in a lucid and chronological order. Identify the age at onset of congestive heart failure to decide whether patient is having congenital or acquired heart disease. In infants, rapid breathing, easy fatigability while feeding, inability to suck vigorously and continuously, failure to thrive and puffiness are recognized clinical features of CHF.

In an older child, assess and grade the degree of dyspnea. Grade I dyspneic while climbing stairs or running for a short distance; Grade II dyspneic while performing daily routine activity; Grade III dyspneic during below average activity, like going to bathroom or walking from one room to the other; and Grade IV when child is dyspneic at rest and is orthopneic. Older child may give history of palpitations (unpleasant sensation of beating of the heart) while in younger children an observant mother may give history of visible precordial pulsations and bulging of precordium.

Ask history of and age at onset of cyanosis, cyanotic spells and squatting or assuming knee-chest position. The "Tet spells" (tetralogy of Fallot spells) are characterized by bouts of excessive crying, agitation, worsening of cyanosis, and rapid breathing. It is associated with rapid drop in oxygen tension because of total occlusion of right ventricle outflow. The child often assumes a compensatory squatting posture with flexion of hips and elbows (akin to sitting on an Indian toilet) to increase systemic resistance and shunt more blood towards the lungs by reducing right-to-left shunt. Stokes Adams attacks may occur due to episodes of ventricular asystole occurring commonly in complete heart block causing sudden syncope which resolves spontaneously within a minute or so. The child collapses and suddenly becomes pale or white and then cyanosed; and as recovery takes place reactive hyperemia causes marked flushing.

Chest pain due to myocardial ischemia is rare in children but can occur due to pericarditis, severe aortic stenosis or regurgitation, mitral valve prolapse, anomalous origin of left coronary artery, complex congenital heart disease, dilated cardiomyopathy and Kawasaki disease. Chest pain due to pericarditis is precordial or retrosternal in location, radiates to the back or left shoulder, is aggravated in supine position and relieved by sitting and leaning forward.

Ask for history of arthritis and migratory arthralgias, chorea and syncope (due to arrhythmia). Chorea is more common in adolescent girls. Look for purposeless jerky movements of limbs and twitchings of face, pronator sign (pronation of hands when they are raised above the head), inability to keep the tongue protruded ("Jack in the box" tongue) and "milkmaid grip" when child is asked to grip the examiner's hand. Epistaxis (acute rheumatic fever, pulmonic stenosis) and hemoptysis (tight mitral stenosis, pulmonary infarction, pulmonary edema) may occur due to underlying cardiac condition. Hoarseness of cry in an infant may occur due to compression of left recurrent laryngeal nerve as a result of dilatation of main pulmonary trunk and pulmonary hypertension due to underlying congenital heart disease. Ask for history of medications and status of penicillin prophylaxis in a patient suspected to have rheumatic heart disease. History of recurrent chest infections is suggestive of left-to-right shunt. Patients with rheumatic fever may give history of recurrent streptococcal sore throats.

Ask family history of consanguinity, congenital heart disease and hypertension among siblings and parents. There is increased risk of congenital and even rheumatic heart disease among relatives as compared to general population. Maternal diabetes mellitus is associated with hypertrophic cardiomyopathy with asymmetric septal hypertrophy, transposition of great vessels and hypoplastic left heart syndrome in the offspring. Ask for maternal history of rubella, mumps and other viral infections and intake of drugs during first trimester of pregnancy which is characterized by organogenesis. Rubella syndrome is associated with patent ductus arteriosus while mumps during pregnancy may be associated with endocardial fibroelastosis in the fetus. Maternal systemic lupus erythematosus (SLE) is associated with increased risk of complete heart block in the offspring.

GENERAL PHYSICAL EXAMINATION

Assess whether child is comfortable or dyspneic, evaluate the severity of dyspnea, posture (orthopnea), physical growth and development. Look for peculiar phenotype (Down syndrome, Turner syndrome, Marfan syndrome, Hurler syndrome, glycogenosis, etc.), malar flush, puffiness and chorea. Table 13.1 outlines common cardiac malformations in association with chromosomal and developmental syndromes.

TABLE 13.1 Common cardiac malformations in association with chromosomal and developmental syndromes

Syndrome	Phenotype	Cardiac abnormalities
Alagille syndrome	Micrognathia, broad overhanging forehead, deep set eyes, cholestasis due to paucity or atresia of bile ducts, butterfly vertebral anomalies, and short distal phalanges. It is an autosomal dominant genetic disorder. Xanthomatosis occurs due to elevation of cholesterol and lipids	Peripheral pulmonic artery stenosis and tetralogy of Fallot are most common
CHARGE association	**C**oloboma, **a**tresia choanae, **r**etarded growth and development, **g**enital hypoplasia, **e**ar anomalies and deafness, facial dysmorphism (broad forehead, square face, facial asymmetry, broad nasal tip, ptosis, arched eyebrows, laterally protruding ears), cranial nerve palsies, and hypocalcemia	75–80% have cardiac defects especially conotruncal anomalies, i.e. tetralogy of Fallot, double outlet right ventricle, truncus arteriosus, and interrupted aortic arch
Cornelia de Lange syndrome	Bushy eyebrows which meet in the midline (synophrys), long curly eyelashes, cleft palate, small nose with anteverted nostrils, long philtrum, downward curving of angle of mouth, microcephaly, and mental retardation	Ventricular septal defect, ASD, pulmonary stenosis, coarctation of the aorta
DiGeorge or CATCH-22 syndrome (Deletion 22 q 11.2)	Fish mouth, hypertelorism, anti-mongoloid slant of eyes, cleft palate or velopharyngeal incompetence, gastroesophageal reflux, nasal speech, attention deficit hyperactivity disorder, hypoplasia or aplasia of thymus and parathyroids, tetany, cell-mediated immune deficiency	Interrupted aortic arch, truncus arteriosus, tetralogy of Fallot and double outlet right ventricle
Down syndrome (Trisomy 21)	Brachycephaly, upward slant of eyes, flat occiput, Brushfield spots, small mouth with protruding fissured tongue, hypotonia, incurved little finger, simian crease, sandal toes and developmental retardation	Endocardial cushion defect, atrio-ventricular canal defects and ventricular septal defect in 50% cases, Fallot's tetralogy without transposition of great arteries
Duchenne's muscular dystrophy	Sex-linked disorder with progressive muscular weakness, hypertrophy of calves due to fatty infiltration, positive Gower's sign, and waddling gait	Cardiomyopathy
Ellis-van Creveld syndrome	Long narrow dysplastic chest (short ribs) and abdomen, multiple frenula of upper lip, cleft lip and palate, defective teeth, natal teeth, postaxial polydactyly of hands, acromesomelic shortening of limbs, fusion of hamate and capitate bones, sparse hair, hypoplastic nails, cone-shaped epiphyses, small pelvic bones, genu valgum, and epispadias	ASD (60%) and single atrium

(contd.)

TABLE 13.1 Common cardiac malformations in association with chromosomal and developmental syndromes (*contd.*)

Syndrome	Phenotype	Cardiac abnormalities
Glycogen storage disease (Pompe's disease)	Marked hypotonia, macroglossia, hepatomegaly, normal mental development, and early death	Cardiomegaly with or without EKG changes (left axis deviation, short PR interval, broad QRS complex)
Holt-Oram syndrome	Deformities of forearm bones due to absent or hypoplastic radius, finger-like triphalangeal or absent thumbs, syndactyly, and polydactyly	Familial ASD, VSD in 50% cases
Hurler syndrome	Coarse features, thick lips and broad nose, cloudy cornea, hepatosplenomegaly or mental retardation	Mitral or aortic regurgitation, coronary artery disease, and mitral valve prolapse
LEOPARD syndrome (lentiginosis)	Multiple lentigines over neck and upper trunk, ocular hypertelorism, growth failure, genital abnormalities and deafness	Pulmonic stenosis, hypertrophic cardiomyopathy, and conduction defects on EKG
Marfan syndrome	Tall stature, long slender arms and fingers/toes, positive "thumb sign*" (tip of the thumb protrudes beyond the ulnar border of the palm when fist is clenched), subluxated lens, lower segment of the body is longer than the upper segment, and arm span is longer than height	Dilatation of aortic root with aortic regurgitation, and mitral valve prolapse
Noonan syndrome	Turner-like phenotype, webbed-neck, hypertelorism with antimongoloid slant of palpebral fissures, pectus excavatum, cryptorchidism and small testes	Pulmonary valvular stenosis or ASD, dysplastic pulmonary valve, peripheral pulmonic stenosis, and hypertrophic cardiomyopathy
Rubella syndrome	Microcephaly, deafness, cataracts, chorioretinitis, and metaphysitis	Peripheral pulmonary artery stenosis, patent ductus arteriosus
Shprintzen-Goldberg syndrome (SGS syndrome)	"Marfanoid habitus", craniosynostosis, long narrow head, hypertelorism, exophthalmos, antimongoloid slant of eyes, high narrow palate, micrognathia, low set ears, microglossia, intellectual disability	Valve regurgitation or prolapse, aortic root dilatation and aneurysm
TAR syndrome	Thrombocytopenia, absent or hypoplastic radii	About one-third have cardiac defects, like TOF, VSD
Trisomy 13–15 (Patau syndrome)	Microophthalmia, coloboma, mid-facial hypoplasia, cleft lip/palate, microcephaly, broad flat nose, micrognathia, low set ears, capillary hemangiomas, simian crease, localized scalp defects, holoprosencephaly, postaxial polydactyly of hands or feet, and flexion deformity of fingers	VSD, ASD, PDA, dextrocardia in 90% cases
Trisomy 17–18 (Edward syndrome)	Microcephaly, dolichocephaly, prominent occiput, small eyes and oral opening, low set ears, micrognathia, short sternum, and clenched hands with overlapping fingers, simian crease, short dorsiflexed first toe, and rocker bottom feet	VSD (90%), PDA (70%), ASD (20%), valvular regurgitation may occur at multiple sites

(*contd.*)

TABLE 13.1 Common cardiac malformations in association with chromosomal and developmental syndromes (contd.)

Syndrome	Phenotype	Cardiac abnormalities
Tuberous sclerosis	Adenoma sebaceum, ashleaf skin macules, shagreen patch, epilepsy, intracranial clacification, and mental retardation	Rhabdomyoma of heart
Turner syndrome (Monosomy X)	Lymphedema of dorsa of hands and feet during neonatal period, triangular face with antimongoloid slant of eyes, broad chest with widely spaced nipples, short webbed neck, low hair line, cubitus valgus, amenorrhea, and short stature	Coarctation of aorta (XO), pulmonary stenosis (XO/XY), and bicuspid aortic valve
VACTERL or VATER association	Vertebral defects, anal atresia, tracheoesophageal atresia with fistula, radial and renal anomalies, and limb defects (radial agenesis)	Around 50% have cardiac defects, VSD is most common
Williams syndrome (Deletion 7 q 11)	Elfin facies, cute mischievous cheerful demeanor, prominent forehead, widely spaced puffy eyes, short pelpebral fissure, upturned nose, stellate iris, long philtrum, wide mouth (ear-to-ear smile), small widely spaced teeth, patulous lower lip, small chin, mental retardation, short stature, hyperacusis and hypercalcemia during infancy	Supravalvular aortic stenosis, pulmonary artery stenosis, stenosis of renal arteries or coronaries

*Thumb sign is absent in homocystinuria, a condition in which other phenotypic features are similar to Marfan syndrome

Pulse Radial pulse is examined with tips of the index and middle fingers by gently compressing the vessel against lower end of the radius. It is difficult to feel the radial pulse in newborn babies and infants. Pulse can be recorded from several other peripheral arteries, like brachial, carotid, femoral, popliteal, posterior tibial and dorsalis pedis. The carotid pulse should be felt in the groove infront of the sternocleidomastoid muscle while auscultating the heart. The presence of carotid thrill with an ejection systolic murmur in the second right intercostal space is diagnostic of aortic stenosis. In coarctation of aorta, femoral pulsations are feeble and delayed as compared to simultaneously felt radial or brachial pulsations. The following characteristics of the pulse should be noted.

Rate (beats/min), volume (thrust), tension (force required to obliterate the pulse), rhythm (volume and rate), character (normal, bounding, collapsing or water hammer type, plateau), pulsus alternans (alternate stronger and weaker beat), pulsus bigeminus (alternate normal and ectopic beat), pulsus paradoxus, pulse on the other side and femorals (volume and temporal relationship with radial pulse) should be assessed (Figure 13.2). Pulse pressure (systolic BP–diastolic BP) is high (>40 mm Hg) in children with aortic regurgitation, patent ductus arteriosus, arteriovenous fistula and thyrotoxicosis. The pulse is low volume with narrow pulse pressue (<25 mm Hg) in patients with aortic stenosis, pericarditis, pericardial tamponade and significant tachycardia. Assessment of vessel wall for its thickness is not important in children.

Look for pulse deficit by simultaneously recording heart rate and pulse rate (ectopics and auricular fibrillations). The pulse may be regularly irregular due to an ectopic beat occurring at a regular interval or it may be irregularly irregular because of atrial fibrillation. Sinus arrhythmia in which pulse rate becomes fast during inspiration and slows during expiration is common and physiological in children (Box 13.1). Pulsus alternans is characterized by alternating strong and weak beats due to severe dysfunction of left

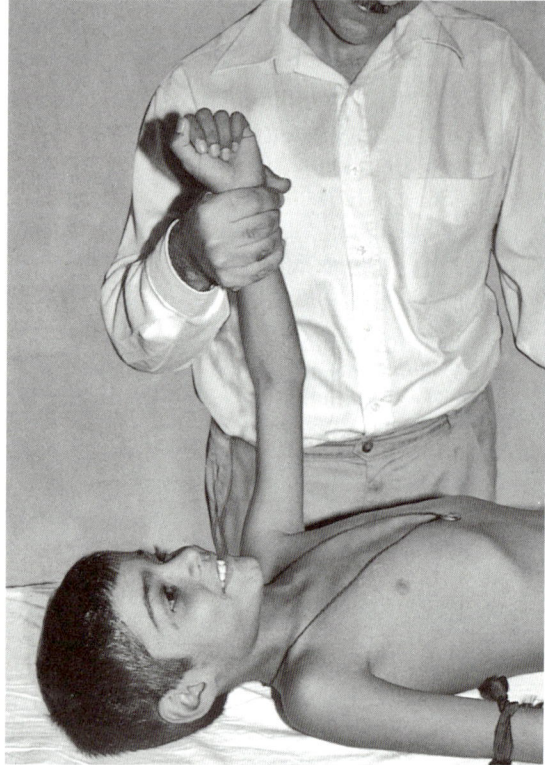

Figure 13.2 Looking for water hammer type of pulse. The patient lies supine with both arms on the sides. The wrist of one hand is so grasped that radial pulse is barely palpable. When arm is lifted up beyond the plane of the body, radial pulse becomes more readily palpable, if it is collapsing in character.

TABLE 13.2 Causes of tachycardia* in children	
Cause	Heart rate (beats/min)
▪ **Tachyarrhythmias**	
□ Supraventricular tachycardia	180–320
□ Atrial tachycardia	120–180
□ Atrial flutter	100–320 (atrial rate 250–400)
□ Ventricular tachycardia	120–240
▪ **Sinus tachycardia**	up to 225
□ Physiological (age-related)	
□ Fever	
□ Exercise	
□ Emotional disturbances (excitement, anxiety, panic attacks)	
□ Anemia	
□ Dehydration	
□ Hypovolemia	
□ Shock	
□ Myocarditis	
□ Cardiac failure	
□ Pulmonary embolism	
□ Thyrotoxicosis	
□ Pheochromocytoma	
□ Hypoglycemia	
□ Autonomic dysfunction	
▪ **Drugs** Atropine, aspirin, β-agonists, amphetamine, theophylline, cyclic antidepressants, methylphenidate, leukotriene modifiers, phenylephrine, azithromycin, fluoroquinolones, thyroxine and cocaine	

*Tachycardia of more than 240 beats/min suggests primary cardiac disease

---

Box 13.1 Causes of irregular pulse

- Sinus arrhythmia
- Atrial extrasystoles
- Ventricular extrasystoles
- Atrial fibrillation
- Atrial flutter with variable response
- Second-degree heart block

Box 13.2 Causes of bradycardia* in children

- Bradyarrhythmias: Sinoatrial block, AV block, complete bundle branch block, sick sinus syndrome, and long QT syndrome
- Athletic child
- Hypothermia
- Hypoxia
- Hypothyroidism
- Acidosis and electrolyte disturbances
- Raised intracranial tension
- Brainstem compression
- Excessive vagal tone
- Drugs and toxins: Digitalis, β-blockers, calcium channel blocker, intravenous calcium therapy, narcotics, clonidine, and organophosphates

*A sinus rate of less than 90 beats/min in neonates and less than 60 beats/min in older children is suggestive of sinus bradycardia

---

ventricle. Tachycardia may occur from a large number of cardiac and systemic conditions (Table 13.2). Bradycardia is diagnosed when sinus rate is less than 90 beats/min in neonates and less than 60 beats/min in older children (*Box 13.2*).

Pulsus paradoxus is a misnomer because it is an exaggeration of physiological finding wherein arterial pressure or pulse volume markedly diminishes or even disappears during deep inspiration. The systolic blood pressure is more than 10 mm Hg lower during inspiration as compared to expiration. In a child who is unable to control his breathing on request, there is an alternative method to look for pulsus paradoxus. Ask the child to breathe normally and record his blood pressure. Note the reading on the manometer when first Korotkoff sound is heard. Allow the mercury to fall slowly until you hear the Korotkoff sounds loudly and continuously which gives a "doubling" effect to the sounds. Note the reading at this point and calculate the difference between first and second reading. A difference of 10–20 mm Hg is equivocal but a difference of more than 20 mm Hg is highly suggestive of pulsus paradoxus. Pulsus paradoxus is classically seen in patients with cardiac tamponade (pericardial effusion, constrictive pericarditis), restrictive cardiomyopathy, severe bronchial asthma, pneumothorax and pleural effusion.

Temperature Fever may occur due to rheumatic activity, bacterial endocarditis, pulmonary infarction, and chest infection. Fever may also occur due to a cause unrelated to the cardiac condition.

Respiratory rate Tachypnea is seen in CHF, anoxic spells, pulmonary emboli and intercurrent respiratory infection.

Blood pressure Mercury or aneroid sphygmomanometer and automatic oscillometric devices are commonly used for recording blood pressure. A sphygmomanometer with a mercury column is more reliable than an aneroid instrument. It is conventionally recorded in the upper arm at the site of brachial artery. The child should be sitting with arm kept at the level of heart or lying comfortably in bed. The appropriate size of the cuff which should cover two-thirds of upper arm (or it should be 20% wider than the diameter of upper arm or width of the cuff should be 40% of the circumference of the arm) should be used. The recommended cuff size in infants below one year of age is 2.5 cm, 1–4 years is 5 cm, 5–9 years is 9 cm and over 10 years is 13 cm. The use of a narrow blood pressure cuff is associated with spuriously high systolic blood pressure reading and vice versa. The cuff is applied snugly over the upper arm by keeping its lower edge at least 2.0 cm above the cubital fossa. The manometer is kept at the same level as the cuff on the arm (heart level) and should be conveniently placed for the observer to view it.

Inflate the pressure in the cuff while palpating brachial pulse. The level at which brachial pulse disappears is a rough estimate of systolic blood pressure. Inflate the cuff further by another 20–30 mm Hg and listen through the diaphragm of stethoscope placed lightly over the brachial artery. Deflate the cuff slowly by decrements of 2–3 mm Hg and the point when Korotkoff sounds are first heard is indicative of systolic blood pressure. When cuff is further deflated, the Korotkoff sounds become abruptly muffled and finally disappear which is taken as an indication of diastolic blood pressure. The blood pressure reading is taken to the nearest 2 mm Hg. At times the Korotkoff sounds do not disappear and in that case muffling of the sounds is taken as the criterion for diastolic blood pressure (Figure 13.3). A child is said to have hypertension, if blood pressure is at or above the 95th centile for age and height

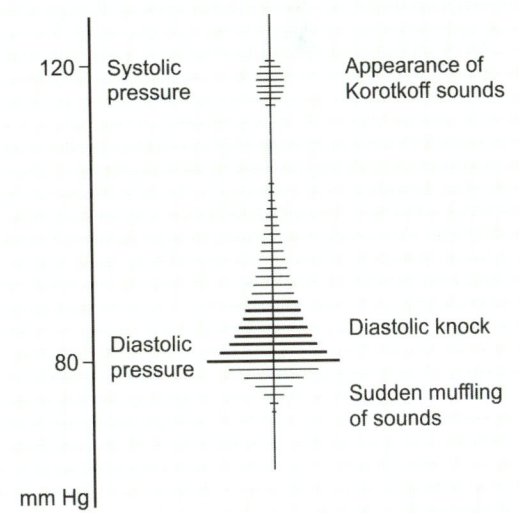

Figure 13.3 The nature of sounds heard during measurement of blood pressure by auscultation method.

TABLE 13.3 Criteria for hypertension

Age	95th centile blood pressure (mm Hg)
Newborn	Systolic 95
7 days	Systolic 105
Up to 2 years	112/74
3–5 years	116/76
6–9 years	122/78
10–12 years	126/82

Hypertension is defined as average systolic blood pressure or diastolic blood pressure ≥95th percentile for sex, age and height on three or more occasions.
For normalized BP percentile table in children, refer to http://www.nhibi.nih.gov/health_pro/guidelines/current/hypertension_pediatric_jnc,4/blood_pressure_tables

(Table 13.3). The blood pressure should be recorded in both the upper and the lower limbs when polyarteritis or coarctation of aorta is suspected.

For recording lower limb blood pressure, child is made to lie in prone position (face down), apropriate-sized cuff is applied over the thigh and stethoscope is placed over the popliteal artery in the popliteal fossa. Normally, the lower limb systolic blood pressure is more by 10–30 mm Hg while the diastolic blood pressure is identical in upper and lower limbs. In coarctation of aorta, the lower limb blood pressure is lower than the upper limb while in aortic regurgitation, the lower limb blood pressure is at least 40 mm Hg higher than the upper limb (Hill sign). The pulse pressure is the difference between the systolic and diastolic blood pressure and is indicative of pulse volume. In aortic regurgitation, pulse pressure is high (≥80 mm Hg) while in aortic stenosis, pulse is feeble with low pulse pressure. Some adolescent children may complain of dizziness on standing due to postural hypotension. Check blood pressure in a relaxed supine position and record again after 2 minutes of standing. When there is ≥20 mm Hg drop in blood pressure on standing, it is suggestive of postural hypotension.

In infants and newborn babies, it is difficult to record blood pressure by the conventional method. Blood pressure can be recorded by *flush method*. Cuff is wrapped around the upper arm, limb is raised vertically and held above the head till palm becomes pale. The pressure in the cuff is raised beyond the expected systolic blood pressure while maintaining the arm in vertical position. The arm is then brought down to the side on the cot and cuff is gradually deflated. The point at which the palm becomes flushed is indicative of systolic blood pressure of the infant. The diastolic blood pressure cannot be recorded by this method. In newborn babies and young infants, it is more convenient and reliable to use non-invasive Doppler system to record the blood pressure. In children, hypertension is usually secondary to renovascular causes. Medical history and physical examination can provide clues to the likely etiology of hypertension (Table 13.4).

Anemia, cyanosis, jaundice (chronic liver congestion, pulmonary infarction, unrelated), lymphadenopathy and edema should be looked for. Differential cyanosis with pink hands and blue feet may occur due to right-to-left shunt through patent ductus arteriosus because of severe pulmonary arterial hypertension. Early and intense cyanosis (first week) should alert to the possibility of "T" diseases, like **T**GA, **T**APVC, **T**ricuspid atresia, **T**runcus arteriosus, **T**otal (critical) PS and **T**ricuspid regurgitation. Pink fingers with blue toes suggest that there is normal connection of great vessels. When there is complete transposition of great vessels, with pulmonary hypertension and reversed flow through the ductus arteriosus, the fingers will be more cyanosed than the toes. Measurement of SaO_2 in the right hand (pre-ductal) should be compared with either foot (post-ductal) to look for differential cyanosis. In newborn babies and infants with cardiac failure, sacral edema and puffiness may be seen while pedal edema is rare.

Nails Marked or drumstick clubbing is seen in children with cyanotic heart disease. Clubbing, splinter hemorrhages, (reddish-brown linear marks along the axis of nails), Osler nodes (tender red nodules over the pulps of fingers and toes due to deposition of immune complexes) and palmar ecchymosis (Janeway's lesions) are indicative of bacterial endocarditis.

TABLE 13.4 Clinical correlates of hypertension in children

Findings	Likely etiology
General	
▫ Tachycardia	Primary HTN, pheochromocytoma, neuroblastoma, hyperthyroidism
▫ Growth retardation and pallor	Chronic renal failure
▫ Elevated BMI	Primary HTN in adolescents
▫ Truncal obesity	Hypercorticism, insulin resistance syndrome
Recognized syndromes	
▫ Acanthosis nigricans (dark patches of skin with velvety texture over axillae, groins, neck and joints)	Insulin resistance due to metabolic syndrome X and PCOD
▫ Cafe au lait spots	Neurofibromatosis
▫ Exophthalmos, tremors, thyromegaly with a murmur, and weight loss	Hyperthyroidism
▫ Elfin facies (prominent forehead, widely spaced eyes, upturned nose, under developed mandible and patulous lips)	Williams syndrome
▫ Webbed neck, widely spaced nipples, short stature, delayed sexual maturation	Turner syndrome
▫ Moon facies, truncal obesity, abdominal striae, acne, and hirsutism	Cushing syndrome
▫ Episodes of pallor, flushing and diaphoresis	Pheochromocytoma
▫ Ambiguous genitalia, virilization, pigmentation	Congenital adrenal hyperplasia
▫ Arthralgias, oral ulcers, skin rash	Vasculitis syndromes
Cardiovascular abnormalities	
▫ Delayed and weak femoral pulses, low blood pressure in the legs and murmur in the left infraclavicular area and below the left scapula	Coarctation of the aorta
▫ Apical heave	Left ventricular hypertrophy
▫ Abdominal bruit	Renal artery stenosis
▫ Pericardial friction rub	Vasculitis, uremia
Abdomen	
▫ Abdominal mass	Wilms tumor, neuroblastoma, pheochromocytoma, hydronephrosis, PKD, bladder neck obstruction
▫ Hepatosplenomegaly	ARPKD
Central nervous system	
▫ Fundoscopy	Hypertensive retinopathy (arteriolar constriction, arteriovenous nicking, vascular wall changes, flame-shaped hemorrhages, cotton-wool spots, yellow hard exudates, optic disk edema)
▫ Focal neurological deficits	Stroke
▫ Retinal hamartoma and hemangioblastomas in various organs	Von Hippel-Lindau syndrome

Abbreviations: ARPKD, autosomal recessive polycystic kidney disease; BMI, body mass index; HTN, hypertension; PCOD, polycystic ovarian disease; PKD, polycystic kidney disease

Skin and joints Look for subcutaneous nodules, erythema marginatum, chorea and swelling of joints which are suggestive of rheumatic activity. However, fortunately chorea and arthritis never coexist. Infants with CHF may have cold sweat on the forehead due to sympathetic overactivity as a consequence of decreased cardiac output. Examine joints and throat for any inflammatory signs.

Neck Internal jugular vein is in direct communication with the right atrium and is best suited for assessment of venous pressure and pulse waveforms. Look for jugular venous pressure (normal or raised), venous and arterial pulsations and thrill. JVP is difficult to evaluate in infants due to short neck. In infants with congestive heart failure, scalp veins may become prominent and engorged. Examine thyroid gland for enlargement and bruit to rule out thyrotoxicosis.

Venous pulsations Venous pulsations in relation to various phases of cardiac cycle are depicated in Figure 13.4. The mechanism for development of various individual waves in the internal jugular veins is shown in Table 13.5. As opposed to arterial pulsations, venous pulsations are not palpable and are less readily visible in an erect posture. Inspiration enhances venous pulsations by increasing venous return to the thorax. They are absent in children with auricular fibrillation, superior mediastinal obstruction and constrictive pericarditis (prominent Y descent). Giant 'a' waves or cannon waves are seen in tricuspid stenosis or atresia, pulmonary stenosis, pulmonary arterial hypertension, Ebstein's disease, nodal rhythm, ectopic beats, and complete heart block. Giant 'v' waves are seen in children with tricuspid regurgitation.

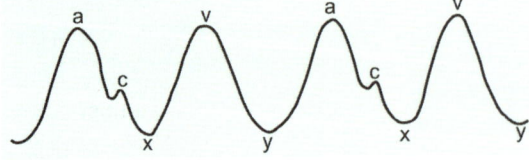

Figure 13.4 The venous pulse has three positive waves; a, c and v and two negative waves or descents; x and y.

TABLE 13.5 The mechanisms for development of individual waves in the internal jugular veins

a wave	Due to right atrial contraction
c wave	Coincides with onset of ventricular systole and results due to the movement of the tricuspid valve into the right atrium as the right ventricular pressure rises
x descent	Due to atrial relaxation
v wave	Due to passive rise in the pressure as venous return to the right atrium continues during ventricular systole while the tricuspid valve is closed
y descent	There is lowering of right atrial pressure as the tricuspid valve opens and the blood rushes into the right ventricle

Liver Examine for liver size, tenderness, pulsations, and hepatojugular reflux (compression of hepatic area is followed by engorgement of neck veins). Hepatojugular reflux is a sign of right ventricular compromise. Heptomegaly is the most reliable sign of CHF in infants.

Spleen Splenomegaly may occur due to bacterial endocarditis or intercurrent infections, such as malaria or septicemia (typhoid fever).

Fundus Roth spots (flame-shaped hemorrhages with "cotton-wool" pale center) may be seen in children with bacterial endocarditis. In aortic regurgitation and patent ductus arteriosus, dancing retinal vessels are characteristic.

Signs of Cardiac Failure

Dyspnea, tachycardia, raised JVP, enlarged tender liver, edema, cardiomegaly and basal crackles are recognized clinical signs of congestive heart failure (CHF). Jugular venous pressure is assessed by visualizing the engorgement of internal jugular veins in the neck. The patient lies supine with neck elevated by 45°. The vertical distance from the angle of Louis (sternal angle) to the imaginary line drawn from the upper end of jugular venous column gives JVP which is measured in centimeters (Figures 13.5 and 13.6). The sternal angle is taken as the reference point because the center of right atrium is located at a depth of 5 cm behind the

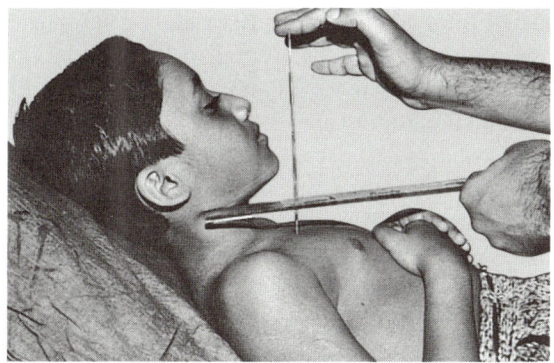

Figure 13.5 Method for evaluation of jugular venous pressure. Child is made to lie in a Fowler's position at an angle of 45°. The level of venous engorgement of jugular vein in relation to angle of Louis is measured with the help of two plastic rulers as shown in the photograph. When JVP is grossly elevated, neck veins may be engorged right up to the angle of jaw even when child sits up.

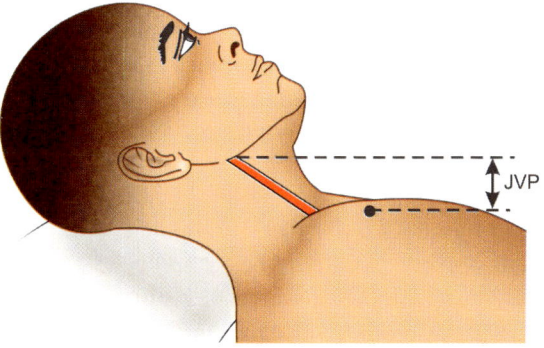

Figure 13.6 Diagrammatic representation of jugular venous pressure (JVP). The child is placed in a reclining position at an angle of 45° so that angle of Louis corresponds to the base of neck or upper margins of the clavicle. In this position, the height of the engorged right internal jugular vein is measured to assess JVP.

sternal angle in any position of the body. When JVP is raised 3 cm above the sternal angle or internal jugular vein is engorged above the level of clavicle, it is abnormal and suggestive of CHF, pericardial effusion, constrictive pericarditis and mediastinal mass. In infants, evaluation of JVP is unreliable due to short neck and pedal edema is uncommon. *Hepatomegaly is the most consistent and reliable sign of CHF in infants.* The central venous pressure can be measured by introducing a needle in the antecubital vein and connecting it to a manometer filled with saline. The normal CVP ranges between 4 and 6 cm H_2O and it is raised in CHF and reduced in hypovolemic shock.

In infants, CHF indicates the presence of severe underlying cardiac abnormality, like severe stenosis or atresia, left-to-right shunt, valvular regurgitation and conditions with transposition physiology. CHF may be aggravated by underlying anemia, infective endocarditis, systemic hypertension and coincidental myocardial disease. The time of onset of CHF is useful to suspect the nature of underlying congenital heart disease (Table 13.6). In most instances of congenital heart disease, CHF usually occurs during first 3–6 months of life. Infact, if there is no CHF during first year of life, it is unlikely to occur till the child is at least 10 years or older.

TABLE 13.6 Time of onset of congestive heart failure in children with congenital heart disease

Age at onset	Cardiac lesion
First 3 days of life	Atresias or critical stenosis of pulmonary, mitral and aortic valves
4 days to 1 week	Hypoplastic left and right heart syndromes, transposition and malposition of great arteries
1–4 weeks	Transposition and malposition complexes, endocardial fibroelastosis, and coarctation of the aorta
1–2 months	Transposition and malposition complexes, endocardial cushion defects, ventricular septal defect, patent ductus arteriosus, total anomalous pulmonary venous connection, and anomalous left coronary artery from pulmonary artery
2–6 months*	Transposition and malposition complexes, ventricular septal defect, patent ductus arteriosus, total anomalous pulmonary venous connection, aortic stenosis, and coarctation of the aorta

*There is sudden fall in pulmonary vascular resistance during 2–6 months of age with aggravation of left-to-right shunt

EXAMINATION OF HEART

Inspection

Bulging precordium (long-standing cardiomegaly), and bulging intercostal spaces (pericardial effusion) should be looked for. There are several thoracic lines of reference used in the examination of the heart to express degree of cardiac enlargement (Figure 13.7).

Precordial pulsations Note whether precordium is quiet (pericardial effusion, endocardial fibroelastosis, Ebstein disease), hyperdynamic or hyperkinetic (anemia, thyrotoxicosis, left-to-right shunt, aortic and mitral regurgitation, etc.). Look for suprasternal and epigastric pulsations, dilated veins over the chest, and collateral arteries. Identify the site of apex beat, if it is visible.

Palpation

Apex beat It is the outermost and lowermost point of palpable impact of cardiac impulse. The apex beat is best palpated with the child sitting and leaning forward. The important landmark for counting the intercostal spaces is the angle of Louis or sternal angle. It is felt as a ridge connecting manubrium sterni with body of the sternum. The rib corresponding to the sternal angle is second rib and space below is the second intercostal space. In preschool children, apex beat is located in the 4th intercostal space just lateral to the midclavicular line. In older children, it is located in the 5th intercostal space inside or over the midclavicular line. Assess whether it is visible or not (look on both sides of chest), its location (up, down, outwards, inwards or right side), and character (normal, feeble, tapping, heaving and hyperkinetic).

Tapping apex is suggestive of palpable S_1 in the mitral area while heaving (forceful, broad and sustained) apex is indicative of left ventricular hypertrophy due to pressure overload. The heaving apex with parasternal lift is graded into 3 grades. Grade 1; mild lifting of fingers and impulse can be obliterated, Grade 2; the lift is significant but not sustained and Grade 3; when lift is forceful and sustained. Hyperkinetic apex beat is characterized by exaggerated ill-sustained thrust of cardiac impulse and is seen in conditions associated with volume overload (anemia, aortic regurgitation, PDA, VSD, MR, thyrotoxicosis). Left parasternal heave (due to right ventricular hypertrophy or conducted impulse from left atrial enlargement) and diastolic shock (palpable S_2) should be looked for. At times right parasternal heave may be felt, if right atrium is hugely dilated (Ebstein disease). Pulsations may be felt over the interscapular and infrascapular region due to dilatation of collateral vessels in children with coarctation of aorta, pulmonary atresia and Blalock-Taussig shunt.

The point of maximal impulse (PMI) is helpful in determining whether the right or left ventricle is dominant. In patients with left ventricular dominance, the impulse is maximal at the apex whereas in right ventricular dominance the cardiac impulse is maximal over the left sternal border.

Thrill Vibratory sensations of heart musculature conducted through the chest wall (like purring of cat) when assessed on palpation is called a thrill. It is associated with a murmur of Grade IV or higher. Note the site and timing of thrill. The presence of a thrill is a more certain evidence of underlying organic disease of the heart as opposed to the

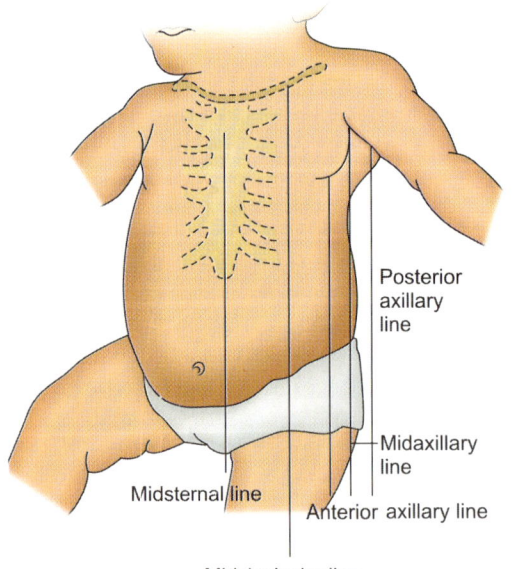

Figure 13.7 Thoracic reference lines used for assessment of cardiac enlargement.

presence of a murmur alone. *Functional murmurs are never associated with a thrill.*

Percussion

It has a limited clinical utility and is used to outline cardiac borders and to assess the heart size. In pericardial effusion, the dullness extends beyond the apex, and there is dullness over the 2nd left intercostal space which disappears when patient sits up, i.e. there is shifting dullness (c.f. pulmonary hypertension). In pulmonary hypertension and dilatation of pulmonary conus, second left intercostal space is dull both in supine and sitting positions. Dullness over second right intercostal space and manubrium sterni may be seen in aortic aneurysm and mediastinal mass (thymus).

Auscultation

There is nothing criminal about the student's use of the stethoscope as a status symbol but your status will suffer, if your symbol lets you down. Admittedly, the most important part of the stethoscope is the part between the ears and your brain!

John Apley

After inspection, it is desirable to auscultate the heart in a sleeping infant before he is frightened or awakened by palpation and percussion (Figure 13.8). Offer a toy, key ring or your finger to the infant while auscultating to prevent him fiddling with the tubing of the stethoscope. The bell type chest piece is better suited for detecting low-frequency or low pitched events (mitral diastolic murmur, third heart sound and gallop rhythm) whereas the diaphragm selectively picks up the high-frequency sounds and murmurs. Good quality stethoscope with short tubes (about 12 inches length) and snugly fitting rubber earpieces, waxless ears and intact drums of an experienced examiner, quiet infant and serene surroundings are crucial correlates for optimal auscultatory yield. Auscultatory findings are subjective and need experience and expertise on the part of physician. Auscultation technology has been revolutionized by introduction of an iStethoscope or digital stethoscope (EKO™) which is connected to a

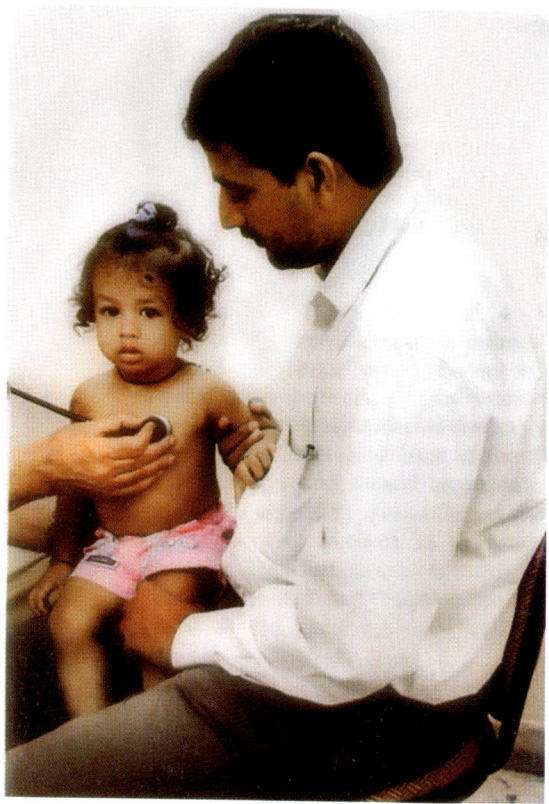

Figure 13.8 Infant is best examined while sitting in the lap of mother or father. Auscultation should be done before doing palpation and percussion.

mobile smartphone or iPhone. The availability of echocardiography has deflated the ego of many a cardiologists. The defeatist attitude, however, should be replaced by the desire to improve and sharpen clinical acumen with the help of available imaging technology.

Mitral (apex), tricuspid (above xiphoid cartilage), 3rd and 4th left parasternal intercostal spaces, pulmonary (second intercostal space adjacent to left sternal border) and aortic (second intercostal space adjacent to right sternal border) area, neck vessels, sides and back of the chest and thyroid gland should be auscultated (Figures 13.9 and 13.10). In patients with dextrocardia, instead of cardiac areas, the specific areas of chest should be auscultated to express the abnormal findings. Auscultation should be done with patient in the supine, upright, and left lateral positions and

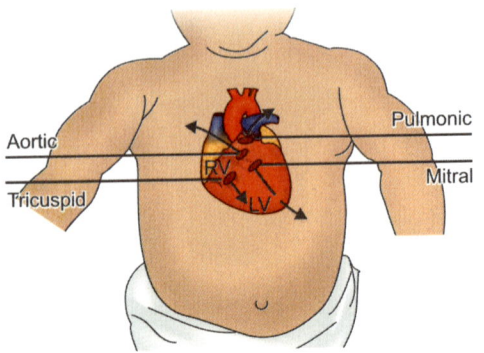

Figure 13.9 Areas for auscultation of heart. The heart sounds follow the direction of blood flow. The four standard cardiac areas project from the anatomical positions of cardiac valves as shown by arrows.

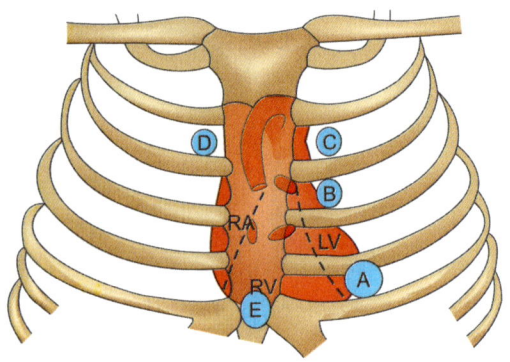

Figure 13.10 Areas of auscultation of heart sounds (A) Mitral area; (B) 3rd and 4th left intercostal spaces; (C) Pulmonary area; (D) Aortic area; (E) Tricuspid area.

leaning forward. It is best to auscultate all areas of the heart for the quality and intensity of heart sounds and murmurs. The findings should be synthesized, reconciled and expressed keeping in mind their character, intensity, "best heard" sites and radiation.

A protocol or a sequence should be developed to describe auscultatory findings:
(i) The first and second heart sounds
(ii) 3rd and 4th heart sounds in diastole
(iii) Clicks and opening snaps
(iv) Pericardial rub
(v) Murmurs in systole and/or diastole

Heart sounds The temporal relationship between events in the cardiac cycle and production of heart sounds and jugular venous pulsations are diagrammatically depicted in Figure 13.11. The events on the two sides of the heart are asynchronous, the left ventricle starts contracting before the right ventricle. The normal first heart sound is low-pitched, louder in intensity, longer in duration and the pause preceding it is longer than that following it. First heart sound (closure of mitral and tricuspid valves) is best studied in the mitral area while second heart sound (closure of aortic and pulmonary valves) is best heard in the pulmonary and aortic areas. The second heart sound has two components; the aortic closure sound (A_2) and the pulmonary closure sound (P_2). During

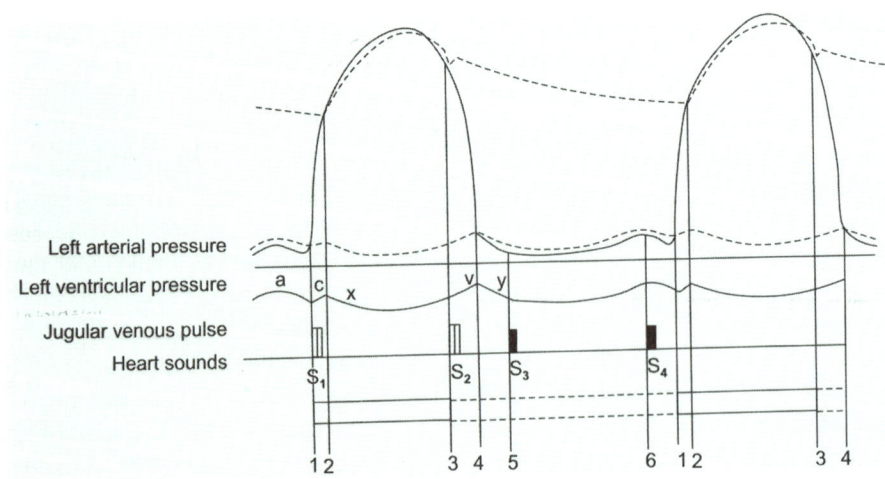

Figure 13.11 The cardiac cycle. Note the temporal relationship of jugular venous pulsations with heart sounds and cardiac systole and diastole.

expiration, the two components are superimposed on each other resulting in a single second heart sound. During inspiratory phase of respiration, A_2 occurs slightly early while P_2 is delayed resulting in split second heart sound or S_2. Second heart sound (P_2) is normally as loud as A_2 and split (especially during inspiration) in children. P_2 is louder than A_2 during 3–6 months of age. Proper evaluation of S_2 provides diagnostic clues in a number of clinical situations (Table 13.7).

TABLE 13.7 Clinical significance of abnormal S_2

Abnormal splitting of S_2
1. *Widely split and fixed S_2*
   - Volume overload (ASD, TAPVR)
   - Electrical delay (RBBB, WPW syndrome type A)
   - Early aortic closure (MR)
2. *Wide and variable split S_2*
   - Pulmonary stenosis
   - Mitral regurgitation
   - VSD
   - Partial anomalous pulmonary venous connection with intact atrial septum
3. *Narrowly split S_2*
   - Pulmonary hypertension
   - Aortic stenosis
4. *Single S_2*
   - Pulmonary hypertension
   - One semilunar valve (PA, AA, PTA)
   - P_2 not audible (TGA, TOF, severe PS)
   - Severe aortic stenosis
5. *Paradoxically split S_2 (delayed aortic closure or early pulmonary closure)*
   - Severe aortic stenosis
   - Left bundle branch block (WPW syndrome)
   - PDA and post-stenotic dilatation of aorta
   - Severe systemic hypertension
   - Aortic regurgitation

Abnormal intensity of P_2
- Increased P_2 (pulmonary hypertension)
- Decreased P_2 (severe PS or pulmonary atresia, TOF, tricuspid stenosis)

ASD: atrial septal defect; TAPVR: total anomalous pulmonary venous return, PS: pulmonary stenosis, RBBB: right bundle branch block, LBBB: left bundle branch block, VSD: ventricular septal defect, MR: mitral regurgitation, PA: pulmonary atresia, AA: aortic atresia, PTA: persistent truncus arteriosus, TGA: transposition of great arteries, TOF: tetralogy of Fallot.

When split is heard both during inspiration and expiration, it is called a wide split. It is designated as a wide and variable split when the degree of splitting varies in inspiration and expiration; and a wide fixed split when it does not vary during inspiration and expiration. In reversed or paradoxical split, P_2 occurs earlier than A_2 (Figure 13.12). The opening of normal cardiac valves do not produce any sound but when they are diseased they may produce ejection clicks. The *opening snap* is a high frequency sound heard in diastole immediately after the second heart sound and is indicative of a stenotic mitral valve with a pliable and mobile anterior leaflet. It is best heard in expiration at the fourth intercostal space over the left lower sternal border.

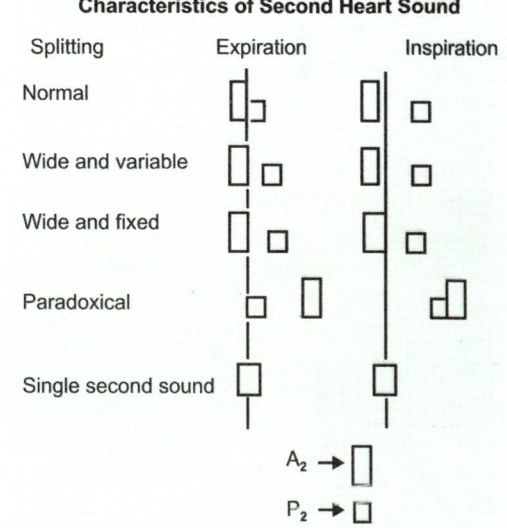

Figure 13.12 Splitting of the second heart sound (S_2). Normally S_2 is single in expiration and split in inspiration due to slightly early A_2 and delayed P_2. Wide and variable S_2 means that the split can be made out during expiratory phase of respiration and during inspiration the A_2 and P_2 interval increases further. Wide and fixed split S_2 means that the A_2 and P_2 interval increases further. In widely and fixed split S_2, both components can be made out during the expiratory phase of respiration, but during inspiration the A_2–P_2 interval becomes less or only single S_2 is heard due to normal inspiratory delay in P_2. The single second sound represents either A_2 (Fallot's physiology) or P_2 (aortic atresia) or a combination of both (Eisenmenger VSD).

Look for intensity of heart sounds, whether relative and absolute, splitting (fixed or variable), 3rd heart sound (triple or gallop rhythm due to rapid filling of ventricles during early diastole), opening snap (snappy sound inside the apex that closely follows the second heart sound due to opening of stiff mitral valve), and ejection or systolic click due to opening of diseased pulmonary and aortic valves (Figure 13.13). Fourth heart sound which represents atrial contraction may be heard in patients with severe pulmonic stenosis, pulmonary hypertension and Ebstein disease. It is a low-pitched sound occurring before S_1 and rarely heard in children. Third and fourth heart sounds are best heard when the patient is turned to the left side and auscultation is done with the bell of the stethoscope. The heart sounds and murmurs should be diagrammatically charted as shown in Figure 13.14. The significance and mechanism of production of abnormal and extra heart sounds is shown in Table 13.8.

Cardiac murmurs They are produced due to turbulence of the blood flow at or near a valve or because of an abnormal communication within the heart. Site of maximum intensity, grade (1–6/6), timing (systolic, diastolic or continuous), character and quality (ejection, holosystolic or pansystolic, decrescendo or crescendo and continuous type) and radiation or conduction should be carefully evaluated (*Box 13.3*). The murmurs are timed in relation to first and second heart sounds and by

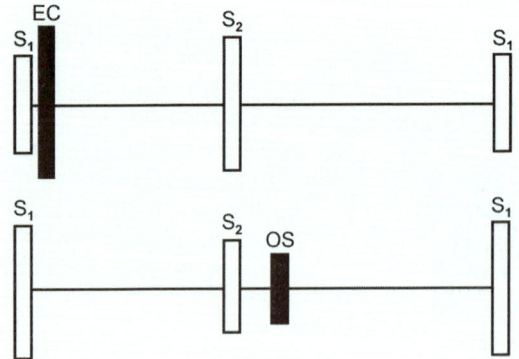

Figure 13.13 Diagram showing temporal relationship between ejection click (EC) and diastolic opening snap (OS) to heart sounds.

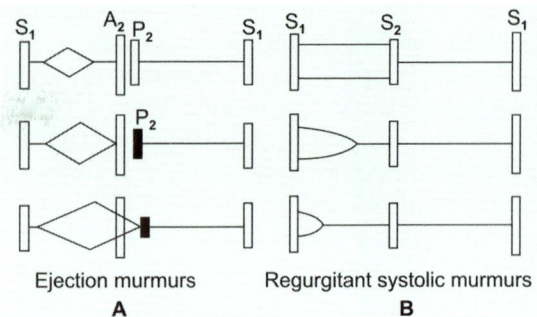

Figure 13.14A and B Diagram showing ejection and regurgitant systolic murmurs. (A) Ejection type systolic murmurs appear after S_1. They are diamond shaped in character with apex of diamond in the early phase of systole in mild stenosis of the semilunar valves (top). With increasing severity of obstruction to flow of blood, the murmur becomes longer and apex of diamond moves towards S_2 (middle). In severe pulmonary stenosis, the murmur may go beyond the A_2 (bottom). (B) Regurgitant systolic murmurs invariably start immediately after S_1 which may be drowned in the murmur and when holosystolic in character they are heard throughout systole all the way up to S_2 (top).

> **Box 13.3 Conduction or radiation of cardiac murmurs**
>
> - Localized murmurs: Mitral stenosis, pulmonary and tricuspid valve lesions
> - Mitral regurgitation: Left axilla and left infrascapular area
> - Aortic stenosis: Carotid arteries and apex
> - Patent ductus arteriosus and pulmonary stenosis: Back
> - Ventricular septal defect: Right sternal edge

simultaneous palpation of apex beat or carotid artery (Figure 13.15). Some murmurs are best heard in certain postures and phases of breathing. Murmurs originating from the right side of the heart increase in intensity during inspiration owing to increase in stroke output of the right ventricle. Conversly murmurs arising from the left side are accentuated during expiration. All murmurs increase in intensity with forceful maneuvers, like hand grip except mitral valve prolapse and idiopathic hypertrophic subaortic stenosis. Positions and maneuvers for best elicitation of certain murmurs are given below.

TABLE 13.8 Significance and mechanism of production of abnormal heart sounds

Timing/sound	Abnormal sound	Features and location	Mechanism	Significance
S_1	Loud	Best heard at the apex	Sudden closure of mitral valve	Mitral stenosis. It is also loud due to nervousness, thyrotoxicosis and exercise
Systole	Ejection click	It is a sharp sound that appears immediately after S_1 and is best heard at the base	Delayed opening of semilunar valves	Aortic or pulmonary stenosis with mobile valves
	Midsystolic click	It is late in onset and best heard at the mitral valve area	Mitral valve prolapse into atrium	Congenital anomaly of the valve in young girls
S_2	Loud	Best heard at the base	Abrupt closure of semilunar valves	Systemic or pulmonary arterial hypertension
	Split	Best heard at the base	Asynchronous closure of aortic and pulmonary valves	Physiological. Refer to Table 13.7 for significance of abnormal S_2
Diastole	Opening snap	Sharp sound appears before first heart sound and is best heard in expiration at the apex	Sudden opening of an abnormal mitral valve	Mitral stenosis with a mobile valve
	3rd heart sound*	Occurs shortly after S_2 and is best heard at the left parasternal region or at the apex	Diastolic distension of diseased myocardium	May be heard in normal children and young adults. Commonly seen due to right or left heart failure
	4th heart sound*	Occurs before S_1 and is best heard in the left parasternal region	Forceful atrial contraction against raised ventricular pressure	Left or right ventricular failure or hypertrophy

*Gallop rhythm: Rapid heart beats with summation of 3rd and 4th heart sounds giving a semblance of a galloping horse.

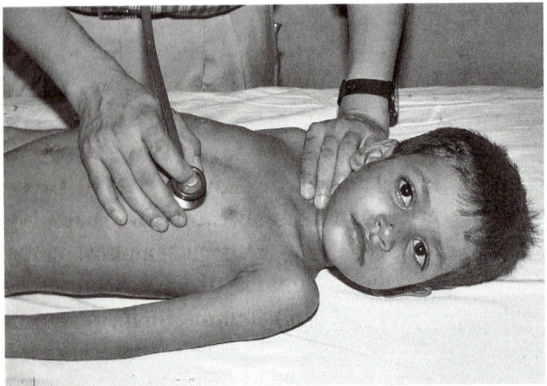

Figure 13.15 Timing of a murmur by simultaneous palpation of carotid artery while auscultating the heart.

Mitral stenosis. Left lateral position (bell of stethoscope).

Aortic regurgitation. Child sitting, leaning forward, and during expiration (diaphragm or chestpiece of stethoscope).

Tricuspid regurgitation. End of deep inspiration.

The intensity of murmur is conventionally graded from I to VI. Grade I: Barely audible; Grade II: Soft but easily audible; Grade III: Loud but not accompanied by thrill; Grade IV: Louder and associated with thrill; Grade V: Audible with stethoscope barely touching the chest; Grade VI: Audible with stethoscope off the chest or naked ear *(Box 13.4)*.

Box 13.4 Grading of murmur*	
Grade I	Soft, audible to an experienced cardiologist
Grade II	Soft but clearly audible
Grade III	Easily audible murmur without any thrill
Grade IV	Loud murmur associated with a thrill
Grade V	Very loud murmur, audible even when diaphragm of stethoscope is barely touching the chest
Grade VI	Audible directly by naked ear or diaphragm lifted off the chest

*The intensity of murmur may not suggest the severity of underlying heart disease. For example, a small VSD may produce a loud flow murmur while a large aortic regurgitation may produce inaudible flow murmur. A neonate with complex congenital cardiac malformation may die without manifesting any significant cardiac murmur. No murmur is usually audible in patients with transposition of the great arteries, double outlet right ventricle, cardiomyopathy and arrhythmias.

The presence of a continuous murmur in an acyanotic patient is a recognized feature of patent ductus arteriosus, rupture of sinus of Valsalva fistula into the right atrium or ventricle, systemic AV fistula, coarctation of aorta, peripheral pulmonary stenosis, aortopulmonary septal defect, anomalous left coronary artery from pulmonary artery, mitral stenosis with small atrial septal defect and venous hum. The continuous murmur must be differentiated from pericardial friction rub. The characteristics of cardiac murmurs are summarized in *Box 13.5*. In prosthetic valves, the opening and closing sounds are louder with a clicking or metallic quality. They may be associated with a midsystolic murmur but presence of a diastolic murmur in association with a prosthetic valve suggests a leak.

Venous hum It may be present in 40–50% of children below the age of 5 years. It is a faint

Box 13.5 Characteristics of the murmur
▪ *Timing*: Systolic, diastolic or continuous
▪ *Character*: Blowing, rumbling, rough and rasping, ejection systolic or "diamond" shaped
▪ *Intensity*: Grade I–VI
▪ *Conduction or selective propagation*: See the *Box 13.3*
▪ *Change with breathing*: Right heart murmurs increase with deep inspiration (tricuspid regurgitation) while left heart murmurs decrease with inspiration.
▪ *Valsalva maneuver**: The murmurs of mitral valve prolapse and hypertrophic obstructive cardiomyopathy increase in intensity
▪ *Change with position*: Most murmurs diminish in intensity on sitting or standing except murmurs of mitral valve prolapse, hypertrophic obstructive cardiomyopathy, aortic regurgitation and soft systolic murmur of acute rheumatic fever
▪ *Exercise*: Most murmurs increase in intensity after exercise except murmur due to hypertrophic obstructive cardiomyopathy and innocent murmurs
▪ *Effect of systemic arterial resistance*: When peripheral vascular resistance is increased by applying blood pressure cuff on both upper arms and inflating it beyond systolic pressure, it increases the intensity of murmurs due to mitral regurgitation, aortic regurgitation and ventricular septal defect

Valsalva maneuver: Ask the child to blow or strain against closed glottis (as if trying to pass a constipated stool) so that intrathoracic pressure goes up

continuous hum best heard at the first or second right interspaces adjacent to the sternum. The hum disappears when neck vessels are obliterated by applying finger pressure just above the medial end of right clavicle.

Pericardial rub It is a leathery to-and-fro, superficial creaky sound, variable in intensity, and heard in both phases of cardiac contraction. It is altered or aggravated when chest piece of stethoscope is more snugly pressed. It is best heard at the base of the heart or inside the apex especially when the patient leans forwards.

DIAGNOSTIC CLINICAL SIGNS OF COMMON CARDIAC CONDITIONS

Mitral Stenosis

Feeble pulse, left parasternal heave, tapping apex, palpable S_2, diastolic thrill, lound S_1 in mitral area, opening snap (occurring shortly after the second heart sound), mid-diastolic rough and rumbling murmur with presystolic accentuation are characteristic clinical findings. Absence of late diastolic accentuation of murmur goes against the diagnosis of significant mitral stenosis. The presystolic component disappears during auricular fibrillation. A loud first heart sound and opening snap indicates presence of a relatively pliable non-calcified valve. The closeness of the opening snap to the second heart sound and duration of diastolic murmur are useful indicators of the severity of mitral stenosis. A short mid-diastolic rumble (Carey-Coomb murmur) due to mitral valvulitis may be heard in patients with acute rheumatic carditis without any established mitral stenosis.

Mitral Regurgitation

Pulse is good volume with wide pulse pressure. Heaving and hyperkinetic apex, systolic thrill in mitral area, muffled or inaudible S_1, with high-pitched pansystolic murmur (murmur starts immediately after the first heart sound and continues up to and through the second heart sound) which is conducted towards the axilla and back. In most cases of mitral regurgitation, a third heart sound is audible at the apex and indicates early rapid filling of the left ventricle.

Mitral Valve Prolapse

It is usually asymptomatic in children and characterized by an apical mid-systolic click, a high frequency usually loud intensity sound with a scratchy quality which is best heard in a sitting or standing position. There may be a mid-late Grade II systolic murmur with a whistling character. The abnormality is commonly seen in young girls who may complain of palpitations. The prevalence of mitral valve prolapse is increased in patients with Duchenne muscular dystrophy, osteogenesis imperfecta, Ehlers-Danlos syndrome, Marfan syndrome, von Willebrand disease, fragile X syndrome and anorexia nervosa.

Tricuspid Regurgitation

Prominent venous pulsations (giant 'v' waves followed by a large 'y' descent) in neck, pulsatile liver, high-pitched pansystolic murmur at lower end of sternum accentuated by deep inspiration are characteristic features. Functional tricuspid regurgitation due to right ventricular failure is associated with third heart sound. It is usually associated with signs of pulmonary hypertension and mitral valve disease.

Aortic Regurgitation

There are features of "aortic run off" like collapsing or water hammer pulse, wide pulse pressure, prominent arterial pulsations, prominent carotid pulsations (Corrigan's sign), pistol shot sounds, forceful heaving apex, decrescendo high-pitched, blowing and early diastolic murmur in the aortic area. In severe aortic regurgitation, nodding of head may occur with each systole (deMusset's sign) due to sudden filling of carotid vessels. The diastolic murmur is best heard with diaphragm of the stethoscope placed over the left upper parasternal area when patient sits up, leans forwards and breathes out. The increased flow of blood across the aortic valve may produce an ejection systolic murmur. The first heart sound is soft and aortic component of the second sound is delayed and accentuated. In severe aortic regurgitation, a low-pitched diastolic flow murmur called Austin-Flint murmur may be audible at the mitral area. This murmur originates from the anterior leaflet of the mitral valve due to the confluence of two streams of blood, i.e. antegrade flow from the left atrium and regurgitation stream from incompetent aortic valve. There is exaggeration of systolic pressure difference between brachial and femoral arteries (Hill's sign). When systolic pressure in the femoral artery is 40–60 mm Hg higher than upper limb pressure, it is indicative of moderate-severe aortic regurgitation.

Aortic Stenosis

Plateau or feeble pulse, narrow pulse pressure, heaving apex, systolic thrill over the aortic area conducted to neck vessels, delayed aortic component of S_2, a "diamond-shaped" ejection systolic murmur conducted to neck vessels are characteristic findings of aortic stenosis. Ejection click may be audible just after the first heart sound in valvular aortic stenosis. The S_2 may be single or paradoxically split and pulse pressure is extremely narrow. In severe aortic stenosis, S_3 and S_4 may be heard. Williams syndrome is characterized by peculiar "elfin facies", hypercalcemia, mental retardation and supravalvular aortic stenosis.

Atrial Septal Defect (ASD Secundum)

Parasternal heave, grade 2–3 ejection systolic murmur over 2nd and 3rd intercostal spaces, and fixed wide splitting of S_2, are diagnostic features of ASD secundum. The murmur is produced by increased flow of blood through the pulmonary valve and not due to left-to-right shunt. The murmur may be widely transmitted all over the chest and may be associated with a delayed diastolic murmur at the lower left sternal border. Cardiomegaly is mild and cardiac failure is rare. Marked cardiomegaly suggests existence of additional lesions, like mitral valve obstruction (Lutembacher syndrome) or mitral regurgitation (ostium primum defect or associated rheumatic mitral regurgitation).

Endocardial Cushion Defect (Ostium Primum Defect)

The defect in the atrial septum is located below the fossa ovalis and is associated with a cleft in the anterior leaflet of the mitral valve. In addition to the findings of ostium secundum listed above, there are additional clinical features suggestive of left ventricular hypertrophy, pansystolic murmur of mitral regurgitation and left axis deviation of more than – 30° on EKG. Congestive heart failure is common in children with common atrioventricular canal. Endocardial cushion defect is common in children with Down syndrome.

Ventricular Septal Defect

Wide pulse pressure, hyperdynamic precordium with forceful apex beat, systolic thrill over left sternal border, pansystolic murmur over left sternal region (3rd to 5th interspace), and masking of both heart sounds are usual clinical findings. S_2 may be split with accentuation of P_2. A third heart sound may be audible at the apex. A diastolic flow murmur in the mitral area may be heard in children with a large defect. Children with VSD become symptomatic around 6–10 weeks of age when pulmonary pressure becomes lowest.

Pulmonic Stenosis

Prominent 'a' waves in jugulars, parasternal heave, wide and variably split S_2, harsh grade 2–5/6 ejection systolic murmur, and systolic ejection click best heard during expiration, are recognized clinical features of pulmonary stenosis. The intensity and duration of the murmur and delay in the pulmonary component of S_2 are suggestive of severity of pulmonary stenosis.

Patent Ductus Arteriosus (PDA)

Collapsing pulse, heaving apex, systolic thrill below the left clavicle, machinery or rolling thunder harsh continuous systolo-diastolic murmur best heard over 2nd left intercostal space, and multiple clicks are recognized clinical findings of PDA. The first sound is accentuated and S_2 is narrowly or paradoxically split with a large left-to-right shunt.

Pulmonary arteriovenous fistulae, coronary arteriovenous anastomoses, aorticopulmonary fenestration and venous hum are also recognized to produce continuous murmurs. Diastolic murmur in the mitral area may appear due to a large blood flow across the mitral valve.

Tetralogy of Fallot

Fallot's tetralogy consists of pulmonary stenosis, ventricular septal defect, right ventricular hypertrophy and over-riding of aorta. Cyanosis, clubbing, anoxic spells, prominent 'a' waves in the jugular venous pulse, mild right ventricular hypertrophy, ejection systolic murmur over pulmonary area, single second heart sound (absent pulmonary component), and absence of congestive heart failure are suggestive of tetralogy of Fallot. Anoxic or cyanotic spells and squatting are common in children with TOF.

Eisenmenger's Syndrome (Eisenmenger Physiology or Tardive cyanosis)

It is characterized by long-standing left-to-right shunt (usually caused by ventricular or atrial septal defect) which leads to development of cyanosis because of pulmonary hypertension as a consequence of prolonged right-to-left shunt. Following advent of echocardiography and early diagnosis of congenital heart disease, the incidence of Eisenmenger's complex has decreased.

The common signs and symptoms include cyanosis, clubbing, bleeding diathesis, hemoptysis, fainting, cardiac failure and infective endocarditis. Apart from clinical features of the underlying cardiac defect, additional manifestations occur due to pulmonary arterial hypertension. There is parasternal impulse and palpable second heart sound over left parasternal region. The pulmonary component of S_2 is accentuated and louder than the aortic component. A constant pulmonary ejection click may be heard both during inspiration and expiration at the second left interspace. A functional pulmonary regurgitation murmur (Graham Steell murmur) may be present along the left sternal border. The prognosis of patients who develop Eisenmenger physiology is extremely grave.

Tricuspid Atresia

Cyanosis, anoxic spells, prominent 'a' waves in jugular veins, presystolic pulsations in the liver, apical impulse of left ventricular type, non-significant or absent cardiac murmur are usual clinical findings. It may be difficult to clinically differentiate these patients from tetralogy of Fallot.

Transposition of Great Vessels

Cyanosis with CHF since early infancy, right ventricular hypertrophy, loud and single S_2 with systolic ejection click, short systolic ejection murmur of pulmonary stenosis or systolic regurgitant murmur of VSD, or absence of murmur are recognized clinical features of transposition of great vessels.

Ebstein Anomaly

Cyanosis, clubbing, dominant 'v' waves in the neck, quiet precordium, left ventricular type apical impulse, normal or split S_1, tricuspid opening snap, triple or quadruple heart sounds (multiple sounds are audible), systolic thrill with mid- or pansystolic murmur at the left sternal border are suggestive of Ebstein's anomaly. There may be delayed short diastolic murmur at the tricuspid area. Both systolic and diastolic murmurs produced at the tricuspid valve may have a scratchy character not unlike a pericardial friction rub.

Coarctation of Aorta

The blood pressure proximal to the stricture, i.e. upper limbs is increased so that blood pressure in the arms is higher than the lower limbs. Femorals are feeble and delayed as compared to simultaneously felt radial or brachial pulsations. Upper arms are stronger and span may be longer than the height. Palms may appear pinker compared to the soles. Collateral vessels connecting the subclavian arteries and intercostal arteries may be seen or felt over the interscapular and infrascapular areas. Collaterals are palpable over the under surface of ribs on the back and along both the borders of scapulae. Precordial examination shows evidences of left ventricular hypertrophy, aortic ejection systolic murmur (due to associated congenital bicuspid aortic valve) and constant ejection click. Ejection systolic or continuous murmur may be audible over the back due to presence of collaterals or flow of blood through the narrow segment of aorta (Suzman sign).

Myocarditis

There is cardiomegaly, marked tachycardia, low-intensity heart sounds with gallop rhythm. At times, a "tic-tac" rhythm in which interval between the first and second heart sounds is equal to or even longer than diastole may be heard. Regurgitant murmur may be produced by gross enlargement of heart with dilatation of the valves. Dysrhythmias in the form of ventricular premature beats or conduction disturbances are common. Evidences of congestive heart failure are usually present.

Functional Cardiac and Extracardiac Murmurs

Transient, nonsignificant murmurs are common during newborn period due to postnatal delay in circulatory adaptation. The closure of ductus and foramen ovale may be delayed. Conversely infants with VSD may not have any murmur during neonatal period which may appear after 4 to 6 weeks of age when pulmonary vascular resistance falls leading to establishment of left-to-right shunt.

The *"functional"* or *"innocent murmurs"* are best heard at the base, are low-pitched and low in intensity, systolic in timing, unassociated with a thrill, often modified by posture of the patient and usually disappear following exercise *(Box 13.6)*. All innocent murmurs are accentuated by high-output states, like fever and anemia, and are associated with normal EKG and skiagram of chest. Anemic children with a cardiac murmur should be reexamined after correction of anemia before any pathologic significance is ascribed to the murmur. Functional murmurs may also occur in children with fever, scoliosis, kyphoscoliosis and pectus excavatum.

Venous hum is best audible at the right infraclavicular and supraclavicular areas as a continuous murmur (louder diastolic component) due to turbulence of blood in jugular system especially in children between 3 and 6 years of age. The murmur is best heard in upright position and disappears when child lies supine or by rotation of the neck. The murmur also disappears, if neck veins are occluded with a finger or by increasing pressure over the chestpiece of stethoscope. *Carotid bruit* may be heard as an early ejection systolic murmur over the carotid arteries. Unlike aortic stenosis, there is no ejection click and no thrill or murmur is heard over the aortic area. In children with coarctation of aorta, look for murmur over the back due to collaterals. Auscultation of skull, liver and lumbar regions is advocated in children with unexplained CHF and hypertension. A continuous or ejection systolic murmur may be audible due to arteriovenous fistula, angiomatous malformation and arterial stenosis.

The murmur is considered as pathological, if child has cyanosis and there are features suggestive of cardiac failure. The presence of heart disease can be suspected on the basis of Nadas criteria *(Box 13.7)*. The presence of one major or two minor criteria is suggestive of underlying heart disease.

Box 13.6 Characteristics of innocent murmurs

- Predisposing factors: Early age, fever, anemia, chest or spinal deformity
- Ejection systolic low-pitched murmur Grade II or less, best heard in upright position. No thrill is palpable.
- Murmur is modified and may disappear after exercise, change of position or rotation of head, occlusion of neck veins or by increasing pressure over the chestpiece of stethoscope
- No diastolic murmur
- S_2 normal
- Normal EKG and X-ray chest

Box 13.7 Nadas' criteria for presence of heart disease

Major	Minor
- Systolic murmur Grade III or more	- Systolic murmur less than Grade III
- Diastolic murmur	- Abnormal second heart sound
- Cyanosis	- Abnormal EKG
- Cardiac failure	- Abnormal X-ray chest
	- Abnormal blood pressure

	Scheme for Presentation
General physical examination	Comfortable, dyspneic (severity or grade), orthopneic, physical growth and development, facial dysmorphism, skeletal deformities, and malar flush. Pulse (rate, volume, rhythm, character, other peripheral pulses including volume and timing of femorals, sleeping pulse rate), temperature, respiratory rate, and blood pressure in both upper and lower limbs. Anemia, cyanosis, jaundice, lymphadenopathy, edema (pedal, facial, sacral), clubbing, splinter hemorrhages, Osler nodes, Janeway lesions, subcutaneous nodules, erythema marginatum, arthritis, chorea, evidences of congestive heart failure, bacterial endocarditis and rheumatic activity.
Inspection	Precordial bulge (costal or intercostal), pulsations over the precordium (normal, hyperdynamic or quiet), neck vessels, suprasternal area and epigastrium, collateral arteries and dilated veins, apex beat visible or not.
Palpation	Site and character of apex beat (normal, tapping, heaving), point of maximal impulse of cardiac contraction, palpable heart sounds, left parasternal heave, and thrills (site and timing in relation to cardiac cycle).
Percussion	Outline of cardiac borders, dullness beyond apex beat, dullness or impaired percussion note over the aortic area (aneurysm), manubrium sterni (mediastinal mass) and pulmonary area (pulmonary conus and pericardial effusion), shifting dullness over pulmonary area on sitting up (pericardial effusion).
Auscultation	Describe the findings in a systematic manner over all the cardiac areas: Mitral, tricuspid, 3rd and 4th left parasternal areas, pulmonary area, aortic area, neck vessels, sides and back of chest, and thyroid gland. Heart sounds, intensity, single or split, variable or fixed splitting of S_2, third heart sound, gallop rhythm, and fourth heart sound. Heart sounds produced by opening of the diseased valves, i.e. opening snap and ejection clicks. Cardiac murmurs: Site of maximum intensity, grade, timing (systolic, diastolic or continuous), character (ejection, pansystolic, crescendo or decrescendo) and conduction or radiation. Describe any functional cardiac and extracardiac murmurs including pericardial and pleuropericardial rubs.

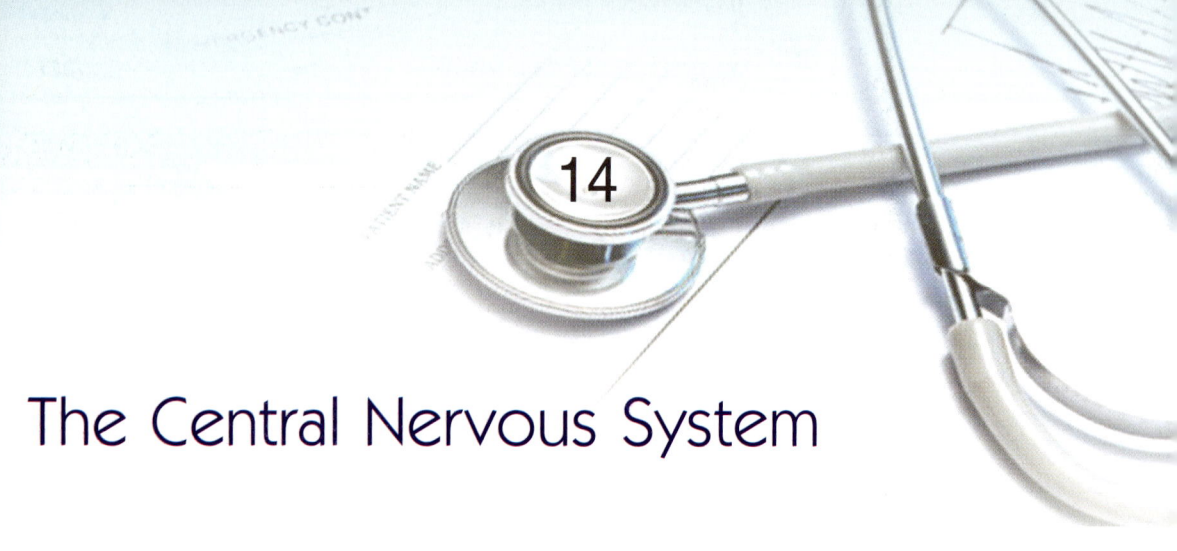

14

The Central Nervous System

The examination and evaluation of the nervous system in children is a daunting task. Some ingenuity, use of special tricks and adoption of non-structured "play attitude" are mandatory to elicit their cooperation and identify various CNS abnormalities. Like other body organs, the central nervous system in children is a dynamic, developing and maturing system. Newborn baby has brain weight of about 70% of an adult, while his body weight is only 5% of an average adult weight. Almost 15% brain growth occurs during the first year of life and about 10% during the remaining preschool years. Developmental disorders due to hypoxia, congenital anomalies and inborn errors of metabolism are by and large limited to children. The possibility of the neurological symptoms being due to a systemic or a metabolic disease rather than CNS disease, is more likely in children than adults.

ANATOMY

The nervous system consists of the brain and spinal cord (central nervous system) and peripheral nerves (peripheral nervous system). The neuron has a cell body and axon which terminates at a synapse and constitutes the functioning unit of the nervous system. Astrocytes provide the structural framework for the neurons and control their biochemical environment and provide the blood–brain barrier. The brain consists of two cerebral hemispheres, each with six functionally specialized lobes (frontal, parietal, temporal, occipital, insula and limbic), the brainstem and cerebellum. The cortical functions of various lobes are listed in Table 14.1. The brainstem consisting of the midbrain, pons and medulla oblongata, contains the nuclei of cranial nerves and all the sensory and motor pathways entering and leaving the cerebral hemispheres. The cerebellum, which lies below the cerebral hemispheres and posterior to the brainstem, is responsible for coordination, posture and steady gait. The brain is covered by three membranes, the outermost dura mater, middle arachnoid and innermost pia mater. The subarachnoid space between the arachnoid and pia is filled with cerebrospinal fluid.

The spinal cord contains afferent and efferent fibers, which are arranged in functionally discrete bundles, are responsible for motor reflexes, sensory information for touch, temperature, pain and proprioception. Peripheral nerves are made up of large myelinated axons and smaller slower unmyelinated axons. The sensory cell bodies of peripheral nerves are situated in the dorsal root ganglia while the motor cell bodies are located in the anterior horn cells of the spinal cord.

HISTORY

Ask for presenting complaints. Identify the precise timing and onset of the neurological disease, whether acute, subacute or insidious. Record the evolution or progression of the disease process. Assess whether the disease is stationary,

TABLE 14.1 Cortical functions of various lobes of the brain*

Areas	Functions
Frontal lobe	Cognition, personality, social behavior, emotional responsiveness, voluntary movements, expressive (Broca's area) speech, sphincters, and primitive reflexes
Parietal lobe	Cortical sensations, language development, spatial awareness, and visual perception (upper fibers of optic radiation)
Temporal lobe	Memory, perception of smell, hearing, vision (lower fibers of optic radiation) and speech (Wernicke's area)
Occipital lobe	Processing and analysis of visual stimuli
Limbic lobe	The limbic system comprises of amygdala, hippocampus, thalamus, hypothalamus, basal ganglia and cingulate gyrus. They control motivation, emotions, learning, memory, behavior, habits and homeostasis
Insular lobe	Consciousness, emotions, perception, self-awareness, cognition and social interactions

* The left and right hemispheres are credited to have different functions and attributes. The left hemisphere (dominant hemisphere) is endowed with masculine characteristics, like cognition, logic, reasoning, analytical skills, language, communication skills, public speaking, mathematical skills, etc. The right hemisphere is credited with feminine or artistic characteristics, like painting, music, dance, poetry, peace, poise, insight, extrasensory perception or intuition, creativity, spirituality, etc. We are all provided with mixed characteristics of both right and left hemispheres in various combinations.

progressive or improving. Ask in detail the developmental status of the child before the onset of the disease. Preceding or concurrent history of fever and its severity should be asked. History of perinatal distress factors and abnormalities, head injury and immunizations before the onset of CNS manifestations should be recorded.

Ask for any history of medications and accidental or suicidal poisoning in a comatosed child. Headache, neck and/or spinal stiffness and photophobia are suggestive of meningeal irritation. Ask for symptoms suggestive of raised intracranial tension, such as headache especially on rising up in the morning, vomiting without preceding nausea, enlargement of head size, and diplopia. Excessive and unexplained high-pitched crying may be the sole symptom of raised intracranial tension (ICT) in infants. Rarely, raised intracranial pressure may cause stretching and compression of intracranial component of vagus nerve leading to development of stridor due to bilateral vocal cord paralysis. The salient components of history are summarized in *Box 14.1*.

Ask for history of syncope or fainting. There is temporary and sudden loss of consciousness and postural tone due to hypotension and cerebral hypoperfusion. The episode is brief in duration

> **Box 14.1 The key points on history**
> - Presenting symptoms
> - Onset: Sudden, subacute, insidious
> - Fever: Preceding or concurrent and its severity
> - Neuromotor development before the onset of CNS disease
> - Evolution: Is condition improving, stationary, slowly progressive or rapidly progressive?
> - Are there any symptoms suggestive of raised intracranial tension and meningeal irritation?
> - Syncope, seizures and their morphology
> - Is there any involvement of special senses and sphincters?
> - Mental status: Alert, irritable, lack of interest, drowsy, stuporose or comatosed
> - Family history of similar disease, epilepsy, tuberculosis, inborn error of metabolism, and consanguinity
> - Etiologic history: Birth weight, gestation, perinatal events, trauma, hypoxic ischemic encephalopathy, hypoglycemia, bleeding, severe jaundice, drugs and toxins, infection or post-infectious degenerative or demyelinating disorder, genetic or metabolic and chromosomal disorder

lasting for 1–2 min. The common correlates include prolonged standing, sudden rising from sitting or lying position, anxiety, emotional stress and acute pain (intramuscular injection in an adolescent girl). Syncope is most commonly due to vasovagal attack

TABLE 14.2 Characteristic features of common conditions mimicking seizures

Condition	Salient features
Syncope	Episode is invoked by Valsalva maneuver, sudden rising from sitting or lying position and acute pain, anxiety and emotional stress especially in adolescent children. The attack may occur because of cardiac arrhythmia. There is transitory loss of consciousness for 1–2 min, pallor, dizziness, bradycardia, cold clammy extremities, and tunneling of vision. A brief period (up to 10 s) of convulsive motor activity may occur when subject remains upright. Headache may occur soon after the syncope.
Psychogenic seizures	The behavior is usually a part of conversion reaction, which occurs in a dramatic way when patient is being watched. There may be side-to-side turning of head, large amplitude shaking movements of limbs, pelvic thrusting, screaming, groaning, moaning, gesturing, and so on. There is no injury or loss of conciousness. The abnormal behavior gradually abates when patient is left alone.
Migraine	There may be visual or auditory aura or photophobia followed by unilateral headache. It may be associated with recurrent abdominal pain and cyclical vomiting, light headedness, scalp tenderness, vertigo, and at times alteration of consciousness may occur. Rarely syncope, seizure and confusional state may occur.
Tics	They are stereotyped, awkward, and repetitive movements of a particular part of the body. The common examples of tics are shrugging of shoulders, blinking of eyes, twisting of neck, or attempts at coughing. They usually occur between 8 and 10 years of age and are more common when a child is tense and anxious.
Breath-holding spells	Breath-holding spells usually occur in children between 6 months and 3 years of age. The child gets angry and throws a temper tantrum or gets hurt, and cries loudly. After a long uninterrupted cry, the child holds his breath in expiration. The child may become blue and rarely the attack may lead to a seizure. After the spell, the child may start crying again and start asking for the same demand that triggered the attack.
Narcolepsy	There is excessive, uncontrollable, daytime episodes of sleep with disturbed night sleep. There may be sudden weakness or loss of muscle tone (cataplexy). At the onset of sleep, there may be vivid hallucinations or feeling of muscle paralysis.
Drug abuse	Intake of psychoactive drugs may be associated with hallucinations and schizophrenia-like reactions.

or autonomic in origin. It may occur due to cardiac causes like tachyarrhythmias, orthostatic hypotension, and ventricular outflow obstruction (severe aortic stenosis, Eisenmenger complex). The miscellaneous causes of syncope include migraine, panic attack, dehydration, hypoglycemia or hysteria.

Enquire details about any seizures, i.e. onset, type, preceding aura, seizure morphology, postseizure phenomenon, frequency of fits, and response to previous treatment. Several disorders may be confused with seizures and should be excluded (Table 14.2). Ask about any disturbances referable to special senses and sphincters. Family history of similar disease, tuberculosis and epilepsy should be enquired. History of consanguinity among parents should be asked.

GENERAL PHYSICAL EXAMINATION

The 'containers' of CNS, i.e. skull and spine should be examined in detail. Look for size, shape, symmetry, swellings, sutures and fontanels of skull. Marked prominence of occiput may signify Dandy-Walker syndrome. In craniosynostosis, there is ridging of sutures. The skull becomes odd-shaped because of cessation of growth of the skull bones at right angle to the prematurely fused sutures. Macewen's sign (cracked pot sound on percussion of skull) should be looked for. It is physiological during early infancy because sutures are open. The bulging of anterior fontanel and prominence of scalp veins are suggestive of raised intracranial pressure. Auscultation and transillumination of skull is useful in selected cases. Auscultate the skull by using the bell of the stethoscope for any intracranial bruits. Transillumination of skull lights up the entire calvarium in hydranencephaly while in Dandy-Walker malformation, the occiput is prominent and transilluminant because of posterior fossa cyst. Look for any operative scars on the spine due to repair of meningomyelocele or over the scalp for placement of ventriculoperitoneal shunt. Face should be examined for any dysmorphism and characteristic facies suggestive of developmental, chromosomal and metabolic disorders. Obesity, sleep disturbances and features of diabetes insipidus are suggestive of hypothalamic disorder.

The skin should be examined for any evidences of neuroectodermal dysplasia, e.g. adenoma sebaceum, strawberry mark on the face, telangiectasia of bulbar conjunctiva or vascular malformation of the retina, café au lait spots, shagreen or ash-leaf spots, etc. (Figures 14.1 to 14.3). Skin rash and petechiae should be looked for. Teeth should be examined for brownish discoloration, blue-line over the gums and Hutchison's teeth. Eyes should be examined for proptosis, corneal opacities, buphthalmos, Kayser-Fleischer ring (golden-green discoloration in the form of crescent in the inner layer of peripheral cornea just inside the limbus), and cataracts.

Record temperature, pulse, respiration and blood pressure. Look for Cushing's response to raised intracranial tension, i.e. bradycardia, elevation of blood pressure and abnormalities in the respiratory pattern.

Trousseau's sign (carpopedal spasms) and nerve irritability (Chvostek's sign) should be looked for in a child with history of tetanic spasms. In Chvostek sign, tapping of facial nerve just anterior to the tragus, results in contraction of the facial muscles with blinking of eyelids and twitching of corner of the mouth. Although a useful sign of tetany, it may be present in normal newborn babies. Carpopedal spasms or Trousseau's sign can be elicited by occlusion of the blood vessels of upper arm with a sphygmomanometer cuff. The cuff is inflated beyond the systolic blood pressure and held

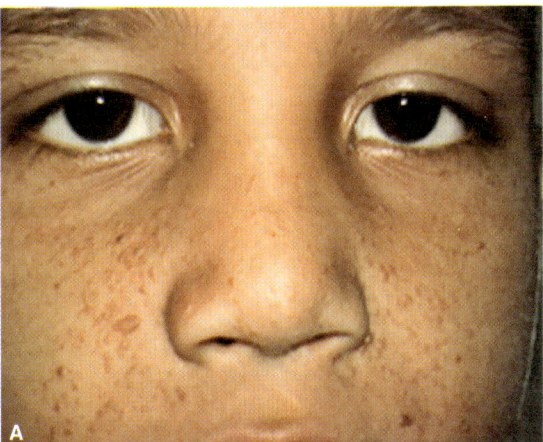 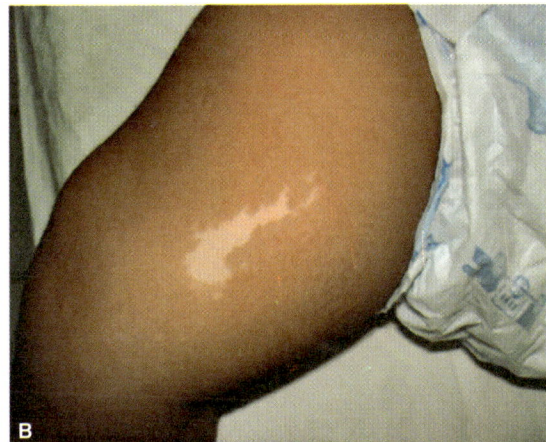

Figure 14.1A and B (A) Typical flesh-colored papulonodular skin lesions of adenoma sebaceum on the cheeks, nose and forehead. (B) Ash-leaf depigmented macule over the thigh. The patient had classical triad of tuberous sclerosis, i.e. epilepsy, adenoma sebaceum and intracranial calcification.

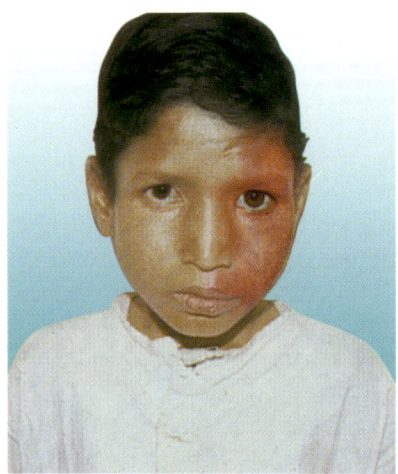

Figure 14.2 Sturge-Weber syndrome. The patient had nevus flammeus on left cheek, typical intracranial calcification ("railroad-track" type) and partial simple seizures on the right side.

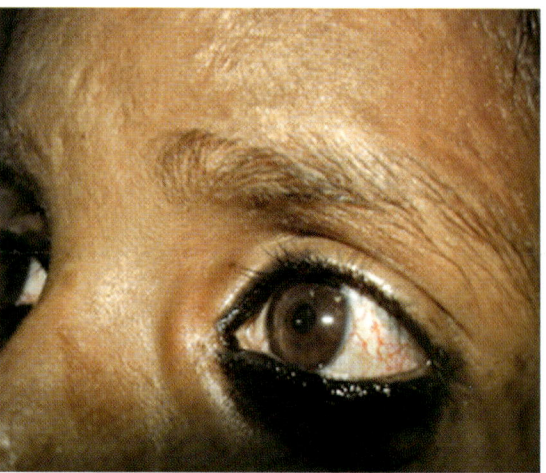

Figure 14.3 Characteristic conjunctival telangiectasia in a child with ataxia telangiectasia.

in place for 3 minutes. The peroneal sign is elicited by tapping the peroneal nerve over the head of the fibula. The sign consists of dorsiflexion and eversion of the foot.

Look for anemia, cyanosis, jaundice, lymphadenopathy, hepatosplenomegaly and abdominal mass. Spine should be examined for any evidences of developmental defects (platybasia, Klippel-Feil deformity, meningocele, pilonidal sinus, tuft of hair, etc.), trauma, Pott's disease, epidural abscess, primary neoplasm or metastatic deposits (Figure 14.4A and B). Sinus tract over the region

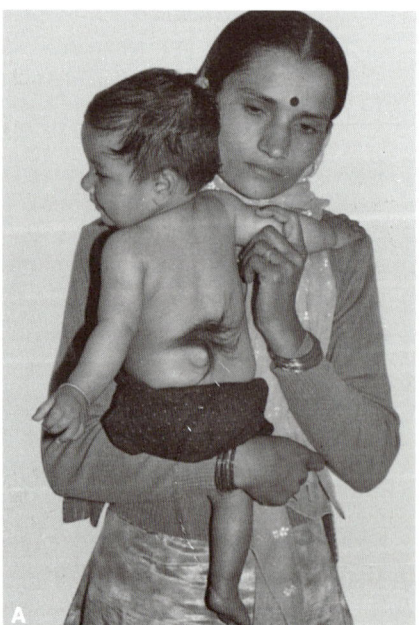 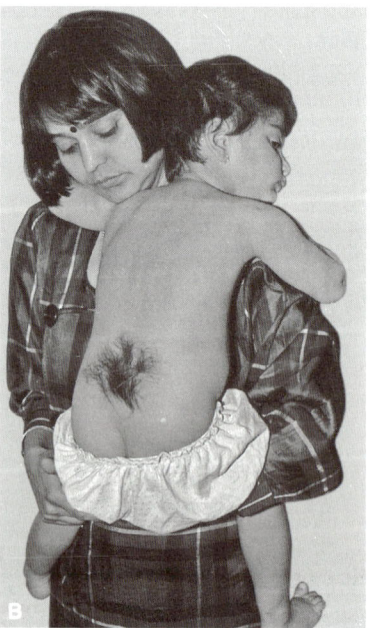

Figure 14.4A and B (A) Hairy nevus on the back with spina bifida occulta. (B) Hairy nevus over the sacrum with diastemetomyelia.

> **Box 14.2 Key points on general physical examination**
>
> - Handedness of the child
> - General appearance, posture, nature of disability, build and nutrition, and anthropometry
> - Skull and spine: Size, shape, sutures, fontanels, Macewen's sign, auscultation, transillumination, and spinal deformities
> - Facial dysmorphism, abnormalities of eyes, ears, nose oral cavity, teeth, and evidences of neuroectodermal dysplasia
> - Anemia, cyanosis, jaundice, hepatosplenomegaly, and abdominal mass
> - Vital signs including Trousseau's sign
> - Evidences of meningeal irritation: Neck rigidity, Kernig's sign, Brudzunski's sign, tripod sign, and photophobia
> - Evidences of raised intracranial pressure: Cushing's response, i.e. bradycardia, elevation of blood pressure and abnormalities in respiratory pattern. Evidences of herniation of hippocampus, i.e. unilateral dilated and fixed pupil, paralysis of upward gaze with involvement of vital centers in brainstem, Macewen's sign and papilledema

> **Box 14.3 Key points on CNS examination**
>
> - Higher mental functions: Level of consciousness, orientation in time and place, memory, emotional status, and speech
> - Developmental screening and handedness of the child
> - Cranial nerves
> - Motor system: Posture, muscle bulk, tone, power, trophic changes, abnormal movements, coordination, deep tendon jerks, and gait
> - Sensory system
> - Superficial reflexes
> - Brainstem signs
> - Cerebellar signs
> - Sphincter disturbances
> - Autonomic dysfunction
> - Localization of the lesion

of dorsal spine and fracture of base of skull may be associated with recurrent pyogenic meningitis. Enquire whether child is right or left handed. The handedness is established around 3 years of age. Left handers have a diffuse representation of language function in the brain and their recovery from aphasia is better compared to right handers. If an infant below 2 years has a preference to use only one limb, it suggests weakness or paralysis of the other limb. The salient components of general physical examination are listed in *Box 14.2*.

EXAMINATION OF CENTRAL NERVOUS SYSTEM

Most pediatricians lack the confidence and are often frustrated while conducting neurological examination of young children. With tact, experience and patience, the neurological examination of an infant should not be an ordeal, rather it should be fun both for the examiner and the patient. Adopt an attitude of play activity in conformity with the age and developmental status of the child. Harness your ingenuity, imagination and tact effectively by literally coming down to the level of the child. Smiling at the infant and speaking in a soft and reassuring tone during the examination are highly effective to elicit cooperation. Attempt should be made to identify all neurological abnormalities, localize the probable site of lesion in CNS and identify the etiology and diagnosis of the disease process. The salient components of CNS examination are summarized in *Box 14.3*.

ESSENTIAL TOOLS

The pediatric neurologist should have colored toys/cubes, reflex hammer, temple bell, flash light with rubber adaptor, fiberglass tape measure, objects for testing stereognosis, tuning fork (128 Hz for vibration sense and 256 Hz for Rinne test), two-point discriminator (measuring divider), development kit, and ophthalmoscope.

HIGHER MENTAL FUNCTIONS

1. *Level of consciousness* The level of consciousness can be clinically classified into six stages: (a) Alert or fully consious, (b) Drowsy but gives response to verbal commands, (c) Semiconscious and gives withdrawal response to pain, (d) Unconscious with flexion of upper limbs and adduction of thumbs into palms and extension of lower limbs to pain (decorticate posture

TABLE 14.3 Coma scales

	Glasgow Coma Scale		Modified Glasgow Coma Scale for under-3 children	
Parameter		Score	*Parameter*	Score
Eye opening			**Eye opening**	
Spontaneous		4	Spontaneous	4
Responds to verbal stimuli		3	Responds to verbal stimuli	3
Responds to pain*		2	Responds to pain*	2
No response		1	No response	1
Best verbal response			**Best verbal response**	
Oriented		5	Coos, babbles, interacts, smiles and consolable	5
Confused		4	Irritable	4
Inappropriate words		3	Cries to pain	3
Incomprehensible sounds		2	Moans to pain	2
No response		1	No response	1
Best motor response			**Best motor response**	
Obeys commands		6	Normal spontaneous movements	6
Localizes pain		5	Withdraws limb on touch	5
Withdrawal of limb in response to pain		4	Withdrawal of limb to pain	4
Flexion response to pain (decorticate posturing)		3	Flexion response to pain (decorticate posturing)	3
Extension response to pain (decerebrate posturing)		2	Extension response to pain (decerebrate posturing)	2
No response		1	No response	1

*Pain is imparted either by a strong pinch, applying pressure on the finger nail with a pencil, squeezing big toe or applying pressure over the supratrochlear notch located on the medial end of upper margin of orbit.
Coma score of <12 suggests severe head injury, score of <8 suggests need for intubation and ventilation and a score of <6 suggests need for intracranial pressure monitoring.

with a lesion above the brainstem or basal nuclei), (e) Unconscious with hyperextension of upper and lower limbs, pronation of upper limbs and plantar flexion of feet (decerebrate rigidity due to lesion in the midbrain between the superior colliculus and pons), (f) Unconscious with no response. A quick and simple way to assess the level of consciousness is to use the **AVPU** scale where **A** stands for alert, **V** for response to voice, **P** for response to pain and **U** for unresponsive to any stimulus. Coma can be quantified by objective coma scales (Table 14.3).

In hysterical coma, the eyes are kept tightly closed and when attempts are made to open them by force, the child would promptly reclose them. The demonstration of nystagmus on cold caloric test (vestibulo-ocular reflex) is suggestive of hysterical or feigned coma. In children with extensive brain damage (due to anoxia, meningitis, encephalitis and near-drowning), coma may be followed by persistent vegetative state or minimally conscious state *(Box 14.4)*.

Box 14.4 States of consciousness

Persistent vegetative state (PVS)
- No awareness of self or environment.
- No sustained reproducible, purposeful or voluntary behavioral response to visual, auditory, tactile or noxious stimuli.
- No language comprehension or expression.
- Mostly intact cranial nerve reflexes.
- Roving nystagmoid eye movements.
- Presence of sleep and awake cycles, often eyes are open during the day.
- Stable unsupported blood pressure and intact respiratory drive.
- Bowel and bladder incontinence.

Minimally conscious state (MCS)
- Patient makes eye contact or turns head when being talked to.
- Almost emotionless state but with eye tracking movements.
- May speak a few words, and may fend off pain.
- Eyes follow a moving person or object.
- Some intelligible verbalization.
- May hold an object or use an object when asked.

The child is awake but gives a blank staring look with roving eye movements and without any response to social interactions. The child remains inattentive, does not speak or show any signs of awareness, pain or pleasure.

2. **Emotional status** Assess behavior, perception and emotional lability. Look for signs of hyperactivity, short span of attention, distractibility and impulsiveness. In children with a psychiatric disorder, mental status examination (MSE) is done to assess several domains of mental functioning. The various parameters include appearance, attitude, behavior, mood, affect, thought process, perception, cognition, insight and judgement.

3. **Memory and orientation** Assess orientation in time, place, person and memory of immediate, recent and past events in children above the age of 5 years. Ask name of the school and its location, names of teachers, father, friends and siblings, day of the week and time and ability to obey simple commands. Tell a brief story and ask the child to repeat. Ask the child to repeat a set of numbers forwards and backwards. A normal 6-year-old can repeat five digits forwards and count three digits backwards while a 10-year-old can count six digits forwards and four digits backwards.

4. **Delusions and hallucinations** Delusion is a false belief which the patient maintains for which there is no evidence. Hallucination is a false signal or impression from the organ of special senses.

5. **Speech** The cortical center for speech production is located in the Broca's area in the left frontal lobe in a right-handed person and vice versa. Other areas of brain concerned with comprehension and production of speech include Wernicke's area (temporal lobe), the tract of nerves (arcuate fasciculus) that connect Broca's and Wernicke's areas and angular gyrus. In all comatosed children, brainstem reflexes, such as pupillary response to light, corneal reflex, oculocephalic and oculovestibular reflexes must be assessed.

(i) *Aphonia or dysphonia* may occur due to paralysis of vocal cords (bulbar paralysis). In children with paralysis of respiratory muscles, the volume or intensity of speech is affected. The child can be asked to blow out a lighted candle from a distance of 5 cm or asked to count from one to hundred in one breath.

(ii) Disorders of cerebral hemisphere may produce sensory (Wernicke's area) or motor (Broca's area) aphasia. Aphasia may affect all modalities of language like speaking, writing, reading and listening because of brain damage. Developmental dyslexia is characterized by slowness in learning to read, mirror-image writing, reading from right to left, poor phonation and clumsy handwriting.

(iii) Disorders of articulation (dysarthria) may lead to several speech defects. Stammering, lalling or baby speech occurs due to psychogenic rather than neurologic causes, scanning or staccato speech (speaks slowly and deliberately in monosyllables as if scanning a line of poetry) and slurring speech when syllables are slurred as if in a state of intoxication, interspersed with explosive monotonous speech, is seen in cerebellar disorders. Spastic dysarthria is seen in children with cerebral palsy and is associated with brisk jaw jerk (pseudobulbar palsy). Bulbar dysarthria due to bulbar palsy (involvement of nuclei of 9th, 10th, 12th cranial nerves in the medulla oblongata which appears like a bulb) is characterized by slurring dysarthria, dysphagia with nasal regurgitation of feeds and accumulation of secretions in the throat.

(iv) Nasal speech occurs due to palatal paralysis or cleft palate. To test for articulation, ask the child to say "ka, pa, ta" first slowly and then as fast as he can. These three words can test the main components of articulation effectively because 'ka' is produced deep in the throat, the word 'pa' is produced by the lips and 'ta' is produced by the tongue and palate. The child with pervasive developmental disorder (autism spectrum disorder) has communication difficulties, like inability to understand the language of others, difficulty in understanding abstract thoughts, riddles and jokes, lack of social interactions or eye contact, gibberish repetitive (echolalic speech) and delayed development of speech or regression of speech.

6. *Automatic neonatal reflexes* The persistence of Moro reflex and palmar grasp beyond 4 to 5 months of age is pathological and indicative of neuromotor retardation.

7. *Doll's eye phenomenon (vestibulo-ocular reflex)* The infant is placed supine, the eyelids are kept open, and head is suddenly turned towards either side. In a comatosed child with intact brainstem, the child's eyes lag behind like a doll, i.e. there is conjugate deviation of the eyes towards the opposite side. The reflex is absent in a normal awake person. Absence of doll's eye phenomenon in a comatosed child is indicative of damage to brainstem due to increased intracranial pressure and transtentorial herniation. It may be associated with unilateral dilated fixed pupil. In a child with metabolic coma, the eyes may be immobile with absent oculocephalic response. The test should not be performed, if there is suspicion of injury to the cervical spine.

Signs of Meningeal Irritation

Look for photophobia, neck rigidity, Kernig's sign, Brudzinski's sign, and tripod sign (Figures 14.5 to 14.7). The signs of meningeal irritation may be absent in infants below 3 months and seriously sick or malnourished children. In a struggling infant, suspend the head beyond the edge of table and then test for neck rigidity. The older child may be asked to touch his chest with the chin without opening the mouth (Figure 14.8). Kernig's sign will be absent, if neck rigidity is due to local causes rather than meningeal irritation. The spinal meningeal irritation causes rigidity of back and child sits with a "poker spine" with extended legs and by

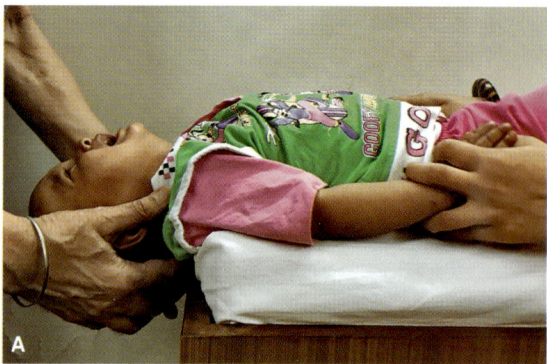
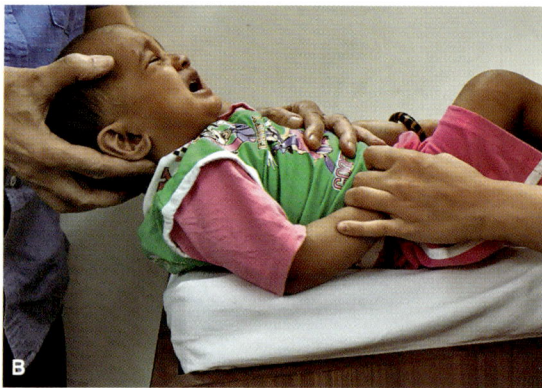

Figure 14.5A and B Examination for neck rigidity. (A) In a struggling infant, head is suspended beyond the edge of table. The infant is likely to relax his neck in this position. (B) The head is then flexed to look for neck rigidity.

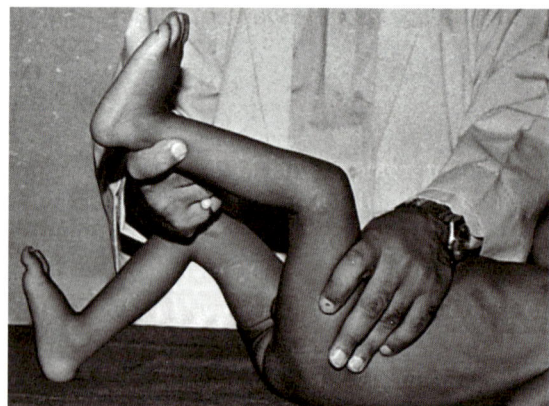

Figure 14.6 Kernig's sign. Hip is flexed to right angle and knee is kept at 90° angle. With the hand placed behind the ankle, examiner tries to extend the knee. Kernig's sign is positive, if there is pain and stiffness of hamstring muscles which limits extension of the knee joint.

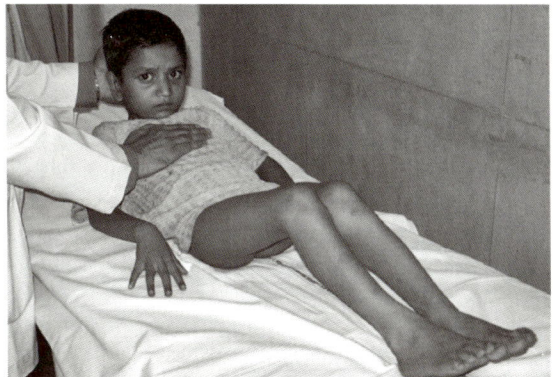

Figure 14.7 Brudzinski's sign. Flexion of neck is followed by flexion of both the lower limbs.

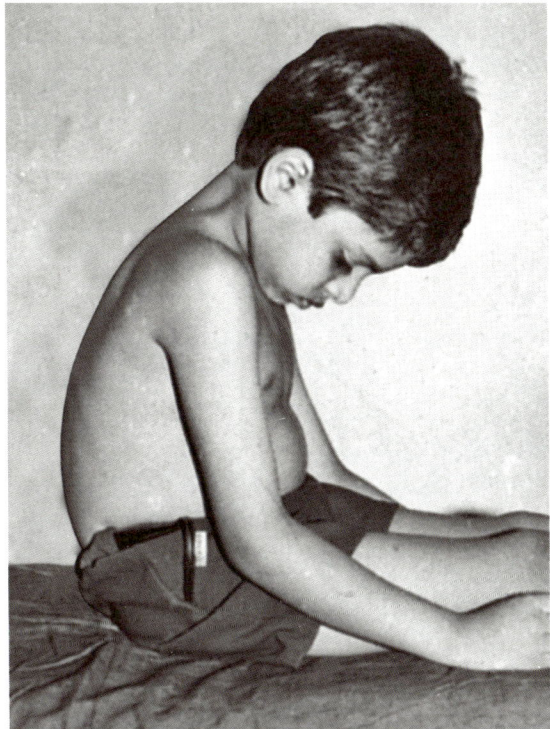

Figure 14.8 Examination for neck rigidity. Older child is asked to sit up and touch his chin to the front of chest without opening his mouth.

supporting the trunk on palms of both hands which are placed on the cot behind the trunk (tripod sign). The child is unable to "kiss the knee" while sitting. Infants with acute poliomyelitis may have positive tripod sign and head drop due to weakness of neck flexors. Refer to Chapter 8 for detailed list of conditions producing neck rigidity. Opisthotonos is characterized by marked neck rigidity with ventral arching of the whole trunk.

Developmental Screening

Developmental status should be assessed on the basis of detailed history and physical examination (refer to Chapter 6). Intelligence and school attainments should be checked in older children. The child may be asked to draw or imitate a circle (3 years), triangle (4 years), square or pyramid (5 years) or draw a man (3 years for drawing a circle and one year each for drawing different parts of the face). Look for evidences of attention deficit hyperactivity disorder (ADHD) in the form of hyperkinetic behavior, short attention span, easy distractibility, motor clumsiness and soft neurological signs.

CRANIAL NERVES

There are 12 pairs of cranial nerves, the optic nerve is really an extension of the brain rather than a peripheral nerve. The precise evaluation of cranial nerves may be difficult due to lack of cooperation in young children. It is useful to assess the cranial nerves in their numerical order, but there are exceptions where nerves are best grouped together and their numbers may not the sequential.

First (Olfactory) Nerve

Anatomy

The receptors of the olfactory nerve are situated deep in the nasal cavity. From these receptors, thin filaments pass centrally through the cribriform plate of the ethmoid to the olfactory bulbs, containing the second order of neurons. These neurons project via the olfactory tract to the ipsilateral medial temporal lobe and amygdala.

Testing

Ask for any defect in the smell and let the blindfolded child identify some common odorous materials, i.e. rose water, peppermint, orange, chocolates, coffee, *ilaichi*, etc. The child with common cold cannot be tested for sense of smell.

Avoid use of irritating substances, like ammonia and acetic acid which may be perceived through fifth nerve. It is difficult to assess the individual nostril separately. Anosmia in children may be seen following fracture of cribriform plate, meningitis, thrombosis of anterior cerebral artery, lead poisoning, hydrocephalus, Kallmann syndrome, Rud syndrome, immotile cilia syndrome and hysteria. When pleasant odors are perceived as unpleasant, it is called parosmia.

Second (Optic) Nerve

Anatomy

The fibers of optic nerve originate from the retina and reach optic chiasma. At this point, the fibers from the inner nasal half of each retina (representing the temporal field) decussate or crossover, while those from the temporal half (nasal field) of retina remain on the same side of optic tract. The optic tract passes through the lateral geniculate body to form optic radiation. The optic radiation starts from lateral geniculate body, goes backwards through the posterior limb of internal capsule to the calcarine cortex of the occipital lobe. In the occipital cortex around the calcarine fissure, the left half of the field of vision is represented in the cortex of right hemisphere and vice versa. The most peripheral part of the visual fields is represented anteriorly in the calcarine cortex and most medial or macular field is represented in the occipital pole (Figure 14.9).

Testing

The following functions of optic nerve should be tested:

(a) *Acuity of vision* In infants above 6 months, look for optokinetic nystagmus by rotating a striped drum infront of the eyes. The presence of opticokinetic reflex confirms integrity of cortical

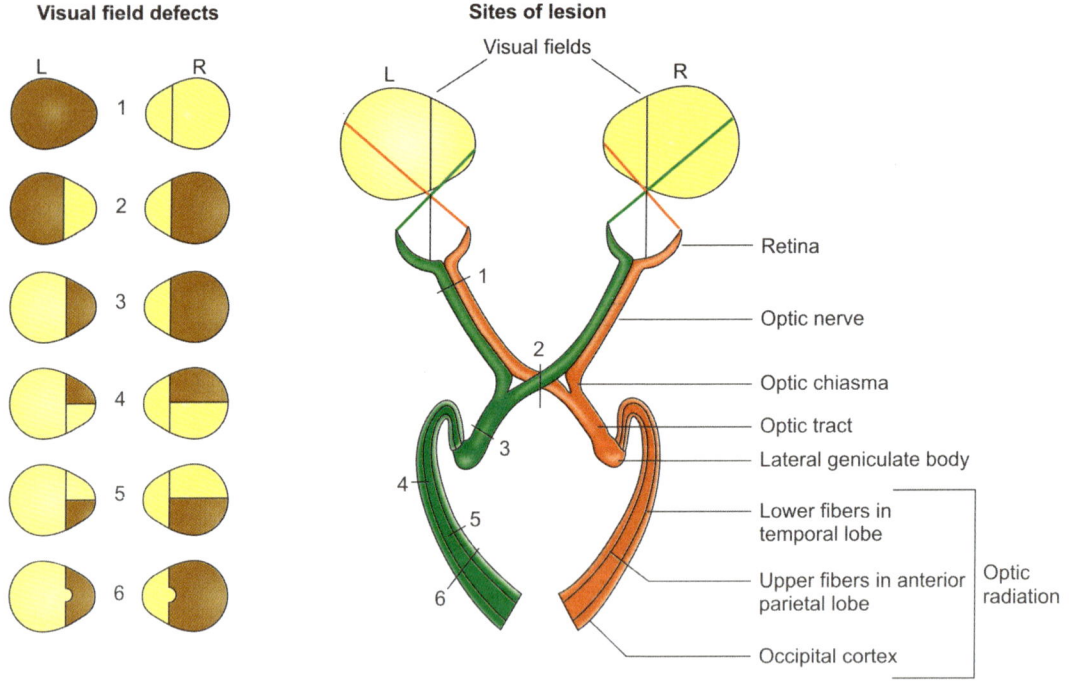

Figure 14.9 Visual field defects. (1) Total loss of vision in one eye because of a lesion of the optic nerve. (2) Bitemporal hemianopsia due to compression of optic chiasma. (3) Right homonymous hemianopsia as a result of a lesion of the optic tract. (4) Upper right quadrantanopsia from a lesion of the lower fibers of the optic radiation in the temporal lobe. (5) Lower quadrantanopsia from a lesion of the upper fibers of the optic radiation in the anterior part of the parietal lobe. (6) Right homonymous hemianopsia with sparing of the macula due to lesion of the optic radiation in the posterior part of the parietal lobe.

vision, while its absence is of no significance. In children above 3 years, vision can be screened by use of E chart or Snellen's picture charts. The Es in the chart have their limbs directed to different directions—up, down, right and left. Visual acuity (V) is recorded according to the formula V=d/D where d is the distance at which patient is able to read the letters and D is the distance at which the letters are readable by a person with normal vision. The patient is positioned at a distance of 6 meters from the test types (d=6) and each eye is tested separately.

In infants, vision is tested by checking blinking response to bright light, turning of head towards diffuse light or following red moving ball or ring. Pupils may be dilated and fixed in optic atrophy; while in cortical blindness, pupillary responses are normal. The visual acuity in a term newborn baby is approximately 6/45, around 6/18 at one year, and it gradually matures to an adult level of 6/6 by the age of 6 to 7 years.

Congenital blindness should be differentiated from global mental retardation. Roving nystagmoid eye movements, persistent squint beyond 6 months of age, absence of optokinetic nystagmus (tested with rotating striped drum), lack of blink response to bright light or to sudden movement of examiner's finger towards infant's eye are suggestive of congenital blindness. A blind infant is extrasensitive to noise and gets easily frightened by sudden noise.

(b) *Field of vision (confrontation test)* It can be tested in children above the age of 3 years. The child sits about 50 cm away from the examiner at the same eye level and is asked to fix the gaze on the nose of the examiner. The examiner places his hands at the lateral limit of his own visual field midway between himself and the patient. The examiner quickly flexes or moves one of the fingers of either hand and child is asked to say "yes" when he is able to see the finger (Figure 14.10). Alternatively an object like a small toy or a bright pen is gradually brought from the periphery towards the field of vision of the eye and child is asked to inform when the object is visualized. Visual field of each eye is tested separately by blocking one eye. The conventional perimetry is

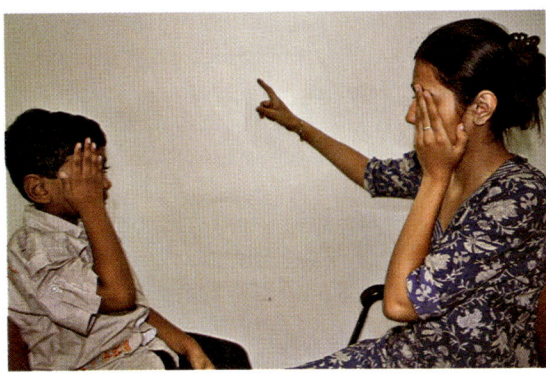

Figure 14.10 Confrontation test for assessment of field of vision. Refer to text for details.

feasible in children only after 8 to 9 years of age. Bitemporal hemianopsia (decreased vision in half of visual field) is characteristically seen due to craniopharyngioma producing lesion in the region of optic chiasma while homonymous hemianopsia (temporal field of one eye and nasal field of opposite eye) occurs due to lesions in optic radiations or visual cortex.

(c) *Color vision* It is difficult to evaluate color vision in children below 3 years. Color blindness is an X-linked disorder and affected boys are unable to differentiate between red and green colors. Ishihara pseudoisochromatic color plates are available for formal assessment of color vision. The child is asked to identify numbers or figures produced by virtue of different colors. About 8% boys and 0.5% girls have congenital X-linked color blindness.

(d) *Fundus examination* Effective pupillary dilatation in children can be achieved by instillation of 10% phenylephrine eyedrops every 5 minutes for a period of 15 to 20 minutes. Better pupillary dilatation can be achieved by additional instillation of 0.5% tropicamide or 1% homatropine eye drops. By holding the ophthalmoscope a few inches from the patient's eye, examine the iris and lens for evidences of iridocyclitis and cataract by using +10 or +12 diopters lens. The ophthalmoscope should then be brought as close as possible to the patient's eye to examine the fundus by using appropriate lens depending upon the refractive error of the patient.

Fundus is the window to the central nervous system. Look for papilledema, papillitis, optic atrophy, chorioretinitis, retinal colobomas (Aicardi syndrome, CHARGE association, Goldenhar syndrome, linear sebaceous nevus, focal dermal hypoplasia), hypertensive retinopathy, retinal hemorrhages, cherry red spot (GM1 gangliosidosis, Tay-Sach disease, Sandhoff disease, sialidosis, infantile Gaucher disease, Niemann-Pick disease, mucolipidosis type 1), retinitis pigmentosa (Laurence-Moon-Biedl syndrome, Refsum disease, neuronal ceroid lipofuscinosis, Cockayne syndrome, abeta-lipoproteinemia, Kearns-Sayre syndrome, Hurlers syndrome), phakomata and choroidal tubercles.

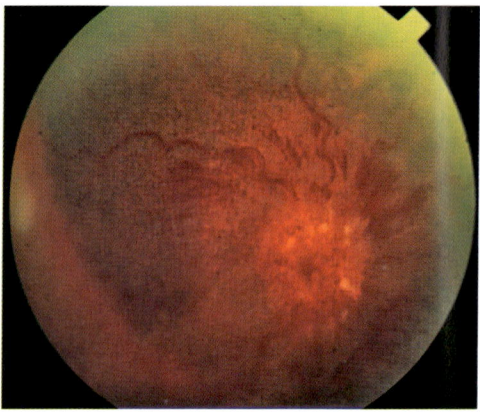

Figure 14.11 Papilledema due to medulloblastoma. Optic disk is elevated with blurred margins and marked hyperemia.

Optic disk is relatively pale in infants. Papilledema and papillitis are characterized by elevated disk with obliteration of physiological cup and blurred edges. The veins are engorged with marked hyperemia and hemorrhages (Figure 14.11). Visual loss in papillitis differentiates it from papilledema. Hypertensive retinopathy is characterized by generalized constriction and irregular narrowing of arterioles, thickening of vessels giving silver-wire appearance, flame-shaped hemorrhages, "cotton-wool patches", retinal edema and papilledema. In primary optic atrophy, the disk is shallow and chalky white with sharp distinct margins (Figure 14.12). There is loss of vision. The disk is dirty-pale with blurred margins in post-papilledematous optic atrophy (Figure 14.13). Unilateral optic atrophy with contralateral papilledema due to frontal lobe tumor is designated as Foster-Kennedy syndrome. Toxoplasmosis is characterized by yellow-white exudates which later turn into pigmented scars, and have a special predilection for macula (Figure 14.14). Focal or generalized "salt and pepper" type of pigmentary mottling is seen in infants with congenital rubella syndrome. Congenital CMV infection is characterized by multifocal atrophic pigmentary lesions over the peripheral areas. Diffuse "salt and pepper" pigmentary changes along with arteriolar attenuation and periphlebitis may be seen in patients with congenital syphilis. Most infants with TORCH infection usually develop optic atrophy,

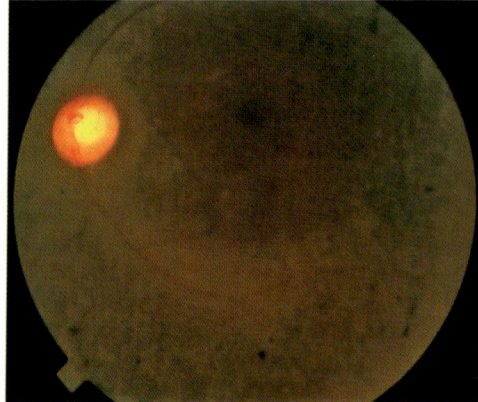

Figure 14.12 Primary optic atrophy in a patient with tuberculous meningitis. The optic disk is chalky white with sharp well-defined edges.

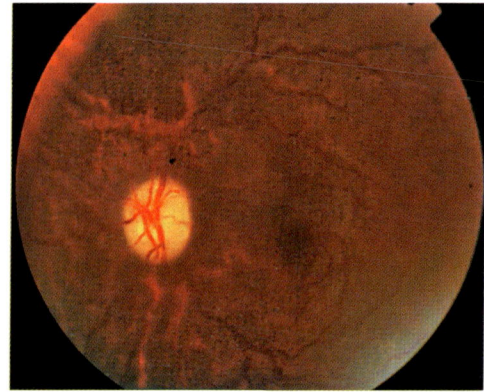

Figure 14.13 Post-papilledematous optic atrophy. The optic disk is dirty-pale with indistinct edges.

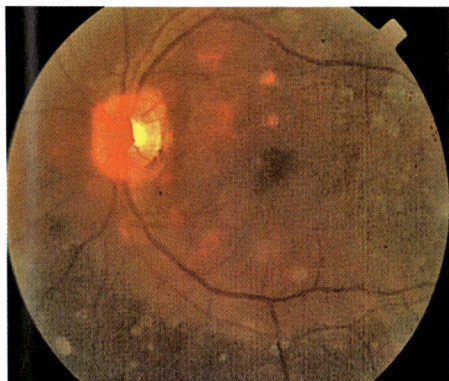

Figure 14.14 Diffuse chorioretinitis due to congenital toxoplasmosis.

strabismus and microphthalmos or bulbar phthisis. In retrobulbar neuritis, "neither the ophthalmologist nor the patient sees anything", because the lesion lies behind the lamina cribrosa. The common causes of retrobulbar neuritis include meningitis, avitaminosis and multiple sclerosis. It may lead to optic atrophy on follow-up.

Third (Oculomotor), Fourth (Trochlear) and Sixth (Abducent) Nerves

Anatomy

The external ocular muscles are supplied by the 3rd, 4th and 6th cranial nerves. All extraocular muscles (including sphincter pupillae and levator palpebrae superioris) are supplied by 3rd nerve except superior oblique which is supplied by the 4th cranial nerve and the lateral rectus by the 6th cranial nerve. The normal functions of various extraocular muscles are shown in Table 14.4.

TABLE 14.4 Functions of extraocular muscles

Muscle	Function
Medial rectus	Adduction
Lateral rectus	Abduction
Superior oblique	Depression, abduction, internal rotation or intorsion
Inferior oblique	Elevation, abduction and external rotation or extorsion
Superior rectus	Elevation
Inferior rectus	Depression

The nuclei of the 3rd, 4th and 6th cranial nerves are located in the brainstem at the level of quadrigemina and extend caudally as the eminentia teres in the floor of 4th ventricle. The nucleus of 3rd nerve is located more anteriorly. Its rostral part (Edinger-Westphal nucleus) supplies parasympathetic fibers to the ciliary muscles and iris. Its caudal part chiefly supplies the extraocular muscles. The nucleus of the 4th nerve is located below the 3rd nerve nucleus. The 6th nerve nucleus is situated in the floor of 4th ventricle at the level of pons. The 3rd and 4th nerves are the only cranial nerves that decussate between their nuclei at their point of emergence dorsally from the brainstem. The 6th nerve emerges between medulla and pons and has a long intracranial course which makes it vulnerable to the effects of raised intracranial tension leading to internal squint or diplopia on lateral gaze (false localizing sign.)

Testing

They are tested together because they are concerned with ocular movements. Diplopia is the most reliable symptom of involvement of any of these nerves. Look for squint, movements of eyeballs, pupils, ptosis, diplopia and nystagmus. Head tilt may occur in order to compensate for the squint. Doll's eye movement phenomenon is used to test the ocular movements in infants. Supranuclear lesions of ocular nerves lead to paralysis of conjugate movements of the eyes.

Paralytic squint should be differentiated from concomitant squint which is characterized by early onset (below 3 years), normal eye movements in all directions, absence of diplopia, identical primary and secondary deviation and defective vision or amblyopia in the deviating eye (Table 14.5).

Oculomotor nerve (third nerve) Its nucleus lies in the midbrain and it supplies all the extraocular muscles of the eye, except external rectus and superior oblique. It also supplies ciliary muscles and levator pelpebrae superioris.

Look for the following abnormalities:
(i) Diplopia or double vision is best seen when child looks towards the side of action of paralyzed muscle.

TABLE 14.5 Salient differences between paralytic and concomitant squints

Feature	Paralytic squint	Concomitant squint
▪ Onset	Sudden	Gradual and insidious
▪ Amblyopia (visual loss)	Uncommon	Common
▪ Diplopia	Common	Absent
▪ Ocular movements	Ocular movements are limited	Ocular movements are normal
Primary and secondary deviations of eyes	Secondary deviation is more than the primary deviation	They are equal
▪ Visual axis*	Varies as gaze is turned to different directions	Constant
▪ False projection**	Common	Absent
▪ Vertigo	May occur	Absent

Visual axis*: A straight line that passes through both the center of the pupil and center of the fovea.
False projection**: Patient is asked to cover the normal eye and then quickly look at an object held infront him.

(ii) Ptosis and pupillary changes may not occur in children who have a nuclear lesion of the oculomotor nerve (Figure 14.15). Bilateral ptosis which becomes worse in the evening is characteristically seen in patients with myasthenia gravis. In Marcus Gunn phenomenon, there is reflex elevation or closure of the ptotic lid in response to swallowing movements of the jaw.

(iii) Pupils should be examined for size, shape, equality of size on two sides, response to light, response to light on opposite side (consensual light reflex), response to accommodation and response to pain (ciliospinal reflex). The pupil is best seen when torch light is shone obliquely over the eye. It is useful to use a hand lens with inbuilt light for assessment of pupillary responses.

(iv) Dilated and fixed pupil is a characteristic feature of oculomotor palsy. There is no response to light and consensual reflex. The consensual reflex is tested by shining light into one eye and noting the contraction of pupil in the other eye. In retrobulbar neuritis, pupillary response to direct light is lost but consensual reflex is maintained. Unilateral dilatation of pupil with deteriorating consciousness should be considered as a sign of unilateral tentorial herniation unless proved otherwise. Dilatation of pupils may occur due to fear, anxiety and medication (atropine). Pupils are normally larger in size in children than in adults and their diameter is normally up to 5 mm.

(v) Pinpoint pupils are seen in children with pontine lesions, head injury, Horner syndrome, and following intoxication with certain drugs especially opioids, barbiturates, phenothiazines, ethanol, phencyclidine, and organophosphate insectiside poisoning.

(vi) Loss of accommodation. The child is asked to look at a far object in the room. The examiner suddenly brings his finger in front of patient's nose, and child is told to look at it. The eyes converge and the pupils should contract on both sides as the child accommodates for the finger.

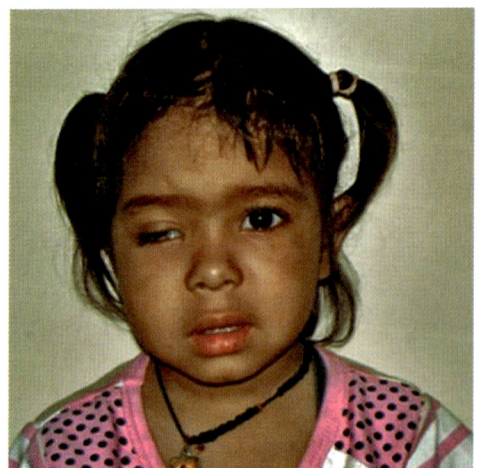

Figure 14.15 Congenital ptosis of the right eye.

The Central Nervous System

TABLE 14.6 Deviation of eyeball due to paralysis of individual eye muscles

Muscle	Nerve	Deviation of eyeball	Diplopia occurs when child looks
Medial or internal rectus	III	Outward or external squint	Towards nose
Superior rectus	III	Downward and inward	Upward and outward
Inferior rectus	III	Upward and inward	Downward and outward
Inferior oblique	III	Downward and outward	Upward and inward
Superior oblique	IV	Upward and outward	Downward and inward
Lateral or external rectus	VI	Inward or internal squint	Towards temple or outward

(vii) Argyll-Robertson pupils are seen in children with neurosyphilis, diabetes mellitus, and Perinaud's syndrome. The pupillary light reflex is lost but the accommodation reflex is preserved.

(viii) The eye is displaced outwards and downwards. There is loss of all movements of the eye and it can only be moved slightly outwards and little downwards.

Table 14.6 depicts deviations of eyeball due to paralysis of individual extraocular muscles. Diplopia occurs when child is asked to look towards the direction where the paralyzed muscle normally moves the eyeball.

Trochlear nerve (fourth nerve) The nucleus lies in the midbrain and it supplies superior oblique muscle. There is slight upward and outward deviation of the eye when trochlear nerve is paralyzed. The downward movements of the eyeball is impaired and child complains of diplopia on looking below the horizontal plane or during adduction of the eye.

Abducent nerve (sixth nerve) Its nucleus lies in the pons and it has a long intracranial course and may get compressed due to raised intracranial tension. It supplies external rectus muscle. The paralysis would cause internal squint and inability to move the eyeball outwards and diplopia occurs on looking outwards **(Figure 14.16)**. The paralysis of 6th nerve may occur due to generalized increase in intracranial pressure as a false localizing sign.

During examination of ocular movements, look for nystagmus **(Figure 14.17)**. The child is asked to look at the examiner's finger which is moved slowly horizontally in either direction and vertically up and down. Note the position of the

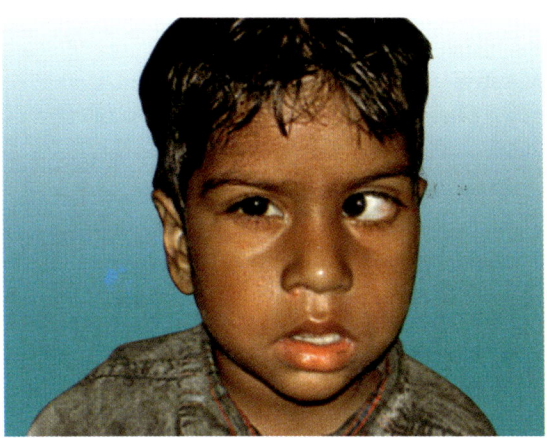

Figure 14.16 Paralytic convergent squint in a child with left 6th nerve palsy. Note that the left palpebral aperture is larger due to concomitant facial palsy.

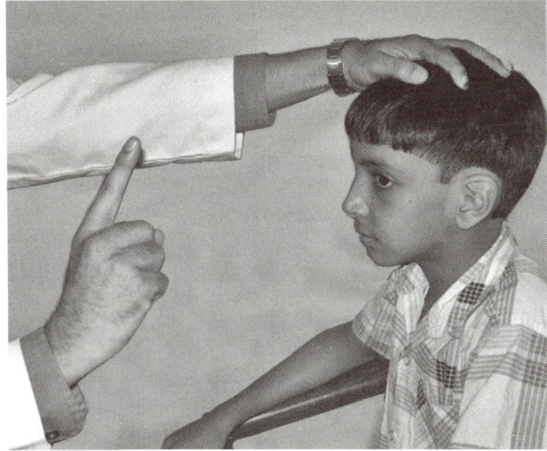

Figure 14.17 Assessment of ocular movements and nystagmus. The child is asked to follow the examiner's finger in horizontal and vertical directions without moving the head.

eye when nystagmus occurs, its character, and direction of fast component. The nystagmus may be fine or coarse, pendular (amblyopia), jerky (vestibular), rotary (labyrinthine), horizontal (cerebellar) and vertical (brainstem).

Syndromes involving 3rd, 4th and 6th Cranial Nerves

A number of syndromes are associated with congenital and acquired disorders of ocular cranial nerves.

Horner syndrome (C8, T1) It is characterized by miosis, ptosis, enophthalmos and lack of sweating over the face on the affected side. The ciliospinal reflex is lost, i.e. pinching of skin of neck is not followed by dilatation of pupil.

Perinaud's syndrome There is paralysis of conjugate upward gaze due to involvement of superior colliculi which may occur due to pineal tumor, hydrocephalus, encephalitis, vascular lesions and disseminated sclerosis. There may be nystagmus, enophthalmos and pupils contract on accommodation but do not respond to light (Argyll-Robertson pupil).

Gradenigo's syndrome There is paralysis of unilateral rectus muscle with tenderness or swelling behind the ipsilateral ear due to inflammatory disease in the petrous bone.

Moebius syndrome There is bilateral paralysis of external recti associated with paresis of facial muscles because of aplasia of the 6th nerve nuclei in the brainstem (Figure 14.18).

Benedikt's syndrome It is characterized by ipsilateral oculomotor palsy with contralateral tremors, ataxia or hyperkinesis of upper extremity because of involvement of 3rd nerve as it passes through the red nucleus.

Weber's syndrome Paralysis of third nerve with contralateral hemiparesis occurs because of involvement of 3rd nerve as it passes through the cerebral peduncles due to lesion in the midbrain.

Pontine crossed paralysis A lesion in the pons involving nucleus of the 7th nerve causes ipsilateral facial paralysis and contralateral spastic paralysis of arm and leg.

Millard-Gubler syndrome It is characterized by ipsilateral 6th and 7th nerves paralysis with involvement of contralateral pyramidal hemiparesis because of lesion in the brainstem.

Foville's syndrome There is ipsilateral 7th nerve palsy with contralateral pyramidal hemiparesis and paresis of lateral gaze due to involvement of para-abducens nucleus.

Fifth (Trigeminal) Nerve

Anatomy

The trigeminal nerve is a mixed nerve having motor and sensory components. It has three branches supplying ophthalmic, maxillary and mandibular regions of the face (Figure 14.19). The sensory root

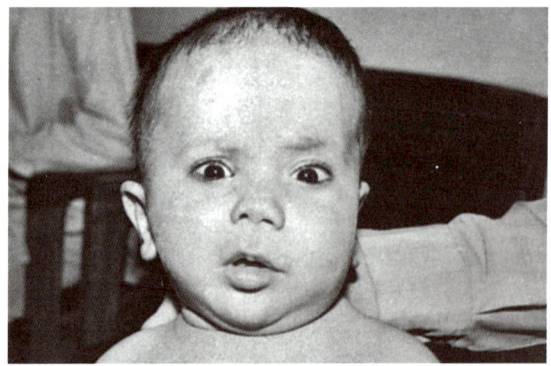

Figure 14.18 Moebius syndrome. Note bilateral paralytic convergent squint and paresis of facial muscles.

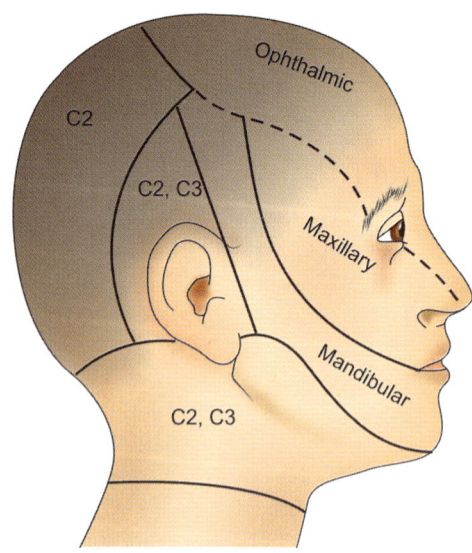

Figure 14.19 Sensory supply of the face by branches of trigeminal nerve and upper cervical roots.

TABLE 14.7 Functions of trigeminal nerve

Branch	Sensory	Motor
Ophthalmic	Bulbar and upper eyelid conjunctiva, lacrimal gland, skin of medial part and tip of nose, upper eyelids, forehead and scalp up to vertex	None
Maxillary	Skin of cheek, front of temple, lower eyelid including conjunctiva, side of the nose, upper lip, upper teeth, upper part of pharynx, roof of mouth, part of soft palate	None
Mandibular	Lower part of the face, lower lip, lower teeth, tongue and part of ear. It also supplies parasympathetic fibers to the salivary glands	All muscles of mastication except buccinators

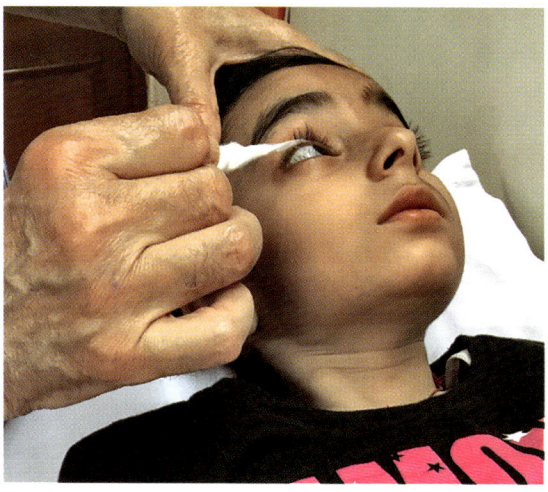

Figure 14.20 Corneal reflex. Ask the child to look in one direction and bring a wisp of cotton from the side to touch the bulbar conjunctiva or cornea. There is a blink response in a normal child.

takes origin from nerve cells in the trigeminal (Gasserian) ganglion and enters the lateral surface of the pons at about its middle. The fibers which conduct impulses for light touch terminate in a large nucleus in the pons which is situated lateral to the motor nucleus near the floor of 4th ventricle. The fibers for pain and thermal sensations enter the bulbospinal tract ("descending" fibers) which extends as low as the 2nd cervical segment of the cord before ascending in the medial lemniscus. The ophthalmic and maxillary divisions of 5th nerve are purely sensory while the mandibular division has both sensory and motor components (Table 14.7).

Testing

(i) Corneal or conjunctival reflex is lost by involvement of either 5th or 7th (efferent fibers for this reflex are carried by the seventh nerve) cranial nerve. Ask the child to look in one direction and bring a wisp of cotton wool from the opposite direction (to avoid visual blink) and gently touch the bulbar conjunctiva or cornea (Figure 14.20). Absence of corneal reflex is suggestive of involvement of either 5th or 7th cranial nerve.

(ii) Sensory loss over scalp, cheek or mandible depending upon which branch is affected. The patient gets a feeling of broken glass or cup on the affected side while drinking.

(iii) Loss of pain sensations over anterior two-thirds of tongue.

(iv) Ask the patient to clench his teeth. The masseters and temporalis muscles do not contract on the paralyzed side.

(v) Ask the patient to open his mouth. The jaw is deviated towards the paralyzed side by the unopposed action of healthy pterygoid muscle. The patient cannot move the jaw from side-to-side.

Seventh (Facial) Nerve

Anatomy

The motor nucleus of facial nerve is situated in the pons lateral to the nucleus of abducens nerve. Efferent fibers loop around the nucleus of 6th cranial nerve before leaving the pons. At the cerebellopontine angle, it is joined by the nervus intermedius. The two then enter the facial canal in the temporal bone exiting the skull through the stylomastoid foramen. The nervus intermedius carries taste sensations from anterior two-thirds of the tongue via lingual and chorda tympani nerves. The afferent fibers originate from the geniculate ganglion and provide secretory fibers to the lacrimal glands via the petrosal nerves. During its course through temporal bone, facial nerve gives off a branch to stapedius muscle which limits the movements of the eardrum and ossicles in response to loud noise. Before it emerges through the stylomastoid foramen, it is joined by the chorda tympani. During its course through the facial canal, the nerve is enclosed in a bony tube and is thus susceptible to trauma and inflammatory edema. After its exit from the stylomastoid foramen, the nerve passes anteriorily through the substance of the parotid gland and divides into a number of branches to innervate all the muscles of the face and scalp (including platysma) except the levator palpebrae superioris.

Testing

(i) Palpebral fissure is wider on the affected side. Affected eye cannot be closed firmly. When attempt is made to forcibly close the eye, the eyeball rolls upwards exposing the sclera (Bell's phenomenon).
(ii) Forehead cannot be wrinkled on the affected side when child is asked to look upwards.
(iii) When the child cries or smiles there is asymmetry of the face and angle of the mouth is pulled up on the healthy side while nasolabial fold is flat on the affected side. The sign can be elicited by asking the patient to show the teeth.
(iv) Ask the patient to whistle or blow. The air leaks from the paralyzed side. Ask him to inflate his cheeks with air under pressure and test the tension on both sides by tapping each cheek with a finger. The air leaks from the mouth more easily from the paralyzed side.
(v) Taste fibers from anterior two-thirds of tongue are carried by chorda tympani branch of 7th nerve (taste over posterior one-third of tongue is supplied by the 9th nerve). The taste is examined with a solution of sugar, salt, lemon and quinine in that order. Taste, salivation and tears may be affected, if lesion lies between the brainstem and origin of chorda tympani in the middle ear.
(vi) Hyperacusis may occur due to involvement of nerve to the stapedius in the facial canal which is supplied by 7th nerve.

In lower motor neuron paralysis (nuclear and infranuclear), the facial palsy is total but in upper motor neuron paralysis (pseudobulbar palsy), eyes and forehead are partially spared and emotional expressions of face are preserved due to bilateral representation of the upper face in the cortex.

The common causes of unilateral infranuclear facial paralysis include Bell's palsy, Ramsay-Hunt syndrome, otitis media, hypertension, meningitis, Kawasaki disease, Lyme disease, sarcoidosis, Henoch-Schönlein purpura and rhabdomyosarcoma of middle ear.

Bilateral facial palsy is difficult to diagnose and gives a mask-like flat or non-expressive appearance to the face. It is a recognized feature of Guillain-Barré syndrome, Moebius syndrome, infantile botulism and various myopathies.

Eighth (Vestibulocochlear) Nerve

Anatomy

There are two components of vestibulocochlear nerve, one supplying the cochlea and serving auditory functions and the other supplying the labyrinth and semicircular canals thus serving the function of equilibrium or balance. Auditory fibers from the vestibular nuclei in the pons and medulla traverse and terminate in the inferior colliculi and medial geniculate bodies. The secondary fibers from these locations pass through the internal capsule to the cortical center for hearing which is located in the temporal lobe. The vestibular fibers originate in the vestibular ganglion and terminate in a group of nuclei in the pons and medulla.

Testing

The nerve has two components—auditory and vestibular. Enquire about any hearing defect, tinnitus, hyperacusis, objective vertigo (vestibular), subjective vertigo (8th nerve, middle ear or brainstem) and dizziness. Ask for response of the child to noise of jet plane, banging of door, music and calling of his name, etc. In infants, assess for startle response, blinking of eyes, sudden change or cessation of activity, change in heart rate, turning of head towards the sound stimulus of a bell, whistle, cup and spoon, cymbals, and squeaky toy or 60 db vocal sound. The sound stimulus should not be visible to the infant and it should not produce a whiff of air (Figure 14.21). In infants, lack of response to sound may occur due to general developmental retardation rather than deafness. If hearing defect is present, ascertain whether it is due to middle ear disease or nerve deafness. Normally the air conduction is better than bone conduction. In middle ear disease, bone conduction is unaffected but air conduction is diminished while in nerve deafness both are affected. This can be evaluated clinically with the help of a tuning fork (256 Hz).

In *Rinne's test,* vibrating tuning fork is placed infront of the ear (air conduction) and then over the mastoid bone (bone conduction). In nerve deafness, both air and bone conductions are proportionately reduced while in conduction deafness bone conduction is retained and becomes better than air conduction. In *Weber's test*, the vibrating tuning fork is placed over the middle of patient's forehead (Figure 14.22). In conduction

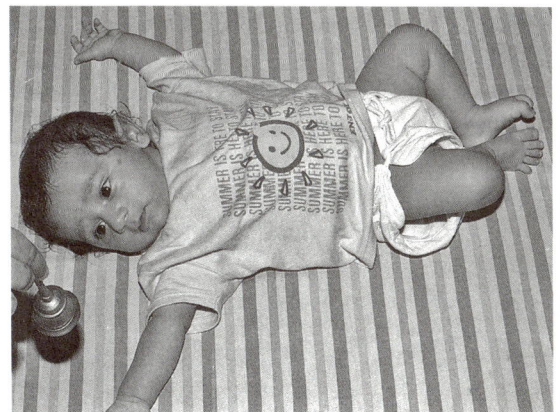

Figure 14.21 Assessment of hearing in an infant with a temple bell.

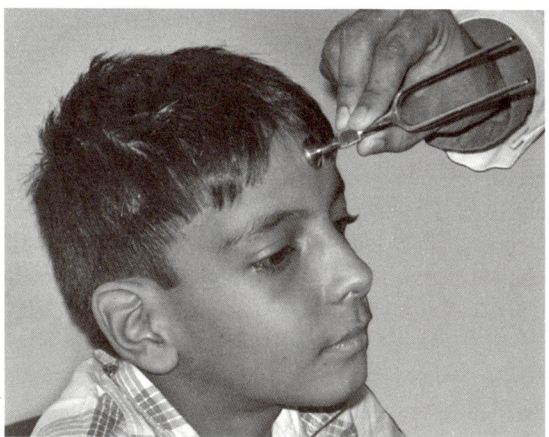

Figure 14.22 Weber's test to differentiate between conduction and nerve deafness. Refer to text for details.

deafness, *Weber's test* is lateralized to the abnormal side; while in nerve deafness, it is lateralized towards the normal side. These tests have been replaced by tympanometry and audiometry.

Audiometric evaluation reveals loss of high tones in children with nerve deafness while middle ear deafness is characterized by loss of hearing capability for low tone sounds. When there is gross hearing loss, there is global loss of all sound frequencies. In young children, hearing is assessed with brainstem auditory evoked responses, evoked otoacoustic emission and behavioral audiometry.

Vestibular dysfunction may manifest as vertigo, giddiness and dizziness. In vestibular disorders, the vertigo is objective but difficult to evaluate in children. The caloric test is more objective but is scary for children. The test should be performed, if auditory canal is free of wax and tympanic membrane is intact. The child's head is kept steady in a semireclining position (30° with pillows). 10 mL of cold water (30°C) is injected into the ear canal and nystagmus recorded on electromyography. Normally cold caloric test produces slow deviation of eyes towards the side of injection with rapid phase of nystagmus away from the side of injection. Instillation of warm water (44°C) produces opposite effect when vestibular system is intact. In cases of vestibular damage (or brain death), cold or hot caloric tests do not produce any nystagmus in the eyes.

Ninth (Glossopharyngeal), Tenth (Vagus) and Eleventh (Accessory) Nerves

Anatomy

The glossopharyngeal, vagus and accessory nerves arise, in order from above downwards, in an elongated nucleus located in the floor of 4th ventricle. They emerge by several roots along the lateral aspect of the medulla oblongata. The spinal component of the accessory nerve emerges from the lateral column of the cord, passing up through the foramen magnum to join its medullary part and then emerging along with it through the jugular foramen. After emerging, its two divisions separate, the medullary or accessory portion joining the vagus nerve and supplying motor fibers to the larynx and pharynx. The spinal portion supplies the sternomastoid and upper part of the trapezius muscle.

The glossopharyngeal nerve is mostly sensory. It carries sensations from the porterior third of tongue and mucous membrane of the pharynx. It supplies motor fibers to the middle pharyngeal sphincter and the stylopharyngeus muscle. It also carries taste fibers from the porterior third of the tongue.

The vagus is a motor nerve for soft palate (with the exception of the tensor palate), pharynx and larynx. It is sensory and motor for the respiratory tract, heart and most of the abdominal viscera via parasympathetic ganglia. The vagal fibers to the soft palate, pharynx and larynx originate in the nucleus ambiguous and traverse through the accessory nerve. The visceromotor and cardio-inhibitory fibers are derived from the dorsal nucleus of the vagus in the floor of the 4th ventricle.

The accessory nerve provides motor functions to the sternocleidomastoid muscle, which extend and rotate the neck, and the trapezius, which is used to shrug the shoulders.

Testing

The child may complain of dysphagia and nasal regurgitation of fluids through the nose and nasal twang of voice due to paralysis of soft palate and pharynx. There is loss of swallowing reflex with drooling of saliva and choking. The gag reflex or pharyngeal reflex is lost. The soft palate is pulled or deviated towards the normal side when child with open mouth is asked to say 'ah'. The bilateral affection of vagus nerve may produce hoarseness of voice or aphonia while unilateral paralysis can be diagnosed on examination of larynx. The left recurrent laryngeal branch of the vagus may be damaged by mediastinal tumor or enlarged pulmonary conus causing stridor and hoarseness of voice due to abductor paralysis. There is loss of sensation of taste over the posterior one-third of the tongue.

The paralysis of accessory nerve results in inability to shrug or elevate the shoulders against resistance and weakness in extension of neck and rotation of chin towards the opposite side.

Twelvth (Hypoglossal) Nerve

Anatomy

The hypoglossal nerve is a purely motor nerve supplying the tongue and the depressor muscles of the hyoid bone. It arises from its nucleus located in the lower part of the floor of 4th ventricle close to the midline. It emerges from the brainstem between the anterior pyramid and the olive.

Testing

The paralysis is characterized by deviation of protruded tongue towards the paralyzed side. The apparent deviation in a patient with facial palsy should be kept in mind. Ask the child to move the tongue from side-to-side and lick inner side of each cheek with it. The tongue is wasted and shows fasciculations in nuclear and infranuclear lesions (Figure 14.23). Bilateral weakness, atrophy and fasciculations of tongue are pathognomonic of Werdnig-Hoffmann disease.

Bulbar paralysis It occurs due to involvement of bulbar nerves or their nuclei (9th, 10th, 11th and 12th cranial nerves) in medulla oblongata. It is characterized by pooling of secretions in the posterior pharynx, drooling of saliva, dysphagia, nasal regurgitation of feeds, dysarthria with nasal twang in the voice. There may be involvement of the medullary respiratory and vasomotor centers

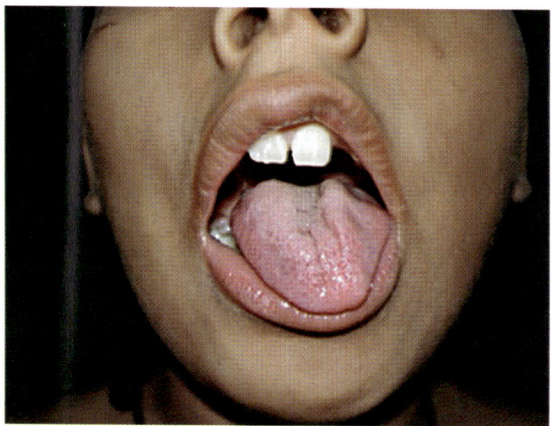

Figure 14.23 Paralysis of hypoglossal nerve on the left side. Note deviation of tongue towards left side with atrophy of left half of tongue.

producing respiratory irregularity and cardiac dysrhythmia. The common conditions causing bulbar paralysis include acute poliomyelitis, pontine glioma, nasopharyngeal carcinoma or sarcoma, Moebius syndrome, Guillain-Barré syndrome, infantile botulism, diphtheritic neuritis, tuberculous meningitis, encephalitis, demyelinating diseases and phenothiazine toxicity.

Pseudobulbar or suprabulbar paralysis It is characterized by difficulty in articulation and swallowing, with pooling of secretions and facial rigidity due to bilateral involvement of corticospinal fibers above the level of brainstem nuclei. In upper motor neuron lesion, the tongue deviates away from the side of lesion. The jaw jerk is exaggerated and there may be evidences of bilateral involvement of corticospinal tract with extensor plantar response. Pseudobulbar paralysis may occur due to encephalitis, quadriparetic cerebral palsy, bilateral cerebral thrombosis, infantile form of Gaucher's disease, glycogen storage disease type II (Pompe disease) and children with acquired immunodeficiency disorder.

MOTOR SYSTEM

Examine upper limbs, trunk and lower limbs in that order.

1. *Posture* The limbs may be placed in an abnormal position due to alterations in muscle tone and power. The paralyzed lower limb is kept in a state of extension and external rotation at the hip. "Pithed frog" position of legs is seen in Werdnig-Hoffmann disease, scurvy and poliomyelitis. Decerebrate rigidity results from brainstem lesion any where between intercollicular level and vestibular nucleus. It is characterized by persistent or episodes of extensor-hypertonia and internal rotation of all the four limbs with opisthotonos. Coma, pinpoint pupils and bilateral Babinski sign may also be present. It is characterized by shortening and lengthening reactions which are modified by tonic neck, labyrinthine (Magnus-de Kleijn) and phasic spinal reflexes. The site of lesion in decorticate rigidity is more cephalad, at the interphase of cerebral hemispheres and diencephalon. It is characterized by flexor hypertonia of upper limbs and extensor hypertonia of lower limbs. Decerebrate rigidity is of graver prognostic significance as compared to decorticate rigidity.

2. *Involuntary movements* Look for abnormal movements and note whether they persist during sleep or disappear.

    (a) *Tremors* Rhythmical oscillations of parts of a limb due to alternate contractions of opposing muscles produce tremors. They may be fine or coarse, static or action or intention tremors. Fine tremors of outstretched hands are seen in anxiety and thyrotoxicosis while more proximal coarse tremors of the outstretched arms and wrists (wing-beating tremors) are seen in Wilson disease (Figure 14.24).

    (b) *Chorea* It is characterized by jerky arrhythmic, irregular semi-purposive movements of a limb or part of a limb almost simulating a bizarre dance. The movements occur at the proximal joints. They are increased by agitation, decreased by voluntary activity and disappear during sleep. If the movements involve one side of the body, it is called hemichorea. They are accompanied by respiratory irregularity and rapid protrusion and retraction of the tongue with "flapping" of its tip (Figure 14.25). There is hypotonia, hyperextensibility of joints and inability to hold the hands above the head with palms extended. The common causes of chorea include Sydenham chorea (rheumatic fever), CNS infections, HIV, herpes simplex, pertussis, diphtheria, varicella, systemic lupus erythematosus, bacterial endocarditis, Behcet disease, benign hereditary chorea, Huntington's disease and chorea due to drugs (levodopa, anticonvulsants, antipsychotics), thyrotoxicosis, polycythemia rubra vera, antiphospholipid syndrome, celiac disease, etc.

(c) *Athetosis* It is characterized by continuous, slow sinuous, writhing movements mostly located over the peripheral or distal parts of the extremities. The patient is unable to maintain the fingers and toes in any one position.

(d) *Dystonia musculorum deformans or torsion spasms* It is characterized by contortions and torsion spasms of wide amplitude involving muscles of neck, trunk and proximal parts of limbs (Figure 14.26). The head, trunk and limbs may be maintained in a bizarre position. Chorea, athetosis and dystonia are produced due to disorders of basal ganglia. It

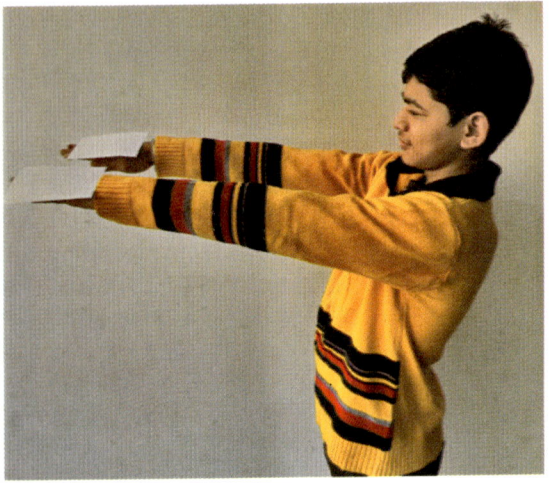

Figure 14.24 Method for elicitation of fine tremors of hands. Place a piece of paper on the dorsum of outstretched hand to look for tremors.

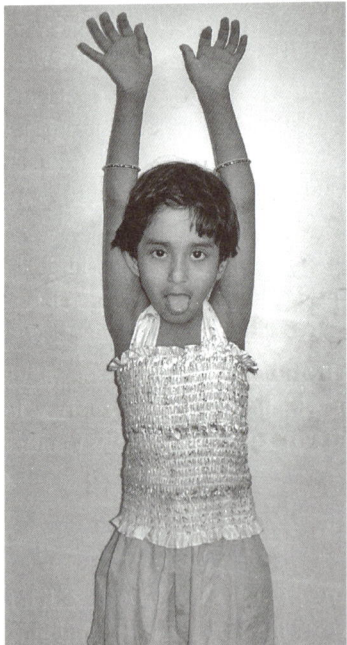

Figure 14.25 Method for examination of child with chorea. The child is unable to maintain the hands above the head and cannot keep the tongue out of the mouth ("Jack in the box" tongue).

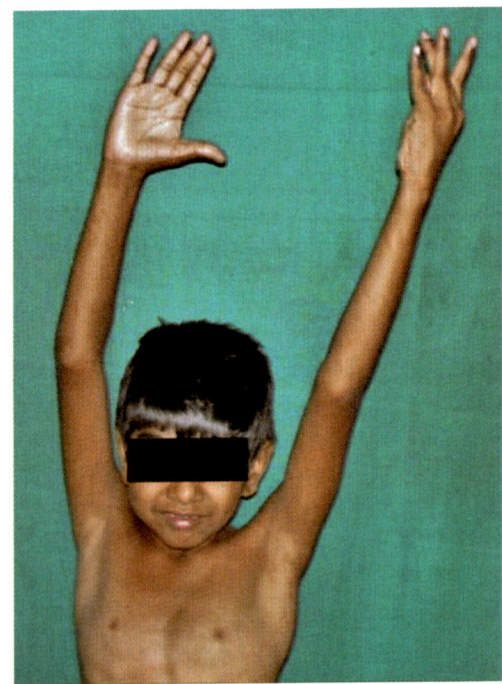

Figure 14.26 Dystonic posturing of left upper limb in a child with basal ganglia infarct. Note twisting of wrist and fingers.

is usually associated with grimacing, grunting and protrusion of tongue. The abnormal movements disappear during sleep and may become less severe during relaxation and volitional activity, like dressing and feeding. The common predisposing conditions include birth asphyxia, birth trauma, kernicterus and encephalitis.

(e) *Hemiballismus* It is characterized by frequent, violent, rapid, swinging movements of proximal joints of one arm or leg which may injure the patient or others. The condition is usually of sudden onset and is extremely disabling and exhausting. It occurs due to a vascular or neoplastic lesion near the vicinity of subthalamic nucleus.

(f) *Myoclonus* It is unpredictable, sudden, rapid jerk or twitch of one or more muscle groups. It is distinguished from chorea by virtue of its abruptness and brevity. It usually occurs due to lesions in brainstem and reticular formation.

(g) *Fasciculations and twitchings* Twitching of muscle fibers of tongue and limbs may occur due to slow degeneration of anterior horn cells or motor nuclei of cranial nerves.

(h) *Tics* Tics or habit spasms are bizarre facial and shoulder movements without any organic disease. They are stereotyped, repetitive movements which are easily produced voluntarily, such as blinking of eyes, pursing of lips, frowning of forehead, twisting of neck, coughing or clearing of throat, jerking of extremities and shrugging of shoulders. They increase in severity during anxiety, tension and nervousness especially when child is being watched and often disappear while concentrating on a job. Gilles de la Tourette syndrome is a rare disorder which is characterized by multiple persistent tics often accompanied by inarticulate cries or barks and compulsive utterances of obscenities. Rett syndrome, which is limited to girls, is characterized by stereotypic tics, like hand washing, rubbing or wringing of hands, clapping, tapping and mouthing automatisms.

(i) *Carpopedal spasms* In tetany due to hypocalcemia or alkalosis, there may be episodes of adduction of thumbs with partial flexion at metacarpophalangeal and interphalangeal joints with flexion of wrist and elbow. The carpal spasm can be induced by inflating the sphygmomanometer cuff worn around the upper arm beyond systolic pressure for about 3 minutes (Figure 14.27). Increased excitability of nerves can be demonstrated by tapping the facial and peroneal nerves. Tapping of facial nerve infront of ear lobe, as it comes out of the stylomastoid foramen, is followed by twitching of facial muscles with each tap (Chvostek sign).

(j) *Asterixis or flapping tremors* may be seen as non-rhythmic, asymmetric, abrupt, brief loss of posture in the outstretched hands. It occurs in decompensated hepatic failure (liver flap), Wilson disease, viremia, poisoning and over dose of hypnotic drugs.

3. **Bulk of muscles** The wasting of muscles is marked in cases of lower motor neuron paralysis. Assess whether it is predominantly affecting proximal or distal groups of muscles and whether involvement is symmetrical or asymmetrical on the two sides. The circumference of the limbs should be measured at identical points identified in relation to reliable bony landmarks, like anterior superior iliac spine, acromion, olecranon, patella, and medial malleolus. In congenital hemiatrophy or hemihypertrophy, all the tissues of the limb including the bones are affected. In Duchenne's muscular dystrophy (DMD) and Becker's muscular dystrophy (BMD), the calf muscles are hypertrophied (Figure 14.28). The salient differences between various muscular dystrophies are shown in Table 14.8.

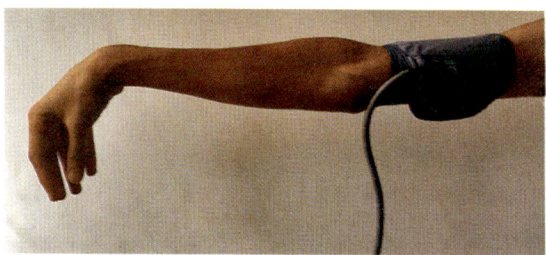

Figure 14.27 Trousseau sign being elicited by inflating the cuff of the sphygmomanometer.

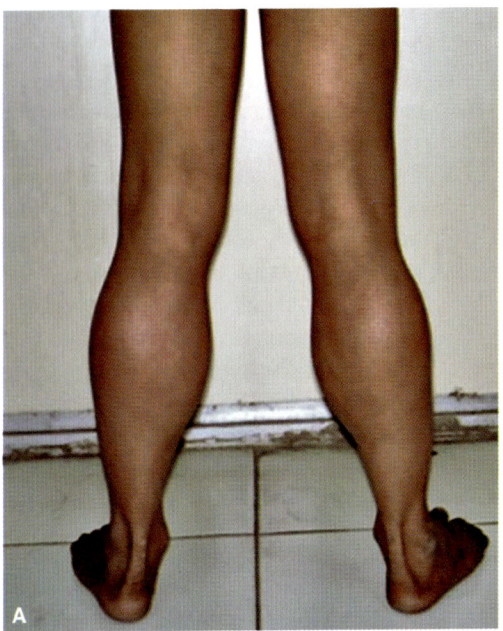
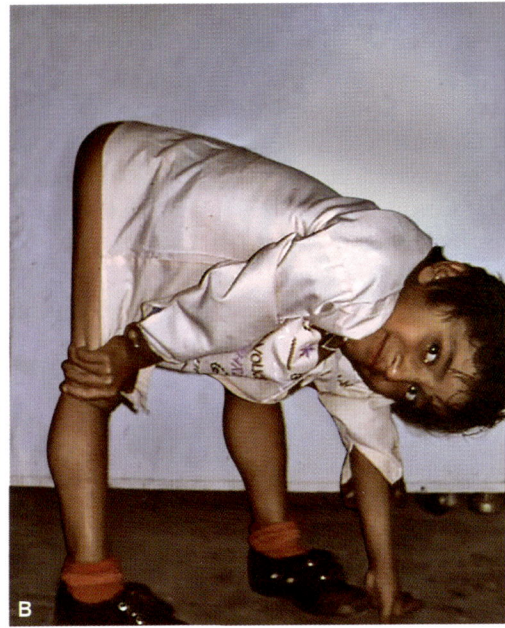

Figure 14.28A and B (A) Bulky calves due to pseudohypertrophy of calf muscles in an 8-year-old boy with Duchenne's muscular dystrophy. (B) Gower sign. The child supports himself in all the four limbs, then climbs up on his own body by placing his hands on the knees and thighs to lift himself.

TABLE 14.8 Clinical features of common muscular dystrophies					
Features	Duchenne	Becker	Facioscapular humeral	Limb-girdle	Myotonic
Inheritance	X-linked recessive	X-linked recessive	Autosomal dominant	Autosomal recessive	Autosomal dominant
Age at onset	Early childhood	Late childhood and adolescence	Adolescence and early adult life	Adolescence and early adult life	Highly variable
Commonly affected muscles	Pelvic and shoulder girdle	Pelvic and shoulder girdle	Face and shoulder girdle	Pelvic and shoulder girdle	Face and distal limbs
Rate of progression	Rapid	Slow	Very slow	Variable	Variable
Associated muscle features	Pseudohypertrophy of calves	Pseudohypertrophy of calves	None	Pseudohypertrophy rarely	Myotonia
Systemic features	Mental retardation, cardiac myopathy with electrocardiographic abnormalities	Occasional	None	None	Mental retardation, heart block, cataracts, hair loss, testicular atrophy, diabetes mellitus

Pelvic girdle involvement is demonstrated by Gower maneuver. Shoulder girdle involvement is characterized by upward displacement of the shoulders and abnormal rotation of the scapulae when child is lifted by placing hands under the axillae and there is spontaneous winging of scapulae

4. *Trophic changes* Look for painless effusion of joints, vasomotor disturbances, bedsores or trophic ulcers, erythema or pigmentary changes.

5. *Muscle tone* The muscle tone is evaluated by (i) looking for abnormal posture of the limb, (ii) palpation of muscles for soft or flabby and stiff feel, (iii) resistance to and range of passive movements at major joints (adductor angle, popliteal angle at foot, heel-to-ear maneuver, scarf sign) and (iv) by shaking the unsupported limb for range and flaility of movements. Refer to Chapters 6 and 15 for assessment of tone in infants. *The tone should be compared on the two sides by maintaining the head in midline.* It may be normal, decreased or increased. In pyramidal lesions, the patient develops claspknife type of spasticity when resistance is most marked at the beginning and end of passive movements. In cerebral diplegia due to pyramidal lesion, the neck and trunk remain relatively hypotonic. The various types of spastic cerebral palsy are shown in Table 14.9. Plastic or lead-pipe type of rigidity is seen due to increased tone of both protagonist and antagonist muscles in patients with extra-pyramidal lesion. The presence of tremors in such a patient leads to cogwheel type of rigidity.

6. *Power of muscles* Assess the motor disability by asking as to which activities of daily living, the child is unable to perform. Whether the child can self-feed, undress and dress himself, look after toilet needs, and comb his hair or not. Apraxia is defined as inability to carry out a well-organized voluntary acitivity on command without having any significant impairment of motor, sensory and coordination function. Watch the manner and dexterity with which an infant holds and manipulates the toy and his responses to what is going around him. During first 2 years, most children are ambidexterous and do not have any preference to use a particular hand. When there is unequivocal preference to use a particular hand during infancy, it should be considered as an earliest manifestation of infantile hemiplegia due to neonatal stroke.

Ask the child to hop on one foot, walk forwards and backwards, toe walk, heel walk, and rise from squatting or lying down position. The active movements at all the joints should be tested without and against varying grades of resistance. The infant should be watched for spontaneous movements. Assess whether weakness is affecting predominantly proximal (myopathy, dermatomyositis, Guillain-Barré syndrome) or distal (peripheral neuropathy) group of muscles and whether it is symmetrical or asymmetrical. In hemiplegia, arm is usually more severely affected than the leg while in tetraparesis or diplegia, lower extremities are usually more affected than the upper.

For assessment of trunk muscles, ask the patient to sit up from supine position without taking support of his arms. When he tries to sit up, watch the umbilicus, whether it deviates upwards, downwards or sidewards (Beevor's sign) and whether any portion of abdomen baloons out. By using various tricks and innovations, test the strength of group of muscles used to execute movements of flexion, extension, adduction, abduction and rotation at various joints beginning from the proximal and going towards the distal joints (Table 14.10). Some of the important individual muscles can be tested as follows:

a. Ask the child to elevate or shrug the shoulders (trapezius).
b. Ask the patient to abduct the arms to horizontal position (deltoid, C5, C6).
c. Ask the patient to flex the elbow with forearm supinated and palm facing upwards (biceps, C5, C6).

TABLE 14.9 Types of spastic cerebral palsy

Hemiplegia. Ipsilateral arm and leg are affected, arm is usually worse affected than the leg.

Diplegia. Both legs are predominantly affected while arms are relatively spared.

Quadriplegia. All the four extremities are affected, legs are worse affected than the arms.

Monoplegia. Only one extremity is affected which is usually the upper extremity. The condition is suspected when infant uses only one arm (hand preference).

TABLE 14.10 Movements at different joints

- *Neck*: Flexion, extension, side ways, and rotation
- *Shoulder*: Abduction, adduction, flexion, and extension
- *Elbow*: Flexion and extension
- *Wrist*: Flexion and extension of the wrist, pronation and supination of the forearm
- *Fingers*: Abduction, adduction of the fingers, apposition of thumb and little finger, and hand grip
- *Trunk muscles*: Flexion extension, lateral bending
- *Hips*: Flexion, extension, abduction, and adduction
- *Knees*: Flexion and extension
- *Ankle*: Dorsiflexion and plantar flexion, inversion and eversion
- *Toes*: Flexion and extension

---

d. Ask the child to extend the arm against resistance (triceps, C7, C8).

e. With the patient sitting at the edge of table, ask him to raise the leg to extend the knee (quadriceps, L2, L3, L4).

f. Patient lies in lateral decubitus and is asked to flex the knee and abduct the hip of superior leg (gluteus medius, L4, L5, S1).

g. Patient lies prone with both the knees flexed and is asked to lift the hips off the bed (gluteus maximus, L5, S1, S2).

h. Patient lies supine and is asked to push down examiner's palm with sole of the foot (gastrocnemius and soleus, L5, S1, S2).

i. Patient lies supine and is asked to dorsiflex the foot against resistance (tibialis anterior, L4, L5, S1).

j. Paralysis of respiratory muscles is characterized by rapid shallow breathing, weak voice or cry, inability to count beyond 10 with a single breath, anxious look and cyanosis. Paradoxical breathing, i.e. retraction of abdomen with each inspiration is suggestive of diaphragmatic paralysis which is often associated with paralysis of deltoid muscles because of identical spinal innervation (C5, C6). In phrenic nerve injury, paradoxical inward movement of ipsilateral abdominal wall occurs with inspiration due to paralysis of diaphragm. The umbilicus moves upwards towards the involved side which is called "belly dancer's sign".

The muscle power is graded as shown in **Table 14.11**.

In *hysterical paralysis*, child makes little effort to execute a movement as evidenced by positive Hoover's sign. The patient lies on his back and examiner puts one hand under the heel of the normal side. The child is asked to elevate the apparently paralyzed leg keeping the knee extended. In genuine hemiplegia, while patient is attempting to raise the paralyzed limb, there is counterpressure from the normal limb. There is no counterpressure or any muscle wasting in hysterical paralysis.

7. **Coordination** Incoordination is pathognomonic of cerebellar dysfunction. The coordination cannot be tested unless child has fair degree of muscle power. Infant's coordination can be tested by offering him small objects or toys by playful interaction.

   (a) *Finger-nose test* is done with eyes open and closed **(Figure 14.29)**. Each arm in turn is drawn out to full abduction and child is asked to alternately touch the tip of his nose and examiner's finger (which is moved to different positions) with the help of tip of his index finger. Look for intention tremors and past pointing (dysmetria).

   (b) *Dysdiadochokinesia*. Inability to perform alternating movements with speed and precision, e.g. supination–pronation

TABLE 14.11 Grading of muscle power

Muscle power	Grade
No flicker or visible muscle contraction	0
Flicker present due to visible muscle contraction	1
Movement of joint possible with gravity eliminated	2
Movement of joint possible against gravity	3
Movement of joint possible against gravity and some resistance	4
Normal full power	5

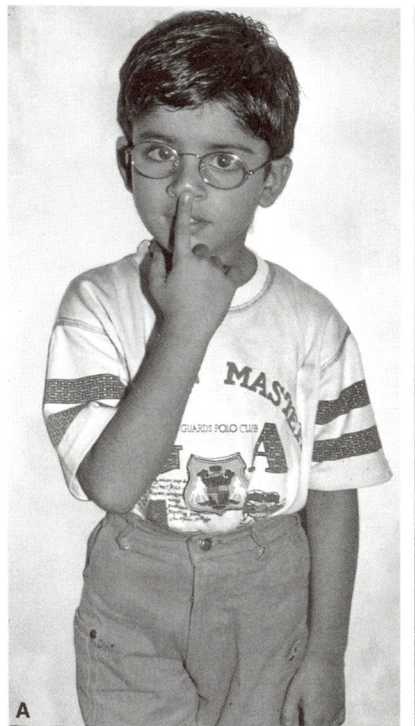
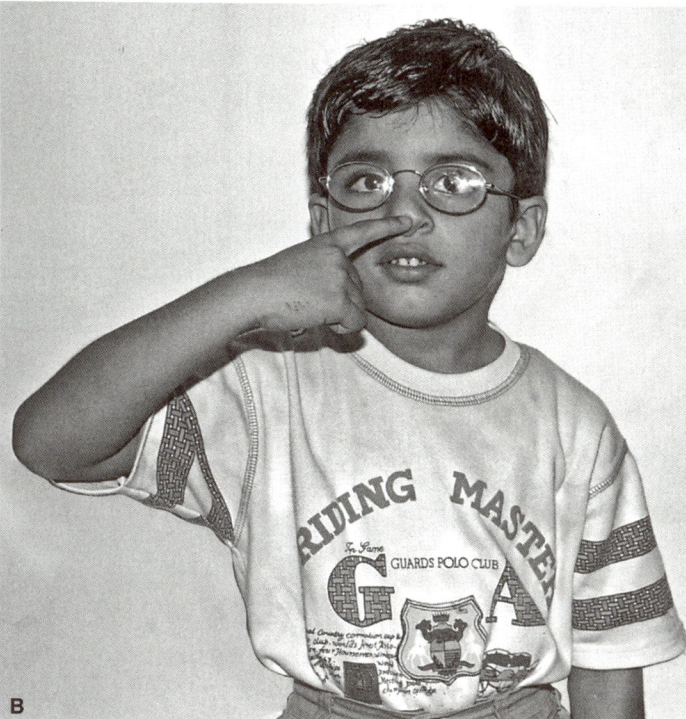

Figure 14.29A and B Finger-nose test. (A) Incorrect method, (B) Correct method. The arm must be drawn out in full abduction away from the plane of the body before touching tip of the nose.

movements, clapping, slapping the thigh with the palm and back of the hand alternately, rapid touching of thumb and little fingers on both sides, etc. Normally children above 5 years of age are able to execute rapid alternate movements with ease and speed.

(c) *Handwriting* record is useful for follow-up to assess the improvement. Ask the patient to draw a line between two converging lines, thread a needle or bead, draw a person, tie shoe laces, etc.

(d) *Rebound phenomenon.* Try to extend the patient's elbow against his biceps contraction and resistance. When wrist is suddenly released, the hand would jerk back suddenly and may hit his face. Positive rebound test is suggestive of cerebellar lesion.

(e) *Heel-knee test* for lower limbs is equivalent of finger-nose test in the upper limbs. In addition, ask the patient to lie in a prone position and maintain his both legs flexed at right angle at the knees. Observe how long the legs can be kept without fatigue and tremors.

(f) *Romberg's sign.* It is not a cerebellar sign but is used to assess loss of position sense (sensory ataxia) in the legs. The patient is asked to stand with feet close together. He is then asked to close the eyes. If Romberg's sign is positive, as soon as the eyes are closed, the patient becomes unsteady and begins to sway and may even fall. The sign is positive in patients with tabes dorsalis and sensory neuropathy.

(g) *Gait*. Ask the patient to "tandem walk" along a straight line with the heel of one foot touching the toes of the other. Make the child walk around a chair, observe his balance on sudden bending of trunk or while taking sudden turn on walking.

8. *Deep tendon reflexes* There are involuntary contractions of muscles when their tendon is tapped with a reflex hammer which causes brisk stretch of the muscles. Tendon reflexes are exaggerated in patients with pyramidal lesion while they are sluggish or absent, if lower motor neurons or muscles are diseased. In muscle disease, tendon reflexes are diminished or absent in accordance with severity of muscle weakness. The patient should be relaxed and free from anxiety or tension when deep jerks are elicited. The attention of the infant should be diverted by offering him a toy or key ring. Look for movements of the limb and visible contraction of the muscle. The spinal segments involved in various deep tendon jerks are given in Table 14.12.

Jaw jerk is elicited by asking the child to relax and open his mouth slightly. The examiner places his index finger on the midpoint of the child's chin and taps it gently with a reflex hammer (Figure 14.30). Easily elicitable jaw jerk is indicative of pyramidal involvement above the level of pons. Exaggerated jaw jerk in a child with evidences of pyramidal involvement in all the limbs indicates that lesion must be higher than the cervical spine. It is commonly seen in patients with pseudobulbar palsy, motor neuron disease and disseminated sclerosis. The techniques for elicitation of other deep tendon jerks are illustrated in Figures 14.31 to 14.37. In newborn babies and infants, middle finger can be used (instead of reflex hammer) to elicit the deep tendon jerks. Deep tendon jerks are rather brisk during infancy. When knee jerk is elicited on one side, crossed adductor

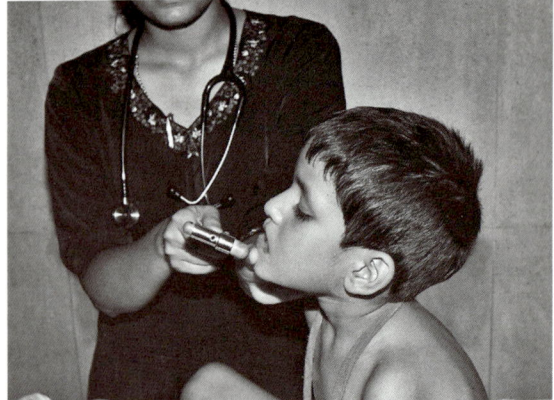

Figure 14.30 Jaw jerk. Refer to the text for details.

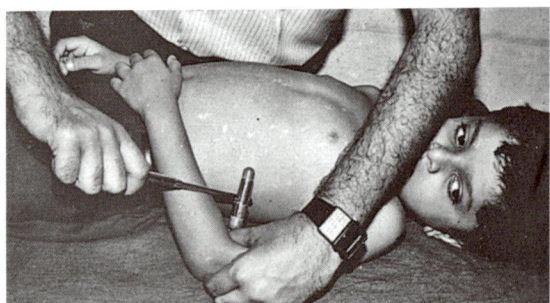

Figure 14.31 Biceps jerk. Thumb or index finger of left hand is placed over the tendon of biceps muscle and tapped with a hammer. Look for flexion of elbow and visible contraction of biceps. For elicitation of all deep tendon jerks, there should be free and easy movements at the wrist joint of the examiner while using a percussion hammer.

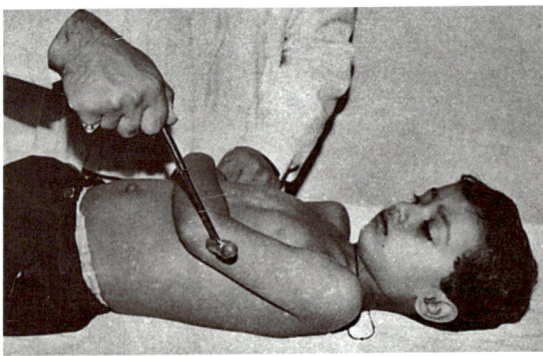

Figure 14.32 Triceps jerk. Elbow is flexed over the chest and tendon of triceps muscle is tapped just above the elbow. Look for extension of elbow and visible contraction of triceps muscle.

TABLE 14.12 Spinal root location of deep tendon jerks	
Reflex	Segmental level
Jaw jerk	Pons
Biceps jerk	C5, C6
Triceps jerk	C7, C8
Supinator or radial jerk	C5, C6
Knee jerk	L3, L4
Ankle jerk	L5, S1, S2

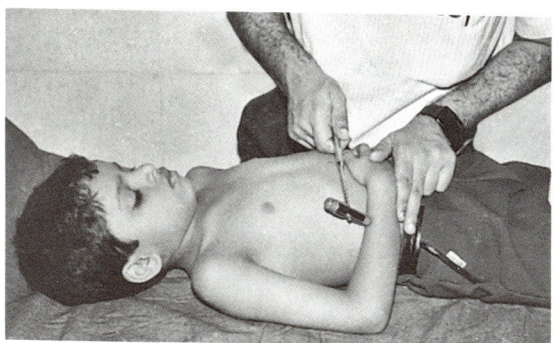

Figure 14.33 Supinator jerk. Tapping of the lower and outer end of forearm is followed by pronation and flexion of forearm and visible contraction of brachioradialis.

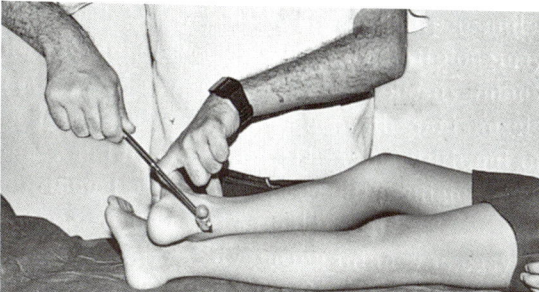

Figure 14.36 Ankle jerk. The leg is externally rotated and knee is slightly flexed to place the foot over the leg. Tapping of tendo-Achilles is followed by plantar flexion which is appreciated by the left hand placed under the sole. There is visible contraction of gastrocnemius muscle.

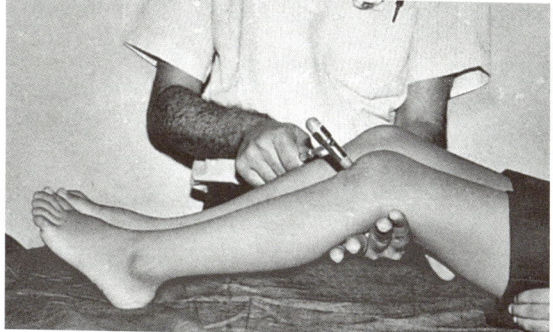

Figure 14.34 Knee jerk. Both knees are semiflexed and supported over the hands or forearm of left upper limb of the examiner. Tapping just below the patella is followed by sudden extension at the knee and visible contraction of quadriceps. Divert child's attention or use reinforcement by asking the child to interlock the flexed fingers of the two hands and pull one against the other. Knee jerk can also be elicited after making the child sit near the edge of a table with both legs hanging freely.

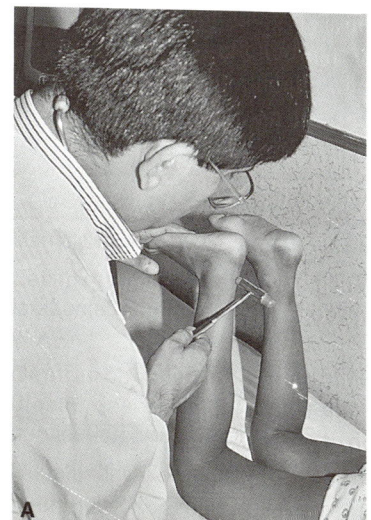

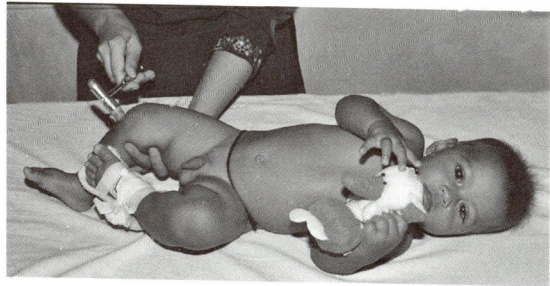

Figure 14.35 Knee jerk. Infant can be offered a key ring or a toy while elicting the knee jerk to divert his attention in order to elicit his cooperation.

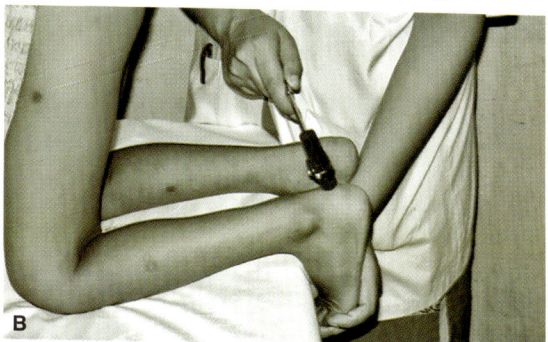

Figure 14.37A and B Alternative methods for elicitation of ankle jerk. (A) The child lies prone and knees are flexed to 90°; (B) The child kneels over the chair or table with feet hanging beyond the edge of the chair or table.

response may be obtained in normal infants. The reacting muscle should be palpated as well as observed for the movement produced. Toe jerks can be elicited in infants by tapping the base or ball of the big toe of the foot. Brisk flexion of toes may be seen in infants with cerebral palsy and progressive degenerative brain disease (Rossolimo sign).

When deep tendon jerks are sluggish, try to elicit them after diverting child's attention or re-enforcement by using Jendrassik maneuver (Figure 14.38). The deep tendon jerks are sluggish or absent when lower motor neurons are involved. In Guillaine-Barré syndrome, the tendon jerks are usually sluggish or absent except when there is acute motor axonal neuropathy (AMAN) when deep tendon jerks are retained and may even be brisk. When deep tendon jerks are exaggerated, look for sustained (at least 8–10 jerks) knee jerks and ankle clonus which are elicited by sudden jerky stretching of tendons (Figures 14.39 and 14.40).

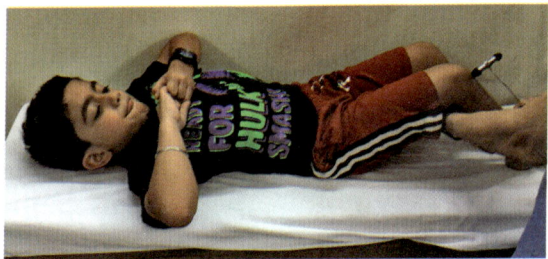

Figure 14.38 Jendrassik maneuver. The child is asked to lock the hands and pull them apart to divert his attention, while deep tendon jerks are being elicited. Alternatively, the child can be asked to clench his teeth.

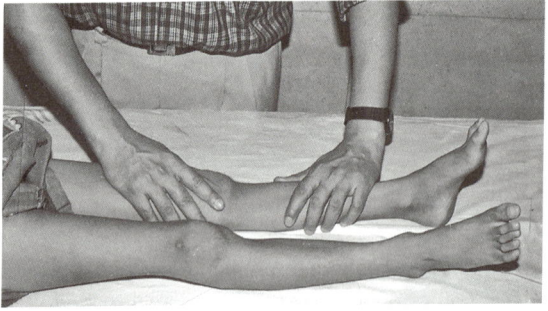

Figure 14.39 Patellar clonus. The patella is held between the thumb and fingers and suddenly pushed towards the foot with a sudden jerk.

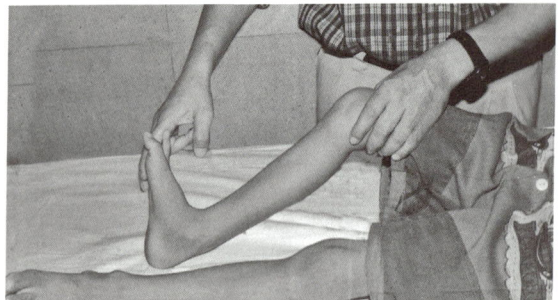

Figure 14.40 Ankle clonus. Knee is lightly flexed and ankle is dorsiflexed with a sudden jerk.

The deep tendon jerks are charted in the file as depicted in Figure 14.41. The tendon jerks are graded as given in Table 14.13.

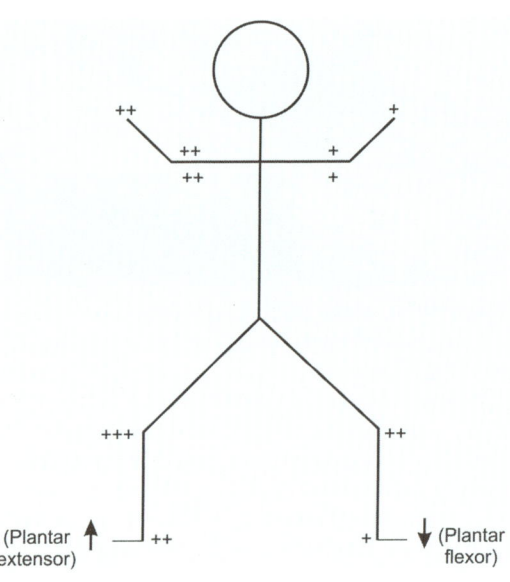

Figure 14.41 Method for diagrammatic recording of deep tendon jerks in the patient's record file.

TABLE 14.13 Grading of tendon reflexes	
Absent even with reinforcement	0
Sluggish	+
Normal	++
Brisk*	+++
Exaggerated and associated with clonus	++++

*Brisk or hyperactive tendon jerks may be associated with or without response in the muscles of adjacent joints or crossed response to the other side.

SENSATIONS

The precise evaluation of sensations is difficult in young children. There are two groups of sensory nerve fibers in the spinal cord. Posterior column carries the information from the same side of the body for stereognosis, i.e. sense of position, weight, shape, size, and vibration. The anterior and lateral columns carry the sensory information for touch, pain and temperature from the opposite side of the body through anterior and lateral spinothalamic tracts. A unilateral lesion of the spinal cord, therefore, results in loss of pain and thermal sensibility below the level of lesion on the opposite side of the body, while on the side of the lesion, in addition to spastic paralysis, there is loss of sense of position, size and vibration (Brown-Sequard syndrome). Look for anesthesia and ask for subjective features of hyperesthesia, i.e. excessive perception of pain and burning sensations wherein child may not tolerate touch or even the weight of the bed sheet. Paresthesias, i.e. sensation of numbness, tingling and crawling of ants is a recognized feature of Guillain-Barré syndrome, systemic lupus erythematosus, transverse myelopathy, tick paralysis, conus medullaris and cauda equina syndromes, Refsum disease and peripheral neuropathy.

Figure 14.42 shows sensory innervation of the skin (dermatomes) over the anterior and posterior aspects of the body.

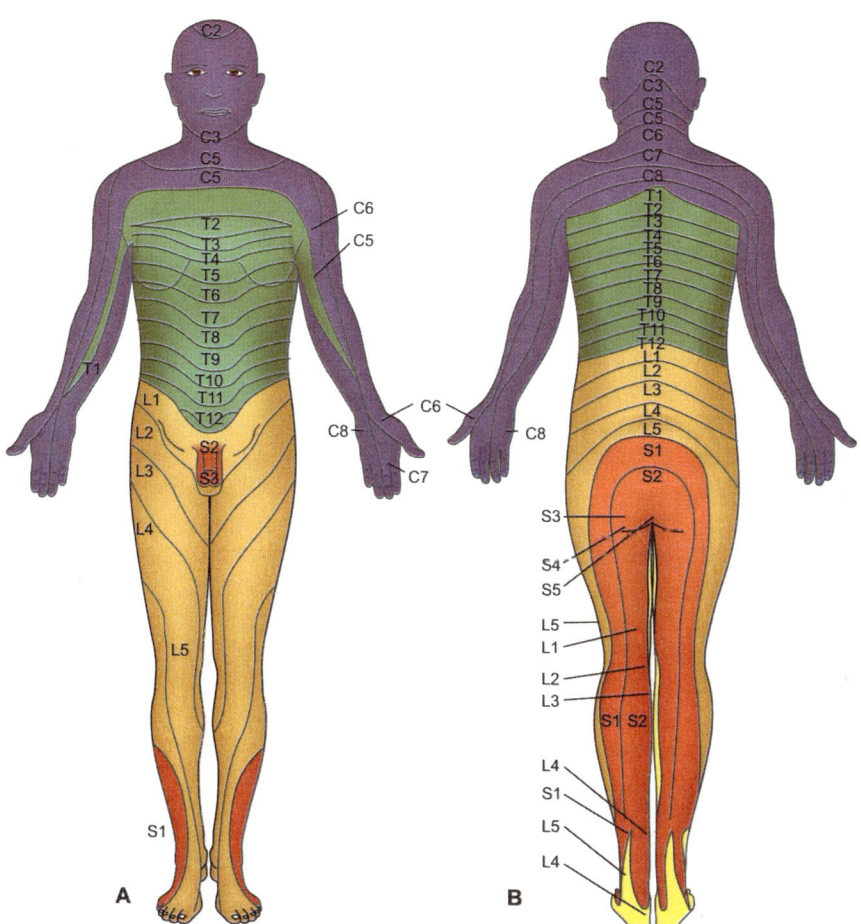

Figure 14.42A and B Sensory innervation of skin (dermatomes). (A) Anterior aspect, (B) Posterior aspect of the body.

1. ***Superficial sensations*** Assess cotton touch, pain (broken wooden spatula or toothpick) and temperature (hot and cold water in metal tubes). Avoid use of sharp pins and needles. Congenital analgia is a recognized feature of congenital indifference to pain, congenital sensory neuropathy, Lesch-Nyhan syndrome, familial dysautonomia, autism spectrum disorder, and Prader-Willi syndrome. These children do not cry when vaccine shots are given and may cause self-mutilation of their fingers or toes.

2. ***Deep sensations*** Sense of pressure, sense of position, sense of movements and vibration sense (128 Hz) are tested. They are impaired in the lower extremities in children with Friedreich ataxia.

3. ***Cortical sensations*** The following signs are useful to assess the loss of cortical sensations.
   (a) *Two-point discrimination.* Two pin pricks up to 1 cm apart with the help of a divider can be normally appreciated.
   (b) *Sensory inattention.* Two mirror spots on the two sides are simultaneously pricked. The patient may not feel the prick on the affected side. When proximal and distal (cheek and hand) parts of the body are touched simultaneously, the patient with parietal lobe lesion may not recognise the distal stimulus due to extinction.
   (c) *Astereognosis.* The child is unable to identify an object by touch (with eyes closed), due to inability to appreciate shape, texture and weight.
   (d) *Graphesthesia.* There is inability to appreciate the figures, and shapes drawn with a pen on the palm and sole of the affected side.

SUPERFICIAL REFLEXES

1. ***Corneal or conjunctival reflex (5th and 7th cranial nerves)*** Touching of cornea or bulbar conjunctiva with a cotton wick is followed by prompt closure of the eye. Ask the child to look in one direction and approach the bulbar conjunctiva from the other side. When sensory reflex arc is disrupted (5th nerve damage), there will be no response from either lid when the affected side is stimulated, and a normal response from both sides when the normal side is stimulated.

2. ***Abdominal reflexes (D6–D12)*** Stroke gently, with a blunt pencil or a key, the four quadrants of the abdomen from periphery towards the midline (Figure 14.43). The underlying muscles in the quadrants would contract and the umbilicus moves in that direction. Abdominal fat of infants may interfere with the response. Avoid too firm pressure hich will elicit deep abdominal reflexes instead. The loss of abdominal reflexes (along with exaggerated deep tendon jerks in the lower limbs) is suggestive of pyramidal lesion above D6 level.

3. ***Cremasteric reflex (L1, L2)*** Stroke the medial aspect of upper thigh and watch for ipsilateral contraction of cremaster muscle. It is usually lost in patients with pyramidal lesion above the level of L1. It is normally exaggerated in infants and may remain intact even when there is a pyramidal lesion. The cremasteric reflex may be absent, if testes are undescended or already retracted and in a case of torsion of testis.

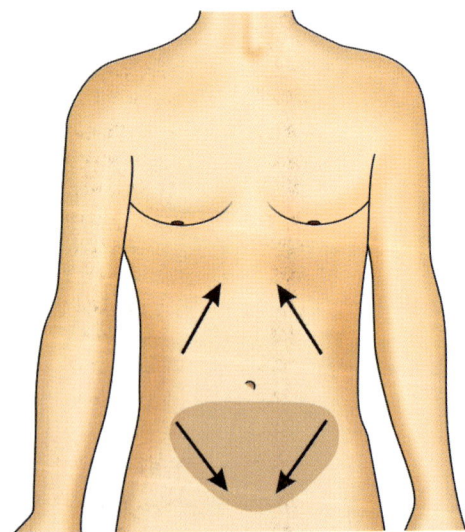

Figure 14.43 Sites and direction of stimuli to elicit the abdominal reflexes.

4. *Anal reflex (S3, S4)* Perianal area is stroked and anal response observed. Anal tone can be assessed by inserting a finger into the anal canal.
5. *Plantar reflex or Babinski response (S1, S2)* The plantar surface of the foot is scratched with thumb's nail, match stick, key or any semi-sharp object along the lateral border of the sole, from heel forwards crossing over the distal ends of the metatarsals towards the base of the great toe. Younger is the child, lighter should be the stimulus. The response may be extensor (positive Babinski) with extension or dorsiflexion of great toe and fanning of small toes, flexor (normal), equivocal or withdrawal (Figure 14.44). In infants up to two years of age, plantar response may be normally extensor on both sides and is associated with eversion of foot and dorsiflexion of ankle. Unilateral extensor plantar response is pathological even during infancy and is suggestive of pyramidal lesion. Extensor plantar response is diagnostic of pyramidal lesion above the level of S1. In addition to conventional technique of elicting plantar response, the following additional techniques may be used to elicit plantar reflex:
   (a) *Oppenheim's sign.* Apply firm pressure over tibia from above downwards to elicit the plantar response.

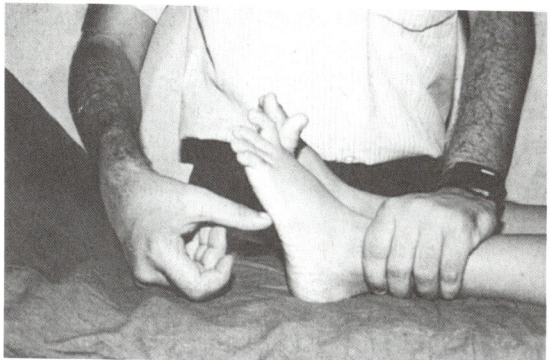

Figure 14.44 Plantar reflex. Typical extensor plantar or positive Babinski response. Refer to the text for details.

   (b) *Chaddock's sign.* Scratch around the lateral malleolus.
   (c) *Gordon's sign.* Firm squeeze of muscles of calf is followed by plantar response.
   (d) *Shaeffer's sign* Achilles tendon is firmly squeezed by the examiners' thumb and index finger to elicit plantar response.
   (e) *Rossolimo sign.* Tap the solar aspect of foot proximal to the big toe (ball of foot). Normally, there is no response. In a pyramidal tract lesion when deep tendon jerks are exaggerated, all the toes are flexed when solar eminence is tapped (Figure 14.45A and B).

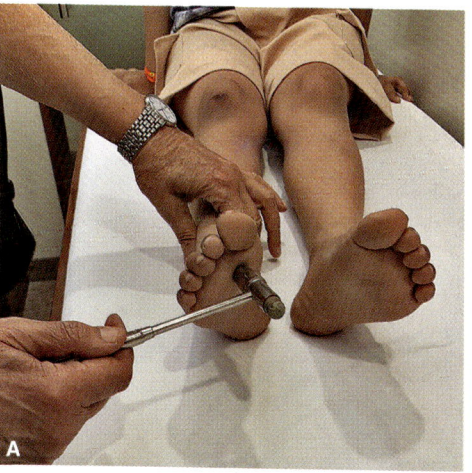
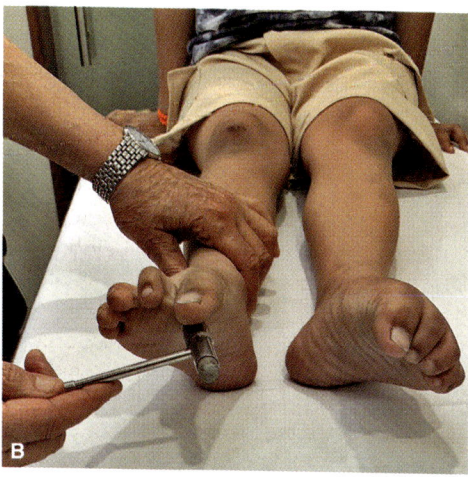

Figure 14.45A and B Rossolimo sign or great-toe reflex. (A) When ball of the big toe is tapped, normally there is no response. (B) When there is brisk flexion of toes with flexion at the ankle, knee and hip joint, it has the same significance as exaggerated tendon reflexes and extensor plantar response.

(f) *Hoffmann's sign* is equivalent of Babinski in the upper limbs. The patient is asked to stretch his hand towards the examiner with palm facing downwards. The middle phalanx of the middle finger of the patient is grasped with the index finger and thumb of examiner's hand (Figure 14.46A and B). A sharp snap or flick is given to the terminal phalanx and nail of patient's middle finger with the thumb of examiner's right hand. Sudden adduction of patient's thumb and flexion of other fingers is indicative of pyramidal lesion above C7.

(g) *Wartenberg's sign.* The child is asked to supinate his hand and flex the fingers like a claw. The examiner locks his flexed fingers with the patient and exerts resistance. Normally, the thumb extends but its terminal phalanx may flex slightly. In pyramidal tract lesion, thumb adducts and flexes strongly towards the palm (Figure 14.47A and B).

6. *Glabellar tap reflex* Tapping of nasion is followed by blink response. The response normally disappears after 3 to 4 taps due to habituation. Persistent uninhibited glabellar tap response is suggestive of diffuse degenerative disorder of CNS.

7. *Palmomental reflex* Scratch or tap the thenar eminence of hand. There is no response normally. Contraction of the mentalis or orbicularis oris muscle on the ipsilateral side is indicative of bilateral frontal lobe lesion.

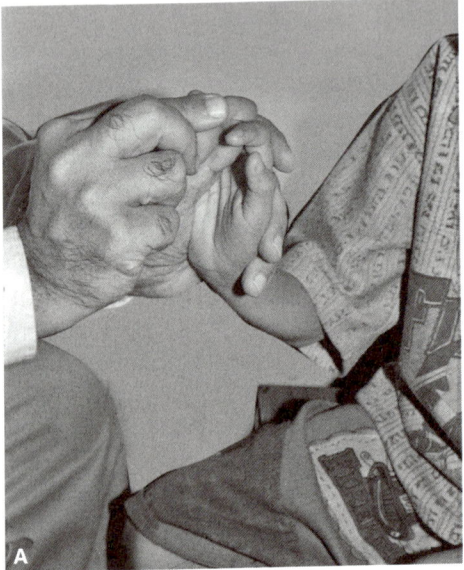

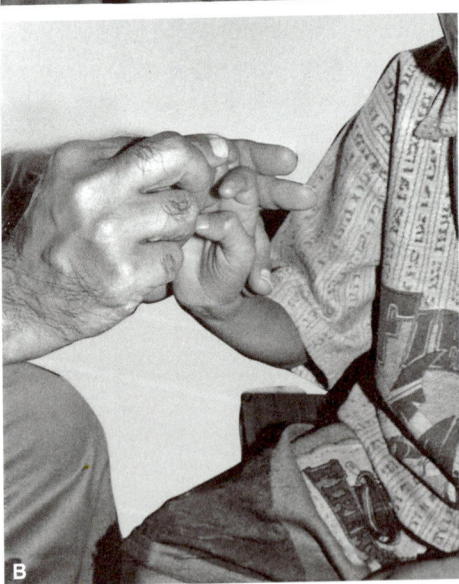

Figure 14.46A and B Hoffmann sign. (A) The sign is negative. (B) Adduction of patient's thumb is suggestive of pyramidal lesion above C7. Refer to text for details.

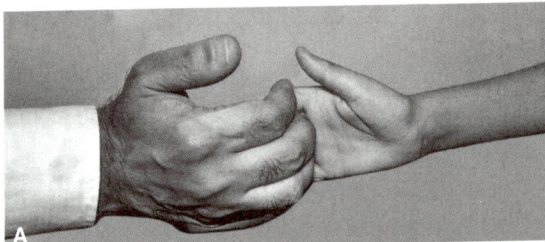

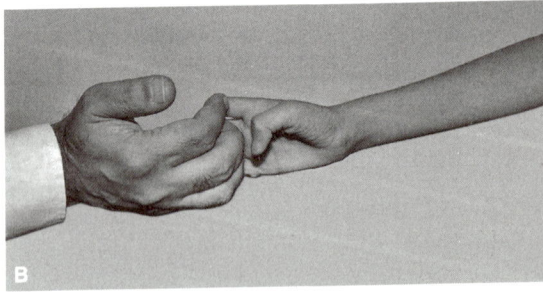

Figure 14.47A and B Wartenberg sign. (A) The sign is negative. (B) Adduction and flexion of the patient's thumb towards palm is suggestive of pyramidal lesion. Refer to text for details.

8. *Grasp reflex* The presence of unilateral grasp reflex in a child with CNS disorder is suggestive of lesion of frontal lobe on the opposite side.
9. *Ciliospinal reflex* When skin of the neck is pinched, the ipsilateral pupil dilates due to stimulation of reflex spinal arc through sympathetic trunk. The absence of ciliospinal reflex is suggestive of deep coma and is used as one of the criteria for brain death.

SPINE AND SPHINCTERS

They must be checked in every patient. The spinal cord ends at the level of lower border of body of first lumbar vertebra (lower border of L3 in the newborn) but meninges are carried as far down as second sacral vertebra. The spinal segments do not correspond numerically with the overlying vertebrae as shown in Table 14.14.

The 10th dorsal arch overlies L1 and L2, eleventh dorsal arch overlies L3 and L4 and twelfth dorsal arch overlies L5 and S1. All the sacral and coccygeal segments are located against the first lumbar vertebra. It should also be remembered that spine corresponds to the next vertebral body below.

The urinary bladder has three neural mechanisms; sacral parasympathetic (S2, S3) which is excitatory or motor, inhibitory sympathetic supply ending at L1, L2 and a voluntary excitatory corticospinal pathway. Cord lesions at the sacral level are associated with urinary retention. After a few weeks, reflex bladder evacuations occur in response to bladder distension.

Neurogenic bladder refers to dysfunction of the urinary bladder due to diseases of the central nervous system, autonomic nervous system or peripheral nerves involved in the control of micturition. Depending upon the site of injury or dysfunction, various types of neurogenic bladder are seen (Table 14.15).

Bowel involvement is usually characterized by constipation and retention of feces irrespective of the level of lesion. The lesion at the sacral level, however, is usually associated with relaxation of external rectal sphincter leading to fecal incontinence.

In diastematomyelia, a bony or fibrocartilaginous septum produces a sagittal division and transfixa-

TABLE 14.14 Identification of spinal segment in relation to the vertebral body

Vertebral body	Spinal segment
Cervical	Add 1
1st–6th Dorsal*	Add 2
7th–9th Dorsal	Add 3
10th Dorsal	L1, L2
11th Dorsal	L3, L4
12th Dorsal	L5 and sacral segments

*Dorsal or thoracic

TABLE 14.15 Clinical features of various types of neurogenic bladder

Type	Spastic or reflexic bladder (UMN)	Autonomous or flaccid bladder (LMN)	Sensory dysfunction of the bladder (LMN)
Site of injury	Corticospinal tract	Cauda equina	Peripheral nerves and afferent sensory limb of bladder spinal reflex
Nature of dysfunction	Bladder empties in response to stretching of the bladder wall (automatic) No inhibition for voiding	Paralysis of bladder musculature	Lack of bladder sensations for urination
Clinical features	Unpredictable and incomplete voiding Incontinence Frequency and urgency of micturition	Inability to void Retention Dribbling due to over-flow	No sensations to void Infrequent and incomplete voiding Large volume of residual urine

UMN: Upper motor neuron; LMN: Lower motor neuron

tion of the spinal cord or cauda equina. The clinical features include delay or difficulty in walking, an abnormal gait, weakness and atrophy of muscles of lower extremity, deformities of feet and urinary incontinence. The caudal regression syndrome is characterized by sacral agenesis with associated abnormalities like a neurogenic bladder, weakness of lower extremities, equinovarus deformities of feet and a frog-like posture. The developmental defect is more common in infants born to diabetic mothers. The salient clinical differences between extramedullary and intramedullary spinal tumors are shown in Table 14.16.

The involvement of lower end of spinal cord and distal spinal nerves produce characteristic syndromes. The conus medullaris syndrome involves T12–L2 spinal segments and is characterized by combined upper motor neuron and lower motor neuron features. The cauda equina (Latin for "horse tail") syndrome occurs due to involvement of spinal nerves and their rootlets extending from L2 through distal lumbar, sacral and coccygeal spinal nerves. It occupies a lumbar cistern, a subarachnoid space inferior to conus medullaris and is characterized primarily by lower motor neuron features (Table 14.17). The common etiological factors for these syndromes

TABLE 14.16 Differences between extramedullary and intramedullary spinal tumors

Features	Extramedullary	Intramedullary
▪ Root pain and spinal tenderness	Common	Rare
▪ Paresthesias	Rare and late	Common and early
▪ Muscle spasms	Common	Rare
▪ Sphincter disturbances	Late	Early
▪ Brown-Sequard syndrome due to hemisection of cord, i.e. ipsilateral motor and proprioceptive impairment and contralateral loss of pain and temperature	May occur	Rare
▪ Pyramidal signs	Prominent	May occur
▪ Sensory dissociation, i.e. there is loss of sensations of pain and temperature while touch is preserved	Absent	Common
▪ Muscle atrophy	Uncommon	Common
▪ Trophic changes	Uncommon	Common
▪ CSF changes due to spinal block	Common	Rare

TABLE 14.17 The salient differences between conus medullaris and cauda equina syndromes

Features	Conus medullaris syndrome	Cauda equina syndrome
Site of lesion	T12–L2 spinal segments	L2-coccygeal nerves
▪ Onset	Sudden and bilateral	Gradual, unilateral or bilateral
▪ Low back pain	Severe and chronic	Moderate and acute
▪ Radicular pain	Mild to moderate	Severe pain with radiation toward back of thighs due to sciatica.
▪ Dysfunction of sphincters	Urinary retention with overflow, atonic anal sphincter with constipation occurs early	Incontinence is common, while urinary retention occurs late.
▪ Sensory symptoms and signs	Symmetrical, bilateral tingling and numbness over perianal area. Sensory dissociation is common	Asymmetric sensory dysfunction involving saddle area. No sensory dissociation.
▪ Motor involvement	Symmetric spastic and/or hypotonic paresis or paralysis of lower limbs. Fasciculations may be present	Asymmetric hypotonic paraplegia with atrophy of muscles. No fasciculations.
▪ Deep tendon jerks	Normal or exaggerated with extensor plantars	Reduced or absent with flexor plantars.

include spinal birth defects, trauma, tumor, infection and disk herniation.

GAIT

Gait of the child should be closely observed to identify any abnormalities. The child should be asked to squat on the floor and watched as he gets up to the standing posture. Gower's sign, wherein child "climbs up his legs" to stand due to weakness of glutei maximi muscles is classically seen in children with Duchenne's muscular dystrophy. Other conditions with positive Gower's sign include centronuclear myopathy, myotonic dystrophy and various conditions associated with weakness of proximal muscles including Becker muscular dystrophy, dermatomyositis and Pompe disease. Difficulty in getting up from the squatting posture is also seen in children with polymyositis, poliomyelitis and Guillain-Barré syndrome. Ask the child to walk on heels and toes, skip on one foot, and climb upstairs. Children above 5 years of age are able to walk on their toes and hop. The ability to skip occurs by 7 years of age and tandem walking is achieved by 9 years. Gait is best evaluated when the child is unaware that he is being watched.

1. *Spastic gait (pyramidal lesion)* There is circumduction and lifting of the leg in the form of an arc at the hip. Hip is elevated on the affected side with slight dragging of the foot and scraping of toes (Figure 14.48).
2. *Stamping gait (posterior column lesion)* The foot is placed on the ground with a thud due to loss of sense of position.
3. *High stepping gait* High steps are taken due to foot drop to avoid tripping of toes. The patient walks cautiously while watching the floor intently. It is seen in children with peripheral neuropathy, poliomyelitis and progressive muscular atrophy.
4. *Ataxic gait or staggering gait or reeling gait (cerebellar lesion)* Patient walks like a drunkard man. The gait is unsteady and uncoordinated and child cannot walk in a straight line or around a chair. Friedreich's ataxia produces combined sensory and cerebellar ataxia.

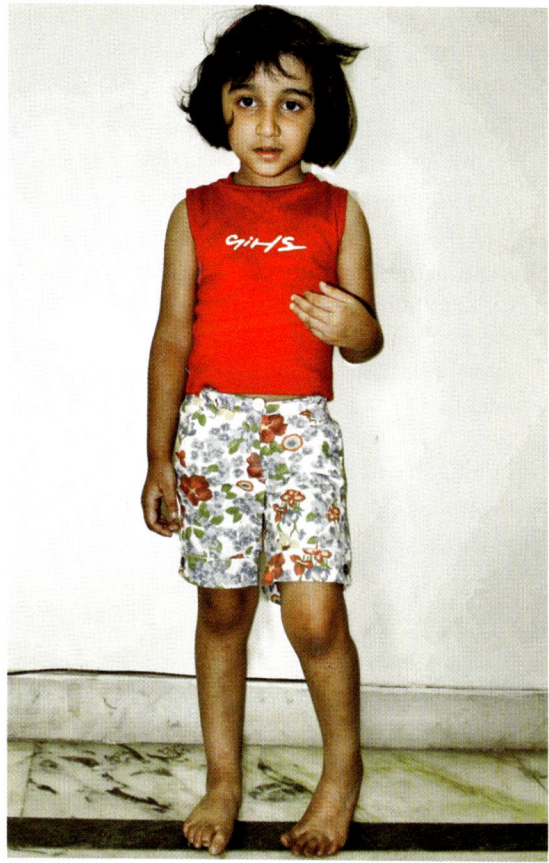

Figure 14.48 Typical stance of the child with hemiplegia on the left side.

5. *Festinent gait (Parkinsonism)* The patient walks with a short, stiff and shuffling steps. The arms do not swing during walking.
6. *Waddling gait* The waddling gait is like the gait of a duck. The trunk is tilted backwards, with an increase in lumbar lordosis, the feet are planted rather widely apart and the body sways from side-to-side as each step is taken. It is seen in patients with Duchenne's muscular dystrophy, bilateral congenital dislocation of hips, bilateral coxa vara (reduction of angle between the shaft and neck of the femur), achondroplasia, Morquio's disease, exstrophy of bladder (pelvic bones are widely separated), bilateral slipped femoral epiphyses, polymyositis, Engelmann's disease (progressive diaphyseal dysplasia) and myelodysplasia.

7. *Scissor gait* It is seen in children with cerebral diplegia due to bilateral adduction and contractures.
8. *Limping gait* may occur due to a variety of neuromuscular and orthopedic disorders of the lower limbs. Refer to Chapter 10 for causes of limping gait.
9. *Astasia abasia* occurs due to hysterical inability to stand and walk. The patient is ataxic and sways from the hips rather than ankles. The ataxia decreases when patient is not watched or attention is diverted by asking him to execute finger-nose test. The hysterical patient does not injure himself. He is not benefitted by holding the wall or furniture unlike a patient with organic ataxia.

CEREBELLAR SIGNS

1. *Muscle tone* is decreased. Power is normal but there is easy fatigability.
2. *Nystagmus* It is characterized by involuntary conjugate movements of the eyes which may be rhythmic (pendular) or non-rhythmic, with a fast and slow component. Nystagmus is defined by the direction of quick phase. It may occur spontaneously (vestibular) or induced by movements of the eyes. Ask the child to follow the movements of the examiner's index finger or a toy, which is quickly moved horizontally or up and down. Keep the finger or toy at the extreme position for a few seconds to see the direction of quick movement and whether nystagmus is transitory or persistent.

   Nystagmus may be horizontal, vertical, rotary or mixed. Coarse, slow, searching, pendular nystagmoid movements are seen in blind children. In cerebellar nystagmus, the fast component is towards the side of lesion. The nystagmoid movements become slow and coarse when eyes are turned towards the side of lesion. In contrast, the fast component of the nystagmus is towards the normal side in vestibular dysfunction and the nystagmus is enhanced when the patient looks in the direction of fast component.
3. Skew deviation of eyes may occur in acute cerebellar lesions. The eye towards the side of lesion is turned downwards and inwards.
4. *Incoordination*. Its presence is assessed by following tests:
   a. Finger-nose test
   b. Dysdiadochokinesia
   c. Ankle-knee test
   d. Handwriting
   e. Rebound phenomenon
   f. Romberg's sign is negative
5. Deep tendon jerks are pendular.
6. Speech is explosive and jerky with scanning of syllables.
7. *Gait is ataxic or reeling in character.* The patient has a tendency to fall towards the side of lesion. The minimal ataxia can be brought out by asking the patient to walk around a chair in both directions, taking sudden turn, sudden flexion of trunk, and by doing sits-stands. Trunkal ataxia is common among children due to involvement of vermis. Heel-to-toe walking and walking along a straight line are particularly difficult in these children. In midline posterior fossa or cerebellar vermis lesion (tonsillar herniation due to Arnold-Chiari malformation), no abnormalities of coordination in upper limbs are detected when patient is lying in bed. However, there will be gross ataxia on walking which should not be misdiagnosed as hysteria.

Autonomic Functions

The autonomic nervous system comprises of central (cortical region, amygdala, hypothalamic and brainstem nuclei) and peripheral (sympathetic thoracolumbar outflow and parasympathetic craniosacral outflow) components. Autonomic dysfunction is evidenced by instability and excessive fluctuations of vital signs, excessive or reduced sweating, areas of skin with blanching or blotchyness, inadequate or absent salivation or lacrimation and sphincteric disturbances. Record the pulse rate at rest and following 6 maximal deep breaths. In normal subjects, the pulse rate should fall by greater than 15 beats/min; while in autonomic dysfunction, pulse rate slows by less than 10 beats/min. In a patient with autonomic dysfunction, the systolic blood pressure may fall greater than 20 mm Hg on standing from recumbent position (orthostatic hypotension).

DIAGNOSIS AND LOCALIZATION OF A CNS DISORDER

Imaging technology (CT scan, MRI) has provided most reliable and non-invasive means for exact localization of the space occupying lesion and other disorders of the CNS. Nevertheless, attempt should be made to identify the following characterstics of the CNS disorder. In order to enhance the clinical acumen, the diagnosis based on clinical evaluation of CNS should be correlated with CT/MRI findings to augment the learning process and improve the clinical skills. The following clinical parameters are useful to identify the site and nature of CNS disorder.

1. Is disease acute or dramatic in onset, subacute or insidious?
2. Is the disorder stationary, progressive or showing slow or fast recovery?
3. Is it upper motor neuron or lower motor neuron disorder? (Table 14.18)
4. Is patient having spinal shock? Sudden and complete transection of spinal cord (traumatic or transverse myelitis) may produce transitory lower motor neuron features due to sudden loss of descending control on the lower motor neurons. There is dramatic onset of flaccid paralysis, areflexia, loss of sensations below the level of lesion, autonomic dysfunction and loss of bowel and bladder control. The state of spinal shock is gradually followed by classical features of upper motor neuron paralysis over a period of few days.
5. Are there any associated clinical features of raised intracranial tension?
6. Is the disease diffuse and generalized or localized to the specific area/s of central nervous system?
7. Is it primarily a white matter disease, gray matter disease or combined?
8. Summarize the positive CNS findings and their probable localization in the CNS. Figure 14.49 provides useful guidelines for localization of the probable site of lesion in the CNS on the basis of abnormal neurological findings and basic knowledge of neuroanatomy.
9. What is the probable nature of the disease and likely diagnostic possibilities? Is it a space occupying lesion, infective, metabolic

TABLE 14.18 Differences between upper and lower motor neuron paralysis

Clinical features	Upper motor neuron paralysis*	Lower motor neuron paralysis**
Power	Reduced	Markedly reduced
Distribution of muscle weakness	Diffuse and symmetrical	Patchy and asymmetrical
Muscle tone	Spasticity	Hypotonia or atonia
Muscle wasting	Minimal or absent	Significant
Deep tendon jerks	Brisk with clonus	Sluggish or absent
Plantars	Extensor	Flexor or absent
Convulsions or involuntary movements	May occur	Fasciculations may be seen
Reaction of degeneration	Absent	Present

*The lesion may be in the motor cortex, internal capsule, brainstem or spinal cord
**The lesion may be anywhere in the spinal reflex arc, i.e. the sensory root, anterior horn cell, anterior spinal root, peripheral motor or sensory nerve, terminal motor end plate or muscle itself.

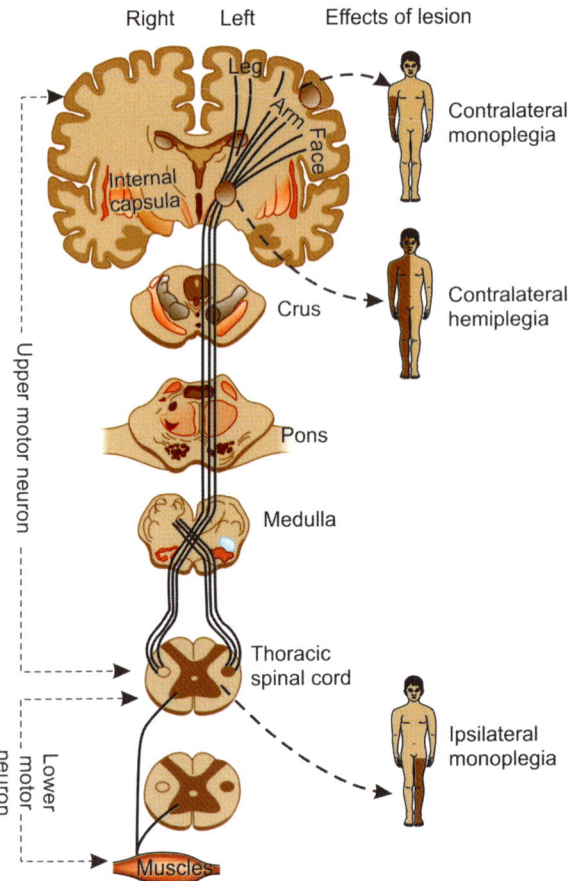

Figure 14.49 Diagram showing location of upper and lower motor neurons and effects of a lesion in different parts of the central nervous system.

or degenerative CNS disorder, vascular phenomenon, anoxic insult, toxic, traumatic, psychological, functional disorder or conduct disorder?

10. Advanced magnetic imaging techniques, like diffusion tensor imaging (DTI), functional MRI (fMRI), real-time MRI, positron emission tomography (PET), magnetic resonance angiography (MRA), MR perfusion (MRP) and MR spectroscopy (MRS) are available for localization and definitive diagnosis of a variety of CNS disorders.

During presentation of the case, the student is asked to summarize important findings of the history and physical examination, localizing neurological features, formulate a differential diagnosis, provide the most likely diagnosis, discuss diagnostic evaluation plan and provide a management protocol.

	Scheme for Presentation
General physical examination	General appearance, level of consciousness, nature of disability, examination of skull for size, shape, symmetry, swellings, anterior fontanel (flat, bulging, pulsatile or non-pulsatile), sutures, Macewen's sign, auscultation for bruit, and transillumination of skull. Examination of spine for deformities, Pott's disease, epidural abscess, primary or metastatic neoplasm, meningomyelocele, tuft of hair, sinus tract, and myelodysplasia. Look for typical facies, facial dysmorphism, evidences of neuroectodermal dysplasia, and abnormalities of teeth. Examine eyes for alignment, proptosis, corneal opacities, buphthalmos, cataracts, pupillary changes, and Kayser-Fleischer ring. Temperature, pulse, respiration, blood pressure (including Trousseau's sign). Anemia, cyanosis, jaundice, lymphadenopathy, hepatosplenomegaly and abdominal mass. Evidences of meningeal signs (neck rigidity, Kernig's sign, Brudzunski's sign, tripod sign, photophobia) and signs of raised intracranial tension, like enlargement of head size, sutural diastasis, bulging anterior fontanel, 6th nerve palsy, Macewen's sign, papilledema, herniation of hippocampus with unilateral dilated and fixed pupil and involvement of vital centers. Record handedness of the child.
Higher functions	Level of consciousness, orientation in time and place, memory (immediate, recent and past), emotional status, delusions and hallucinations, speech, brainstem automatic reflexes and cortical release reflexes.
Developmental screening	Developmental status before the onset of neurological symptoms, developmental age, developmental quotient and clinical grades of mental subnormality (normal, dull normal, educable in ordinary school, educable in a special school, trainable but not educable), status of special senses, i.e. vision and hearing.
Cranial nerves	Describe abnormal findings pertaining to involvement of cranial nerves, unilateral or bilateral, whether upper motor or lower motor neuron type.
Motor system	Describe findings in the upper limbs, trunk and lower limbs. Posture of limbs, abnormal movements, fasciculations and twitchings, wasting, trophic changes, muscle tone (normal, increased, spastic or rigid, decreased), power, nature of disability affecting daily routines of living, can he walk, stand or sit, getting up from supine or sitting position, strength in various groups of muscles, i.e. flexors, extensors, abductors, adductors and rotators and some important individual muscles. Is weakness affecting proximal or distal groups of muscles? Is it symmetrical or asymmetrical motor disability? Coordination (finger-nose test, dysdiadochokinesia, handwriting, rebound phenomenon, heel-knee test, gait, etc.) deep tendon jerks (normal, sluggish, absent, brisk, exaggerated, with or without ankle and knee clonus). Describe gait, walking around a chair, sit-stands, walking upstairs, toe walking, heel walking, Romberg's sign, etc.
Cerebellar signs	Decrease in muscle tone, nystagmus, skew deviation of eyes, incoordination, ataxic gait, and pendular jerks.
Sensations	Superficial, deep and cortical sensations.
Superficial reflexes	Corneal or conjunctival reflex, abdominal reflexes, anal reflex, plantar reflex (flexor, extensor or positive Babinski response, withdrawal response, equivocal). Hoffmann's sign, glabeller tap reflex, palmomental reflex, grasp reflex, ciliospinal reflex.
Autonomic dysfunction	Sphincteric disturbances, instability and wide fluctuations of vital signs, postural hypotension, changes in salivation, lacrimation and sweating.

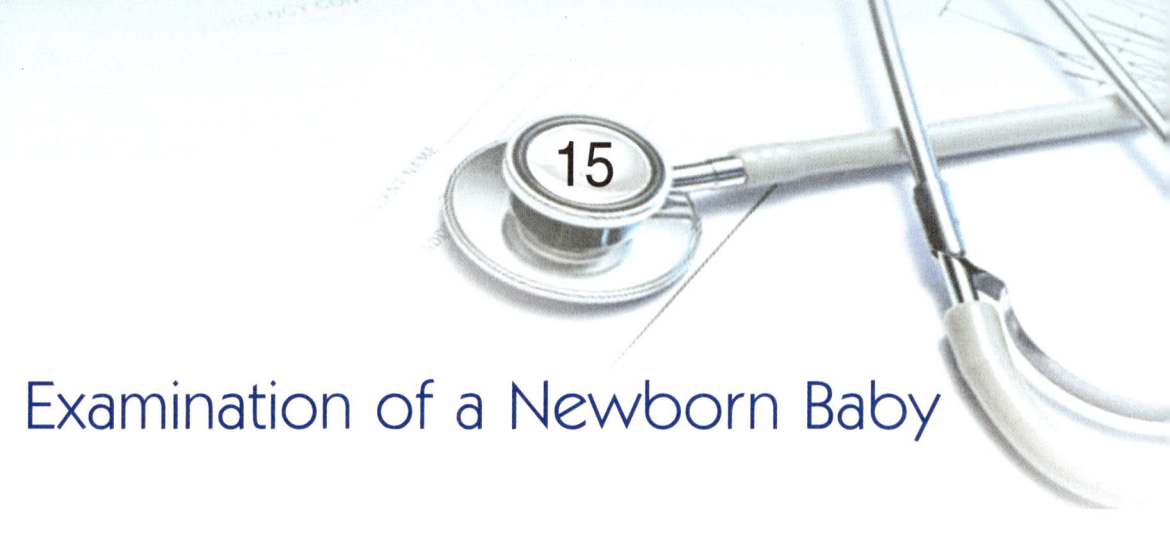

15
Examination of a Newborn Baby

HISTORY

Just as children are not mini-adults, the neonates are not mini-children. They have unique health problems and a different clinical approach is followed for their clinical evaluation. It must be remembered that a newborn baby is around 9 months old at birth unless prematurely born. Neonatology is not a system-limited speciality, it deals with all the systems of a newborn baby (up to 28 days of life). A detailed history regarding diseases suffered by the mother and drugs taken during pregnancy should be elicited (Table 15.1).

Basic Indicators

Health and wellbeing of a fetus is dependent upon the health and nutrition of the mother (not the father!) because she is both the seed as well as the soil wherein baby is nurtured for nine months. Ask whether it was a natural pregnancy or *in vitro* fertilization (IVF) with or without surrogacy. The date of birth, gestational age and birth weight should be recorded. The gestational age is calculated from the first day of the last menstrual period till the date of birth and is expressed in completed weeks and days. For example, gestation of 32 completed week plus 6 days is expressed as $32^{6}/_{7}$ weeks. The education, occupation and economic status of parents should be enquired. Age of the mother is important because young mothers (<18 years) are likely to produce low birth weight babies and have an increased risk of delivery

TABLE 15.1 Review of maternal and perinatal history

Family history
History of hereditary, metabolic, chromosomal and developmental disorders.

Maternal history
Duration of marriage, age, blood group, chronic illnesses, like diabetes mellitus, hypertension, renal disease, cardiac disease, lung disease, endocrinal disorder, systemic lupus erythematosus, bleeding disorder, CNS or psychological disorder, sexually transmitted diseases including herpes and HIV, TORCH screening, etc.

Previous obstetrical history
Gravidity, parity, abortions, stillbirths, neonatal deaths (with possible causes), prematurity, LBW or growth retarded babies, obstructed labor, cesarean section, congenital malformations and history of blood transfusion.

Current pregnancy
Natural pregnancy or IVF, gestational age, weight gain, excessive vomiting, bleeding, polyhydramnios/oligohydramnios, ultrasound examination, diagnostic and therapeutic procedures done during pregnancy. History of pregnancy-induced hypertension, pre-eclampsia, infections (UTI, diarrhea/dysentery, malaria and tuberculosis), surgery, drugs of abuse and medications (hormones, glucocorticoids, tocolytic agents and antibiotics) during pregnancy.

Labor and delivery
Fetal distress, presentation, mode of delivery, duration of rupture of membranes, duration of labor, amnionitis, amniotic fluid (volume, clear or meconium-stained), anesthesia/analgesia given during labor. Apgar score, resuscitation required and any abnormalities of placenta.

hazards while elderly mothers (>35 years) are at an increased risk to have babies with congenital malformations and chromosomal disorders.

Previous Obstetrical History

The gravidity (number of all conceptions including abortions, stillbirths, etc. with possible causes) and parity (number of live births) should be recorded. The interval between successive pregnancies and their outcome should be enquired. History of recurrent abortions and stillbirths is suggestive of incompetent cervical os, diabetes mellitus, syphilis and Rh-isoimmunization. Gestational maturity, birth weight, congenital malformations; obstructed labor, and mode of delivery of previous babies should be recorded. The neonatal course, unusual manifestations and outcome of previous babies should be ascertained.

Prepregnancy Health Status

Maternal systemic disorders, like heart disease, hypertension, bronchial asthma, chronic renal disease, tuberculosis and anemia, are associated with increased risk of abortions, stillbirths, intrauterine growth retardation, premature births and increased perinatal mortality rate. History of maternal endocrinal disorders, such as diabetes mellitus, thyrotoxicosis, myxedema and hyperparathyroidism should be asked. Systemic lupus erythematosus may be associated with complete heart block in the fetus. Chronic undernutrition of the mother during childhood and adolescence leads to short stature (<145 cm) and low adult weight (<40 kg) which are associated with increased risk of low birth weight babies. History of sexually transmitted diseases including herpes, syphilis and HIV should be checked. Rhesus blood group should be identified because of potential risk of Rh-isoimmunization, if Rh-negative mother is carrying an Rh-positive fetus. Tetanus toxoid and rubella vaccination status should be checked.

Course of Pregnancy

The adequacy and quality of antenatal care received should be ascertained. First trimester of pregnancy is characterized by embryogenesis. Diseases suffered and drugs taken during current pregnancy should be recorded. Ask for history suggestive of maternal rubella, cytomegalovirus and toxoplasmosis which are manifested by fever, skin rash and posterior cervical lymphadenopathy. Ask history of petechiae or thrombocytopenia during pregnancy. The abnormalities reported on antenatal ultrasound scans should be recorded. In a malformed or sick baby, a detailed history of medications taken during pregnancy should be recorded because they may produce unusual clinical manifestations in the newborn baby (Table 15.2).

Maternal ABO and rhesus blood type, indirect Coombs' titer (if mother is Rh-negative), hemogram, VDRL and whenever indicated, carrier status for hepatitis B virus and HIV and TORCH screening should be checked. The diagnostic and therapeutic procedures undertaken during pregnancy should be recorded.

Dietary intake, especially during second half of pregnancy, is crucial to ensure optimal growth of the fetus. During an uncomplicated pregnancy, most Indian mothers gain between 6 and 10 kg body weight. History of pregnancy-induced hypertension with or without urinary abnormalities is associated with placental dysfunction, intrauterine growth retardation, perinatal hypoxia, and birth asphyxia. Ask for history of bleeding during pregnancy whether due to abruptio placentae or placenta previa. The quantity of amniotic fluid should be checked. *Oligohydramnios* may be associated with prolonged rupture of membranes and chorioamnionitis. It is associated with placental dysfunction, postmaturity, renal agenesis, polycystic or multicystic dysplastic kidneys, and obstructive uropathy. It is commonly associated with toxemia of pregnancy and maternal medications with prostaglandin inhibition and ACE inhibition. *Polyhydramnios* (amniotic fluid >2 liters) is associated with maternal diabetes mellitus, syphilis, pre-eclamptic toxemia and fetal congenital malformations, such as open neural tube defects, anencephaly, ectopia vesicae, gastroschisis, esophageal atresia, duodenal/jejunal atresia, diaphragmatic hernia, Down syndrome, twins and hydrops fetalis. Meconium-stained liquor amnii in

TABLE 15.2 Common neonatal disorders and malformations due to maternal medications during pregnancy

Neonatal disorders	Drugs
1. Congenital malformations	Thalidomide, haloperidol, progestin-estrogen combination, synthetic progestins, diethyl stilbestrol, clomiphene, valproic acid, diphenyle hydantoin, trimethadione, carbamazepine, lithium carbonate, isotretinoin, finasteride, tetracyclines, streptomycin, cortisone, irradiation, imipramine, antimitotic agents, sedatives, warfarin, quinine vitamins A and D, live vaccines, etc.
2. Vitamin K-dependent bleeding manifestations	Phenobarbitone, primidone, phenytoin, carbamazepine, salicylates, dicumarol derivatives.
3. Thrombocytopenia or thrombocytopathy	Thiazides, quinine and salicylates.
4. Seizures	Narcotic withdrawal syndrome, accidental injection of local anesthetic agent into fetal scalp, chlorpropamide, and propranolol.
5. Cretinism	Antithyroid drugs, ^{131} iodides, lithium carbonate, and povidone-iodine.
6. Deafness	Quinine, streptomycin aminoglycoside, chloroquine, thalidomide
7. Jaundice	Vitamin K, long-acting sulfonamides, nitrofurantoin, primaquine, oxytocin, salicylates, bupivacaine.
8. Intrauterine growth retardation	Addictive drugs or substance abuse, smoking, alcohol, caffein, tetracyclines, propranolol, labetolol, statins and ACE inhibitors.
9. Drug withdrawal syndrome	Morphine, pethidine, diazepam, alcohol, and barbiturate addiction.
10. Cerebral depression and hypotonia	Pethidine, morphine, anesthetic agents, diazepam, barbiturates, magnesium sulfate, ethyl alcohol, and tensilon.

a vertex presenting baby is indicative of fetal distress or fetal diarrhea due to listeriosis.

Labor and Delivery

History of chorioamnionitis, prolonged rupture of membranes (>24 hours) and unclean or too many vaginal examinations are recognized markers of intrauterine bacterial pneumonia. Chorioamnionitis is diagnosed on the basis of maternal fever plus any two of the five clinical parameters like maternal leukocytosis, fetal and maternal tachycardia, uterine tenderness and foul smelling liquor. Prolonged labor (>18 hr first stage, and >6 hr second stage) and difficult delivery are associated with increased risk of birth asphyxia and birth trauma. Determine whether the baby was delivered vaginally following spontaneous labor or after induction/augmentation with oxytocin. Ask for history of instrumentation (forceps, vacuum), or operative delivery (elective or emergency cesarean section). Check whether any evidences of fetal distress were present during labor. Evidences of cephalopelvic disproportion, cord around the neck or cord prolapse, etc. should be noted. Analgesics and anesthetics used during labor can adversely affect the fetus.

Neonatal History

Ask whether baby cried immediately after birth or was asphyxiated. Details regarding Apgar score should be checked in case of institutionalized delivery. If 1-minute Apgar score is low, it should be checked at 5 minutes and 10 minutes. Determine whether baby was kept in the NICU or roomed-in with the mother. General activity and history of feeding during first week should be asked. Ascertain the passage of first urine (upper limit is 48 hours) and stools (upper limit is 24 hours) after birth. Urine may cause discoloration of diaper in certain metabolic disorders. Red diaper syndrome is a benign condition due to excretion of excessive uric acid or overgrowth of *Serratia marcescens*, black staining of diaper on exposure to air due to alkaptonuria and blue diaper because of Hartnup disease and tryptophane gastrointestinal malabsorption syndrome. An occasional vomiting on the first day of life is common and is of no significance. Ask for history of inactivity, severe jaundice, seizures and feeding difficulties during neonatal period.

History of Present Illness

Ask and assess the chief complaints as told by the mother or attendant in a chronological order. The newborn babies manifest nonspecific symptoms due to a variety of disorders. They have a limited capacity to produce specific symptoms. Refusal of feeds, lethargy and inactivity are common manifestations due to several neonatal disorders. *The nature of predisposing or associated conditions is more crucial to make a diagnosis in a newborn baby.* Assess the predisposing factors (gestational maturity, birth weight, birth asphyxia, prolonged rupture of membranes, etc.), age of onset, and evolution of symptoms. The common neonatal conditions include birth trauma, asphyxia, respiratory distress syndrome, jaundice, septicemia, bleeding manifestations, inborn errors of metabolism and congenital malformations.

Preterm babies are vulnerable to develop a variety of disorders including hyaline membrane disease, metabolic disorders, hypothermia, infections, necrotizing enterocolitis, intraventricular hemorrhage, patent ductus arteriosus, retinopathy of prematurity, etc. Neonates are known to manifest a large number of minor developmental peculiarities and physiological problems which need to be identified to offer reassurance and advice to the mother. On the other hand, when a neonate is genuinely sick, he cannot be managed on an ambulatory basis and must be admitted in a hospital providing level II or intensive neonatal care.

Family History

Ask for the family history of developmental and metabolic disorder. History of neonatal deaths in sibship or family should be asked. History of a similar disorder in a previous sibling should be ascertained. History of consanguinity among the parents should be asked.

Immunizations

Check whether BCG, hepatitis B and oral polio vaccines have been taken or not. Maternal status of tetanus toxoid vaccination should be enquired.

PHYSICAL EXAMINATION

Examination should be conducted in a warm and comfortable room with the baby completely undressed and placed on a flat surface at a height convenient for the physician. A good source of light should be available and examiner's hands should be clean and warm. The detailed examination in a term healthy baby is conducted routinely at birth, within 24 hours or next day, and at the time of discharge. The key timings for examination of newborn babies are shown in *Box 15.1*.

The baby should be examined in detail whenever there is any evidence of abnormality or illness. The newborn baby is best examined one hour after the feed. Before the feed, the baby may be crying or cranky due to hunger and when a baby is examined soon after the feed, it may lead to vomiting and aspiration.

Examination at Birth

The aim of examination of the baby at birth is to ensure and assess that lungs have expanded and the air passages are not obstructed, and to make an early diagnosis of life-threatening congenital malformations and birth injuries.

Apgar Scoring System

Despite its limitations, Apgar scoring system is coventionally used to assess the condition of the baby at birth (Table 15.3). It is no longer used for

---

Box 15.1 Key timings for examination of newborn babies

- At birth
- Daily assessment in the lying-in ward
- Examination at the time of discharge
- Examination of sick babies in the NICU as often as required
- Healthy babies for anthropometry and immunizations in the well child clinic
- Follow-up of NICU babies or unwell babies in the specialized clinic

TABLE 15.3 Apgar scoring system

Criteria	Score		
	0	1	2
Breathing	Nil	Slow, gasping	Crying
Heart rate/min	Nil	Up to 100	More than 100
Muscle tone	Flaccid	In-between	Flexed
Reflex response*	Nil	Grimace	Cough, sneeze or cry
Color	Blue	Peripheral cyanosis	Pink

*By inserting a catheter in the nostrils or tactile stimulation

taking decision for resuscitation of a baby. The 5-min Apgar score is a useful marker of neuromotor status of an asphyxiated baby. The most crucial items in the Apgar scoring system are breathing and heart rate because muscle tone, response to reflex stimulus and color are dependent upon cardiorespiratory status. Time taken by the baby to produce first cry after birth should be noted. Ask whether amniotic fluid was clear or meconium-stained.

SCREENING FOR CONGENITAL MALFORMATIONS

The maternal history should be screened for any ingestion of teratogenic and goiterogenic drugs, irradiation and viral infections during first trimester of pregnancy. The existence of polyhydramnios in the mother should alert the pediatrician to the possibility of obstruction in the upper intestinal tract. About 25% cases of esophageal atresia and 75% cases of obstruction of the duodenum and upper jejunum are associated with polyhydramnios. In fact, one out of every seven cases of polyhydramnios are associated with upper intestinal obstruction. Oligohydramnios, on the other hand, may be associated with bilateral renal agenesis, obstructive uropathy and Potter facies. Family history of any developmental anomalies should be enquired. A quick but complete examination should be conducted with the following scheme in mind.

Birth weight and gestational age The incidence of anomalies in preterm babies is twice in frequency compared to term appropriate-for-gestational age babies. In small-for-dates (especially hypoplastic) babies, the incidence of anomalies is 10 to 20 times higher. A thorough examination and observation of these babies is essential for early diagnosis of anomalies.

Single umbilical artery and palmar crease The cut end of the cord should be inspected for number of the vessels. Normally there are two umbilical arteries and a single umbilical vein. A single umbilical artery, which has an incidence of around 0.8%, is associated with internal congenital malformations in 15 to 20% of cases. The commonly associated malformations include esophageal atresia, imperforate anus and genitourinary anomalies. Single palmar crease should alert one to make a thorough search for additional anomalies.

Hypoplasia of the depressor anguli oris muscle The asymmetric crying facies due to congenital hypoplasia of the depressor anguli oris muscle (DAOM) should be looked for because these infants are likely to have additional associated anomalies in over 20% of cases. During crying, angles of the mouth and mandible are pulled down with flattening of the nasolabial fold on the normal side due to unopposed action of DAOM (Figure 15.1). Cardiovascular anomalies and congenital dislocation of hips are most commonly associated.

Orifice counting and their patency The anomalies are concentrated around orifices. Look for cleft lip, cleft palate and ectopic or closed anus. The patency of esophagus should be checked by

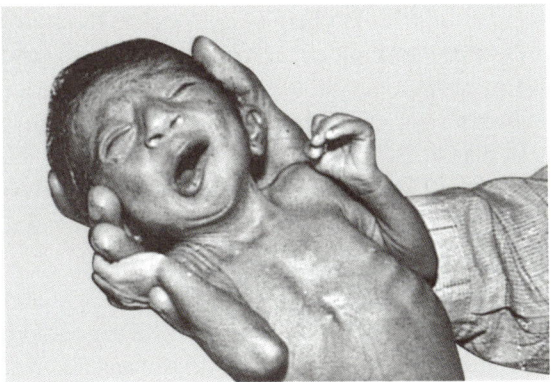

Figure 15.1 Asymmetric crying facies with hypoplasia of the depressor anguli oris muscle on the left side.

passing a stiff rubber catheter into the stomach in the situations listed below. Some pediatricians recommend this procedure routinely in all babies.

(i) Small-for-dates baby
(ii) Single umbilical artery
(iii) Polyhydramnios
(iv) Maternal diabetes mellitus
(v) Frothiness and drooling of saliva
(vi) Choking while feeding

When the catheter has reached the stomach, the gastric contents should be aspirated. If gastric aspirate exceeds 20 mL, it is strongly suggestive of high intestinal obstruction.

Evidences of respiratory difficulty The surgical causes of respiratory distress should be excluded and an urgent X-ray chest should be taken.

Midline lesions on the back and front Cleft lip, cleft palate, spina bifida, meningomyelocele, pilonidal sinus, ambiguous genitalia, hypospadias, exomphalos, etc. should be looked for (Figure 15.2). Cleft palate may occur as an isolated defect or may occur in association with ventricular septal defect and several syndromes, like trisomy 13, trisomy 18, mandibulofacial dysostosis, Wolf-Hirschhorn syndrome, velocardiofacial syndrome and Pierre-Robin syndrome. Submucous cleft of the palate can be missed unless carefully looked for a thin and transparent defect in the palate. A bifid uvula also indicates a submucous cleft of the palate which requires surgery.

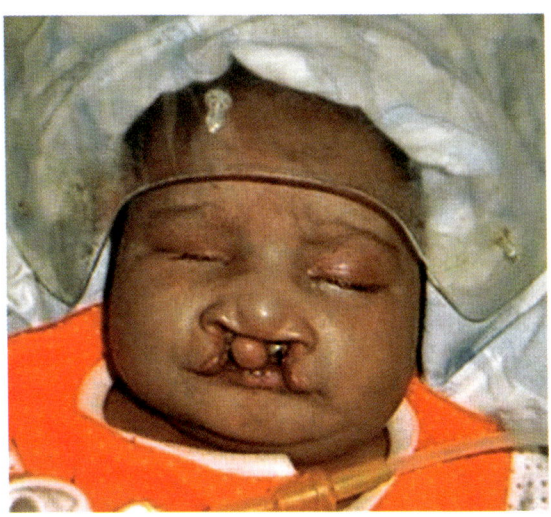

Figure 15.2 Bilateral cleft lip and cleft palate. The infant had associated ventricular septal defect.

Routine systemic examination Abdomen should be palpated for any masses and heart examined for its position and murmurs. 'Dextrocardia' due to pushing of the heart, in association with respiratory difficulty, is suggestive of left-sided pneumothorax and diaphragmatic hernia. Look for musculo-skeletal anomalies and evidences of congenital amputations due to amniotic bands (Figure 15.3).

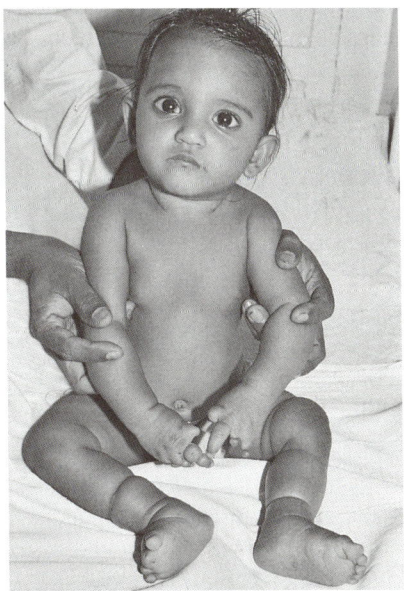

Figure 15.3 Amputation of digits and deep grooves over the legs due to amniotic bands.

First-day Examination

The main purpose of first-day examination is to record anthropometric measurements, to make sure that no anomalies have been overlooked, to enquire about feeding behavior and to look for onset of jaundice. History of frothiness, choking and vomiting during feeds should be asked for and evaluated. Enquiry should be made regarding the time of passage of first meconium (up to 24 hours) and urine (up to 48 hours). Some infants may cry before passing urine due to unpleasant sensation of a full bladder, become quiet or dazed while passing urine and resume crying after evacuation due to discomfort of wet diaper. This is a normal pattern and should not be mistaken with bladder neck obstruction.

Vital signs The vital signs in healthy term babies include median heart rate of 140/min, respiratory rate 40/min, blood pressure 60/40 mm Hg and core body temperature of 36.5°C to 37.0°C. It is easy and convenient to remember that in a healthy term infant, respiratory and heart rates are twice while blood pressure is one-half of an healthy adult. A persistent heart rate of more than 200 per minute in a quiet baby is suggestive of paroxysmal atrial tachycardia while a heart rate consistently below 80 beats per minute suggests complete heart block. Bradycardia in newborn babies is a recognized feature of asphyxia, hypothermia, hypothyroidism, raised intracranial tension, hypertension and hyperkalemia.

Instead of febrile response, hypothermia is more commonly associated with septicemia especially in preterm babies. Fever may occur in term babies having Gram-positive infections or meningitis. Skin temperature can be assessed reliably by touch alone with some experience. In a healthy baby, trunk should feel warm to touch and soles and feet should be reasonably warm and pink. When trunk is warm but soles and feet are pale and cold, it suggests that baby is in cold stress and his ambient temperature should be raised, and baby should be adequately clothed. Breathing should be recorded in a quiet baby at least one to two hours after a feed. Blood pressure may be recorded with flush method or with the help of a Doppler. In infants with adequate tissue perfusion, the baby is pink and warm without any mottling of skin, the difference between central and peripheral skin temperature is less than 1.5°C, and capillary refill time over the upper chest is less than 2 sec (Figure 15.4 A and B) and urine output is adequate (at least 1.0 mL/kg/hr).

General behavior Look for color, respiration, movements of limbs and their posture, general alertness and activity of the child. Excessive sleepiness or irritability is indicative of an infective, metabolic or CNS disorder. Persistent unconsolable high-pitched crying is suggestive of meningitis. Routine neurological examination or even elicitation of Moro response is unnecessary, if the baby is active and feeding normally. Onset of jaundice within 24 hours of age is indicative of Rhesus or ABO hemolytic disease of the newborn.

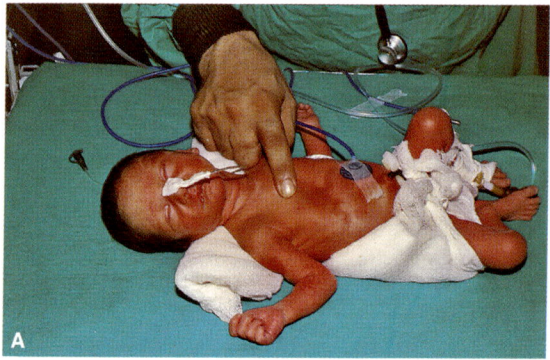
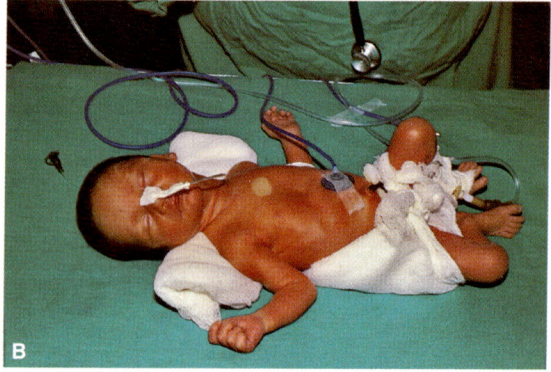

Figure 15.4A and B Assessment of tissue perfusion. (A) Blanch the skin of upper chest by firm pressure with a finger. (B) Blanching disappears by capillary refill within 2 seconds, if tissue perfusion is satisfactory.

Assessment of pain A number of acronyms are used to assess the severity of pain in term and preterm neonates. The clinical tools used for assessment of acute pain include PIPP (premature infant pain profile), NPASS (neonatal pain agitation and sedation scale), NIPS (neonatal infant pain scale), and CRIES scale (**c**rying, **r**equirement of oxygen, **i**ncrease in vital signs, **e**xpression, and **s**leeplessness). The subjective criteria of pain include grimace, crying and behavior of the neonate while objective criteria include heart rate, blood pressure, oxygen saturation and salivary cortisol levels.

Anthropometry

Birth weight should be recorded at birth as soon as the baby is stable and preferably during first 24 hours of life. The birth weight and gestation of the child is plotted on the intrauterine growth chart to identify whether the baby is appropriate-for-dates, small-for-dates, or large-for-dates (Figure 15.5). Occipitofrontal head circumference, chest circumference at nipples and crown heel length on an infantometer are recorded. The head circumference should preferably be taken after 24 hours of birth when caput succedaneum and over-riding of sutures would have disappeared. In a term baby, head circumference is around 34–35 cm with a crown-heel length of 48–50 cm. Ponderal index (weight in grams/(length in cm)^3 × 100) should be calculated. The PI is usually less than 2 in asymmetric small-for-dates babies compared to ponderal index of more than 2 in term AGA infants and symmetric SFD babies.

Gestational Assessment

Assess gestation by physical and neurological examination, if menstrual history is unavailable or uncertain. As gestation proceeds, the baby grows and matures physically and neurologically. The anthropometric measurements such as weight, length, head and chest circumference are unreliable parameters of maturity because they may be adversely affected by intrauterine growth retardation. Head circumference and length are relatively spared in a baby with intrauterine malnutrition as compared to weight and chest circumference.

Grouping of Babies into Preterm and Term

In a baby with unknown gestation, assessment of the maturity of the baby on the basis of physical characteristics alone is fairly reliable. This simple approach helps in deciding whether the baby should be roomed-in with the mother or kept in the special care nursery but does not permit classification of the baby on the basis of birth weight and gestational age. The preterm baby (less than 37 weeks) shows most of the following characteristics:

Anthropometry In preterm babies, birth weight is usually less than 2500 g (term small-for-dates babies may also be low birth weight), crown heel length <47 cm and head circumference of <33 cm and head size is usually more than 3 cm bigger than the chest circumference.

Sole creases In a preterm baby, there is a single deep crease over anterior one-third of the sole or no

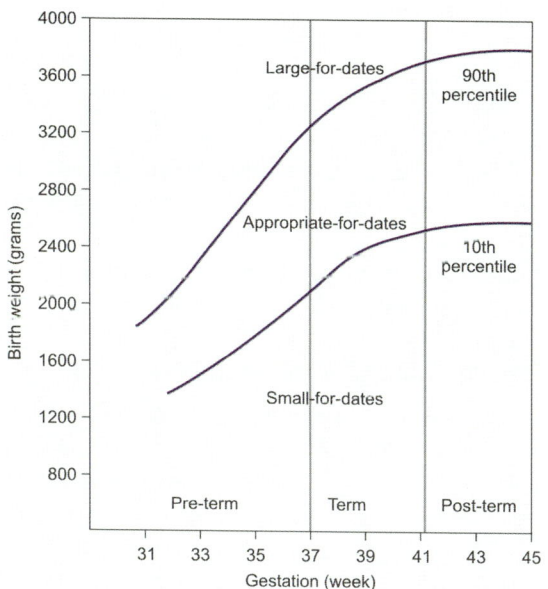

Figure 15.5 Intrauterine growth chart to classify the babies at birth. *Adapted from* Singh M, Giri SK, Ramachandran K. *Indian Pediatr* 1974, 11:475

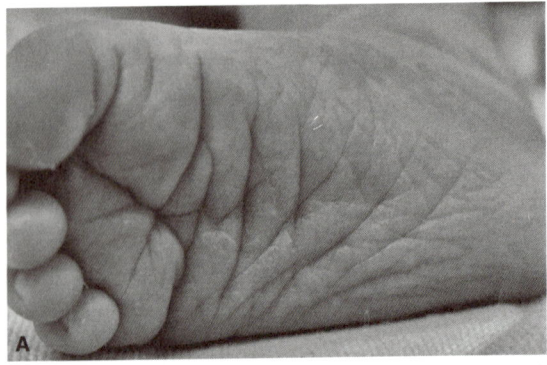
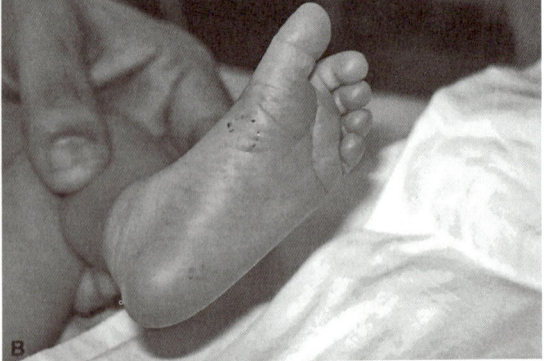
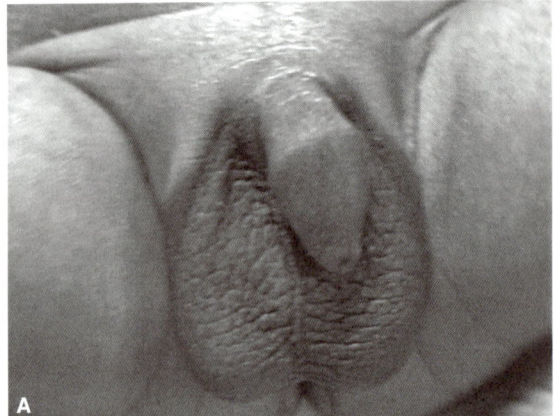
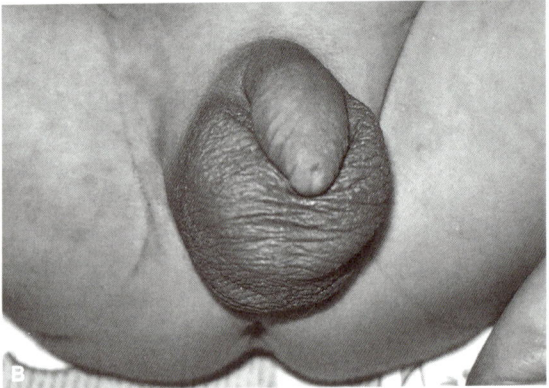

Figure 15.6A and B Sole creases. (A) Deep sole creases covering two-thirds of sole are indicative of term gestational maturity while sperficial sole creases or single deep sole crease (B) is seen in preterm babies.

Figure 15.7A and B Male genitals. Scrotum is fully developed and at least one testis is descended in a term infant (A). In a preterm baby, scrotum is small with a few or no rugosities and testes are undescended (B).

deep crease. The sole may be full of superficial creases (Figure 15.6A and B).

Genitals In male babies, both the testes are at the external ring or above and scrotum is small with scanty rugosities (Figure 15.7A and B). In girls, labia majora are widely separated, the labia minora is fully exposed and clitoris is hypertrophied (Figure 15.8A and B).

Breast nodule Breast nodule is less than 5 mm and nipple is small or absent. In small-for-dates babies, breast tissue may be deficient or absent even when they are gestationally fully mature.

Ear cartilage Cartilage is deficient and even absent at places and on folding the external ear, the recoil may be poor (Figure 15.9A and B).

Hair Brownish-black fuzzy or woolly in appearance with no difficulty in identifying the individual hair fibers (Figure 15.10A and B).

Depending upon the degree of immaturity, the preterm babies may have shiny and oily plethoric skin, plenty of lanugo and edema. Neurologically, they are less alert, hypotonic and various neonatal reflexes may be absent or incomplete.

Precise Estimation of Gestational Age

The physical characteristics outlined above are very reliable to differentiate between preterm and term babies but are of limited value to assess the precise gestation of the babies. On the other hand, neurological parameters are more reliable for precise delineation of gestational maturity of preterm babies, while they are of limited predictive value in relatively mature babies. The neurological assessment is based on four clinical criteria.

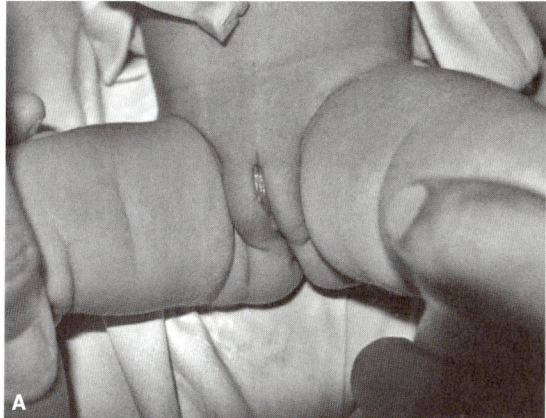
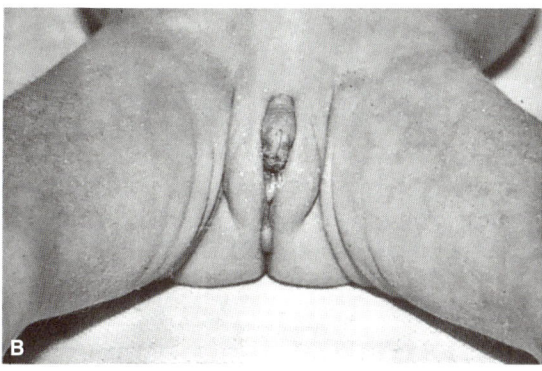

Figure 15.8A and B Female genitals. Labia majora completely cover the labia minora in a term baby (A). In a preterm baby, labia majora are widely separated and labia minora are exposed (B).

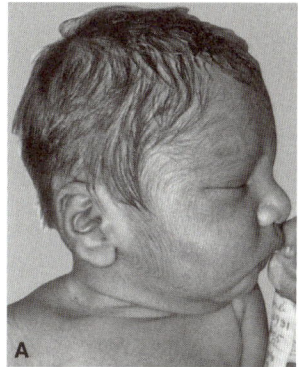
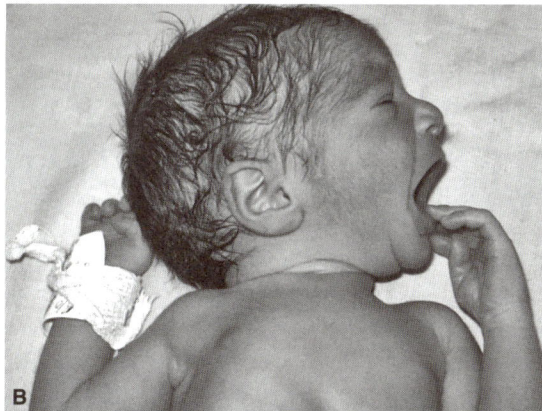

Figure 15.10A and B Scalp hair. The hair are black and silky in appearance in a term baby (A). They are woolly and fuzzy wherein individual hair fibers can be seen in a preterm infant (B).

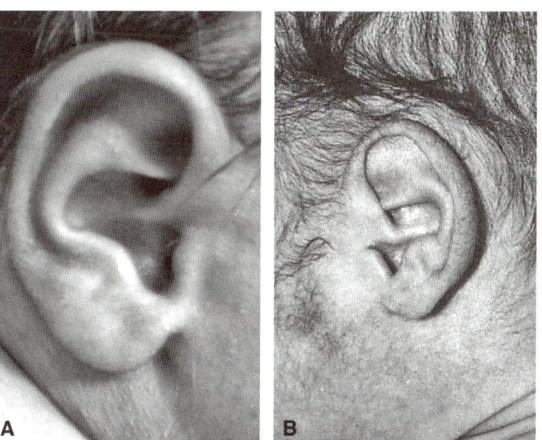

Figure 15.9A and B Ear cartilage. The ear is well shaped and has a firm cartilage in a term infant (A). In a preterm baby, ear is soft, flat and poorly formed with no or minimal recoil (B).

a. *Muscle tone* The muscle tone progressively increases *in utero* as maturity proceeds. The tone in newborn baby is assessed by three parameters.
   (i) Posture or attitude
   (ii) Passive tone is evaluated by assessing popliteal angle and scarf sign **(Figures 15.11 and 15.12).**
   (iii) Active tone is assessed by traction response and recoil **(Figures 15.13A and B).**

b. *Joint mobility* The degree of flexion at ankle and wrist (square-window) is limited in preterm babies because of relatively greater stiffness of joints in early gestation **(Figures 15.14A and B).** As term approaches, the joints become more flexible and mobile to allow for easy moulding during delivery.

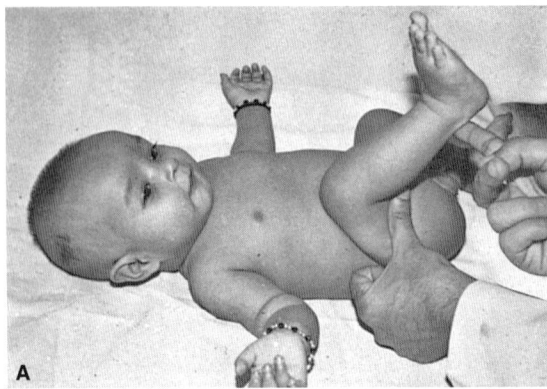
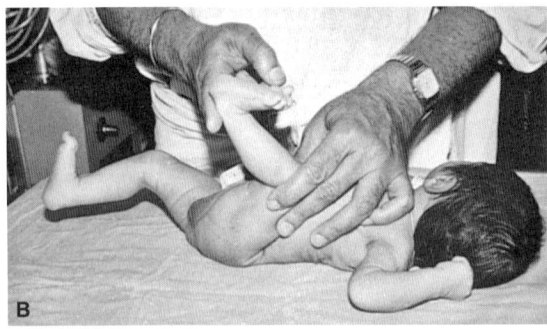
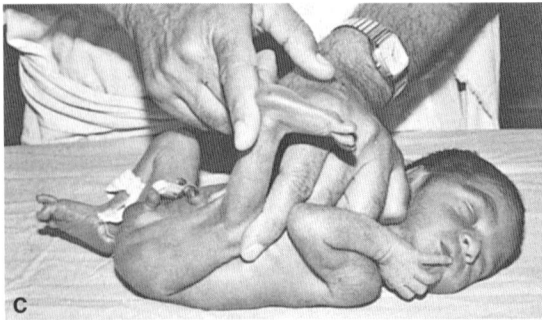

Figure 15.11A to C Popliteal angle. Thigh is held in knee-chest position and examiner tries to extend the knee with gentle pressure behind the ankle. The angle is 90° or less in a term infant (A), 120° among 33–36 weeks infants (B) and almost 180° in an infant less than 32 weeks (C).

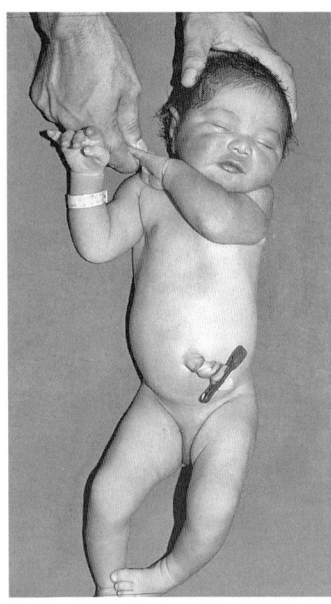

Figure 15.12 Scarf sign. The baby lies supine and head is maintained in the midline. Arm is held by the hand and pulled across the chest towards the opposite shoulder. In a preterm baby, elbow readily goes beyond the midline of chest.

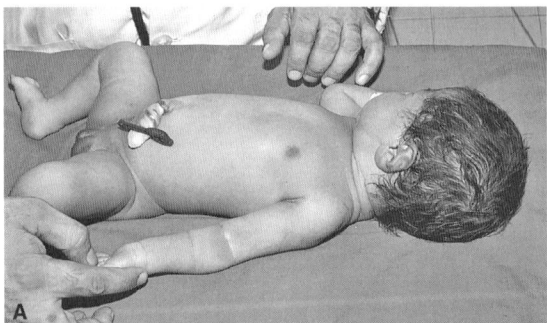
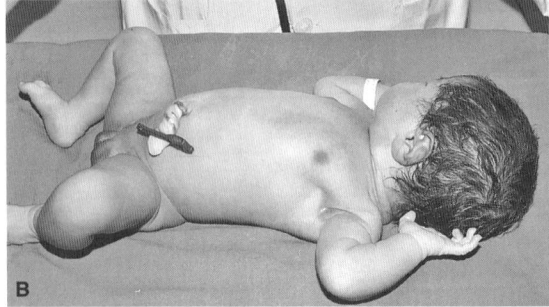

Figure 15.13A and B Arm recoil. The arm is extended and brought close to the trunk (A). When released, it briskly recoils or flexes in a term infant (B).

c. *Automatic reflexes* They appear at specific ages of gestational maturity. Moro reflex appears as early as 28–30 weeks but lacks complete adduction phase till 38 weeks of gestation. Pupillary response to light is present after 30 weeks and infant may turn his head towards diffuse light during 32–36 weeks of gestation. Grasp response makes its appearance around

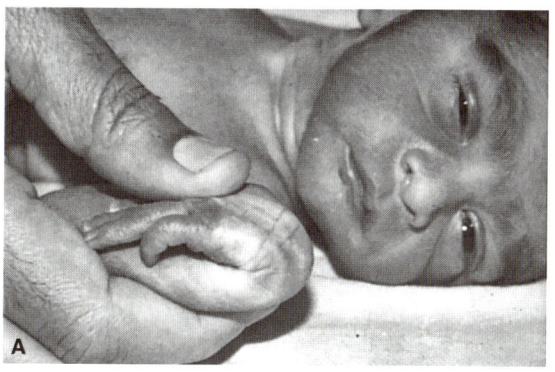 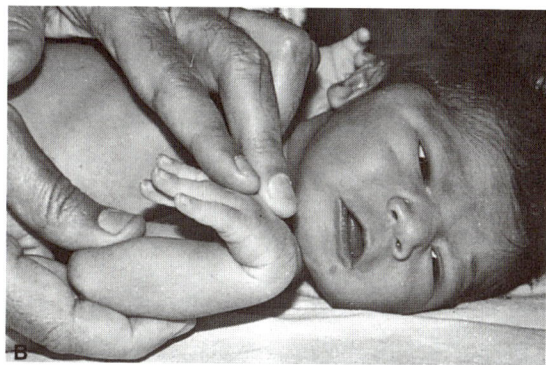

Figure 15.14A and B Square window. Hand is flexed on the forearm between thumb and index finger of the examiner and angle between the palm and volar aspect of the forearm is measured. In a term baby, wrist can be flexed to touch the palm with the front of forearm (A). The joints are relatively stiff in a preterm baby which limits flexion at the wrist (B).

30 weeks but a strong grasp is elicitable only after 36 weeks. Neck flexors are able to contract in response to traction around 33 weeks of maturity. Rooting and coordinated sucking efforts are present by 34 weeks of gestation.

d. *Fundus examination* The disappearance of the anterior vascular capsule of the lens has been used to assess the gestational age of the infant with a gestation of less than 28 weeks. After 34 weeks of maturity, anterior capsular vessels are almost completely atrophied with graded changes in babies between 28 and 34 weeks of gestation. Ophthalmic examination is, however, technically cumbersome in newborn babies due to physiological photophobia and lack of cooperation.

In view of a rather wide overlap in the time of appearance and persistence of various physical and neurological criteria, many workers have evolved scoring systems by using the combined maturity score of physical and neurological criteria for assessment of gestation. Table 15.4 outlines one such simplified scoring system for assessment of gestation. The assessment should be made on babies with a normal Moro response, because neurologically damaged and severely ill babies would be grossly under scored on neurological assessment. The babies with severe intrauterine growth retardation may also be under scored to some extent due to its adverse effects on the development of breast tissue and muscle tone. On the basis of combined physical and neurological scores, the expected gestational age of the baby can be read from Table 15.5 with a predictive error of ±2 weeks.

A number of other scoring systems based on physical and neuromotor evaluation are used for gestational assessment. A revised Ballard score is widely used in clinical practice and is credited to have greater accuracy for assessment of gestational age in extremely premature infants (Table 15.6).

GENERAL PHYSICAL EXAMINATION

Minor Developmental Peculiarities

Examine the skin for toxic erythema or urticaria neonatorum, milia (yellow-white papules on the nose due to blocked sebaceous glands), acne neonatorum, stork bites or salmon patches (capillary ectasia over the upper eyelids, glabella and nape of the neck), capillary hemangiomata, and mongolian blue spots over the butocks and sacral region (Figures 15.15 and 15.16). Subconjunctival hemorrhage over the outer canthus of eye, Epstein pearls (epithelial inclusion cysts as white papules one on either side of median raphe of hard palate) and sucking callosity as a rounded cornified plaque at the center of upper lip are commonly seen in healthy term infants. Gingival cysts and Bohn's nodules over the alveolar ridge of maxillary gums

TABLE 15.4. Scoring system for assessment of gestational age

Criteria	Score*			
	0	1	2	3
I. PHYSICAL				
Skin texture Test by inspection and pinching	Very thin and gelatinous	Smooth, medium thickness with superficial peeling	Thick with peeling and cracking over hands and feet	—
Lanugo Examine on the back	Nil or scanty	Abundant lanugo	Thinning lanugo at places	Scanty lanugo with areas of baldness
Plantar creases Assess after stretching the skin	Nil	Faint red marks over anterior half of sole	Deep indentations over anterior 1/3rd to 1/2 of sole	Deep indentations throughout the sole
Breast nodule Test by holding the breast tissue between thumb and index finger	Nil	Breast tissue less than 5 mm on one or both sides	Breast tissue 5–10 mm	Breast tissue more than 10 mm diameter
Ear firmness Assess by palpation	Pinna feels soft and easily folded into bizarre shapes	Soft but some recoil is present	Some cartilage is felt along the edge and recoil is instant	Pinna firm with a definite cartilage throughout and instant recoil
Genitalia Male	Neither testis in scrotum	At least one testis in the inguinal canal and can be pulled down into the scrotum	At least one testis present in the scrotum	—
Female	Labia majora are widely separated and labia minora protruding	Labia majora partly cover labia minora	Labia majora completely cover the labia minora	—
II. NEUROLOGICAL				
Posture Observe with infant quiet and in supine position	Arms and legs extended	Beginning of flexion of hips and knees, but arms are extended	Stronger flexion of legs and some flexion of arms	Legs flexed and abducted while arms completely flexed

(contd.)

TABLE 15.4. Scoring system for assessment of gestational age (contd.)

Criteria	Score*			
	0	1	2	3
Arm recoil In a supine infant, the flexed forearm is extended by pulling at hand and then it is released	No recoil or only random movements	Arm returns to incomplete flexion or sluggish response	Arm briskly returns to full flexion	—
Popliteal angle** With infant in a supine position, the thigh is held in the knee-chest position by supporting the thighs with examiner's left hand. The leg is then extended by gentle pressure with examiner's right hand index finger placed behind the ankle and popliteal angle is measured	180°	180°–150°	150°–120°	120°–90°
Head lag With the infant lying in supine position, the baby is grasped at elbows and slowly pulled towards sitting position. During the procedure, the position of the head in relation to trunk is observed	Complete head lag	Partial head lag	Able to maintain head in line with the body	Brings head anterior to the body
Glabellar tap Tap sharply at glabella (mid-point between eyebrows) and look for closure of the eyes	Absent	Weak response	Brisk response	—
Physical score = 0–16	Neurological score = 0–13		Combined total score = 0–29	

*Whenever, a criterion, physical or neurological, tested bilaterally gives a different score on the two sides, the mean score should taken.
**Popliteal angle may be unreliable in babies born by breech presentation.
(Reproduced from Singh M, Razdan K, Ghai OP. Modified scoring system for assessment of gestational age in the newborn. *Indian Pediatr* 1975, 12:311)

TABLE 15.5 Relationship between combined total score with gestational age

Combined total score	Gestation (weeks)
9	28
10	29
11	30
12	31
13	32
15	33
16	34
18	35
19	36
20	37
23	38
25	39
≥26	40

are common and disappear spontaneously over next few weeks. Some infants may be born with incisor teeth which may have to be removed, if they are loose or cause feeding difficulty. Genuine tongue-tie is uncommon and is characterized by a tight fibrous frenulum, notch at the tip of the tongue and inability to protrude the tongue beyond the margins of the lips. Tongue-tie seldom interferes with sucking or causes delay in the onset of speech.

Mastitis neonatorum is characterized by enlargement of breasts in fullterm infants of both sexes on third or fourth day of life due to the effect of transplacentally transferred maternal hormones. Withdrawal type of vaginal bleeding on third or fourth day may be seen in female infants and is of no pathological significance. Hymenal tags and slimy mucoid vaginal discharge are extremely common. Hydrocele due to collection of fluid in one of the scrotal sacs is common and usually disappears spontaneously during first three months of life. In male infants, foreskin of penis cannot be retracted due to physiological phimosis. Bowing of legs (genu varus) is common in healthy neonates. After first birthday, it is replaced by physiological knock kness. A detailed "head to toes" examination should be performed.

Head Examine for caput succedaneum, cephalhematoma, forceps marks, encephalocele and widely separated or closed sutures. Caput succedaneum is a localized edema of the scalp over the presenting part of the head following vaginal delivery. It pits on pressure, crosses the suture lines, is non-fluctuant and disappears within 1–2 days. In contrast, cephalhematoma is a subperiosteal collection of blood which appears a few hours after birth as a large cystic swelling limited by suture lines (Figure 15.17). It tends to resolve slowly over a period of few days or weeks and may leave a calcified edge. It may aggravate the severity of physiological jaundice. Rarely, a large hematoma may occur under the occipitofrontalis aponeurosis (subgaleal hematoma) leading to periorbital and periauricular edema, anemia, jaundice and hemorrhagic shock. Unlike subperiosteal or cephalhematoma, subeponeurotic hemorrhage (subgaleal hematoma) is not limited by suture lines.

Anterior fontanel varies in size between 2 and 3 cm while posterior fontanel is small (admits finger tip) and usually closes by 2 months of age. In preterm, small-for-dates and hydrocephalic babies, head circumference is more than 3 cm bigger than the chest. The size, shape and symmetry of skull may be altered by craniosynostosis. Cradle cap over the scalp is common due to crusting of sebum. Craniotabes or softening of skull bones which can be pressed like a table tennis ball is suggestive of prematurity, hydrocephalis, congenital rickets, congenital syphilis and osteogenesis imperfecta. It should be looked for some distance away from the sutures.

Face Yellow-white papules on the nose due to retention of sebum (milia) are present in most term babies and disappear spontaneously. Typical acne-like lesions may be seen over the forehead, nose and cheeks at birth in term babies due to transplacental passage of maternal androgens to the fetus. Salmon patches or stork marks or nevus

TABLE 15.6 New Ballard scoring system for assessment of gestation of extremely premature babies

PHYSICAL MATURITY

	-1	0	1	2	3	4	5
Skin	Sticky, friable, transparent	Gelatinous, red, translucent	Smooth, pink, visible veins	Superficial peeling and/or rash, a few veins	Cracking, pale areas, rare veins	Parchment, deep cracking, no vessels	Leathery, cracked, wrinkled
Lanugo	None	Sparse	Abundant	Thinning at places	Bald areas	Mostly bald	
Plantar surface	Heel-toe length 40–50 mm (−1) <40 mm (−2)	<50 mm, no creases	Faint red marks	Anterior transverse crease only	Creases on anterior 2/3rd	Creases over entire sole	
Breast	Imperceptible	Barely perceptible	Flat areola, no bud	Stripped areola, 1–2 mm bud	Raised areola, 3–4 mm bud	Full areola, 5–10 mm bud	
Eyes/ears	Lids fused loosely (−1), tightly (−2)	Lids open, pinna flat, stays folded	Slightly curved pinna; slow recoil	Well-curved pinna, soft but with ready recoil	Formed and firm pinna with instant recoil	Thick cartilage, stiff ear	
Genitals							
Male	Scrotum flat, smooth	Scrotum empty, faint rugae	Testes in upper canal, rare rugae	Testes descending, a few rugae	Testes in scrotal sacs, good rugae	Testes pendulous, deep rugae	
Female	Clitoris prominent, labia flat	Prominent clitoris, small labia minora	Prominent clitoris, enlarging labia minora	Labia majora and minora equally prominent	Labia majora large, minora small	Labia majora completely cover clitoris and labia minora	
					Total physical maturity score		

(contd.)

TABLE 15.6 New Ballard scoring system for assessment of gestation of extremely premature babies (contd.)

NEUROMUSCULAR MATURITY

Sign	-1	0	1	2	3	4	5
Posture							
Square window (wrist)	>90°	90°	60°	45°	30°	0°	
Arm recoil		180°	140–180°	110–140°	90–110°	<90°	
Popliteal angle	180°	160°	140°	120°	100°	90°	<90°
Scarf sign							
Heel to ear maneuver							

Total neuromuscular score

Maturity rating

Score	Weeks
-10	20
-5	22
0	24
5	26
10	28
15	30
20	32
25	34
30	36
35	38
40	40
45	42
50	44

Adapted from Ballard JL, Khoury JC, Wedig K, et al. New Ballard Score, expanded to include extremely premature infants. J Pediatr 1991;119:417–423.

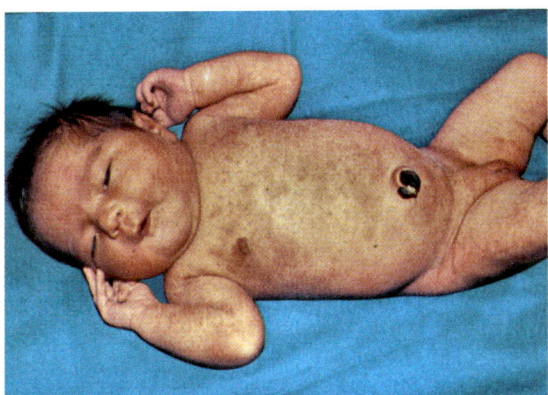

Figure 15.15 Toxic erythema. Erythematous skin rash with central pallor appears on the face and trunk in healthy term babies on second or third day of life. It spontaneously disappears after 2 to 3 days of life.

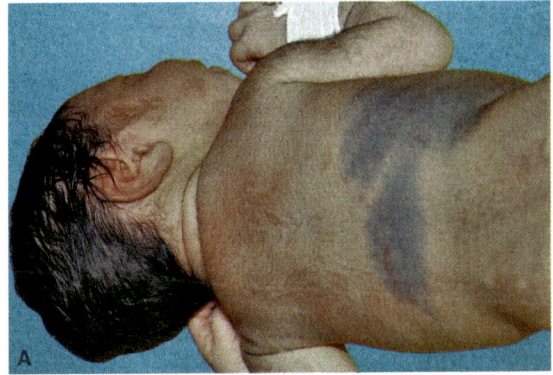

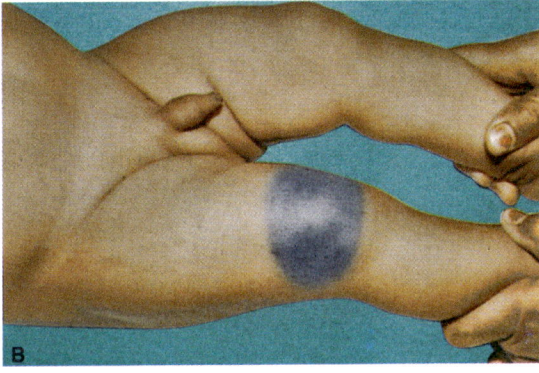

Figure 15.16A and B Mongolian blue spots. They are characteristically present over the back or sacral area (A) but may occur on any part of the body (B). They have no clinical significance and spontaneously disappear by 6 months to one year of age.

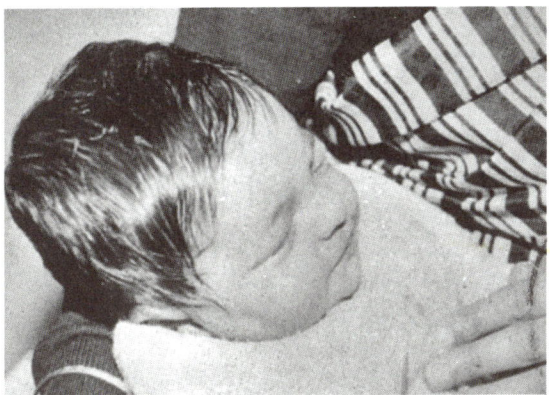

Figure 15.17 Cephalhematoma over the right parietal region. The swelling is subperiosteal, fluctuant and limited by the suture lines.

flammeus are pinkish-gray sparse capillary hemangiomata commonly located at nasal bridge, upper eyelids and nape of the neck. They invariably disappear after a few months.

Look for abnormal facies or dysmorphism by paying due attention to size, shape and position of ears, distance between two eyes and their alignment, size of the oral opening and tongue, shape of the nose and its bridge, shape of lips and size of philtrum and chin size in profile. Recheck for cleft palate. The characteristic constellation of micrognathia, retrognathia, glossoptosis and cleft palate of Pierre Robin syndrome should be looked for (Figure 15.18). Eyes should be examined for conjunctivitis, subconjunctival hemorrhage, corneal haziness, cataract, white reflex and glaucoma. The watering (epiphora) or persistent wetness of one or both eyes may occur due to obstructed nasolacrimal duct. Hairy pinna is characterstically seen in infants of diabetic mothers (Figure 15.19).

Look for preauricular skin tag anterior to the auricle which may be associated with renal anomalies. Preauricular pit or sinus is uncommon and is of no significance.

Neck Short neck with webbing is a recognized feature of Turner syndrome. "Sternomastoid tumor" is a hard swelling over the middle of anterior border of either sternomastoid muscle due to calcified hematoma which may cause torticollis. It usually resolves by passive movements and

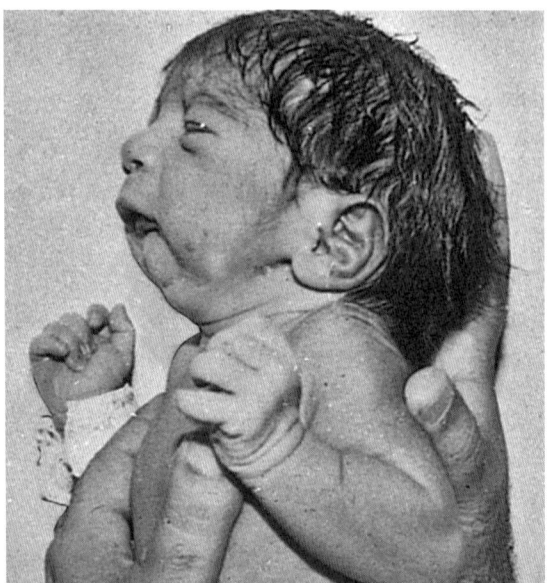

Figure 15.18 Pierre Robin syndrome. Note marked micrognathia and retrognathia. There was associated cleft palate and glossoptosis.

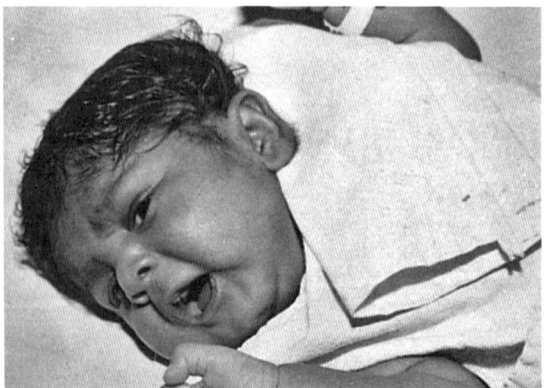

Figure 15.19 Hairy pinna in a large-for-dates baby of a diabetic mother.

physiotherapy of the neck. Look for goiter, cyst or branchial fistula, and lymphangioma. Thyroglossal duct cyst or sinus is located in the midline of the neck while branchial cleft cysts are located at the anterior border of the sternocleidomastoid muscle. Cystic hygroma is a compressible, spongy transilluminant mass which may invade thorax causing respiratory distress. Intertrigo due to fungal infection is common in the neck. Examine clavicles for any callus and crepitus due to fracture.

Skin Examine for jaundice, cyanosis, petechiae, lanugo hair, birth marks, hemangiomata, rashes and evidences of dysmaturity. Toxic erythema or urticaria neonatorum is common in term babies during first week of life. Erythematous skin rash with central pallor appears on the face on second or third day of life and spreads to the trunk and extremities in next 24 hours. It disappears spontaneously after 2–3 days without any treatment. The rash should be differentiated from pyoderma, transient pustular melanosis and congenital syphilis. Congenital syphilis is characterized by maculopapular exfoliative or vesiculobullous skin eruptions involving palms and soles. Perioral ulceration (rhagades) and perianal condylomata should be looked for. Look for evidences of congenital ichthyosis (Figure 15.20).

Transient neonatal pustular melanosis is rare and is characterized by superficial fragile pustules mainly over the chin, neck, forehead, back and buttocks. Pustules are formed due to subcorneal collection of neutrophils with a few eosinophils. They are asymptomatic but may persist up to 3 months.

There is cephalopedal progression of yellow discoloration of skin as the level of serum bilirubin rises. The clinical jaundice manifests on the face at a serum bilirubin level of 5 mg/dL. The yellow staining of trunk indicates serum bilirubin of 10–15 mg/dL, but when soles and palms are yellow-stained, the serum bilirubin is likely to be more than 15 mg/dL.

Spine Spina bifida, meningocele, meningomyelocele, pilonidal sinus and tuft of hair should

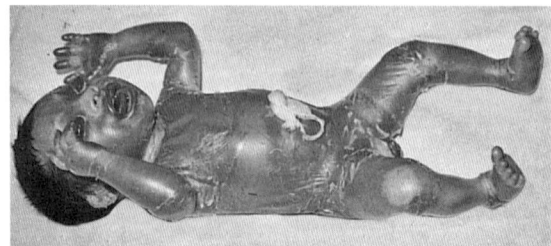

Figure 15.20 Collodion baby. The skin appears like cellotape and is tightly stretched. There is eversion of eyelids (ectropion), lips (eclabium) and characteristic fish-like oral opening.

be looked for. Sacral dimple or pit should not be confused with pilonidal sinus.

Extremities Club feet and minor varus or valgus deformities should be looked for. Talipes equinovarus is characterized by plantar flexion (equinus) and inversion (varus) of the ankle and adduction of forefoot. In talipes calcaneovalgus deformity, the ankle is dorsiflexed and foot is abducted and everted. It should be differentiated from congenital vertical talus (rocker-bottom foot), in which foot is fixed in plantar flexion with a reversed arch. Look for anomalies of digits (oligodactyly, polydactyly, syndactyly), genu recurvatum and arthrogryposis multiplex congenita. Bowed legs are normal during early infancy. Look for any fracture of clavicle, humerus and femur.

SYSTEMIC EXAMINATION

Abdomen and Genitalia

Umbilical cord dries and falls between 5 and 10 days after birth. The separation of cord is delayed in preterm babies, infants with cell-mediated immunodeficiency disorder and because of local infection. Look for any discharge from umbilicus, whether it is watery (urine), purulent or serosanguinous. Umbilical granuloma is characterized by pale irregular granulation tissue while umbilical polyp is pedunculated with a bright-red glistening appearance. Polyp may have a small central opening with watery or fecal discharge due to communication with a urachal cyst or omphalomesenteric duct.

Abdominal examination in a newborn baby is often unsatisfactory unless the baby is quiet or asleep and while taking a feed, otherwise the abdomen becomes tense during palpation. To relax abdominal wall, the infant is supported with a soft pillow in a semi-reclining position or a supine infant is slightly lifted off the cot by holding at both the ankles. Liver edge is normally felt 2 cm below the costal margin. Spleen tip and occasionally lower poles of kidneys, especially the right, may be palpable by an experienced neonatologist. However, if spleen and kidneys are easily palpable, it is abnormal. Bimanual palpation for kidneys can be done with one hand by placing the fingers over the loin while thumb searches for the kidney with gentle, steadily increasing pressure subcostally in a posterior and cephalad direction. *The presence of an abdominal mass in a neonate should be considered as malignant unless proved otherwise.*

Obstructive uropathy is characterized by three abdominal massess (two kidneys and distended bladder) and large over hanging wrinkled skin of abdominal wall (Figure 15.21). The prune belly syndrome is characterized by triad of lax abdominal musculature, cryptorchidism and floppy dysmorphic urinary tract with vesicoureteral reflux. Genitals should be examined for any anatomical abnormalities, undescended testes and hydrocele. In about 1.0% of baby boys, the testicles descend only partially or not at all. In a term infant, scrotum is large, pendulous, darkly pigmented and testes are easily palpable due to absence of cremasteric reflex at birth. Inguinal hernia is more common on the right side because processus vaginalis closes earlier on the left side. As opposed to umbilical hernia, inguinal hernia must be operated within 4–6 weeks of diagnosis because of high incidence of

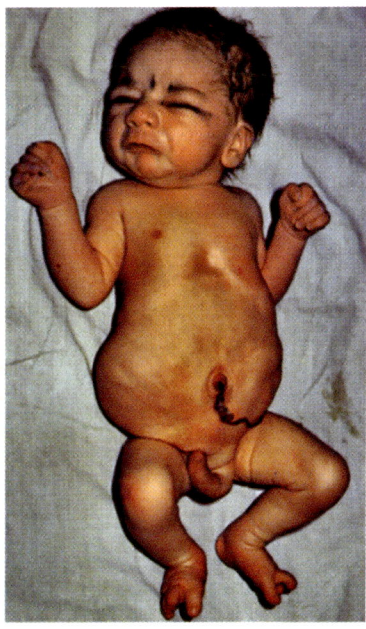

Figure 15.21 Prune belly syndrome. Note a large phallus due to dilated urethra.

incarceration during infancy. Hydrocele should be looked for but its excision should be delayed till 6 months of age because most of them get resorbed spontaneously. Look for opening of urethra to exclude epispadias and hypospadias. Ambiguous genitalia with "salt losing syndrome" (vomiting, diarrhea, dehydration and shock) is suggestive of congenital adrenal hyperplasia.

Cardiovascular System

Developmental cardiac defects are present in about 1 in 200 of newborn babies and about two-thirds of these manifest in the neonatal period. Radial pulse is difficult to palpate in neonates. Examine brachial and femoral pulses for rate, rhythm and volume. Check for any difference in the volume of brachial and femoral pulses, and radiofemoral delay as a marker of coarctation of aorta. Auscultate for any cardiac murmur or abnormalities of heart sounds. It is desirable to use a stethoscope with small-sized chestpiece for auscultation of newborn babies. There is physiological tachycardia and 'tic tic' rhythm due to equal duration of systolic and diastolic phases. Transient cardiac murmur may be heard in 2 to 8% of normal babies during first 48 hours of life. The significant or pathological cardiac murmur is usually loud, grade III or more and may be associated with an ejection click and abnormalities of the second heart sound. The presence of a murmur is not essential for the diagnosis of heart disease. In a severely symptomatic newborn baby, the presence of a soft and insignificant murmur or absence of murmur usually signifies a serious underlying heart disease. Infact, 20% of infants dying of heart disease in the neonatal period may not have a murmur. In infants with left-to-right shunt, murmur may appear after several days or weeks when pulmonary vascular resistance falls and shunt becomes significant. *Therefore, a murmur in the neonatal period does not necessarily indicate the presence of cardiac malformation while absence of a murmur does not rule out congenital heart disease.*

Look for evidences of cyanosis and congestive cardiac failure. The cyanosis due to right-to-left shunt becomes worse when the baby cries. Marked cyanosis in the absence of any respiratory difficulty is highly suggestive of cyanotic heart disease. When arterial oxygen saturation (SaO_2) is less than 90% in a stable baby without any respiratory distress, it is suggestive of congenital heart disease which should be ruled out by 2D electrocardiography with color flow Doppler. Clubbing may appear after 3–6 weeks in cyanotic babies. Tachypnea, tachycardia, progressive hepatomegaly, edema (or sudden weight gain) and cardiomegaly are recognized features of cardiac failure in a newborn baby. Jugular venous pressure is unreliable and difficult to evaluate in a newborn baby due to short neck. The common causes of cardiac failure on the basis of age at onset are listed in Table 15.7.

TABLE 15.7 Common causes of heart failure on the basis of age at onset

Fetal causes
Anemia. Erythroblastosis (Rh-isoimmunization), fetomaternal transfusion, parvovirus B19 infection (hydrops fetalis), and hypoplastic anemia.
Arrhythmias. Supraventricular tachycardia, ventricular tachycardia, and complete heart block.

First 48 hours
Premature infants. Fluid overload, patent ductus arteriosus, bronchopulmonary dysplasia, and hypertension.
Full-term infants. Asphyxial cardiomyopathy, systemic AV fistula, viral myocarditis, polycythemia, sepsis, hypoglycemia, hypocalcemia, complete heart block, congenital thyrotoxicosis, and fluid overload.

First week of life
Critical aortic/pulmonary stenosis, hypoplastic left heart syndrome, transposition of great vessels with intact ventricular septum, obstructed total anomalous pulmonary venous connection, coarctation of aorta, and Ebstein anomaly.

Second week of life
Large ventriculoseptal defect, atrioventricular septal defect, large PDA, unobstructed total anomalous pulmonary venous drainage, and truncus arteriosus.

1–2 months of life
Large L–R shunts, transposition and malposition complexes, anomalous left coronary artery from pulmonary artery, and aorta–pulmonary window.

Respiratory System

In the absence of respiratory difficulty or any other complaints, such as cough or feeding problem, the routine examination of chest is unnecessary and often non-contributory. Cough is an uncommon symptom in newborn babies and may occur due to meconium aspiration syndrome and pneumonia especially due to *Chlamydia trachomatis*. Look for tachypnea, dyspnea, grunting and retractions of chest. Recessions occur readily especially in preterm babies because of soft ribs. Stridor may occur due to upper respiratory tract obstruction. Over inflated barrel-shaped chest because of obstructive emphysema is seen in infants with meconium aspiration syndrome. A number of scoring systems are available to clinically assess the severity of respiratory distress (Table 15.8 and Figure 15.22). Respiratory failure is diagnosed when there is increasing respiratory distress with low arterial oxygen saturation on pulse oximetry

TABLE 15.8 Modified Downes scoring system for assessment of severity of respiratory distress

Parameter	Score		
	0	1	2
Respiration (rate/min)	<60	60–80	>80
Cyanosis	No cyanosis in room air	No cyanosis in 40% oxygen	Requiring more than 40% ambient oxygen
Retractions	Nil	Mild	Moderate to severe
Grunting	Nil	Audible with stethoscope	Audible without stethoscope
Air entry	Good	Decreased	Barely audible

Source: Downes JJ, Vidyasagar D, Boggs TR, Morrow GM. *Clin Pediatr* 1970; 9(6):325–331.

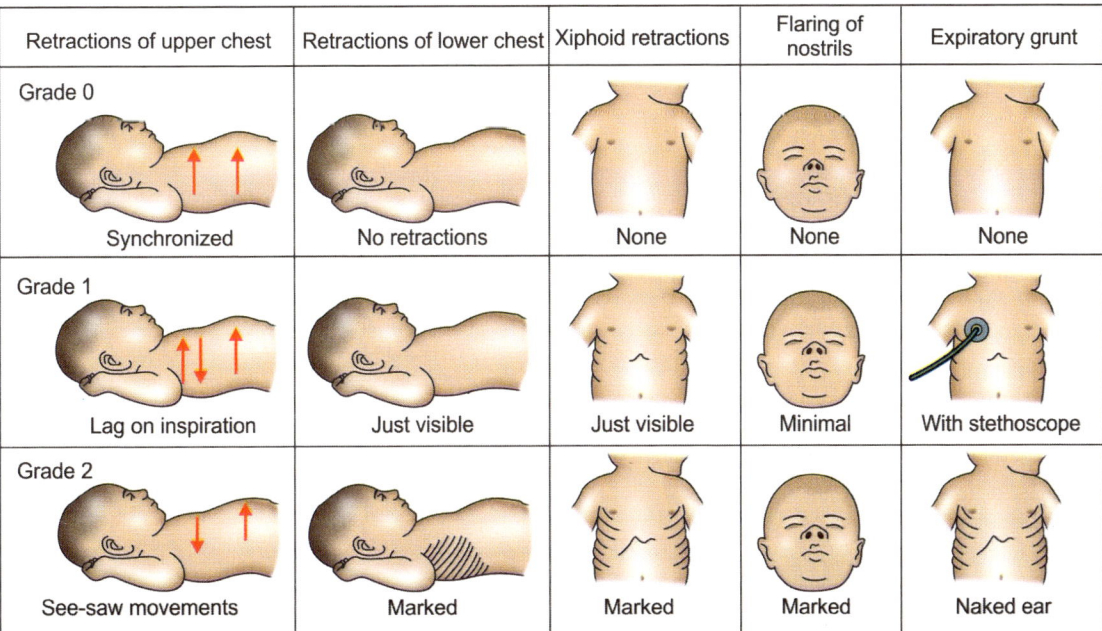

Figure 15.22 Silverman–Anderson retraction score. A score of >6 is indicative of impending respiratory failure. (*Source*: Silverman WA, Anderson DH. *Pediatrics* 1956; 171(1):1–10).

(SpO$_2$ ≤93%), low partial pressure of oxygen in arterial blood (PaO$_2$ ≤60 mm Hg) and/or high partial pressure of carbon dioxide (PaCO$_2$ ≥45 mm Hg) with respiratory acidosis (pH ≤7.2). The neonate may become unresponsive, apneic and cyanosed.

Decreased movements of chest on one side are seen in association with pneumothorax, diaphragmatic hernia, pleural effusion and hypoplasia of lungs. Diaphragmatic hernia is characterized by flat or scaphoid abdomen, reduced chest movements and/or bowel sounds usually in the left hemithorax with displacement of the mediastinum and heart to the opposite side. The auscultation of chest is not always rewarding in newborn babies due to cross-conduction of adventitious sounds. In infants with respiratory distress due to pulmonary causes, the underlying cause is suspected on the basis of associated or predisposing conditions rather than any specific clinical signs (Table 15.9). In all seriously sick neonates, skiagram of the chest is mandatory irrespective of clinical symptoms and signs referable to the respiratory system.

Central Nervous System

Brain in newborn babies functions mostly at a subcortical level because babies born without cerebral hemispheres are indistinguishable in their behavior from normal babies and cerebral motor defects do not generally manifest in the neonatal period. Therefore, the neurological examination has a limited localizing value for cerebral lesions during the neonatal period. The lack of cooperation and proper 'state'* of the baby poses practical difficulties. Therefore, emphasis is laid on thorough observation which is likely to be most informative and least disturbing to the infant. The neurological examination is best performed about two hours after the last feed when baby is in 'state' 3 or 4 but normal babies remain in these 'states' only for 10 to 15% of the time. The examination should never be attempted immediately after the feed because some babies may vomit, if they are handled or disturbed. Most babies fall asleep after a feed.

Purpose of Neurological Examination

Routine neurological examination in a healthy term baby is unnecessary. The information regarding activity, general behavior and feeding behavior of the baby as reported by the mother, absence of any abnormalities of skull and spine and symmetry of spontaneous movements of limbs on the two sides are enough to rule out any significant neurological abnormality. There is no need to elicit Moro reflex in apparently normal babies. In general, a detailed neonatal neurological examination is usually done for the following purposes.

1. Diagnosis of an acute neurological illness.
2. Prognosis for future neuromotor development following perinatal hazards and neurological illness.
3. Assessment of gestational age.

The common symptoms of neurological disorder in a newborn baby include irritability, frank or subtle seizures, high-pitched crying, drowsiness, inability to suck (despite gestational maturity of >34 weeks), bulging anterior fontanel, lack of movements of the limb(s) and seizures. Hypoxic ischemic encephalopathy and metabolic disorders are common causes of seizures in a newborn baby. Age at onset of seizures provides useful clue to the underlying cause of seizures (Table 15.10).

General Observations

The 'containers' of central nervous system (skull and spine) should be carefully examined to exclude

---

*Brazelton's 'states' of wakefulness in a neonate.
State 1. Deep sleep with eyes closed, regular respirations, no movements.
State 2. Light sleep with eyes closed, occasional movements of eye lids, lips, fingers, etc. and irregular respirations (REM sleep).
State 3. Eyes open with no gross movements (quiet wakefulness).
State 4. Eyes open with gross body movements and "cooing" sounds.
State 5. Eyes open or closed and baby is crying.

TABLE 15.9 Common pulmonary causes of respiratory distress in neonates

Condition	Age at onset	Associated or predisposing conditions
- Prenatal and natal aspiration (including meconium aspiration syndrome)	At birth	Post-maturity, small-for-dates, placental dysfunction, fetal distress, meconium-stained liquor, birth asphyxia, and tracheoesophageal fistula
- Intrauterine pneumonia	1–2 days	Prolonged rupture of membranes, foul smelling liquor, peripartal fever with tender uterus, and fetal hypoxia.
- Postnatal aspiration	First week	Preterm, untrained nurses, cleft palate, micrognathia, glossoptosis, and esophageal atresia with tracheo-esophageal fistula.
- Hyaline membrane disease	1–6 hours	Immaturity, birth asphyxia, cesarean section, Rh-isoimmunization, and maternal diabetes mellitus
- Transient tachypnea of the newborn	1–6 hours	Near term baby, cesarean section, and maternofetal transfusion
- Pneumothorax	1–7 days	Aggressive resuscitation, meconium aspiration syndrome, assisted ventilation, hypoplastic lungs, and staphylococcal pneumonia
- Massive pulmonary hemorrhage	First week	Small-for-dates, cold injury, disseminated intravascular coagulation, and hyperosmolar sodium bicarbonate bolus
- Bronchopulmonary dysplasia	2–3 weeks	Prolonged assisted ventilation, PDA, over infusion, and oxygen-dependence
- Pleural effusion	At birth	Hydrops fetalis
- **Congenital malformations**		
▫ Upper respiratory passages	At birth	Choanal atresia, Pierre Robin syndrome, nasopharyngeal tumor, laryngeal stenosis and web, goiter, and vascular rings
▫ Esophageal atresia with tracheoesophageal fistula	First day	Polyhydramnios, single umbilical artery, preterm or small-for-dates baby
▫ Diaphragmatic hernia	At birth	Oligohydramnios, and hypoplasia of ipsilateral lung
▫ Pulmonary agenesis	At birth	Potter facies, oligohydramnios, single umbilical artery
▫ Pulmonary lymphangiectasis	At birth	Lymphedema, chylous ascites, and anomalous pulmonary venous drainage
▫ Lobar emphysema	Variable	Tracheomalacia, and aspiration
▫ Cysts and tumors	Variable	Extrapulmonary teratoma, and neuroblastoma
▫ Asphyxiating thoracic dystrophy (Jeune syndrome)	At birth	Hypertension, polydactyly, hepatic and renal dysfunction, retinal dystrophy

TABLE 15.10 Causes of seizures on the basis of age at onset

First day
Hypoxic-ischemic encephalopathy, cerebral contusion, 'first day' hypocalcemia, pyridoxine dependency, and accidental injection of local anesthetic into fetal scalp

Between day 1 and 3
Intracranial hemorrhage, hypoglycemia, narcotic withdrawal, and inborn error of metabolism

4th to 7th day
Tetany, meningitis, TORCH infections, developmental malformations, kernicterus, and benign neonatal seizures

1–4 weeks
Late-onset hypocalcemia, sepsis, progressive hydrocephalus, herpes encephalitis, inborn error of metabolism, cerebral dysgenesis, and epileptic syndromes

any traumatic or developmental defects. Skin should be examined for any ectodermal dysplasia which may be associated with CNS abnormalities.

'*State*' of the baby and nature of cry should be recorded. High-pitched shrill cry may signify the presence of cerebral irritability.

Skull The occipitofrontal circumference should be measured after 24 hours of birth when molding and over-riding of sutures have disappeared. Abnormalities of shape, symmetry and swellings (cephalhematoma and encephalocele) should be looked for (Figure 15.23). 'Setting sun' sign may be normally seen in some neonates. If persistent and exaggerated, it suggests hydrocephalus and kernicterus. It is suggestive of raised intracranial tension with compression of orbital plate or brainstem irritation.

During the first 48 hours, skull bones overlap each other because of molding. A wide range of normal variations in the size of anterior fontanel and sutural separation makes their interpretation difficult. Hydrocephalus should be suspected when head circumference is more than 95th percentile for the gestation or postnatal age. Sagittal suture may be separated up to 0.50 to 0.75 cm during the first fortnight due to the rapid growth of the brain outstripping the bony growth of the calvarium.

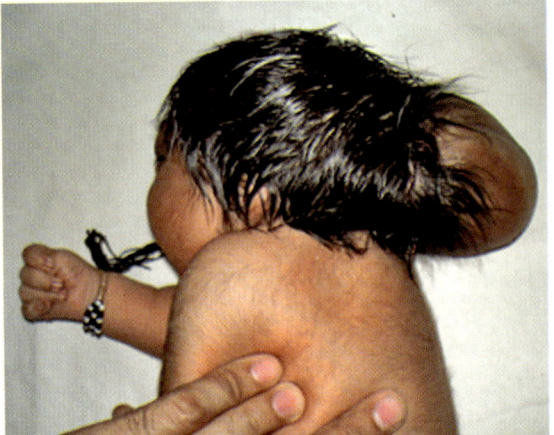

Figure 15.23 Occipital encephalocele in a neonate. Note the associated microcephaly and short neck.

Generally, squamoparietal sutures are not separated except in hydrocephalus but may be open in preterm and small-for-dates babies without hydrocephalus. A ridge at metopic suture (midline on forehead) is normal while sutural ridges at other places suggest craniosynostosis. Auscultation of skull may reveal a bruit in infants with arteriovenous fistula or angiomatous malformation.

Transillumination of skull should be done as a routine in all cases. The torch should be fitted with a circular tightly fitting rubber foam ring over its front end to ensure close contact of the torch to the baby's scalp. Cold-light transilluminator can be used for assessment of transillumination of skull. Normally, the halo of light around the rim of the illuminator extends up to 1 cm in the occipital region and about 2 cm in the frontal region in term babies. Excessive transillumination is seen whenever there is abnormal collection of fluid at any intracranial site within 1 cm of the inner table of skull. When there is large collections of fluid and in infants with hydrancephaly and porencephaly, the whole skull may glow with light.

Spine Exclude spina bifida and associated anomalies, tuft of hair, dermal sinus, fracture of the spine, etc.

Cranial nerves Evaluation of cranial nerves is rather difficult in a newborn baby. For examination of second and eighth cranial nerves, refer to the section on special senses. For examination of third, fourth and sixth cranial nerves, the baby should be held on the arm by supporting the head in your palm. The baby is likely to open his eyes spontaneously look towards the source of diffuse light. Ptosis and inability to close the eye should be looked for. Doll's eye movements should be tested to detect any ocular palsy. Transient nystagmoid movements may be seen in normal neonates. For fifth and seventh cranial nerves, tap the nasion. The eyes close. This evaluates movements of the upper face (Figure 15.24). Rooting reflex gives information regarding the lower half of the face (Figure 15.25). Asymmetry of the face on crying is a useful sign of facial palsy. In partial facial palsy or congenital absence of depressor anguli oris muscle, mandible alone may deviate or is pulled down on the normal side as the baby cries. Corneal reflex is absent when trigeminal nerve is affected. Look for nasal regurgitation during feeds and elicit the gag reflex for testing ninth and tenth cranial nerves. Asymmetry of tongue is seen due to involvement of the twelfth nerve. Fasciculations of tongue are characteristically seen in infants with Werdnig-Hoffmann disease.

Fundus The examination of fundus is of limited value in a newborn baby. Satisfactory pupillary dilatation can be achieved with a mixture of phenylephrine 0.1% and tropicamide or cyclopentolate 0.2% eyedrops. The optic disk is normally pale and devoid of foveal reflex during the first three months of life. Papilledema as a sign of raised intracranial tension is rare because rising tension is easily buffered by sutural diastasis. Retinal hemorrhages are commonly encountered but are of no clinical significance. Large subhyaloid hemorrhages are seen in infants with intracranial bleeding in the subarachnoid and subdural spaces. Choroido-retinopathy is suggestive of certain intrauterine infections. Indirect ophthalmoscopy is recommended for screening of retinopathy of prematurity (ROP).

Special Senses

They can be tested only during 'states' 3 to 4, otherwise the interpretation is unreliable.

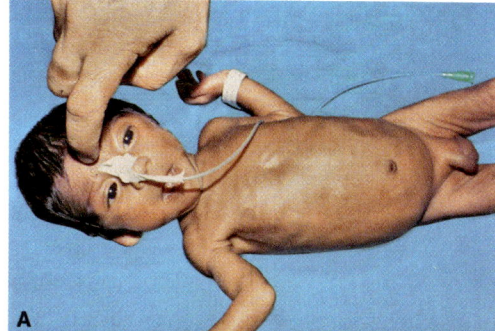
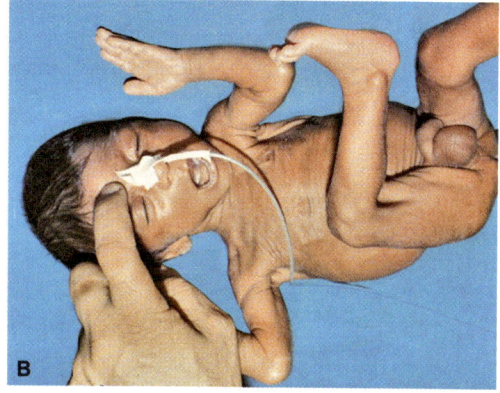

Figure 15.24A and B Glabellar tap. Sudden tapping of nasion (A) is followed by prompt closure of both the eyes (B).

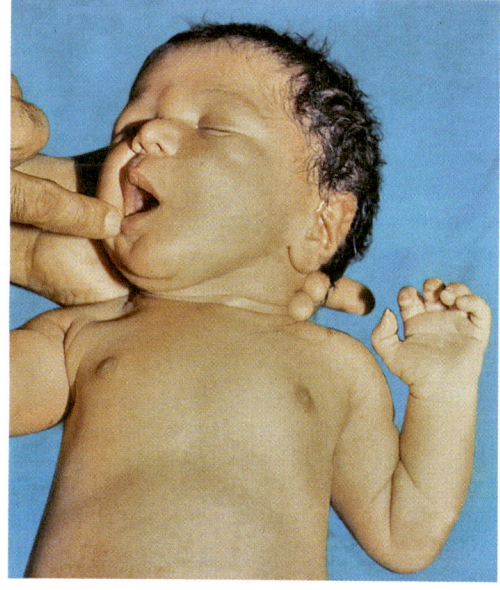

Figure 15.25 Rooting reflex. The baby opens the mouth when cheek is touched near the angle of the mouth.

Vision The visual fixation and attention must be assessed with due patience and care because these are the only functions at birth which indicate the integrity of cerebral hemispheres. The visual acuity in a term newborn baby is around 6/45 and it gradually matures to an adult level of 6/6 by the age of 6–7 years. The vision can be tested as follows:
(i) The baby responds to strong light by blinking.
(ii) Head turns towards diffuse light after 32 weeks of gestation.
(iii) The baby shows attention or follows moving red ball after 34 weeks of gestation.
(iv) Opticokinetic nystagmus is present.

Pupils Their size and reaction to light should be recorded. Pupils do not react to light in babies less than 29–31 weeks of gestation, during raised intracranial tension and posterior fossa compression. Pupils may be dilated and fixed in infants with optic atrophy or retinal detachment; while in cortical blindness, pupillary responses are preserved. In a newborn baby, the dilated pupils give poor prediction regarding the side or site of intracranial hemorrhage. Examine pupils with the help of an ophthalmoscope light. Look for red reflex in both the eyes with the help of +10 diopter lens of an ophthalmoscope from a distance of 10 inches from the infant's eyes. The presence of "red reflex" rules out any serious abnormalities in the anterior and posterior chambers of the eye. The presence of "white pupil" or leukocoria is suggestive of cataract, retinoblastoma, persistent pupillary membrane, vitreous opacity and retrolental fibroplasia due to ROP.

Hearing Clinical examination for hearing in the newborn is not reliable. The baby is watched for the following responses, after giving a sound stimulus of a bell or 60 db vocal sound. Look for startle response, blinking of eyes, sudden change in the activity of the baby with greater alertness and change in the heart rate and breathing pattern or rate.

The positive response, both for visual attention and hearing, signify lack of any generalized neurological disturbance. Negative response, however, is of little significance because many variables may affect it. There is a need to do repeated assessments to evaluate the integrity of vision and hearing. A formal hearing test (BERA, OAE) should be done at the corrected age of 3 months.

Motor Functions

Spontaneous movements The range and symmetry of spontaneous movements should be observed. Watch and record in detail any tremors (jitteriness) and convulsions. Subtle seizures are common in preterm babies and may consist of jerking of the eyes, blinking, staring look, sucking or chewing movements. The seizures are usually multifocal clonic, tonic or myoclonic in type.

Muscle tone The normal term neonate is rather hypertonic while preterm babies are usually hypotonic. Increase or decrease in muscle tone must be significant before it is regarded as abnormal. Differences in muscle tone between the two sides of the body have greater localizing value. *The baby's head must be kept in the midline, while assessing the muscle tone, otherwise tonic neck posture may influence muscle tone unequally on the two sides.* Look for popliteal angle and heel to ear maneuver in the lower limbs and scarf sign in the upper limbs, for assessment of muscle tone.

Avulsion of brachial nerve roots may occur during difficult breech extraction or shoulder impaction. In Erb's palsy (C5, C6), affected arm hangs limply, and is kept adducted and internally rotated with elbow extended (Figure 15.26). When lower cervical roots are affected (Klumpke's palsy),

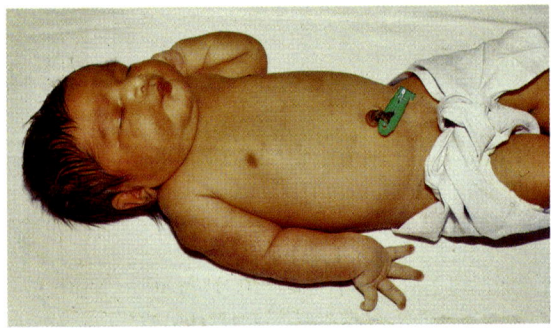

Figure 15.26 Erb's palsy on the right side in a large-for-dates baby of a mother with diabetes mellitus.

there is wrist drop due to flaccid paralysis of hand with absent palmar grasp. The presence of miosis, ptosis, and anhidrosis (Horner's syndrome) though uncommon is suggestive of associated damage to the cervical sympathetic chain of the first thoracic root.

Tendon jerks The deep tendon jerks are rather variable in neoantes and are generally brisk. Index or middle finger can be used to elicit deep tendon jerks in newborn babies. Knee jerk in the newborn is normally followed by contraction of adductors of both hips (crossed adductor spread). Ankle clonus may elicit up to eight jerks in normal babies, but if 10 to 12 uninterrupted jerks are obtained, it is abnormal. The tendon jerks are of poor diagnostic utility except in infants with peripheral nerve and spinal cord injuries.

Primitive Reflexes

The newborn babies have a large number of primitive or automatic reflexes. It is time consuming and tiring both for the baby and the physician to elicit all of these automatic reflexes. The following reflexes are useful for clinical purposes and one should observe whether the response is sluggish, normal or exaggerated and symmetric or asymmetric.

Stepping reflex The infant steps up when held upright with dorsum of the feet touching the edge of a table. The reflex is present at birth and may disappear after 4 weeks to 4 months.

Moro reflex Moro reflex or startle response is the most useful. The baby is held supine by the examiner on the right arm and hand. The flexed head is suddenly allowed to drop by about 30°. A positive response consists of rapid abduction and extension of upper limbs and opening of hands followed by slower adduction and flexion or embrace equivalent (Figure 15.27). The infant may cry. The response can also be elicited by pulling a supine infant by holding at both wrists (as in traction response). When angulation occurs between the head and trunk, the hands are sharply released to cause sudden extension of neck (Figure 15.28).

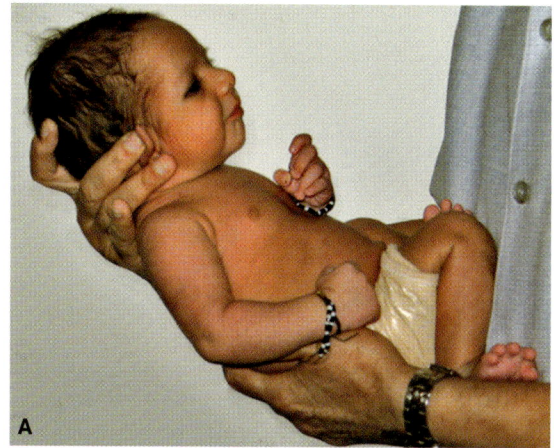
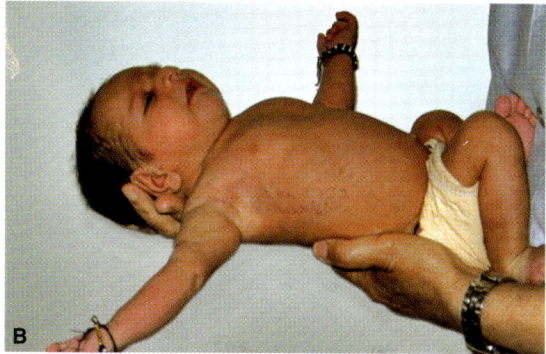

Figure 15.27A and B Moro reflex. The baby is held over the arm and neck is flexed (A). Sudden extension of neck is associated with flexion and abduction of upper limbs (B) followed by adduction or embrace response. Moro reflex should be brisk, complete and symmetrical on two sides.

The response may be depressed or absent in infants with cerebral depression. Exaggerated or jumpy response may be obtained in cases of cerebral irritability. The Moro reflex may be incomplete in babies, with a gestation of less than 35 weeks. Asymmetric Moro response may suggest brachial palsy and fracture of clavicle or humerus. In babies with kernicterus, the Moro response is often characteristic. The sudden extension of arms is not followed by flexion component but often accompanied with downward rolling of eyeballs ('setting sun' sign), lid lag and a peculiar grin. Exaggerated startle reaction to sound is seen in infants with Tay-Sachs disease, GM1 gangliosidosis, Sandhoff disease, progressive cerebral degeneration and blindness.

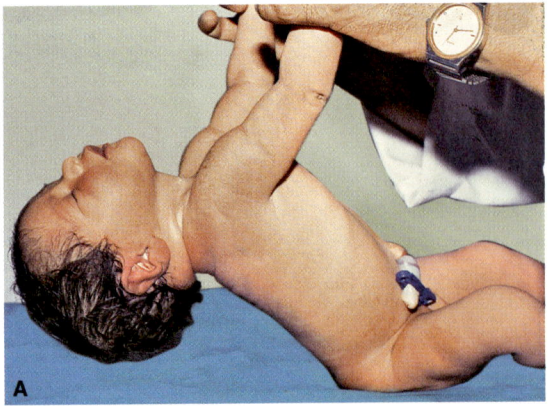

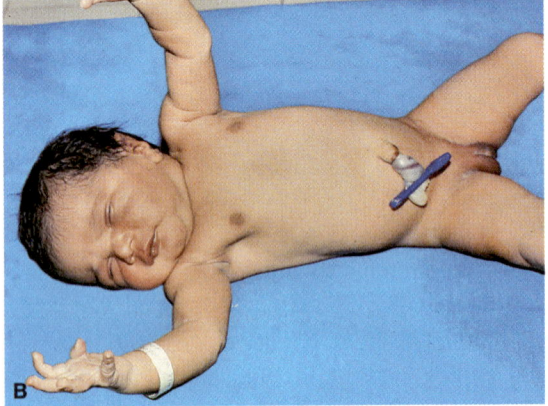

Figure 15.28A and B Moro reflex. The supine baby is lifted off the cot by gently holding at the wrists (A). The baby is suddenly released to elicit the Moro response (B). Moro reflex can also be elicited by sudden banging of the cot or producing a loud noise though it is rather more traumatic and unpleasant for the baby.

Glabellar tap Tapping of nasion is followed by closure of eyes in infants above 30 weeks of gestation (Figure 15.24).

Rooting and sucking responses Stimulation of angle of mouth or lips initiates rooting and sucking in infants above 34 weeks gestation. The mother or nurse's report regarding feeding behavior of the baby is more informative.

Tonic neck reflex When the baby's head is turned to one side, the ipsilateral arm and leg get extended while contralateral limbs are flexed (Figure 15.29). The asymmetric tonic neck reflex disappears after 2 to 3 months. If a baby constantly or persistently maintains the tonic neck posture, it

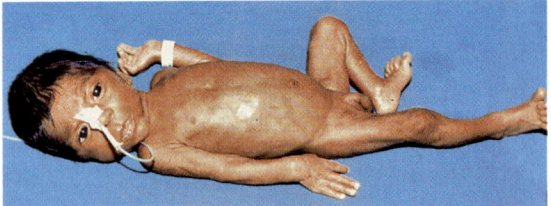

Figure 15.29 Tonic neck reflex. The baby assumes asymmetrical posture when head is turned to one side. The limbs facing the head are extended while the limbs on the opposite side are flexed.

is abnormal and may signify as a marker of future development of cerebral palsy.

Traction reflex The supine baby when pulled up by holding at the wrists, his ability to flex the arms and neck should be observed.

Galant reflex In ventral suspension, stroking of the paravertebral region of the back is followed by contraction of the spine and movement of the pelvis on the stimulated side. The reflex is present at birth and disappears between 2 and 6 months.

Palmar and plantar grasp The finger is placed on the palmar surface of the fingers or plantar surface of toes of the baby to elicit grasp or flexion of digits. Stroke the dorsum of the hand to persuade the baby to open the fist.

Parachute reflex The baby is held in ventral suspension and is suddenly brought down toward the table top. There is brisk extension and abduction of the upper limbs with extension of fingers as if to break the fall. It is a protective reflex and appears around 8 to 9 months of age and never disappears. The reflex is absent in infants with spastic type of cerebral palsy.

Most primitive reflexes disappear between 4 and 5 months of age and their persistence is considered as an early sign of cerebral palsy.

Infants with fetal hypoxia or birth asphyxia should be assessed for severity of hypoxic-ischemic encephalopathy (HIE) by Sarnat staging system (Table 15.11). *The occurrence of seizures within 36 hours of age usually heralds the onset of hypoxic-ischemic encephalopathy (HIE).* Brainstem involvement is ominous and characterized by

TABLE 15.11 Clinical staging of hypoxic-ischemic encephalopathy by Sarnat staging system

Features	Stage I	Stage II	Stage III
Consciousness	Hyperalert	Lethargic	Comatosed
Posture	Mild distal flexion	Strong distal flexion	Intermittent decerebration
Muscle tone	Normal	Hypotonic	Flaccid
Tendon reflexes	Brisk	Exaggerated	Absent
Myoclonus	Present	Present	Absent
Sucking	Active	Weak	Absent
Moro response	Exaggerated	Incomplete	Absent
Grasping	Normal	Exaggerated	Absent
Oculocephalic reflex (Doll's eyes)	Normal	Over reactive	Reduced or absent
Pupils	Dilated and reactive	Constricted	Variable
Respiration	Regular	Periodic	Apneic attacks
Heart rate	Normal	Bradycardia	Variable
Seizures	Absent	Common	Uncommon
EEG	Normal	Low voltage periodic/or paroxysmal	Periodic, isoelectric

Adapted from Sarnat HB, Sarnat MS. Neonatal encephalopathy following fetal distress. Arch Neurol 1976, 33: 695–705.

irregularity of breathing, apneic attacks, changes in pupillary size and dysconjugate eye movements, poor sucking and swallowing with pooling of secretions in the oral cavity.

Sensory Functions

Sensory testing is of limited value in the newborn. The response to painful stimuli should be assessed, if injury or disease of peripheral nerves or spinal cord is suspected. The anal reflex must be elicited in infants with neural tube defects.

Examination of Hips

The hip joints should be examined for evidences of developmental dysplasia of hips (DDH). About 1 to 2 per 1000 babies are likely have DDH, which need early recognition and treatment to prevent limping and chronic disability of hip joint. The condition is more common in girls especially first born, breech presentation, post-dated and is often associated with oligohydramnios. There may be family history of the condition and infant may have other associated postural deformities especially in the feet. The classical signs of dislocation are not seen in the neonatal period. The instability of the hip joint is best detected by a modified Ortolani/Barlow maneuvers as described below.

The infant is placed on his back with legs facing the examiner. The baby should be undressed from waist downwards. The examination should be performed with care, gentleness and warm hands. Infant should be calm, relaxed and adequately fed. The examiner tries to assess whether the hip is dislocated or it is unstable and dislocatable. For examination of the left hip, the examiner steadies the infant's pelvis between the thumb of his left hand placed on the symphysis pubis and the fingers under the sacrum (Figure 15.30). The left thigh is flexed by keeping the knees bent. It is grasped by examiner's right hand by placing middle finger on the outerside over the greater trochanter and thumb on the inner side of the thigh opposite the lesser trochanter.

In the first maneuver, the examiner assesses whether the hip is dislocated or not (Ortolani or

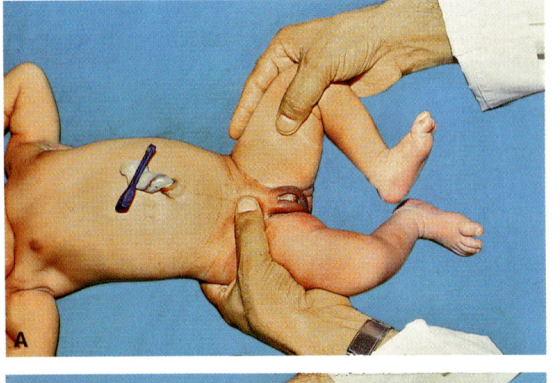
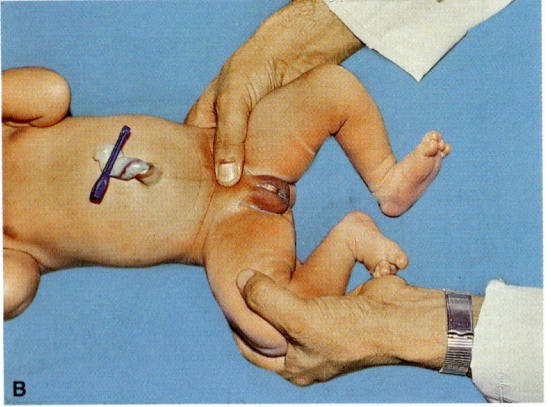

Figure 15.30A and B Examination for assessment of congenital dislocation of left hip. The examiner steadies the pelvis of the baby with his left hand. (A) Backward and outward pressure is applied at the knee and lesser trochanter to dislocate the hip. (B) Abduction of hip is associated with a palpable or audible "clunk" when femoral head re-enters the acetabulum. Refer to the text for details.

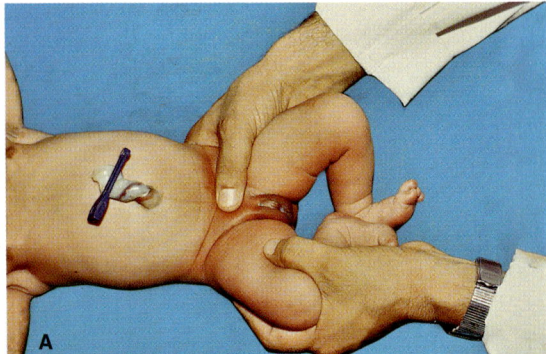
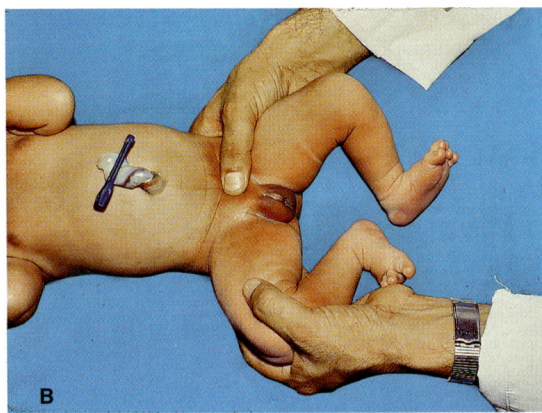

Figure 15.31A and B Examination for assessment of congenital dislocation of right hip. The role of examiner's hands is reversed. Refer to the text for details.

reduction test). The pressure is applied over the greater trochanter with the middle finger by abducting the hip and lifting the thigh upward in an attempt to relocate the displaced femoral head back into the acetabulum. If the head is felt to move (usually not more than 0.5 cm) into the acetabulum with or without a palpable and/or audible 'clunk', it confirms the presence of dislocation. If dislocation is not present, an effort is then made to test for subluxation (dislocatability) of the hip by Barlow test (stress test). With the thumb placed on the inner side of the thigh, backward and outward pressure is applied to the head of the femur in an attempt to dislocate it. If the femoral head is felt to move backwards over the rim of acetabulum, for a distance of 0.5 cm, with or without a palpable or audible clunk, the hip is said to be dislocatable. The right hip is examined by reversing the role of examiner's hands (Figure 15.31). The ligamentous clicks without movement of the head of the femur in or out of the acetabulum may be elicited in 5–10% of hips and should be disregarded.

Auscultatory method It is based on the principle that the vibrations of tuning fork placed on the greater trochanter cannot be transmitted to the pubic symphysis on the dislocated side. The chestpiece of the stethoscope is placed on the pubic symphysis and the foot of the vibrating tuning fork is placed on the greater trochanter on either side one after the other (Figure 15.32). There is poor transmission of vibrations of the tuning fork when femoral head

Examination of a Newborn Baby

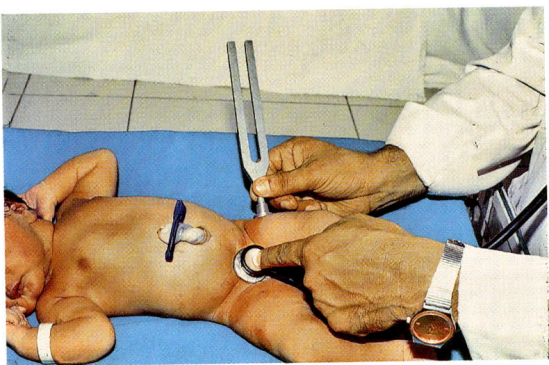

Figure 15.32 Auscultatory method for assessment of congenital dislocation of hips. Refer to the text for details.

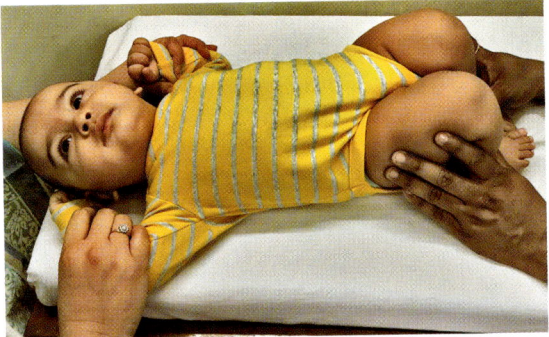

Figure 15.33 Galeazzi test. Infant is made to lie supine and both knee joints and hips are flexed with feet held flat on the cot or examination table. Note left hip is at a lower position due to posterior dislocation.

is dislocated. The "dislocatable" femoral head cannot be identified by this method. In bilateral congenital dislocation of hips, the transmission of vibrations of tuning fork would be adversely affected on both sides.

Older Infants (>3 months)

In infants with untreated congenital dislocation of hips, there may be asymmetry of gluteal and thigh folds, shortening of affected limb and limitation of abduction of the affected hip. The Allis' sign or Galeazzi test may be positive, i.e. in a supine child when both knee joints and hips are flexed and feet are held flat on the cot, the knee on the affected side will be at a relatively lower level due to posterior dislocation of hip (Figure 15.33).

Infants with untreated unilateral DDH are likely to manifest with limping and toe walking on affected side while bilateral DDH is associated with increased lumbar lordosis, prominent buttocks and a waddling gait. Infants suspected to have DDH should undergo dynamic ultrasound examination of hip joint by a skilled pediatric radiologist.

DAILY "CLINICAL SCREENING" OF THE BABY

Between first day examination and the day of discharge, detailed examination is unnecessary and may in fact be harmful for the baby because of risk of introducing infection. The baby-mother dyad should be approached twice a day to enquire about any feeding problems, vomiting, bowel disorders and to assess and allay the anxiety of the mother regarding various developmental peculiarities which may attract her attention. The age of onset and intensity of jaundice should be assessed. Any evidences of superficial infections, such as conjunctivitis, pyoderma, umbilical sepsis and oral thrush should be looked for.

EXAMINATION AND SCREENING AT DISCHARGE

A detailed examination of the baby at the time of discharge is essential to make sure that no anomalies and birth injuries have been missed and initial lactational and feeding difficulties have been surpassed. Careful auscultation of the heart is essential because previously detected functional murmur may no longer be audible and new murmurs may appear any time during the neonatal period.

Pulse oximetry According to recommendations of American Academy of Pediatrics (AAP), all newborns should undergo pulse oximetry screening before discharge. The screening should be done after 24 hours of age or shortly before discharge, if baby is less than 24 hours of age. The measurement of oxygen saturation should be done in the right hand and either of the foot. The screening is considered 'negative' and the baby is declared 'passed', if the SpO_2 is 95% or greater in both right hand and either foot and the difference between

SpO_2 of right hand and foot is ≤3%. The screening is 'positive' and baby is declared 'failed', if the oxygen saturation is less than 90% in any one extremity, or less than 95% in both the extremities, or there is absolute oxygen saturation difference of more than 3% between the right hand and either foot on three consecutive measurements taken one hour apart. The "failed" infants should undergo 2D echocardiography to exclude congenital heart defect.

Hearing Evoked otoacoustic emission (EOAE) testing can be done with a handheld device that produces soft clicks to measure the echoes emitted by the eardrum.

Screening for inborn error of metabolism Blood samples should be taken on special filter papers for screening of newborns for certain inherited metabolic disorders. There is a lack of uniform policy for routine screening of neonates in various NICUs in India.

The mother should be advised about feeding, vitamins and iron supplements, general cleanliness, immunizations and given an appointment for visit to the Well Baby Clinic. High-risk babies discharged from the NICU should be followed up for developmental assessment and detailed examination of central nervous system and special senses in a Special Developmental Clinic.

SICK BABIES IN THE NICU

Babies are looked after in the neonatal intensive care unit (NICU) when a baby is extremely preterm, critically sick, malformed or when mother is unwell or unwilling to look after the baby. Check perinatal events and nature of resuscitation provided. Look for various life-threatening conditions, like RDS, seizures, sepsis, jaundice, bleeding manifestations and shock. Ask for history of procedures, like CPAP, assisted ventilation and its duration, whether received surfactant or not, oxygen dependency, thoracostomy, simple or exchange blood transfusion. The NICU protocol should be followed for routine ultrasound examination of brain and indirect ophthalmoscopy for ROP.

Check the vital signs on the monitor. Assess hemodynamic stability including activity, color, capillary refill time by pressing over the sternum. Is the baby having any respiratory distress or apneic attacks? Is the baby tolerating the enteral feeds without any abdominal distension or gastric residuals. The baby should be screened for sepsis, patent ductus arteriosus, necrotizing enterocolitis and intraventricular hemorrhage. Is the daily weight gain velocity of the baby satisfactory? The baby should be screened daily to look for clinical criteria to assess the well-being of the baby in the NICU (*Box 15.2*).

Box 15.2 Cot-side criteria indicating that a preterm baby is healthy

- Baby is alert, active and pink.
- Vital signs are stable.
- Trunk is warm to touch and extremities are reasonably warm and pink.
- No respiratory distress and apneic attacks.
- Baby is tolerating enteral feeds without any vomiting and abdominal distension.
- Daily weight gain is 1.0–1.5% of the body weight, i.e. 10–15 g/kg per day.

Scheme for Presentation	
Maternal health and family history	Maternal education, occupation, socioeconomic status, age, weight and height, nutritional status, any chronic or systemic disease, endocrinal disorder, sexually transmitted diseases (STDs), blood group, immunization status and history of consanguinity. Family history of hereditary, metabolic, chromosomal and developmental disorders.
Obstetrical history	Gravidity (number of conceptions), parity (number of live births), history of abortions, stillbirths, and neonatal deaths (with possible causes), mode of delivery and any complications at birth, previous birth of LBW and preterm babies and infants with congenital malformations or genetic defects and severe jaundice.

(contd.)

	Scheme for Presentation (*contd.*)
Pregnancy details	Natural pregnancy or *in vitro* fertilization (IVF), with or without surrogacy, single or multiple babies, illnesses or difficulties during pregnancy, and medications taken. Dietary intake and weight gain during pregnancy. History of anemia, pregnancy-induced hypertension (PIH) and toxemia of pregnancy, abnormalities of liquor amnii (oligohydramnios or polyhydramnios) and Rh-isoimmunization. Status for screening of STDs like syphilis, HIV, HBV and TORCH infections should be checked. Gestational maturity, growth and abnormalities of the fetus on antenatal ultrasonography including fetal biophysical profile.
Labor and delivery	Duration of labor, timing of rupture of membranes, history of fetal distress, evidences of amnionitis and mode of delivery, whether spontaneous, instrumental or operative delivery (elective or emergency cesarean section).
Examination of the baby at birth	Single born or multiple gestation (twin, triplet, quadruplet), gestational age, birth weight and sex. Amniotic fluid clear or meconium-stained, time of first cry and Apgar score. Look for any congenital malformations, birth injuries, respiratory distress or difficulty in breathing and number of umbilical arteries. Timing of passage of first urine, and meconium should be noted. Onset of jaundice, its severity and duration should be recorded. Nature of feeding and any feeding difficulties should be looked for. Rule out congenital dysplasia of hip(s).
Evaluation of a sick baby	The main symptoms with their duration, activity and feeding behavior of the infant should be recorded.
General appearance	Alertness, activity or irritability, excessive crying or sleepiness, color (circumoral grayness, jaundice, pallor), breathing difficulty or apneic attacks, whether extremities are warm or cold to touch.
Vital signs	Temperature, breathing rate, heart rate and blood pressure, capillary refill time, any apneic attacks.
Anthropometry	Preterm, term, and location of birth weight on the intrauterine growth chart. Weight, occipitofrontal head circumference and length.
General physical examination	Head size, swellings, sutures, edema, facial dysmorphism, developmental abnormalities, abnormalities of skin, spine and extremities, presence of pallor, cyanosis and jaundice.
Abdomen and genitalia	Look for umbilical discharge, granuloma, polyp and hernia. Abdomen may be scaphoid, normal or protuberant. Look for enlargement of liver, spleen, kidneys and presence of any mass. Genital abnormalities, inguinal hernia, hydrocele, and undescended testis should be looked for.
Cardiovascular system	Cyanosis, shock, evidences of cardiac failure, abnormalities in the peripheral pulsations and arterial oxygen saturation on pulse oximetry. Record heart rate, rhythm, heart sounds and any murmur.
Respiratory system	Respiratory distress, grunting, stridor, cough and apneic attacks are suggestive of involvement of the respiratory system. Displacement of mediastinum with bulging of hemithorax is suggestive of pneumothorax and diaphargmatic hernia.
Central nervous system	Head size, swellings and abnormalities in the spine. "State" of the baby and primitive reflexes. Ectodermal dysplasia of skin should be looked for because it may be associated with CNS abnormalities. Size of the anterior fontanel and whether it is flat or bulging. Cranial nerves and fundus examination to look for retinal hemorrhages, chorioretinopathy and retinopathy of prematurity (ROP). Vision and hearing of the infant should be assessed. Spontaneous movements of limbs, muscle tone and deep tendon jerks. Abnormalities in sensations, anal and cremasteric reflex.

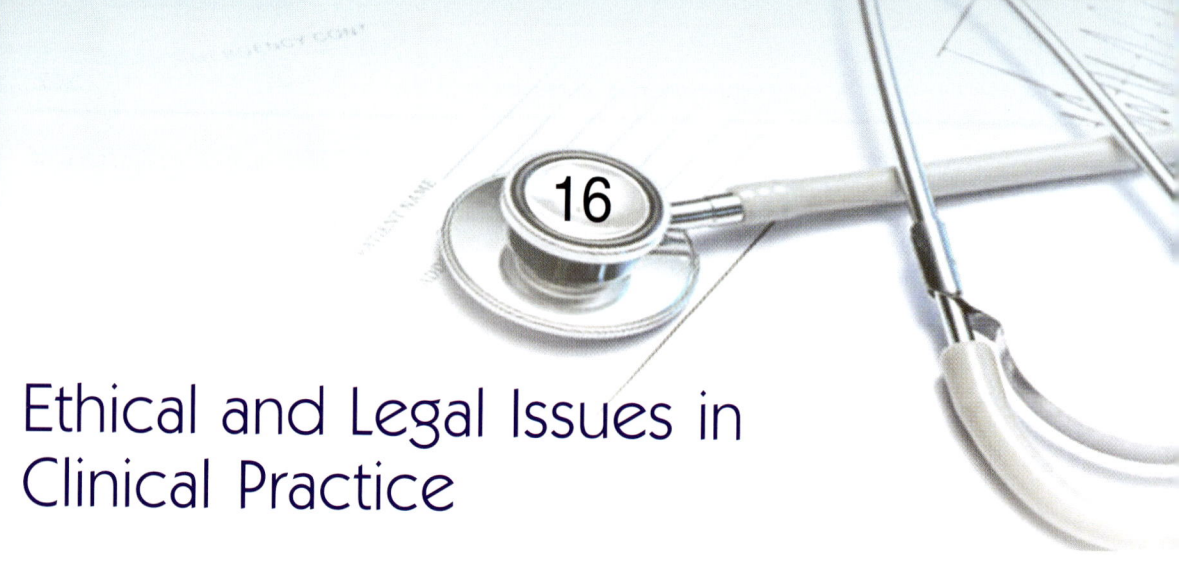

Ethical and Legal Issues in Clinical Practice

"........what is not negotiable is that our profession exists to serve the patient, whose interests come first. None but a saint could follow this principle all the time but so many doctors have followed it so much of the time that the profession has been generally held in high regard."

Sir Theodore Fox

Medicine is regarded as a noble profession because physicians are charged with the supreme responsibility of maintaining health and preserving life of their fellow human beings. There is an age old faith, trust and respect towards physicians in Indian culture. The doctor is often viewed as a demi-god and his advice is usually considered as a gospel truth without any doubt and misgivings. This imposes an onerous responsibility on the part of physician to be ethical, up-to-date and honest in his approach and dealings with his patients. Physicians are both morally and legally accountable to the society. The legendary bond of faith between the doctor and patient is best summed up by Charaka: *"No other gift is greater than the gift of life. The patient may doubt his relatives, his sons and even his parents, but he has full faith in his physician. He gives himself up in the doctor's hands and has no misgivings about him. Therefore, it is the physician's duty to look after him as his own."*

Due to rapid strides in medical technology over the years, medical care of sick children have unfolded complex medical, social, ethical, philosophical, moral and legal issues. It is a sad reality that physicians are allowing technology to de-humanize medicine. The focus of medicine has gradually shifted from the whole patient to his systems, organs, tissues, cells and even DNA! Several physicians have fallen into the trap of treating the disease (rather than the patient) and his laboratory reports rather than viewing the patient in the wider context of his individuality and social milieu. It is a sad reality that the art of medicine is being sacrificed at the altar of scientific advances and technology boom.

THE CONSUMER PROTECTION ACT

"The people who trust their doctor and surrender themselves to his care are more likely to recover than those who approach medicine with distrust, fear and antagonism".

Anonymous

The physicians are both morally and legally accountable to the society. The doctors are expected to provide efficient and effective medical services to the best of their capabilities in a humane and compassionate manner. The doctors are liable under the existent criminal laws for providing poor quality of medical services and negligence. But the legal procedure is time-consuming, expensive and tedious to get speedy justice. The medical councils have failed in their responsibility and obligations to serve as watchdogs to identify and penalize medical practitioners indulging in professional misconduct and various malpractices. In order to rectify this anomaly and ensure speedy compensation to the aggrieved party, the Supreme Court has decreed that the medical practitioners, like other professionals, shall be liable to pay compensation under the purview of 1986 Consumer Protection Act (CPA). When a physician or hospital provides services free of charge to all patients, the CPA cannot be invoked for claiming any damages. Otherwise, both the acts of negligence as well as the "deficiency in service" or "substandard services" are covered under the ambit of CPA. The Supreme Court has conceded to the contention of the Indian Medical Association, that the summary trial of CPA should be limited to only gross or glaring acts of medical negligence. The complex and technical cases of medical negligence shall be handled, as before, by the civil or criminal courts in accordance with the prescribed procedure and with the help of an expert testimony.

In a recent judgment, the Supreme Court has opined that doctors cannot be charged as criminals for the death or disability of patients under their care unless there is an evidence for a gross and glaring professional neglect. In order to reduce the menace of criminal proceedings against doctors on frivolous grounds and provide healing touch to the deteriorating doctor–patient relationship, the Supreme Court of India has made an historic judgement on February 10th, 2010 which states, *"..... It is the bounden duty of the civil society to ensure that the medical professionals are not unnecessarily harassed by the complainant who uses the criminal process as a tool for pressurizing the medical professionals and hospitals for extracting uncalled for compensation. It would not be conducive to the efficiency of the medical profession, if a doctor is to administer medicine with a halter around his neck".*

Most academic bodies and state medical councils believe that the CPA is unjustified because medical service is neither a commodity nor a contract. It is impossible to predict the outcome of medical therapy or surgical procedure due to a large number of biological variables because no two human beings are alike. It is argued that the cost of medical care would escalate because the doctors may indulge in "defensive medicine" (with unnecessary laboratory tests and diagnostic procedures) and they would also try to recover the costs paid for their indemnity insurance. In order to avoid litigation, the doctors may refuse to treat critically sick patients or patients with complex medical problems. The absence of any court fee and stamp duty may lead to filing of frivolous cases. The lack of any expert technical advice to the consumer courts may adversely affect the process of making rational decisions. Above all, it is argued that the CPA would erode the doctor–patient relationship of trust and faith which is crucial for promotion of healing and speedy recovery. It is indeed a paradox that medical councils have no powers to penalize unqualified medical practitioners or quacks because they do not come under the purview of CPA!

The consumer activists, on the other hand, strongly believe that the CPA would tame the doctors to improve their accountability and credibility. They believe that doctors are providing services, like other experts and they ought to have updated medical information and technical competence to handle their patients with due confidence and efficiency. Medicine is already working like a commercial industry and the cost of medicare is sky rocketing in order to recover the exhorbitant cost of medical education obtained from private medical colleges and the financial outlay for the purchase of high-tech equipment.

It is true that most patients do not suspect the competence and technical expertise of doctors because it is assumed that a qualified doctor is competent. But patients do want a doctor who would listen to them, analyze their medical and psychosocial problems and they should have the option to see the same doctor to establish a relationship of trust and confidence and are assured of continuity of care. Patients want a competent,

> **Box 16.1 Common causes of malpractice litigations against doctors under CPA***
>
> - Lack of proper communication.
> - Instigation by "legal/eagles" and jealous professional "friends".
> - Rude, inconsiderate, unsympathetic and arrogant behavior of the doctor.
> - Unsatisfactory and unfriendly hospital ethos and lack of life-saving equipment, drugs and oxygen.
> - Substandard, defective and malfunctioning medical equipment.
> - Unsatisfactory medical record keeping.
> - Indiscriminate use of high-tech expensive investigations and procedures.
> - Lack of clear, and unambiguous expert opinion.
> - Lack of knowledge and expertise.
>
> *Based on a study conducted by Association of Consumer Action Safety and Health (ACASH)

caring and concerned doctor and not merely a highly evolved technocrat. In a study conducted by Association of Consumer Action Safety and Health (ACASH), it has been found that lack of proper communication is indeed the most common reason for taking recourse to CPA *(Box 16.1)*.

Even in the highly litigious society of the USA, it has been found that most patients sue their doctors because of lack of communication rather than due to lack of expertise and medical knowledge. The commonest trigger and annoyance on the part of litigant is always an evasive, unconcerned, insensitive and lackadaisical behavior of the doctor. The technical issues are exploited (often with the help of jealous co-professionals) merely to support the allegations and grievances. Other important reasons for seeking compensation include excessive cost of medical care, lack of basic infrastructure, defective or malfunctioning life-saving medical equipment (Ambu bags, ventilators, suction equipment, oxygen) and lack of accountability of health care professionals in most government and public sector hospitals.

Guidelines for making Ethical Decisions

"Thou shall behave and act without arrogance and with undistracted mind, humility and constant reflection. Thou shall pray for the welfare of all creatures……"
Charak Samhita

Ethical decisions are based on five principles of *beneficence, non-malificence, parental autonomy, correct medical facts* and *justice*. Beneficence ensures that doctors should be the best advocates of their patients and promote their best interests in accordance with the age old Hippocratic tradition. The physicians should be concerned with saving life and they should avoid doing any wilful harm to their patients, i.e. there should be non-malificence in their diagnostic and therapeutic interventions. Florence Nightingale also said that the first dictum of patient care is *"do no harm"*. Almost 1000 years ago, according to Manu's code of conduct for the physicians, it was ordained that you should *"Dedicate yourself entirely for helping the sick, even though this may be at the cost of your own life. Never harm the sick, not even in thoughts…. May the gods help you if you follow this rule. Otherwise may the gods be against you"*.

The autonomy and wishes of parents should be honored and they should be taken into confidence while making a decision regarding their medical care through a process of informed consent. The correct ethical decisions are based on sound medical facts. The principle of justice demands that we seek the morally correct distribution of resources, ensure cost-effectiveness of therapeutic interventions by balancing medical benefits and burdens to the family and society. The principle of justice and fairness is often sacrificed in a developing country because due to lack of resources even essential medical care may be denied to indigent patients. The steps in ethical decision making process are shown in **Figure 16.1**.

A large number of other factors and considerations are taken into account while making a decision in case of children with life-threatening medical disorders. Is there a reasonable chance of survival of the child with the available technology or efforts are likely to be futile? Would the quality of life be worthwhile, if the child survives with aggressive management? Can the family afford expensive intensive care management? Should we be concerned with the best interests of the child alone or global interests of the family, society and state? Also there are likely to be cultural

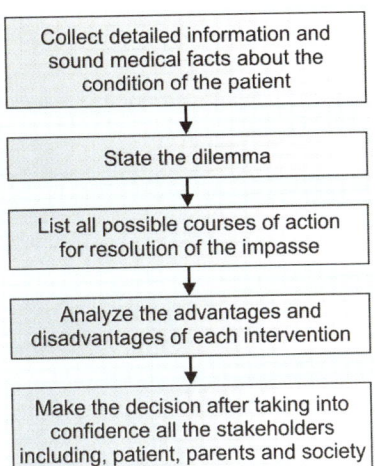

Figure 16.1 The ethical decision-making process.

Box 16.2 Professional qualities, duties and attributes of a pediatrician

- Dress smartly, exhibit pleasant demeanor and greet the child/parent with a smile.
- Be humble, honest, trustworthy and open, and act with integrity and without any ulterior motive.
- Care and welfare of the patient should be the topmost priority.
- Protect and promote the health of the children in the community.
- Be a good listener and establish cordial doctor–patient and doctor–parent relationship.
- Be up-to-date in knowledge and skills and provide good standard of evidence-based medical care.
- Treat children as children and respect the dignity of the patients and their parents.
- Be humane, compassionate and responsive to the needs of children and their parents.
- Never make a slighting remark against the professional colleagues.
- The physicians should not allow the technology to further dehumanize medicine and they must treat children not only with their heads but also with their hearts.
- The physician must strive to become a good human being before he or she can become a good doctor!

considerations, the fertility of the couple, the concept of destiny or will of God, the doctor-knows-the-best attitude, socioeconomic status, education of parents, gender of the child, social support system and national priorities. It is unfortunate but true that in a developing country, economic and social realities may out weigh and override ethical considerations.

Obligations of Doctors Towards their Patients

The professional qualities and attributes of a pediatrician are listed in **Box 16.2**. The physician should provide not merely cure but holistic care to all patients with due competence, consideration and compassion. The physician is not duty bound to treat each and every patient seeking his services. But, he or she has a moral obligation to provide emergency care to his regular patients as and when it is sought. However, in the absence of a pre-existing relationship, physician is not duty-bound to provide care to every patient unless no other physician is available in the nearby vicinity in the event of a dire emergency. When a physician finds himself technically incompetent to handle the medical problem, he should make a referral to an appropriate consultant after discussing with the family. Patients should be handled in a technically appropriate, transparent and efficient manner without unnecessary laboratory investigations.

Physicians are ethically obliged to provide competent and humane care to all patients including those with HIV infection. The information obtained during the course of clinical evaluation should be kept as a guarded secret by the physician. The information should only be released with due consent of the patient or when sought by the Court of Law. However, when a patient is suffering from a notifiable disease, physician is duty bound to bring it to the attention of public health authorities. The sense of duty towards a patient and society should take precedence over undue concern for monetary compensation or rewards.

Essential and Relevant Investigations

There is no denying the fact that a large number of unnecessary investigations are being undertaken because of the lure of "cuts" being offered by the ever mushrooming diagnostic centers in the country. It is a sad reality that laboratory investigations have become a substitute for taking a detailed history and conducting a complete physical examination. At times, the excessive and unnecessary investigations are justified as a safeguard against the increasing trend of seeking legal action by the consumers. It is not uncommon to see that most cases of headache are investigated by doing a CT scan of brain but without doing any ophthalmologic and ENT evaluation. Every case of cerebral palsy is investigated by doing a CT scan and MRI of the brain which has no diagnostic or therapeutic implications. Some pediatricians are known to monitor the extent of hepato-splenomegaly with the help of serial ultrasound examinations of the abdomen instead of doing a careful physical examination.

In private hospitals, doctors are vying with each other to generate revenue for the hospital by fair or foul means because that is the sole criteria of their survival in the system. *The practice of ordering a routine battery of tests in every patient must be condemned.* Instead, the choice of investigations must be individualized in every patient depending upon the diagnostic possibilities based on a detailed clinical evaluation. It is important that only those investigations should be undertaken which are likely to provide a clue or confirmation of a diagnosis or provide guidelines for rational management and prognosis of the disease process.

Unethical Practices

There is increasing commercialization and gradual decline of human values at all levels of our society. The common correlates and types of unethical medical practices are listed in **Box 16.3**. It is true that doctors are also human beings but medicine should not be considered merely as another profession but rather a mission in life. Because of exorbitant cost of medical education in the private sector, upcoming doctors may resort to unethical practices to make a quick buck or try to become rich overnight in order to pay back their loan or debt. Unlike many other professions, medical profession has a long incubation period of protracted studies (graduate, postgraduate, postdoctoral, skill development and clinical experience) before a decent regular job can be bagged or clinical practice is established. A number of national and international academic bodies and councils have provided moral guidelines and code of conduct for an acceptable and dignified professional conduct of physicians. The following medical practices are considered as unjustified and unethical.

> **Box 16.3 Common correlates and types of unethical medical practices**
> - Change of social values with an urge to become "rich overnight".
> - Doctors are competing with each other to create revenue for the corporate hospital by fair or foul means.
> - Exhorbitant cost of medical education in the private sector and need to earn fast to pay back the loan.
> - Unnecessary diagnostic studies to get the "cuts" or the laboratory is owned by the physician.
> - "Kickbacks" for referrals.
> - Superfluous medical procedures, like endoscopies and biopsies.
> - Needless hospital admissions.
> - Unnecessary surgical procedures or even surgical operations.
> - Self-promotion through advertisements.

1. Self-advertisement, glorification, display of large signboards, self-aggrandizement and claims of miracle therapies in lay press are common unethical practices. A medical practitioner is permitted to make a formal announcement in press regarding the start of private practice, intimate the change of address, temporary non-availability and date of resumption of practice for the information of his clients.
2. Physicians can charge a reasonable professional fee depending upon their seniority and expertise but should not indulge in unfair practices, like receiving "cuts" from their specialist colleagues for referring patients to them.
3. Due to deluge of diagnostic facilities and cut throat competition, many laboratories are enticing the physicians by offering "kickbacks" to them to refer patients for investigations. It is a sad reality, that in order to make quick money, many unnecessary or irrelevant investigations are ordered and they are justified or legitimized in the garb of a safeguard against the viles and vagaries of Consumer

Protection Act. The practice of ordering a battery of tests merely to receive gratification or "cuts" from the laboratory is unethical and is strongly condemned.
4. Unnecessary admissions of patients to the hospital for treatment or undertaking a diagnostic or surgical procedure which is unwarranted, is unethical.
5. During our clinical practice, we screen a large number of prescriptions and investigations conducted by our colleagues. We must review them without arrogance and with due humility without making any adverse remarks or exhibiting it through our body language. We must treat our doctor colleagues as members of a big family and we should never utter a disparaging word or remark against our professional colleagues. Sir William Osler has extolled that *"Never let your tongue say a slighting word of a colleague"*.
6. Medicine should be practiced with conscience and dignity and without any greed or commercial motive. It is unethical and a criminal offence to abet "female feticide" by prenatal determination of sex by ultrasonography. Nothing should be done in our day-to-day dealings and practice which hurts our inner voice or conscience in order to prevent guilt feelings and remorse.
7. It is unethical to take any overt or covert sexual liberties or exhibit misconduct with patients or their attendants whether in thought, behavior or action.
8. It is unethical and fraudulent to issue false medical certificates or disability certificates for financial considerations. The physician should provide true information with a sense of fairness, honesty and integrity.
9. Public and patients should not be blackmailed or put into inconvenience by striking work or adopting work-to-rule mandates by doctors in the government institutions to get their demands fulfilled under duress. Instead of harassing the patients, they should harness the support of public to get their just demands fulfilled. The Government of India has brought the medical services under the ambit of Essential Service Maintenance Act (ESMA) to put a curb against the menace of strikes by doctors.
10. It is unethical, illegal and immoral to trade the body organs for transplantation for pecuniar or financial considerations.
11. It is unscrupulous and dishonest for physicians to receive courtesies, favors and gifts from manufacturers and suppliers of equipment and pharmaceutical companies. The Medical Council of India has issued guidelines and directives to promote ethical relationship between doctors and companies producing health care products (Table 16.1).

TABLE 16.1 Medical Council of India's directives to promote ethical practices

Gifts	A medical practitioner shall not receive any gift from any pharmaceutical or allied health care industry.
Travel	No travel within or outside the country, either for self and/or family member/s for attending conferences, seminars, workshops, CME programs, etc. can be sponsored by a health care company.
Hospitality	Hotel accommodation for the doctor and/or family member/s by the pharmaceutical or medical equipment company is strictly prohibited.
Cash or monetary gains	Doctors cannot receive any financial incentives under any pretext from the pharma houses or companies dealing with nutritional products and medical equipment. Funding for medical research can be received only through approved institutions by modalities and guidelines laid down by the government of India.
Endorsements	Individual doctors as well as professional and academic associations are banned to endorse and promote any health care products.

12. Research must be conducted with fairness, sincerity and with due safeguards to the study subjects. The medical profession should ensure safety and efficacy of new technologies and informed consent must be taken before recruiting patients for therapeutic interventions and drug trials. Fraud in research either by plagiarization or "quantum jugglery" are condemned and punished for professional misconduct. The researcher should not misrepresent ideas of others as his own.

The violation of any of the MCI directives shall be considered as "Misconduct" and, therefore, can invite penalties in the form of temporary or protracted suspension or cancellation of medical registration. However, the implementation of these guidelines is a major challenge for the Medical Council of India or recently launched National Medical Commission (NMC).

Withholding or Withdrawal of Life Support

Cardiopulmonary resuscitation (CPR) is withheld, if a patient is terminally sick or it is believed that the available therapies are likely to be futile and in the event of survival there will be virtual or total loss of cognition for any meaningful existence (Box 16.4). Humanistic teachings in general and philosophies of the major religions of the world recognize that there comes a time in the care of every patient when it is appropriate for the doctor to stop further attempts to unnecessarily prolong the process of dying. The policy of passive euthanasia is followed by withholding CPR, life-saving surgery, assisted ventilation, dialysis, vasopressors, administration of blood and blood products and expensive antibiotics. Instead of continuation of life-prolonging therapies, it is desirable to provide palliative care to relieve pain and suffering.

The decision to withhold or withdraw life support should be taken after due deliberations among various experts by taking the family into confidence through the process of informed consent. The decision should be recorded in the case file along with full medical justifications and should be duly signed by the parent or surrogate. This approach is duly approved by the professional and academic bodies of the world. The policy is logical and rational and is aimed at reducing the suffering and misery of both the dying patient and his close relatives. But it lacks legal sanction and protection. There is a need to accord legal sanctity to the act of passive euthanasia in order to avoid unnecessary litigations. The procedure manual in the PICU should outline the details of admission policies, indications for withdrawal and withholding of life support.

Communication and Doctor–Patient Relationship

"A person may have learnt a great deal and still be an exceedingly unskillful physician, who awakens little confidence in his powers. The manner of dealing with patients, art of winning their confidence, soothing and consoling them, or drawing their attention to serious matters ... all this cannot be learnt from books..."

— **John Apley**

Effective communication is essential to establish good doctor–patient/parent relationship. It is indeed the key to build confidence, faith and trust of the parents to augment the process of healing. Most parental complaints of mismanagement originate due to lack of communication or because of abrasive, arrogant or callous attitude of the doctor or member for the healthcare team rather than due to lack of skills or faulty technical management of the patient. We should not judge, belittle or argue with parents. The patients and parents must feel at all times that they are being

---

Box 16.4 Indications for do-not-resuscitate (DNR) orders

- Advanced metastatic malignancy
- Multisystem end-stage organ failure
- Severe irreversible CNS disorder, trauma, bleeding and tumor
- Severe and untreatable underlying neuromotor disability
- Persistent vegetative state
- Brain dead*

*This is an indication for withdrawal of life support

> **Box 16.5 Benefits of good doctor–patient/parent communication**
>
> - Better confidence, trust and faith of the physician.
> - Reduced anxiety and greater satisfaction of the patients and parents.
> - Better cooperation of the child during physical examination.
> - Provision of holistic care rather than mere cure.
> - Involvement of parents in decision making.
> - Better compliance to therapeutic options.
> - Better health outcomes and reduced length of hospital stay.
> - Reduced risk of intolerance and vandalism against health care professionals.
> - Reduced risk of malpractice litigations.

treated with due courtesy and consideration. Humility, concern, empathy and compassion are crucial to generate faith and provide emotional support to the family. Even if the enquiry or query of the parents is illogical, repetitive and irritating, we must respond with due grace, sensitivity, equanimity and calmness without any hurry, anger or arrogance. *Communication is indeed the most vital link to strengthen doctor–patient relationship.* The virtues and benefits of good doctor–patient communication are listed in **Box 16.5**.

It is an amazing fact that most parents are grateful even when we are unable to save the life of their child especially when we showed concern, care and compassion and parents and relatives were made to perceive that whatever was humanely possible was done for the care of their child. It is important to communicate "with" parents by literally coming down to their level and by maintaining an eye-to-eye contact. We should be careful and tactful not only in deciding "what to tell" the parents but also "how to tell it". The parents should be told about the condition of the child in a simple, easily understandable language. We should try to be pragmatic and honest in communicating true status of the child but nevertheless try to keep the hope alive which has tremendous healing capabilities. In a critically sick child, always give a guarded prognosis which can be tempered with hope, will power and godly benevolence. We should not allow technology to further dehumanize medicine and try to resurrect the declining image of the medical profession. It is desirable that all the medical and nursing colleges in the country should initiate regular education programs in the fields of social and behavioral sciences, art of communication and medical ethics for graduate and postgraduate medical and nursing students.

Chronic or Incurable Disease

When a child is suffering from an incurable disease or an affliction which is likely to have lifelong disability, the parents are likely to respond with disbelief, anger, shock or feeling of hopelessness. The bad news should preferably be conveyed to both the parents simultaneously in a relaxed atmosphere with due concern, compassion and empathy. Parents and attendants have emotional feelings and we should never say, "nothing can be done", because something can always be done. The facts should be explained in a simple language without any medical jargon. The nature of disease, likely prognosis, available therapeutic interventions, cost of care, etc. should be explained. We should allow the parents to ventilate their feelings and concerns and try to answer their queries in an honest and unambiguous manner. We should try to follow the well-known philosophy, *"talk less and listen more"*, that is why God has given us one mouth and two ears! We should be pragmatic but not pessimistic and always keep the hope alive which is a great healing force and remember that miracles do happen.

We should be careful and diplomatic in conveying the nature of the disease without hurting parental sentiments. Instead of saying bluntly that "your child is mentally retarded", it is preferable to say that your child is slow or having developmental delay. In our society, it is important to provide spiritual dimension to their tragedy by saying that *"God has chosen you to provide care and comfort to your special child because you are so compassionate, caring and sensitive human being"*. The family should be encouraged to join the Self Help Associations of Parents of children having the same medical problem. It is useful to form a network and learn from each other by sharing mutual concerns and difficulties and by effective utilization of available technologies and services of specialists. It is important that normal children in the family are not neglected, instead they should be involved in the care of the "special child".

The End-of-Life Issues

> "Death is certain for the born and rebirth is inevitable for the dead. You should not, therefore, grieve over the inevitable".
> **The Bhagavad Gita**

Despite all the technological advances, *medicine cannot achieve immortality*! We are all destined to die and death indeed is the ultimate truth of life. But death is always unacceptable especially when life is cut short in the bud without fulfillment of purpose of existence or when it is due to unnatural causes. It is easier to face death when it is anticipated and family is adequately prepared for the eventuality.

Pediatricians face several situations in clinical practice wherein a child is diagnosed to have a potentially fatal disease (AIDS, malignancy, genetic disorder) or develops an acute life-threatening disorder or dies suddenly in the emergency room due to polytrauma or road accident. The news of an incurable or difficult-to-manage intractable disease should be given to both the parents in a relaxed manner with due consideration and compassion. Parents must be given an opportunity to ask questions and ventilate their feelings and you must listen attentively and provide appropriate answers to relieve their anxiety, concerns and worries.

It is controversial as to how much information should be given to the child and whether he or she should be taken into confidence and told about the nature of the disease or it should be kept as a guarded secret. By and large, it depends upon the age, inquisitiveness, sensitivity and emotional maturity of the child whether he should be told about the nature of disease or not. We should seek the advice of parents in this matter. The news about the "bad or lethal" disease should never be conveyed bluntly like a bolt from the blue. We should be honest and pragmatic in our approach and the news of "gloomy prognosis" must be tempered with due optimism and godly benevolence to keep the hope alive in order to augment the process of healing. *It is important to keep in mind that nature, time, patience, faith, hope, prayer, positive thinking and willpower have tremendous healing capabilities and they should be effectively harnessed in our day-to-day clinical practice.* It is important that we should not only provide state-of-the-art care to the critically sick child but also make the parents and attendants perceive that whatever was humanly possible, it was done for their child.

The family should be prepared emotionally and spiritually before declaration of death. The news of death should be conveyed with utmost compassion but in no unmistakable term that the child has died despite our best intents and efforts. Acceptance of death becomes difficult when a child dies in the Emergency Department because of an acute life-threatening disease or road accident. A large number of emotions, like anger, hostility, shock, grief, guilt, denial, and depression, need to be handled with poise, sympathy and utmost care so that reality is accepted with due grace as a will of God or nature's ordain and as a matter of fact or destiny. If CPR is being provided (where DNR is not applicable), the parent or attendant should be escorted to the rest room and allowed to ventilate his/her feelings. The family's wishes for religious support (amulets, mantras, holy water, etc.) and ceremonies and their desire that the death should occur in the familiar atmosphere of home rather than hospital, should be honored as far as possible. When a child is conscious and dying, the parents should be at his bedside holding his hand and talking with him to allay his fears and assist him to express his concerns, desires and emotions. Silent listening and support at this stage is valued more than unnecessary talking.

During the emotionally surcharged atmosphere of the process of dying, some resident doctors and nurses may feel extremely frustrated, upset and demoralized because of their inadequacy and inability to save life despite sincere and maximal efforts. They also need emotional support, guidance and advice to avoid unnecessary identification and attachment with the family. They should be encouraged and assisted to learn the art of detachment, imperturbability and poise at all odds. After taking relevant postmortem biopsies, family should be approached with caution and tact to seek permission for autopsy. We should never give an impression to the parents that autopsy is needed for making a correct diagnosis but it is required for helping science and society regarding the prevention of disease among contacts and siblings and for possible genetic counseling.

After completing urgent formalities, a death certificate should be prepared. The family should be provided with necessary courtesy, compassion and conveyance for a dignified journey of the dead child to the mortuary or home. The coping of death of a child in the hospital is a painful and challenging experience but one that can also provide respect for humanity and life. Death deflates our ego and teaches us humility and provides strength to face and accept the greatest reality and truth of life with equanimity and grace.

Organ Transplantation

The enaction of Human Organ Transplant Act by the Indian Parliament in 1994 has opened opportunities for cadaveric transplant of heart, liver, kidneys, pancreas, etc., which should be fully exploited. The possibility of a positive contribution through their tragedy with the hope that their child may see the world or live through some body else's eyes or organs, may be accepted with enthusiasm. The issue of organ donation should not be broached, if there are well-recognized contraindications for donation of organs, such as primary immunodeficiency disorder, genetic defect, HIV, HBsAg-positivity, viremia and septicemia. Xenotransplantation (animal-to-human transplant) of cells, tissues and organs with or without genetic engineering is fraught with serious hazards of transmission of animal viruses, rejection, social injustice, moral and religious considerations.

Violence against Doctors

Intolerance and resentment against doctors is an emerging global phenomenon but India seems to lead the world in violence against doctors. According to World Health Organization, about 8–38% health care workers suffer physical violence at some point in their careers. Many more are verbally abused or threatened. Public is behaving like health sector terrorists and media is exploiting the situation by promoting the mandate, "*A muderer is innocent till proved guilty but a doctor is guilty till proved innocent*". There is a need to arrest the development of further distrust between doctors and their patients and attendants, otherwise it will compromise all achievements of medical science, and adversely affect the healing capabilities of doctors.

Rude and aggressive behavior of the parents or attendants, and arrogant and lackadaisical approach of the doctor, is the root cause of intolerance and violence against doctors. Most cases of violence occur in the emergency department and intensive care areas. These areas are the face of medical care and must be provided with adequate staff, infrastructure and life-saving drugs and functional equipment at all times. *There should be no delay in attending to a critically sick patient.* Doctors should handle patients with due empathy and concern. The training of doctors should not focus on writing prescriptions alone, they must be trained in the art of communication, bedside manners and medical ethics. According to our scriptures, physicians should see and visualize God in every human being (*Aham Brahmasmi*) and feel honored that we have been given the supreme responsibility to serve Him.

It is possible to reduce the incidence of intolerance and violance against doctors but difficult to eliminate it completely. The hospitals must have adequate infrastructure, facilities and staff to handle emergencies without delay and with due confidence and skills. The security of health care providers should be improved by having adequate number of security guards, frisking facilities, extensive CCTV network and availability of "Quick Response Team" to handle unruly mob.

Laws to prevent violence against doctors do exist but they need to be made more stringent and implemented properly. The government should establish fast track courts to provide justice within 3 months when any incidence of violence and vandalism against health care providers is brought to their notice. In case of any perceived "medical neglect" or grievances, the public should handle the situation in a civilized manner and seek redressal through Medical Protection Act and available legal avenues.

The Optimism and Hope

The declining image of the medical profession needs a moral boost and rejuvenation through a process of soul searching and ethical cleansing in the light of existent social realities. The continuing process of erosion of doctor–patient relationship and trust due to insensitive and commercialized attitude of some physicians and over demanding attitude of educated and well-informed internet-savvy parents, needs to be checked against further disintegration. In view of the fact that services of the doctors have been included in the purview of Consumer Protection Act for redressal of grievances and grant of compensation by the consumer courts, it is essential for the doctors to be more cautious, considerate and ethical in their dealings with their patients to avoid any litigations. The revolution in technology is no substitute for the over-riding need for trust and communication which indeed is the key to maintain an ideal doctor–patient relationship.

It is desirable that all medical and nursing colleges in the country should initiate regular education programs in the field of social and behavioral sciences, art of communication and medical ethics for graduate and postgraduate medical and nursing students. The teachers must serve as role models to infuse and enthuse the qualities of compassion, sensitivity and genuine concern towards patients and their attendants. We should not allow the technology to further dehumanize medicine and we must treat our patients not only with our heads but also with our hearts. The world needs caring and concerned physicians, and not merely curing and commercial robots who lack the sensitivity and deny the healing virtues of human touch. Ethics and grievances committees should be established in all hospitals and they should serve as watchdogs to monitor and maintain the sanctity of all ethical decisions. All attempts should be made to improve the doctor–patient/parent relationship and reduce the triggers for intolerance and violence against doctors. It is nice to have an up-to-date knowledge and be a well-informed doctor but above all it is much nicer to be a good human being in order to provide global and holistic care and not merely cure to our patients. The physicians should make concerted efforts to resurrect the declining medical image, master the sublime art of medicine and acquire the divine gift of healing.

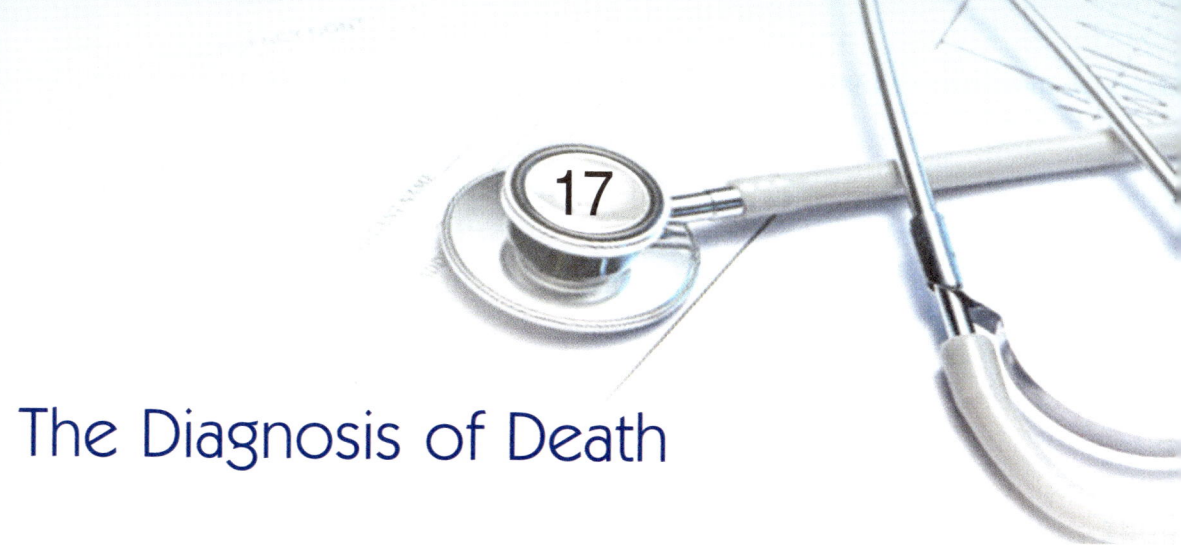

The Diagnosis of Death

Despite advances in medical technology, the medical science can never achieve immortality. Death indeed is the ultimate truth of life and we as pediatricians are quite used to facing children with acute catastrophic life-threatening diseases and terminal illnesses. Many critically sick children are supported by artificial life-sustaining measures, like vasopressors and mechanical ventilation in whom criteria of brain death are used to declare them as dead even when their heart is beating. The prolonged and unnecessary maintenance of a "dead" child on a life support system is an extremely stressful experience for the parents and expensive for the state. Accurate timing of brain death is also important to harness the organs of children, whose parents are willing, for cadaveric transplant of heart, lungs, liver and kidneys. Following the enaction of Human Organ Transplant Act by many countries, it is legally justified to remove organs from brain dead patients who are still having heart beats.

Death is diagnosed when child has sustained either (1) irreversible cessation of circulatory and respiratory functions or (2) there is irreversible cessation of all functions of the entire brain including the brainstem. *Irreversible coma and apnea must coexist, for the diagnosis of brain death.* After the brain is dead and spontaneous respirations have ceased, the heart may continue to beat, if mechanical ventilation maintains adequate oxygenation of blood.

HISTORY

The probable cause of coma should be ascertained to ensure that there is no remediable or reversible condition. Identify and exclude any potentially reversible toxic and metabolic disorder, use of sedative-hypnotic drugs or paralytic agents, hypothermia, drowning, hypoxia, trauma, electrocution, hypotension and surgically correctable condition.

CESSATION OF CIRCULATION AND BREATHING EFFORTS

Vigorous cardiopulmonary resuscitation (CPR) should be continued for at least 30 minutes while continuously monitoring vital signs. Absence of heart beats and spontaneous respiratory efforts during an appropriate period of observation (at least 30 min) is a satisfactory criteria of clinical death. When a patient is attached to an ECG monitor, flat tracings are indicative of cellular death. The diagnosis of cessation of breathing poses practical difficulties in babies on a ventilator. The ventilator can be periodically switched off and spontaneous respiratory movements are watched. It is essential to maintain $PaCO_2$ of the patient around 60 mm Hg or 20 mm Hg above the normal baseline value (so that there is enough drive for the respiratory center) before the ventilator is switched off.

BRAIN DEATH

The current legal definition of death requires clinical evidences of irreversible brainstem death.

The three essential criteria of brain death include coma, absence of brainstem reflexes and apnea. Hypotension, hypothermia and metabolic disturbances that could affect the neurological examination must be corrected before evaluation of brain death. Sedatives, anticonvulsants and neuromuscular blockers should be discontinued for a reasonable time period, based on the elimination half-life of the pharmacologic agent, before conducting the neurologic examination for brain death. The clinical criteria for brain death are listed in Table 17.1. In deeply comatosed patients (absence of facial grimace on firm pressure over the supraorbital region), on assisted ventilation and advanced life support system, it is futile to continue with life support measures, if neurologic functions have irreversibly ceased. When brain death occurs, patients lose their brainstem reflexes in a rostral-to-caudal direction and the medulla oblongata is the last part of the brain which ceases to function. The cessation of neurologic functions is assessed by evaluation of following brainstem reflexes.

(a) **Pupillary response to light** The pupils should be dilated (4–8 mm) at midposition and fixed on both sides without any response to bright light. A magnifying glass with inbuilt light can be used to assess pupillary response to light. It is mediated by components of the optic and oculomotor nerves located in mesencephalon.

(b) **Corneal reflex** The corneal reflex should be absent. The corneal reflex is elicited by touching the cornea with a wisp of cotton and observing the reflex closure of the eyelids. It is mediated by sensory (5th nerve) and motor (7th nerve) components having neuroanatomic centers within pons.

(c) **Oculocephalic reflex or 'Dolls' head-eye-movements** are elicited by rotation of the patient's head from one side to the other or up and down with eyelids held open. In a comatosed child with intact brainstem, when head is turned to one side and maintained in that position for a few seconds, there are conjugate movements of both the eyes to the opposite side. When oculocephalic reflex is affected, there is either no conjugate movements of the eyeballs or there are dysconjugate movements.

(d) **Vestibulo-ocular reflex** The tympanic membranes must be intact and there should be no local trauma or cerumen (wax) in the ear canal before this reflex is elicited. Head should be kept raised at 30° to the horizontal plane, unless contraindicated by cervical spinal

TABLE 17.1 Clinical criteria for brain death in children

- Irreversible coma
- Absence of motor responses to pain
- Absence of pupillary responses to light and pupils are fixed at midposition (4–8 mm)
- Absence of corneal reflexes
- Absence of caloric responses (vestibulo-ocular reflex)
- Absence of gag reflex or coughing in response to tracheal suctioning
- Absence of sucking and rooting reflexes in a term neonate
- Absence of respiratory drive at a $PaCO_2$ of 60 mm Hg or 20 mm Hg above the normal baseline values
- *The observation period between two evaluations is based on the child's age. The second neurologic assessment should be done by a different attending physician but second apnea testing should be done by the same physician.*
  (i) Term baby up to 30 days: 24 hours
  (ii) >30 days to <18 years: 12 hours
  (iii) >18 years: Interval is optional
- *Confirmatory tests* (EEG and radionuclide cerebral blood flow).
  (i) When clinical examination and apnea testing cannot be completed safely due to the underlying medical condition.
  (ii) When there is uncertainty about the result of neurological examination.
  (iii) When medication effect is present.
  (iv) To reduce the inter-examination observation period.

Adapted from Nakagawa TA, Ashwal S, Mathur M, Mysore MR, et al. Guidelines for the determination of brain death in infants and children. An update of the 1987 Task Force Recommendations. *Crit Care Med* 2011, 39(9):2139–55.

injury. About 20 mL ice-cold water is slowly injected into each auditory canal and directed towards the tympanic membrane. When caloric response is intact there is tonic deviation or nystagmoid movements of both eyes towards the side being stimulated. *The absence of any response is indicative of brainstem dysfunction.* Both oculocephalic and oculovestibular reflexes are mediated by fibers from the vestibular portion of the 8th nerve with nuclei in the pons. From these pontine centers, impulses are conveyed to the 6th nerve nucleus through internuclear synapses, causing lateral movements of the eyes towards side of stimulus. Synapses exist between 6th nerve nucleus and 3rd nerve nucleus through medial longitudinal fasiculus coursing through pons and mesencephalon, resulting in medial deviation of the eyes on the contralateral side.

(e) *Facial response to pain* There is no facial grimace when a firm pressure is applied over the supraorbital nerve, temporomandibular joint or nail bed of a finger.

(f) *Oropharyngeal reflex* The gag reflex and cough reflex response to suction of oropharynx and trachea should be absent. The tracheal catheter should be advanced up to the level of carina followed by one or two suction attempts.

(g) *Absence of respiratory drive* The patient should be preoxygenated by giving 100% oxygen for 5–10 minutes before initiating apnea test. There is no spontaneous breathing even when $PaCO_2$ is kept around 60 mm Hg or 20 mm Hg above the normal baseline value. The protocol for apnea test is shown in Table 17.2.

Observation Period

It must be remembered that spinal segmental responses and deep tendon jerks may persist even in the presence of brain death. The brainstem reflexes should be elicited in all comatosed children before disconnecting the ventilator. The criteria for brain death are not well-defined in preterm babies. In newborn babies, two EEGs taken 24 hours apart should show electrocerebral silence or dynamic scan (133 xenon CT or PET) should demonstrate absence of cerebral blood flow for more than one hour. The cessation of all brain functions must persist for at least 24 hours in infants up to one month, and 12 hours for infants older than one month. The observation period may be reduced, if the EEG demonstrates electrocerebral silence or the cerebral radionuclide study does not visualize cerebral arteries. The children with potentially reversible conditions, such as hypoxia, narcotic poisoning, carbon monoxide exposure, electrocution, exposure to severe cold, neuromuscular blockade, metabolic conditions, drowning and trauma should be watched for a longer period of time. Hypothermia following drowning or exposure to cold may be associated with a state of "suspended animation" and is the commonest cause of erroneous diagnosis of death.

TABLE 17.2 Protocol for apnea testing

- Core body temperature should be >36°C
- Systolic or mean arterial blood pressure should be within the normal range for the age
- Ventilator is adjusted to provide normocarbia ($PaCO_2$ 35–45 mm Hg)
- Patient is preoxygenated with 100% FiO_2 for ≥10 minutes
- Draw an arterial blood sample for baseline blood gases
- Provide oxygen through T-piece with CPAP at 10 cm H_2O
- Connect a pulse oximeter
- Disconnect ventilator and leave the patient off the ventilator for 8–10 minutes
- Observe the patient for spontaneous respiratory movements
- Measure PaO_2, $PaCO_2$ and pH at the end of 8–10 minutes and reconnect the patient to the ventilator
- Record your observations and comments

*The diagnosis of brain death is confirmed, if there are no respiratory movements at $PaCO_2$ of ≥60 mm Hg or when it is raised ≥20 mm Hg above the baseline $PaCO_2$ of the patient on two occasions.

Adapted from Machado C, Perez J, Pando A. Brain death diagnosis and apnea test safety. *Ann Indian Acad Neurol* 2009, 12(3):197–200.

Confirmatory Tests

The diagnosis of brain death is primarily clinical by evaluation of coma, apnea and brainstem reflexes. No ancillary tests are required, if clinical tests of brain death are unequivocal. Rarely, confirmatory laboratory tests are undertaken to confirm the diagnosis of death (Table 17.3). The ancillary studies may be required when (1) clinical assessment or apnea testing cannot be completed, (2) findings of clinical examination are equivocal, (3) if a medication effect is present, or (4) to reduce the inter-examination observation period.

Brainstem evoked responses, radioisotope [Technetium (Tc 99m) exametazime] scintigraphy, bolus cerebral angiography, xenon CT, digital subtraction angiography, visualization of cerebral arterial pulsations by real-time transcranial ultrasonography are reliable criteria of brain death but they are of limited practical utility. Four-vessel intracranial angiography is diagnostic of cessation of circulation to the brain but it is cumbersome. Electroencephalography with a minimum of 8 electrodes should demonstrate electrical silence for at least 30 minutes. Doppler determination of cerebral blood flow velocity and evoked potentials are being investigated for the diagnosis of 'brain death'. The treating physician must, however, satisfy himself with reasonable certainty that the patient's vital functions pertaining to heart, lungs and even brain have irreversibly ceased before the tragic news of death is communicated to the parents. In a rare instance of a patient showing sign(s) of life at the time of funeral, may lead to dire consequences of medical negligence on the part of a physician and health care establishment. The probable cause of death including predisposing or underlying conditions should be recorded in the death certificate.

TABLE 17.3 Confirmatory tests for diagnosis of brain death

- **Electroencephalography**
  Recordings are obtained for at least 30 minutes with a 16- or 18-channel instrument. Interelectrode impedance should be between 100 and 10,000 Ω. The integrity of the entire recording system should be tested. The distance between electrodes should be at least 10 cm. The sensitivity should be increased to at least 2 µV for 30 minutes with inclusion of appropriate calibrations. The high-frequency filter setting should not be set below 30 Hz, and the low-frequency setting should not be above 1 Hz.
  Electroencephalography should demonstrate a lack of reactivity to intense somatosensory or audiovisual stimuli.

- **Somatosensory evoked potentials (SSEP)**
  Median nerve is stimulated by mild electrical shocks and its response in the brain is assessed by an electrode placed on the patients' head. The absence of brain signals indicates that the brain is no longer able to receive neural messages.

- **Cerebral angiography**
  The contrast medium should be injected under high pressure in both anterior and posterior circulations. No intracerebral filling should be detected at the level of entry of the carotid or vertebral artery to the skull. The external carotid circulation should be patent. The filling of the superior longitudinal sinus may be delayed.

- **Transcranial Doppler ultrasonography (TCD)**
  There should be bilateral insonation. The probe should be placed at the temporal bone above the zygomatic arch or the vertebrobasilar arteries through the suboccipital transcranial window. The abnormalities should include a lack of diastolic or reverberating flow and documentation of small systolic peaks in early systole. A finding of a complete absence of flow may not be reliable owing to inadequate transtemporal windows for insonation.

- **Cerebral scintigraphy or radionuclide brain scan [Technetium (Tc 99m) exametazime].**
  The isotope should be injected within 30 minutes after its reconstitution. A static image of 500,000 counts should be obtained at several time points, i.e. immediately, between 30 and 60 minutes later, and at 2 hours.
  A correct intravenous injection may be confirmed with additional images of the liver demonstrating uptake of the isotope (optional).
  Brain death is confirmed, if there is no radionuclide localization in the middle cerebral, anterior cerebral and basilar artery territories of the cerebral hemispheres (hollow skull phenomenon). No tracer is seen in the superior sagittal sinus although minimal tracer may come from the scalp.

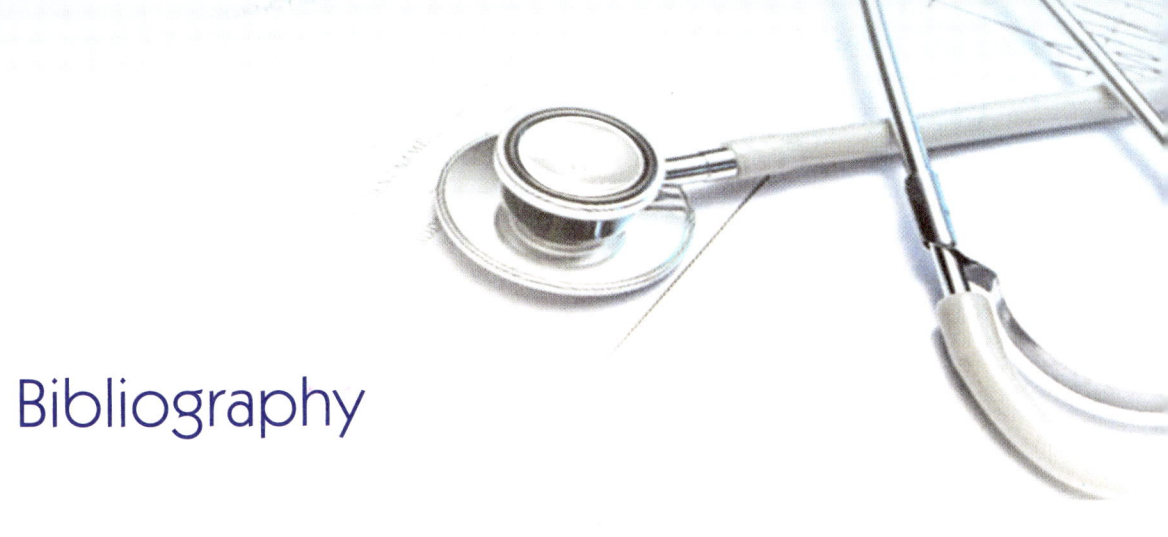

Bibliography

1. Aase JM. Diagnostic Dysmorphology. *Plenum Publishing Co, New York,* 1990.
2. Aase JM. Diagnostic Dysmorphology for the Pediatric Practitioner. *Pediatric Clinics of North America* 1992, 39:135–156.
3. Algranati P. The Pediatric Patient. An approach to History and Physical Examination. *Williams and Wilkins, Baltimore,* 1992.
4. Apley J, Mackeith RM. The Child and his Symptoms. *Blackwell Scientific Publications, Oxford,* 1962.
5. Apley J. The Child with Abdominal Pains. *JB Lippincott, London,* 2nd edition, 1975.
6. Apley J. Paediatrics. *Bailliere Tindall, London,* 2nd edition, 1979.
7. Athreya BH, Silverman B. Pediatric Physical Diagnosis. *Appleton-Century-Crofts, Norwalk,* 1985.
8. Barness LA. Manual of Pediatric Physical Diagnosis. *Year book Medical Publishers, Chicago,* 4th edition, 1972.
9. Bickerstaff ER, Spillane JA. Neurological Examination in Clinical Practice. *Oxford University Press, London,* 5th edition, 1993.
10. Burnside JW. Adams' Physical Diagnosis. *The Williams and Wilkins Co., Baltimore,* 15th ed. 1974.
11. Daniels L, Worthingham C. Muscle Testing Techniques by Manual Examination. *WB Saunders Co., Philadelphia,* 3rd edition, 1972.
12. Davenport WH. The Good Physician: A Treasury of Medicine. *The MacMillan Company, New York,* 1962.
13. Douglas G, Nicol F, Robutson C. Macleod's Clinical Examination. *Churchill Livingstone, New York,* 12th edition, 2009.
14. Gilbride KE. Developmental testing. *Pediatric Review* 1995, 16:338–345.
15. Glynn M, Drake WM. Hutchison's Clinical Methods. *Elsevier Philadelphia,* 24th edition, 2017.
16. Goldbloom RB. Pediatric Clinical Skills. Elsevier Philadelphia, 4th edition, 2011.
17. Gorlin RJ, Pindborg JJ, Cohen MM. Syndromes of the Head and Neck. *McGraw-Hill Book Co, New York,* 2nd edition, 1976.
18. Green M. Pediatric Diagnosis. Interpretation of symptoms and signs in infants, children and adolescents. *WB Saunders Co, Philadelphia,* 6th edition, 1998.
19. Gunn VL, Nechyba C. The Harriet Lane Hand-book. A Manual for Pediatric House Officers. *Elsevier, New Delhi,* 16th edition, 2002.
20. Houghton AR, Gray D. Chamberlain's Symptoms and Signs in Clinical Medicine. An Introduction to Medical Diagnosis. *Butterworth-CRC Press,* 13th Edition, 2010.
21. Illingworth RS. Basic Development Screening. *Blackwell Scientific Publications,* 4th edition, 1988.
22. Illingworth RS. Common Symptoms of Disease in Children. *Blackwell Scientific Publications, Oxford,* 9th edition, 1988.
23. Illingworth RS. The Normal Child. *Churchill Livingstone,* Edinburgh. 10th edition, 1991.
24. Jones KL, Jones MC, Campo Mdel. Smith's Recognizable Patterns of Human Malformations. *Elsevier, Philadelphia,* 7th edition, 2013.

25. Khadilkar V, Yadav S, Agrawal KK, Tamboli S, Bannerjee M, *et al*. Revised IAP growth charts for height, weight and body mass index for 5–18 years old Indian children. *Indian Pediatrics* 2015, 52:47–55.
26. Morgan WL, Engel GL. The Clinical Approach to the Patient. *WB Saunders Co, Philadelphia*, 1969.
27. Paine RS, Oppe TE. Neurological Examination of Children. *William Heinemann Medical Books* Ltd., 1966.
28. Park MK. Pediatric Cardiology for Practitioners. Elsevier, 6th edition, 2014.
29. Pomeranz AJ, Fairley JA. The systematic evaluation of the skin in children. *Pediatric Clinics of North America* 1998, 45, 49–63.
30. Rosser T. Pediatric Neurology: A Case-based Review. *Lippincott Williams and Wilkins, Philadelphia,* 2007.
31. Sarkar M, Mahesh DM, Madabhavi I. Digital clubbing. *Lung India* 2012, 29(4):354–362.
32. Singh M. Care of the Newborn. *CBS Publishers & Distributors Pvt Ltd,* New Delhi, 8th edition, 2015.
33. Singh M. Communication as a bridge to build a sound doctor-patient/parent relationship. *Indian J Pediatr* 2016, 83(1):33–37.
34. Singh M. Intolerance and violence against doctors. *Indian J Pediatr* 2017, 84(10):768–773.
35. Singh M. Medical Quotations by Eminent Physicians and Philosophers. *CBS Publishers & Distributors Pvt Ltd., New Delhi,* 4th edition, 2016.
36. Singh M. The art, science and philosophy of child care. *Indian J Pediatr* 2009, 76:171–176.
37. Singh M. The art and essence of child care: Personal perspective. *Sri Lanka J Child Hlth* 2016, 45(3):203–213.
38. Singh M. The art, essence and philosophy of newborn care. *Indian J Pediatr* 2014, 81(6):552–559.
39. Staheli LT. Fundamentals of Pediatric Orthopedics. 4th Ed. *Lippincott-Williams and Wilkins Publishers, Philadelphia,* 2007.
40. Stockman JA. Difficult Diagnosis in Pediatrics. *WB Saunders Co, Philadelphia,* 1990.
41. Tandon R. Bedside Approach in the Diagnosis of Congenital Heart Diseases. *BI Churchill Livingstone, New Delhi,* 1998.
42. Thureen PJ, Deacon J, Hernandez JA, Hall D. Assessment and Care of the Well Newborn. *WB Saunders, Philadelphia,* 2nd edition, 2005.
43. Vakil RJ, Golwalla AF, Physical Diagnosis. A Textbook of Symptoms and Signs. *Media Promoters and Publishers Pvt Ltd., Bombay,* 16th edition, 2017.
44. Verbov J, Morley N. Color Atlas of Pediatric Dermatology. *MTP Press Ltd,* 1983.
45. Wijdicks EFM. The diagnosis of brain death. *New England Journal of Medicine* 2001, 344:1215–1221.
46. Zuberbuhler JR. Clinical Diagnosis in Pediatric Cardiology. *Churchill Livingstone, New York,* 1982.

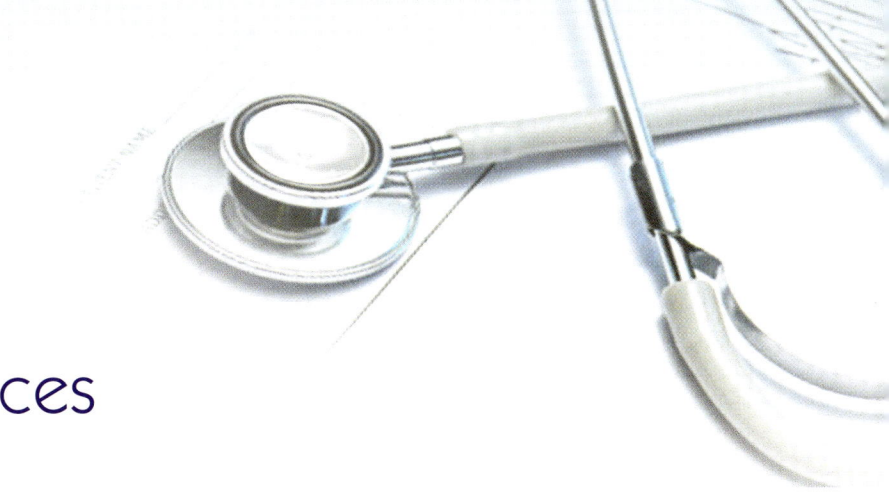

Appendices

APPENDIX I. Weight, length and volume conversion tables

Weight equivalents		Height and weight conversion factors	
Apothecary	Metric	To convert	Multiply by
1 grain	64.799 (say 60) mg or 0.06 g	Inches to centimeters	2.54
15 grain	1000 mg or 1.0 g	Inches to meters	0.0254
60 grain (1 dram)	4 g	Feet to meters	0.3048
8 dram (1 oz)	30 g	Pounds to kilograms	0.4535
1 pound (16 oz)	454 g	Kilograms to pounds	2.2
2.2 pounds	1 kg		

Liquid measures				
	Metric			
Apothecary	Exact	Approximate	Household measures*	
1 minim (drop)	0.059 mL	0.06 mL	Teaspoon	5 mL
15 minims	0.885 mL	1.0 mL	Tablespoon	15 mL
60 minims (1 fl dram)	3.7 mL	4.0 mL	Cup or katori	150 mL
8 fl dram (1 fl oz)	29.6 mL	30.0 mL	Glass	250 mL or 8 oz
16 fl oz (1 pint)	473.2 mL	500.0 mL		
32 fl oz (1 quart)	946.4 mL	1000.0 mL		
1 gallon	3785.6 mL	4 quarts or 4000 mL		

*They are not standard in size and may widely vary in their volume

APPENDIX II. Temperature equivalents

Celsius	Fahrenheit	Celsius	Fahrenheit
35.0	95.0	38.6	101.4
35.4	95.7	39.0	102.2
35.8	96.4	39.4	102.9
36.0	96.8	39.8	103.6
36.4	97.5	40.2	104.3
36.8	98.2	40.6	105.1
37.0	98.6	41.0	105.8
37.4	99.3	41.4	106.5
37.8	100.0	41.8	107.2
38.2	100.7	42.0	107.6

The normal body temperature of 98.4°F corresponds to 36.9°C. To convert Fahrenheit to Celsius subtract 32 and divide by 1.8. To convert Celsius to Fahrenheit multiply by 1.8 and add 32.

APPENDIX III. Calculation of approximate body surface area from weight and height in children with normal physique

Weight range (kg)	Approximate body surface area (m²)
1–5	(0.05 × weight) + 0.05
6–10	(0.04 × weight) + 0.10
11–20	(0.03 × weight) + 0.20
21–40	(0.02 × weight) + 0.40

Lowe's formula: Body surface area (m²) = $\sqrt[3]{\text{weight}^2 \text{ (kg)} \times 0.1}$

Costeff's formula: Body surface area (m²) = $\dfrac{4w + 7}{w + 90}$ where w is weight in kg

Mostellar's formula: Body surface area (m²) = $\sqrt{\dfrac{\text{height (cm)} \times \text{weight (kg)}}{3600}}$

DuBois formula: Surface area (m²) = $0.007184 \times W \text{ (kg)}^{0.425} \times H \text{ (cm)}^{0.725}$

The average body surface area (m²) of a neonate is 0.25, 2 yr: 0.5, 9 yr: 1.07, adult woman 1.6 and man 1.9.

APPENDIX IV. Recommended daily requirements of balanced diet for Indian children (grams)

Food stuffs	1–3 years	4–6 years	7–9 years	10–12 years	13–18 years**
Cereals	150	200	250	320	400–450
Pulses	40–50*	50–60*	60–70*	60–70*	60–70*
Green leafy vegetables	50	75	75	100	100
Other vegetables, roots and tubers	30	50	50	75	150
Fruits	50	50	50	50	50
Milk	200–300*	200–250*	200–250*	200–250*	200–250*
Fats and oil	20	25	30	35	35–50
Meat, fish or eggs	30	30	30	30	60
Sugar and jaggery	30	40	50	50	50

Adapted from Nutritive Values of Indian Foods, Eds. Gopalan C, Rama Sastri BR, Balasubramanian SC, ICMR 1980.
*Higher values refer to vegetarian subjects.
**Requirements are higher in adolescent boys than girls.

APPENDIX V. Chronology of human dentition

Teeth	Primary or deciduous teeth*			
	Eruption		Shedding	
	Mandibular	Maxillary	Mandibular	Maxillary
Central incisors	5–7 months	6–8 months	6–7 years	7–8 years
Lateral incisors	7–10 months	8–11 months	7–8 years	8–9 years
Canines	16–20 months	16–20 months	9–11 years	11–12 years
First molars	10–16 months	10–16 months	10–12 years	10–11 years
Second molars	20–30 months	20–30 months	11–13 years	10–12 years

Teeth	Secondary or permanent teeth*			
	Calcification		Eruption	
	Begins at	Complete at	Mandibular	Maxillary
Central incisors	3–4 mo	9–10 yr	6–7 yr	7–8 yr
Lateral incisors	Mand. 3–4 mo	10–11 yr	7–8 yr	8–9 yr
	Max. 10–12 mo	12–15 yr	9–11 yr	11–12 yr
Canines	4–5 mo	12–13 yr	10–12 yr	10–11 yr
First premolars	18–21 mo	12–14 yr	11–13 yr	10–12 yr
Second premolars	24–30 mo	9–10 yr	6–7 yr	6–7 yr
First molars	Birth	14–16 yr	12–13 yr	12–13 yr
Second molars	30–36 mo	18–25 yr	17–22 yr	17–22 yr
Third molars	Mand. 8–10 yr Max. 7–9 yr			

Mand: mandible, Max: maxilla, mo: months, yr: years
There are wide variations in the age at eruption of the teeth which is genetically determined. Delayed or advanced dentition is poorly correlated both to the nutritional status and neuromotor development of the child.
*Milk teeth or primary teeth are white in color and have a smooth edge in contrast to permanent teeth, which have an ivory-white or off-white color and have a finely serrated edge.

APPENDIX VI. Predicted average peak expiratory flow rates (PEFR) on the basis of height in normal children*

Height (in)	Height (cm)	PEFR (L/min)	Height (in)	Height (cm)	PEFR (L/min)
43	109	147	56	142	320
44	112	160	57	144	334
45	114	173	58	147	347
46	117	187	59	149	360
48	122	214	60	152	373
49	124	227	61	154	387
50	127	240	63	159	413
51	129	254	64	162	427
52	132	267	65	164	440
53	134	280	66	167	454
54	137	293	67	170	467
55	139	307			

*At 100 cm height, average PEFR is about 100 L/min. For every 10 cm increase in height, add 50 L/min to get an approximate PEFR value. When PEFR is less than 80% of the predicted average or patient's known highest PEFR when he is well, it indicates that patient is unwell.
Adapted from Voter KZ, McBride JT. Diagnostic tests of lung function. *Pediatrics in Review* 1996, 17(2):53–63.

APPENDIX VII. Vital signs in children of various ages

Age	Heart rate (beats/min.)	Respiratory rate (beats/min.)	Blood pressure systolic/diastolic (mm Hg)
Premature	120–170	40–70	55–75/35–45
0–3 mo	100–150	35–55	65–85/45–55
3–6 mo	90–120	30–45	70–90/50–65
6–12 mo	80–120	25–40	80–100/55–65
1–3 yr	70–110	20–30	90–105/55–70
3–6 yr	65–110	20–25	95–110/60–75
6–12 yr	60–95	14–22	100–120/60–75
≥12 yr	55–85	12–18	110–135/65–85

Source: Kleigman RM *et al*. Nelson Textbook of Pediatrics. 19th Ed, WB Saunders, Philadelphia, 2011.

APPENDIX VIII. Blood pressure by percentiles of height in boys and girls of age 3 to 18 years

Age (yrs)	BP percentile	Systolic BP (mm Hg) By percentiles of height							Diastolic BP (mm Hg) By percentiles of height						
		5	10	25	50	75	90	95	5	10	25	50	75	90	95
3	50	90	91	94	98	101	104	106	58	59	61	63	66	68	69
	90	99	101	104	107	111	114	116	70	71	73	76	78	80	81
	95	102	104	107	111	114	117	119	74	75	77	80	82	84	85
	99	109	111	114	117	120	124	126	81	82	84	87	89	90	92
4	50	96	97	98	100	101	103	103	62	62	63	64	65	66	67
	90	106	106	108	109	111	112	113	72	73	74	75	75	76	77
	95	109	110	111	113	114	116	117	75	76	77	79	79	80	80
	99	116	117	118	119	121	122	123	81	82	83	84	85	86	86
5	50	93	95	97	99	101	104	105	61	62	63	65	66	68	68
	90	100	101	103	106	108	110	114	73	73	75	76	78	79	80
	95	103	104	106	108	111	113	117	76	77	78	79	81	83	83
	99	114	116	119	123	126	129	131	83	83	85	86	88	89	90
6	50	98	99	100	102	103	105	105	65	66	67	68	69	70	71
	90	109	110	111	113	114	116	116	76	77	78	79	80	81	82
	95	113	114	115	117	118	120	120	79	80	81	82	83	84	85
	99	114	115	117	119	120	122	123	85	86	87	88	89	90	91
7	50	97	98	100	102	104	106	107	65	66	67	68	69	70	71
	90	109	111	112	114	116	118	119	77	77	78	80	81	82	83
	95	114	115	116	118	120	122	123	80	81	82	83	84	85	86
	99	120	121	123	125	127	128	119	87	87	88	90	91	92	93
8	50	102	103	105	106	108	110	111	66	67	68	70	71	73	74
	90	112	113	114	116	118	119	120	76	76	78	79	81	82	83
	95	115	116	118	119	121	123	124	79	79	81	82	84	85	86
	99	120	120	122	124	125	127	128	84	85	86	88	89	91	92
9	50	102	103	104	105	107	108	109	68	69	70	71	71	72	73
	90	112	113	115	116	118	119	120	78	79	79	80	81	82	83
	95	116	117	119	120	122	123	124	79	82	83	83	84	85	86
	99	125	125	126	127	128	129	130	87	87	88	89	90	91	91
10	50	106	106	107	107	108	109	109	69	70	71	72	73	74	75
	90	116	116	117	118	119	119	120	79	80	81	82	84	85	85
	95	120	120	121	122	122	123	123	83	83	84	86	87	88	89
	99	125	126	127	128	129	130	131	89	89	90	92	93	94	94
11	50	105	106	107	108	109	111	111	70	71	72	73	74	75	76
	90	113	114	115	116	117	118	119	78	79	80	81	82	83	84
	95	116	117	118	119	120	122	122	81	81	82	83	84	85	86
	99	121	122	124	125	127	128	129	86	86	87	88	89	90	91

(Contd.)

(Contd.)

Age (yrs)	BP percentile	Systolic BP (mm Hg) By percentiles of height							Diastolic BP (mm Hg) By percentiles of height						
		5	10	25	50	75	90	95	5	10	25	50	75	90	9
12	50	107	107	108	110	111	112	113	71	72	73	73	74	75	75
	90	117	118	119	120	122	123	124	81	82	83	83	84	85	86
	95	121	122	123	124	125	127	127	85	85	6	87	87	88	89
	99	127	128	130	131	133	135	136	90	91	91	92	93	94	94
13	50	107	107	108	109	111	112	112	71	71	72	72	73	73	74
	90	117	118	119	120	121	122	123	80	81	81	82	82	83	83
	95	121	122	123	124	125	126	127	83	84	84	85	85	86	86
	99	129	130	131	133	134	135	136	90	90	91	91	92	92	92
14	50	109	110	111	113	114	115	116	71	72	73	74	75	75	76
	90	120	121	122	123	125	126	127	81	81	82	83	84	85	85
	95	124	125	126	127	129	130	131	84	84	85	86	87	88	88
	99	133	134	135	136	138	139	140	90	90	91	92	93	93	94
15	50	113	114	114	115	116	116	117	73	74	75	75	76	77	78
	90	125	125	126	126	127	127	128	82	83	83	84	85	86	87
	95	129	129	130	130	131	131	132	85	85	86	87	88	89	89
	99	137	138	138	139	140	140	141	90	91	91	92	93	94	94
16	50	115	116	116	117	117	118	118	75	76	76	76	76	76	77
	90	127	127	128	129	129	130	130	85	85	85	85	86	86	86
	95	131	132	132	133	133	134	134	88	88	88	88	89	89	89
	99	140	140	141	142	142	143	144	93	93	93	94	94	94	94
17	50	114	115	115	116	117	118	118	75	75	76	77	78	79	79
	90	126	126	127	128	129	130	130	05	0C	C	07	00	09	09
	95	130	131	131	132	133	134	134	88	89	90	90	91	92	92
	99	141	141	142	143	144	145	146	93	94	95	96	97	98	98
18	50	111	112	115	117	120	122	123	74	75	75	75	75	75	75
	90	127	128	131	133	136	138	139	88	88	88	88	88	89	89
	95	133	134	136	139	141	143	145	92	92	92	92	93	93	93
	99	148	149	150	151	152	153	154	99	100	100	100	100	100	100

Adapted from Krishna P, Prasanna Kumar KM, Desai. N, Thennarasu K. Blood pressure reference tables for children and adolescents of Karnataka. *Indian Pediatr* 2006, 43:491–501.
Use appropriate cuff size that covers two-thirds of upper arm.
Blood pressure (BP) should be measured in the right arm of a seated child.
BP measurement by auscultation with a mercury-containing sphygmomanometer is the gold standard.
Interpretation of blood pressure (BP) readings:
BP is classified as systolic BP (SBP) and diastolic BP (DBP) percentiles for age, sex and height. If SBP or DBP is more than 90th percentile, recheck twice at the same office visit before interpreting results.
Normal BP: SBP and DBP <90th percentile.
Prehypertension: SBP or DBP ≥90th to <95th percentile or BP >120/80 mm Hg to <95th percentile. Keep a watch and institute weight management.
Stage 1 hypertension: SBP and/or DBP ≥95th to ≤99th percentile plus 5 mm Hg. Recheck after 1–2 weeks and start treatment, if BP level remains high.
Stage 2 hypertension: SBP and/or DBP >99th percentile plus 5 mm Hg. Start treatment immediately.

APPENDIX IX. Norms for stretched penile length and testicular volume (mean ±SD)

Age	Penis (cm)	Testicular volume (mL or cm^3)
30 weeks	2.5 ±0.4	
34 weeks	3.0 ±0.4	
Term	3.5 ±0.4	
0–5 months	3.9 ±0.8	
6–12 months	4.3 ±0.8	
1–2 years	4.7 ±0.8	
2–3 years	5.1 ±0.9	1.8 ±0.1
3–4 years	5.5 ±0.9	
4–5 years	5.7 ±0.9	
5–6 years	6.0 ±0.9	
6–7 years	6.1 ±0.9	
7–8 years	6.2 ±1.0	
8–9 years	6.3 ±1.0	
9–10 years	6.3 ±1.0	
10–11 years	6.4 ±1.1	3.5 ±0.2
Adult (erect)	13.3 ±1.6	16.5 ±2.3*

Adapted from Goodman RM and Gorlin RJ, The Malformed Infant and Child, *Oxford University Press, New York, 1983*
Note: The stretched penile length is measured from pubic bone to the tip of the glans. Testicular volume is measured with the help of Prader orchidometers. Ultrasonographic evaluation is more reliable but it overestimates the testicular volume because of the inclusion of the scrotal skin and the epididymis. The volume of testis is calculated by elipsoid equation: $W^2 \times L \times 0.52$ wherein W is width and L is length of testis.
*Ovoid shape with an average measurement of 3 cm anterior-posterior × 2–4 cm (transverse) × 3–5 cm (length).

APPENDIX X. WHO standards for weight-for-age percentiles of boys (birth to 5 years)

Year : Month	Months	3rd	15th	Median	85th	97th
0.0	0	2.5	2.9	3.3	3.9	4.3
0.1	1	3.4	3.9	4.5	5.1	5.7
0.2	2	4.4	4.9	5.6	6.3	7.0
0.3	3	5.1	5.6	6.4	7.2	7.9
0.4	4	5.6	6.2	7.0	7.9	8.6
0.5	5	6.1	6.7	7.5	8.4	9.2
0.6	6	6.4	7.1	7.9	8.9	9.7
0.7	7	6.7	7.4	8.3	9.3	10.2
0.8	8	7.0	7.7	8.6	9.6	10.5
0.9	9	7.2	7.9	8.9	10.0	10.9
0.10	10	7.5	8.2	9.2	10.3	11.2
0.11	11	7.7	8.4	9.4	10.5	11.5
1.0	12	7.8	8.6	9.6	10.8	11.8
1.1	13	8.0	8.8	9.9	11.1	12.1
1.2	14	8.2	9.0	10.1	11.3	12.4
1.3	15	8.4	9.2	10.3	11.6	12.7
1.4	16	8.5	9.4	10.5	11.8	12.9
1.5	17	8.7	9.6	10.7	12.0	13.2
1.6	18	8.9	9.7	10.9	12.3	13.5
1.7	19	9.0	9.9	11.1	12.5	13.7
1.8	20	9.2	10.1	11.3	12.7	14.0
1.9	21	9.3	10.3	11.5	13.0	14.3
1.10	22	9.5	10.5	11.8	13.2	14.5
1.11	23	9.7	10.6	12.0	13.4	14.8
2.0	24	9.8	10.8	12.2	13.7	15.1
2.1	25	10.0	11.0	12.4	13.9	15.3
2.2	26	10.1	11.1	12.5	14.1	15.6
2.3	27	10.2	11.3	12.7	14.4	15.9
2.4	28	10.4	11.5	12.9	14.6	16.1
2.5	29	10.5	11.6	13.1	14.8	16.4
2.6	30	10.7	11.8	13.3	15.0	16.6
2.7	31	10.8	11.9	13.5	15.2	16.9
2.8	32	10.9	12.1	13.7	15.5	17.1
2.9	33	11.1	12.2	13.8	15.7	17.3
2.10	34	11.2	12.4	14.0	15.9	17.6
2.11	35	11.3	12.5	14.2	16.1	17.8

(Contd.)

(Contd.)

Year : Month	Months	3rd	15th	Median	85th	97th
3.0	36	11.4	12.7	14.3	16.3	18.0
3.1	37	11.6	12.8	14.5	16.5	18.3
3.2	38	11.7	12.9	14.7	16.7	18.5
3.3	39	11.8	13.1	14.8	16.9	18.7
3.4	40	11.9	13.2	15.0	17.1	19.0
3.5	41	12.1	13.4	15.2	17.3	19.2
3.6	42	12.2	13.5	15.3	17.5	19.4
3.7	43	12.3	13.6	15.5	17.7	19.7
3.8	44	12.4	13.8	15.7	17.9	19.9
3.9	45	12.5	13.9	15.8	18.1	20.1
3.10	46	12.7	14.1	16.0	18.3	20.4
3.11	47	12.8	14.2	16.2	18.5	20.6
4.0	48	12.9	14.3	16.3	18.7	20.9
4.1	49	13.0	14.5	16.5	18.9	21.1
4.2	50	13.1	14.6	16.7	19.1	21.3
4.3	51	13.3	14.7	16.8	19.3	21.6
4.4	52	13.4	14.9	17.0	19.5	21.8
4.5	53	13.5	15.0	17.2	19.7	22.1
4.6	54	13.6	15.2	17.3	19.9	22.3
4.7	55	13.7	15.3	17.5	20.1	22.5
4.8	56	13.8	15.4	17.7	20.3	22.8
4.9	57	13.9	15.6	17.8	20.5	23.0
4.10	58	14.1	15.7	18.0	20.7	23.3
4.11	59	14.2	15.8	18.2	20.9	23.5
5.0	60	14.3	16.0	18.3	21.1	23.8

Source: de Onis M, Garza C Onyango AW, Martorell R. WHO child growth standards. *Acta Paediatrica (Suppl)* 2006, 450:1–110 and www.who.int/childgrowth/standards/en/.

APPENDIX XI. WHO standards for weight-for-age percentiles of girls (birth to 5 years)

Year : Month	Months	3rd	15th	Median	85th	97th
0.0	0	2.4	2.8	3.2	3.7	4.2
0.1	1	3.2	3.6	4.2	4.8	5.4
0.2	2	4.0	4.5	5.1	5.9	6.5
0.3	3	4.6	5.1	5.8	6.7	7.4
0.4	4	5.1	5.6	6.4	7.3	8.1
0.5	5	5.5	6.1	6.9	7.8	8.7
0.6	6	5.8	6.4	7.3	8.3	9.2
0.7	7	6.1	6.7	7.6	8.7	9.6
0.8	8	6.3	7.0	7.9	9.0	10.0
0.9	9	6.6	7.3	8.2	9.3	10.4
0.10	10	6.8	7.5	8.5	9.6	10.7
0.11	11	7.0	7.7	8.7	9.9	11.0
1.0	12	7.1	7.9	8.9	10.2	11.3
1.1	13	7.3	8.1	9.2	10.4	11.6
1.2	14	7.5	8.3	9.4	10.7	11.9
1.3	15	7.7	8.5	9.6	10.9	12.2
1.4	16	7.8	8.7	9.8	11.2	12.5
1.5	17	8.0	8.8	10.0	11.4	12.7
1.6	18	8.2	9.0	10.2	11.6	13.0
1.7	19	8.3	9.2	10.4	11.9	13.3
1.8	20	8.5	9.4	10.6	12.1	13.5
1.9	21	8.7	9.6	10.9	12.4	13.8
1.10	22	8.8	9.8	11.1	12.6	14.1
1.11	23	9.0	9.9	11.3	12.8	14.3
2.0	24	9.2	10.1	11.5	13.1	14.6
2.1	25	9.3	10.3	11.7	13.3	14.9
2.2	26	9.5	10.5	11.9	13.6	15.2
2.3	27	9.6	10.7	12.1	13.8	15.4
2.4	28	9.8	10.8	12.3	14.0	15.7
2.5	29	10.0	11.0	12.5	14.3	16.0
2.6	30	10.1	11.2	12.7	14.5	16.2
2.7	31	10.3	11.3	12.9	14.7	16.5
2.8	32	10.4	11.5	13.1	15.0	16.8
2.9	33	10.5	11.7	13.3	15.2	17.0
2.10	34	10.7	11.8	13.5	15.4	17.3
2.11	35	10.8	12.0	13.7	15.7	17.6

(Contd.)

(Contd.)

Year : Month	Months	3rd	15th	Median	85th	97th
3.0	36	11.0	12.1	13.9	15.9	17.8
3.1	37	11.1	12.3	14.0	16.1	18.1
3.2	38	11.2	12.5	14.2	16.3	18.4
3.3	39	11.4	12.6	14.4	16.6	18.6
3.4	40	11.5	12.8	14.6	16.8	18.9
3.5	41	11.6	12.9	14.8	17.0	19.2
3.6	42	11.8	13.1	15.0	17.3	19.5
3.7	43	11.9	13.2	15.2	17.5	19.7
3.8	44	12.0	13.4	15.3	17.7	20.0
3.9	45	12.1	13.5	15.5	17.9	20.3
3.10	46	12.3	13.7	15.7	18.2	20.6
3.11	47	12.4	13.8	15.9	18.4	20.8
4.0	48	12.5	14.0	16.1	18.6	21.1
4.1	49	12.6	14.1	16.3	18.9	21.4
4.2	50	12.8	14.3	16.4	19.1	21.7
4.3	51	12.9	14.4	16.6	19.3	22.0
4.4	52	13.0	14.5	16.8	19.5	22.2
4.5	53	13.1	14.7	17.0	19.8	22.5
4.6	54	13.2	14.8	17.2	20.0	22.8
4.7	55	13.4	15.0	17.3	20.2	23.1
4.8	56	13.5	15.1	17.5	20.4	23.3
4.9	57	13.6	15.3	17.7	20.7	23.6
4.10	58	13.7	15.4	17.9	20.9	23.9
4.11	59	13.8	15.5	18.0	21.1	24.2
5.0	60	14.0	15.7	18.2	21.3	24.4

Source: de Onis M, Garza C Onyango AW, Martorell R. WHO child growth standards. *Acta Paediatrica (Suppl)* 2006, 450:1–110 and www.who.int/childgrowth/standards/en/.

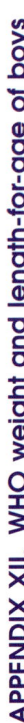

APPENDIX XII. WHO weight and length-for-age of boys

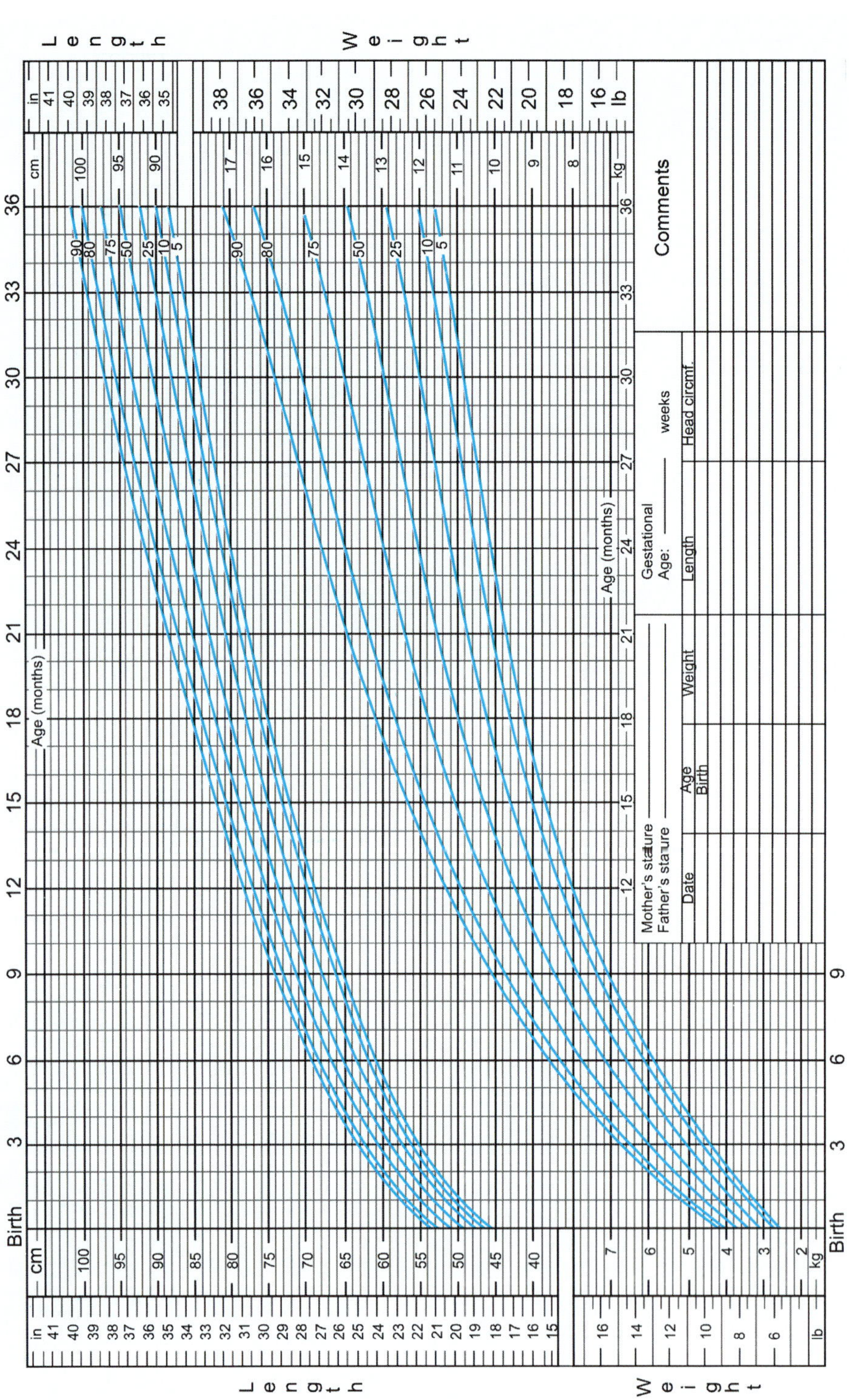

APPENDIX XIII. WHO weight and length-for-age of girls

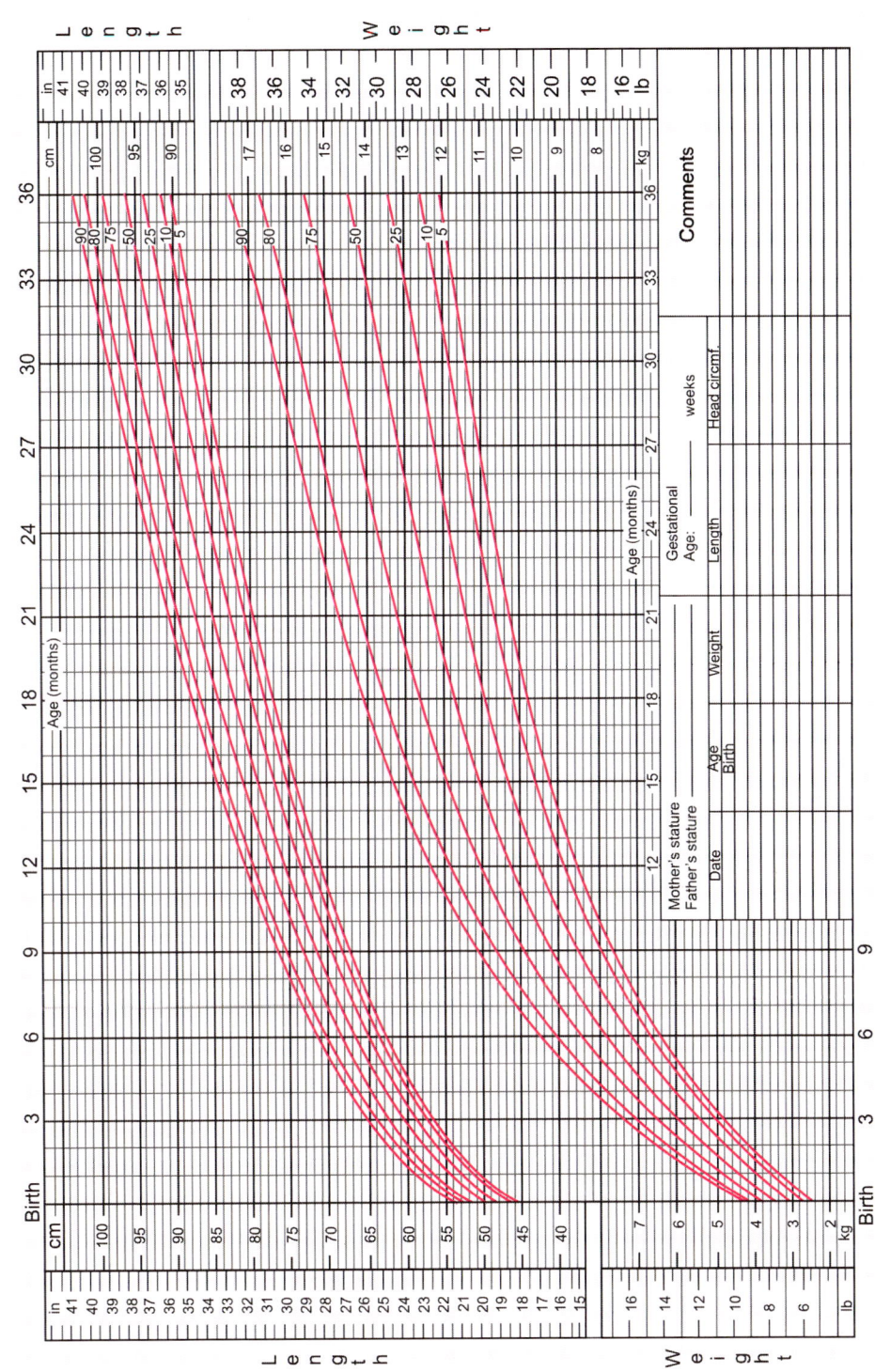

APPENDIX XIV. WHO Length or height-for-age for boys (birth to 5 years)

Length-for-age of boys from birth to 2 years (percentiles)						
Year : Month	Months	3rd	15th	Median	85th	97th
0.0	0	46.3	47.9	49.9	51.8	53.4
0.1	1	51.1	52.7	54.7	56.7	58.4
0.2	2	54.7	56.4	58.4	60.5	62.2
0.3	3	57.6	59.3	61.4	63.5	65.3
0.4	4	60.0	61.7	63.9	66.0	67.8
0.5	5	61.9	63.7	65.9	68.1	69.9
0.6	6	63.6	65.4	67.6	69.8	71.6
0.7	7	65.1	66.9	69.2	71.4	73.2
0.8	8	66.5	68.3	70.6	72.9	74.7
0.9	9	67.7	69.6	72.0	74.3	76.2
0.10	10	69.0	70.9	73.3	75.6	77.6
0.11	11	70.2	72.1	74.5	77.0	78.9
1.0	12	71.3	73.3	75.7	78.2	80.2
1.1	13	72.4	74.4	76.9	79.4	81.5
1.2	14	73.4	75.5	78.0	80.6	82.7
1.3	15	74.4	76.5	79.1	81.8	83.9
1.4	16	75.4	77.5	80.2	82.9	85.1
1.5	17	76.3	78.5	81.2	84.0	86.2
1.6	18	77.2	79.5	82.3	85.1	87.3
1.7	19	78.1	80.4	83.2	86.1	88.4
1.8	20	78.9	81.3	84.2	87.1	89.5
1.9	21	79.7	82.2	85.1	88.1	90.5
1.10	22	80.5	83.0	86.0	89.1	91.6
1.11	23	81.3	83.8	86.9	90.0	92.6
2.0	24	82.1	84.6	87.8	91.0	93.6

Height-for-age of boys from 2 to 5 years (percentiles) (Contd.)

Year : Month	Months	3rd	15th	Median	85th	97th
2.0	24	81.4	83.9	87.1	90.3	92.9
2.1	25	82.1	84.7	88.0	91.2	93.8
2.2	26	82.8	85.5	88.8	92.1	94.8
2.3	27	83.5	86.3	89.6	93.0	95.7
2.4	28	84.2	87.0	90.4	93.8	96.6
2.5	29	84.9	87.7	91.2	94.7	97.5
2.6	30	85.5	88.4	91.9	95.5	98.3
2.7	31	86.2	89.1	92.7	96.2	99.2
2.8	32	86.8	89.7	93.4	97.0	100.0
2.9	33	87.4	90.4	94.1	97.8	100.8
2.10	34	88.0	91.0	94.8	98.5	101.5
2.11	35	88.5	91.6	95.4	99.2	102.3
3.0	36	89.1	92.2	96.1	99.9	103.1
3.1	37	89.7	92.8	96.7	100.6	103.8
3.2	38	90.2	93.4	97.4	101.3	104.5
3.3	39	90.8	94.0	98.0	102.0	105.2
3.4	40	91.3	94.6	98.6	102.7	105.9
3.5	41	91.9	95.2	99.2	103.3	106.6
3.6	42	92.4	95.7	99.9	104.0	107.3
3.7	43	92.9	96.3	100.4	104.6	108.0
3.8	44	93.4	96.8	101.0	105.2	108.6
3.9	45	93.9	97.4	101.6	105.8	109.3
3.10	46	94.4	97.9	102.2	106.5	109.9
3.11	47	94.9	98.5	102.8	107.1	110.6
4.0	48	95.4	99.0	103.3	107.7	111.2
4.1	49	95.9	99.5	103.9	108.3	111.8
4.2	50	96.4	100.0	104.4	108.9	112.5
4.3	51	96.9	100.5	105.0	109.5	113.1
4.4	52	97.4	101.1	105.6	110.1	113.7
4.5	53	97.9	101.6	106.1	110.7	114.3
4.6	54	98.4	102.1	106.7	111.2	115.0
4.7	55	98.8	102.6	107.2	111.8	115.6
4.8	56	99.3	103.1	107.8	112.4	116.2
4.9	57	99.8	103.6	108.3	113.0	116.8
4.10	58	100.3	104.1	108.9	113.6	117.4
4.11	59	100.8	104.7	109.4	114.2	118.1
5.0	60	101.2	105.2	110.0	114.8	118.7

APPENDIX XV. WHO length or height-for-age of girls (birth to 5 years)

Length-for-age of girls from birth to 2 years (percentiles)

Year : Month	Months	3rd	15th	Median	85th	97th
0.0	0	45.6	47.2	49.1	51.1	52.7
0.1	1	50.0	51.7	53.7	55.7	57.4
0.2	2	53.2	55.0	57.1	59.2	60.9
0.3	3	55.8	57.6	59.8	62.0	63.8
0.4	4	58.0	59.8	62.1	64.3	66.2
0.5	5	59.9	61.7	64.0	66.3	68.2
0.6	6	61.5	63.4	65.7	68.1	70.0
0.7	7	62.9	64.9	67.3	69.7	71.6
0.8	8	64.3	66.3	68.7	71.2	73.2
0.9	9	65.6	67.6	70.1	72.6	74.7
0.10	10	66.8	68.9	71.5	74.0	76.1
0.11	11	68.0	70.2	72.8	75.4	77.5
1.0	12	69.2	71.3	74.0	76.7	78.9
1.1	13	70.3	72.5	75.2	77.9	80.2
1.2	14	71.3	73.6	76.4	79.2	81.4
1.3	15	72.4	74.7	77.5	80.3	82.7
1.4	16	73.3	75.7	78.6	81.5	83.9
1.5	17	74.3	76.7	79.7	82.6	85.0
1.6	18	75.2	77.7	80.7	83.7	86.2
1.7	19	76.2	78.7	81.7	84.8	87.3
1.8	20	77.0	79.6	82.7	85.8	88.4
1.9	21	77.9	80.5	83.7	86.8	89.4
1.10	22	78.7	81.4	84.6	87.8	90.5
1.11	23	79.6	82.2	85.5	88.8	91.5
2.0	24	80.3	83.1	86.4	89.8	92.5

Height-for-age of girls from 2 to 5 years (percentiles) (Contd.)						
Year : Month	Months	3rd	15th	Median	85th	97th
2.0	24	79.6	82.4	85.7	89.1	91.8
2.1	25	80.4	83.2	86.6	90.0	92.8
2.2	26	81.2	84.0	87.4	90.9	93.7
2.3	27	81.9	84.8	88.3	91.8	94.6
2.4	28	82.6	85.5	89.1	92.7	95.6
2.5	29	83.4	86.3	89.9	93.5	96.4
2.6	30	84.0	87.0	90.7	94.3	97.3
2.7	31	84.7	87.7	91.4	95.2	98.2
2.8	32	85.4	88.4	92.2	95.9	99.0
2.9	33	86.0	89.1	92.9	96.7	99.8
2.10	34	86.7	89.8	93.6	97.5	100.6
2.11	35	87.3	90.5	94.4	98.3	101.4
3.0	36	87.9	91.1	95.1	99.0	102.2
3.1	37	88.5	91.7	95.7	99.7	103.0
3.2	38	89.1	92.4	96.4	100.5	103.7
3.3	39	89.7	93.0	97.1	101.2	104.5
3.4	40	90.3	93.6	97.7	101.9	105.2
3.5	41	90.8	94.2	98.4	102.6	106.0
3.6	42	91.4	94.8	99.0	103.3	106.7
3.7	43	92.0	95.4	99.7	103.9	107.4
3.8	44	92.5	96.0	100.3	104.6	108.1
3.9	45	93.0	96.6	100.9	105.3	108.8
3.10	46	93.6	97.2	101.5	105.9	109.5
3.11	47	94.1	97.7	102.1	106.6	110.2
4.0	48	94.6	98.3	102.7	107.2	110.8
4.1	49	95.1	98.8	103.3	107.8	111.5
4.2	50	95.7	99.4	103.9	108.4	112.1
4.3	51	96.2	99.9	104.5	109.1	112.8
4.4	52	96.7	100.4	105.0	109.7	113.4
4.5	53	97.2	101.0	105.6	110.3	114.1
4.6	54	97.6	101.5	106.2	110.9	114.7
4.7	55	98.1	102.0	106.7	111.5	115.3
4.8	56	98.6	102.5	107.3	112.1	116.0
4.9	57	99.1	103.0	107.8	112.6	116.6
4.10	58	99.6	103.5	108.4	113.2	117.2
4.11	59	100.0	104.0	108.9	113.8	117.8
5.0	60	100.5	104.5	109.4	114.4	118.4

APPENDIX XVI. Revised IAP body weight (kg) centiles and standard deviations for boys and girls (5–18 years)

Revised IAP weight (kg) centiles and standard deviations for boys (5–18 years)

Age	3	10	25	50	75	90	97	SD
5.0	13.2	14.3	15.6	17.1	19.0	21.3	24.2	3.2
5.5	13.8	15.0	16.5	18.2	20.3	22.9	26.1	2.9
6.0	14.5	15.8	17.4	19.3	21.7	24.6	28.3	3.6
6.5	15.3	16.8	18.6	20.7	23.3	26.6	30.8	3.8
7.0	16.0	17.6	19.6	21.9	24.9	28.6	33.4	4.2
7.5	16.7	18.5	20.7	23.3	26.6	30.8	36.2	4.9
8.0	17.5	19.5	21.9	24.8	28.5	33.2	39.4	5.7
8.5	18.3	20.5	23.2	26.4	30.5	35.7	42.6	6.5
9.0	19.1	21.5	24.3	27.9	32.3	38.0	45.5	6.3
9.5	19.9	22.4	25.6	29.4	34.3	40.5	48.6	7.0
10.0	20.7	23.5	26.9	31.1	36.3	43.0	51.8	7.9
10.5	21.6	24.6	28.3	32.8	38.5	45.8	55.2	8.3
11.0	22.6	25.9	29.8	34.7	40.9	48.7	58.7	8.9
11.5	23.8	27.3	31.6	36.9	43.5	51.8	62.5	9.3
12.0	24.9	28.7	33.3	39.0	46.0	54.8	66.1	10.0
12.5	26.1	30.2	35.1	41.2	48.6	57.8	69.5	10.6
13.0	27.5	31.8	37.0	43.3	51.1	60.7	72.6	11.3
13.5	29.0	33.6	39.1	45.7	53.8	63.6	75.6	11.4
14.0	30.7	35.5	41.3	48.2	56.4	66.3	78.3	12.1
14.5	32.6	37.7	43.7	50.8	59.1	69.1	80.9	11.6
15.0	34.5	39.8	45.9	53.1	61.6	71.5	83.1	12.1
15.5	36.1	41.6	47.9	55.2	63.6	73.4	84.7	11.2
16.0	37.5	43.1	49.5	56.8	65.2	74.8	85.8	12.2
16.5	38.7	44.4	50.9	58.2	66.6	76.1	86.8	12.6
17.0	39.8	45.6	52.1	59.5	67.8	77.1	87.5	12.3
17.5	40.8	46.7	53.2	60.6	68.7	77.8	88.0	12.3
18.0	41.8	47.7	54.3	61.6	69.7	78.4	88.4	11.3

Revised IAP weight (kg) centiles and standard deviations for girls (5–18 years)

Age	3	10	25	50	75	90	97	SD
5.0	12.3	13.4	14.8	16.4	18.5	21.3	25.0	2.5
5.5	13.0	14.3	15.7	17.6	19.9	22.9	27.0	3.5
6.0	13.7	15.1	16.7	18.7	21.3	24.6	29.1	3.4
6.5	14.4	15.9	17.7	19.9	22.7	26.3	31.2	4.1
7.0	15.1	16.8	18.7	21.2	24.2	28.2	33.4	4.4
7.5	15.9	17.7	19.9	22.5	25.9	30.1	35.7	4.8
8.0	16.7	18.7	21.1	24.0	27.6	32.2	38.1	5.2
8.5	17.5	19.7	22.3	25.5	29.5	34.4	40.7	6.4
9.0	18.5	20.9	23.7	27.2	31.5	36.7	43.4	6.4
9.5	19.5	22.1	25.3	29.0	33.6	39.3	46.3	6.9
10.0	20.7	23.5	26.9	31.0	36.0	42.0	49.4	7.7
10.5	22.0	25.1	28.8	33.2	38.4	44.8	52.6	8.3
11.0	23.3	26.7	30.7	35.4	41.0	47.7	55.9	8.5
11.5	24.8	28.4	32.6	37.6	43.6	50.6	59.1	9.1
12.0	26.2	30.0	34.5	39.8	46.0	53.4	62.1	9.0
12.5	27.6	31.6	36.3	41.8	48.2	55.8	64.8	9.7
13.0	28.9	33.1	37.9	43.6	50.2	57.9	67.1	9.4
13.5	30.2	34.4	39.4	45.1	51.8	59.7	69.0	9.8
14.0	31.3	35.6	40.6	46.4	53.2	61.1	70.4	9.6
14.5	32.3	36.6	41.7	47.5	54.3	62.2	71.4	9.4
15.0	33.1	37.5	42.5	48.4	55.1	62.9	72.1	9.6
15.5	34.0	38.3	43.3	49.1	55.8	63.5	72.5	8.7
16.0	34.7	39.1	44.0	49.7	56.3	64.0	72.8	8.7
16.5	35.5	39.8	44.7	50.3	56.9	64.4	73.1	9.2
17.0	36.2	40.5	45.3	50.9	57.3	64.7	73.3	8.8
17.5	36.9	41.1	46.0	51.5	57.8	65.0	73.4	9.5
18.0	37.6	41.8	46.6	52.0	58.2	65.3	73.5	10.2

Source: Khadilkar V, Yadav S, Agrawal KK, Tamboli S, Bannerjee M, *et al*. Revised IAP growth charts for height, weight and body mass index for 5–18 years old Indian children. *Indian Pediatrics* 2015, 52:47–55.

APPENDIX XVII. Revised IAP height (cm) centiles and standard deviations for boys and girls

Revised height (cm) centiles and standard deviations for boys

Age	3	10	25	50	75	90	97	SD
5.0	99.0	102.3	105.6	108.9	112.4	115.9	119.4	5.7
5.5	101.6	105.0	108.4	111.9	115.4	119.0	122.7	5.3
6.0	104.2	107.7	111.2	114.8	118.5	122.2	126.0	5.6
6.5	106.8	110.4	114.0	117.8	121.6	125.4	129.3	5.5
7.0	109.3	113.0	116.8	120.7	124.6	128.6	132.6	5.9
7.5	111.8	115.7	119.6	123.5	127.6	131.7	135.9	5.7
8.0	114.3	118.2	122.3	126.4	130.5	134.8	139.1	6.3
8.5	116.7	120.8	124.9	129.1	133.4	137.8	142.2	6.1
9.0	119.0	123.2	127.5	131.8	136.3	140.7	145.3	6.4
9.5	121.3	125.6	130.0	134.5	139.1	143.7	148.3	6.4
10.0	123.6	128.1	132.6	137.2	141.9	146.6	151.4	6.8
10.5	125.9	130.5	135.2	139.9	144.7	149.5	154.4	6.5
11.0	128.2	133.0	137.8	142.7	147.6	152.5	157.5	7.6
11.5	130.7	135.6	140.6	145.5	150.5	155.6	160.6	7.3
12.0	133.2	138.3	143.3	148.4	153.5	158.6	163.7	8.1
12.5	135.7	141.0	146.2	151.4	156.5	161.1	166.8	7.9
13.0	138.3	143.1	149.0	154.3	159.5	164.7	169.9	9.0
13.5	140.9	146.4	151.8	157.2	162.4	167.6	172.7	8.4
14.0	143.4	149.0	154.5	159.9	165.1	170.3	175.4	9.0
14.5	145.8	151.5	157.0	162.3	167.6	172.7	177.7	7.8
15.0	148.0	153.7	159.2	164.5	169.7	174.8	179.7	7.9
15.5	150.0	155.7	161.2	166.5	171.6	176.5	181.4	6.6
16.0	151.8	157.4	162.9	168.1	173.1	178.0	182.7	7.2
16.5	153.4	159.1	164.5	169.6	174.5	179.3	183.8	6.7
17.0	155.0	160.6	165.9	171.0	175.8	180.4	184.8	6.9
17.5	156.6	162.1	167.3	172.3	177.0	181.5	185.8	6.1
18.0	158.1	163.6	168.7	173.6	178.2	182.5	186.7	6.9

Revised height (cm) centiles and standard deviations for girls

Age	3	10	25	50	75	90	97	SD
5.0	97.2	100.5	103.9	107.5	111.3	115.2	119.3	5.4
5.5	99.8	103.2	106.8	110.5	114.4	118.3	122.5	5.7
6.0	102.3	106.0	109.7	113.5	117.4	121.5	125.6	5.8
6.5	104.9	108.7	112.5	116.5	120.5	124.6	128.7	5.5
7.0	107.4	111.4	115.4	119.4	123.5	127.7	131.9	6.1
7.5	110.0	114.1	118.2	122.4	126.6	130.8	135.0	6.0
8.0	112.6	116.8	121.1	125.4	129.6	133.9	138.1	6.2
8.5	115.2	119.6	124.0	128.4	132.7	137.0	141.3	6.8
9.0	117.8	122.4	126.9	131.4	135.8	140.2	144.5	6.9
9.5	120.5	125.2	129.9	134.4	138.9	143.3	147.6	6.6
10.0	123.3	128.1	132.8	137.4	142.0	146.4	150.8	7.8
10.5	126.1	130.9	135.7	140.4	145.0	149.5	153.9	7.3
11.0	128.8	133.7	138.6	143.3	147.9	152.4	156.8	7.9
11.5	131.5	136.4	141.2	145.9	150.6	155.1	159.6	7.1
12.0	134.0	138.9	143.7	148.4	153.0	157.5	162.0	7.0
12.5	136.3	141.1	145.8	150.5	155.1	159.6	164.1	6.7
13.0	138.2	142.9	147.6	152.2	156.8	161.3	165.9	6.9
13.5	139.9	144.5	149.1	153.6	158.2	162.7	167.2	6.0
14.0	141.3	145.8	150.2	154.7	159.2	163.7	168.2	6.6
14.5	142.4	146.8	151.1	155.5	160.0	164.5	169.0	5.9
15.0	143.3	147.5	151.8	156.1	160.5	165.0	169.5	6.6
15.5	144.1	148.1	152.1	156.6	160.9	165.3	169.8	5.9
16.0	144.7	148.6	152.7	156.9	161.2	165.6	170.1	6.1
16.5	145.2	149.1	153.1	157.2	161.4	165.7	170.2	6.4
17.0	145.1	149.5	153.4	157.4	161.6	165.9	170.4	6.5
17.5	146.2	149.8	153.6	157.6	161.1	166.0	170.5	6.7
18.0	146.6	150.2	153.9	157.8	161.9	166.1	170.6	6.6

APPENDIX XVIII. IAP body mass index percentiles for boys and girls (5–18 years)

IAP body mass index percentiles for boys

Age	3	5	10	25	50	23* Eq(71)	27* Eq(90)	SD
5.0	12.1	12.4	12.8	13.6	14.7	15.7	17.5	1.6
5.5	12.2	12.4	12.9	13.7	14.8	15.8	17.6	1.5
6.0	12.2	12.5	12.9	13.7	14.9	16.0	17.8	1.8
6.5	12.3	12.5	13.0	13.8	15.0	16.1	18.0	1.8
7.0	12.3	12.6	13.1	13.9	15.1	16.3	18.2	1.9
7.5	12.4	12.7	13.2	14.1	15.3	16.5	18.5	2.2
8.0	12.5	12.8	13.3	14.2	15.5	16.7	18.8	2.5
8.5	12.6	12.9	13.4	14.4	15.7	17.0	19.2	2.8
9.0	12.7	13.0	13.5	14.5	15.9	17.3	19.6	2.6
9.5	12.8	13.1	13.7	14.7	16.2	17.6	20.1	2.8
10.0	12.9	13.2	13.8	14.9	16.4	18.0	20.5	3.1
10.5	13.0	13.3	14.0	15.1	16.7	18.3	21.0	3.2
11.0	13.1	13.5	14.1	15.4	17.0	18.7	21.5	3.2
11.5	13.2	13.6	14.3	15.6	17.3	19.1	22.1	3.3
12.0	13.3	13.8	14.5	15.8	17.7	19.5	22.6	3.4
12.5	13.5	13.9	14.6	16.0	17.9	19.8	23.0	3.6
13.0	13.6	14.0	14.8	16.3	18.2	20.2	23.4	3.5
13.5	13.7	14.2	14.9	16.5	18.5	20.5	23.8	3.7
14.0	13.8	14.3	15.1	16.7	18.7	20.8	24.2	3.7
14.5	14.0	14.5	15.3	16.9	19.0	21.1	24.5	3.5
15.0	14.2	14.7	15.5	17.2	19.3	21.4	24.9	3.7
15.5	14.4	14.9	15.8	17.4	19.6	21.7	25.2	3.4
16.0	14.6	15.1	16.0	17.7	19.9	22.0	25.5	3.7
16.5	14.9	15.4	16.3	18.0	20.2	22.4	25.8	3.8
17.0	15.1	15.6	16.6	18.3	20.5	22.6	26.0	3.8
17.5	15.4	15.9	16.8	18.6	20.8	22.9	26.3	3.6
18.0	15.6	16.2	17.1	18.9	21.1	23.2	26.6	3.2

IAP body mass index percentiles for girls

Age	3	5	10	25	50	23* Eq(75)	27* Eq(95)	SD
5.0	11.9	12.1	12.5	13.3	14.3	15.5	18.0	1.4
5.5	11.9	12.2	12.6	13.4	14.4	15.7	18.3	1.7
6.0	12.0	12.2	12.7	13.5	14.5	15.9	18.6	1.7
6.5	12.1	12.3	12.8	13.6	14.7	16.1	18.9	2.0
7.0	12.1	12.4	12.8	13.7	14.9	16.4	19.3	2.1
7.5	12.2	12.5	12.9	13.9	15.1	16.6	19.7	2.2
8.0	12.3	12.6	13.1	14.0	15.3	16.9	20.1	2.3
8.5	12.3	12.7	13.2	14.2	15.6	17.2	20.5	2.7
9.0	12.4	12.8	13.3	14.4	15.8	17.6	21.0	2.7
9.5	12.5	12.9	13.5	14.6	16.1	18.0	21.4	2.8
10.0	12.7	13.1	13.7	14.9	16.5	18.4	21.9	2.9
10.5	12.8	13.2	13.9	15.2	16.8	18.8	22.5	3.1
11.0	13.0	13.4	14.1	15.5	17.2	19.3	23.0	3.1
11.5	13.2	13.7	14.4	15.8	17.6	19.8	23.6	3.3
12.0	13.4	13.9	14.7	16.1	18.0	20.2	24.1	3.2
12.5	13.7	14.2	15.0	16.5	18.4	20.7	24.7	3.2
13.0	13.9	14.4	15.2	16.8	18.8	21.1	25.2	3.3
13.5	14.1	14.6	15.5	17.1	19.1	21.5	25.6	3.5
14.0	14.3	14.9	15.7	17.3	19.4	21.8	25.9	3.4
14.5	14.5	15.1	16.0	17.6	19.7	22.0	26.2	3.3
15.0	14.7	15.2	16.1	17.8	19.9	22.3	26.3	3.4
15.5	14.9	15.4	16.3	18.0	20.1	22.4	26.4	3.1
16.0	15.0	15.6	16.5	18.2	20.3	22.6	26.5	3.1
16.5	15.2	15.8	16.7	18.4	20.4	22.8	26.6	3.2
17.0	15.4	16.0	16.9	18.6	20.6	22.9	26.7	3.0
17.5	15.5	16.1	17.1	18.7	20.8	23.1	26.7	3.1
18.0	15.7	16.3	17.3	18.9	21.0	23.2	26.8	3.6

SD; standard deviation *23 and 27 adult equivalent BMI charts by IAP have 3rd, 5th, 10th, 25th, 50th percentiles and 23 adult equivalent (71st and 75th percentiles for boys and girls, respectively) and 27th adult equivalent (90th and 95th percentiles for boys and girls, respectively. Based on IAP BMI charts, underweight is defined as BMI below 3rd percentile, overweight as above 23 adult equivalent and obese as above 27 adult equivalent.

APPENDIX XIX. Head circumference-for-age of boys from birth to 5 years

Head circumference-for-age of boys from birth to 5 years (percentiles)						
Year : Month	Months	3rd	15th	Median	85th	97th
0.0	0	32.1	33.1	34.5	35.8	36.9
0.1	1	35.1	36.1	37.3	38.5	39.5
0.2	2	36.9	37.9	39.1	40.3	41.3
0.3	3	38.3	39.3	40.5	41.7	42.7
0.4	4	39.4	40.4	41.6	42.9	43.9
0.5	5	40.3	41.3	42.6	43.8	44.8
0.6	6	41.0	42.1	43.3	44.6	45.6
0.7	7	41.7	42.7	44.0	45.3	46.3
0.8	8	42.2	43.2	44.5	45.8	46.9
0.9	9	42.6	43.7	45.0	46.3	47.4
0.10	10	43.0	44.1	45.4	46.7	47.8
0.11	11	43.4	44.4	45.8	47.1	48.2
1.0	12	43.6	44.7	46.1	47.4	48.5
1.1	13	43.9	45.0	46.3	47.7	48.8
1.2	14	44.1	45.2	46.6	47.9	49.0
1.3	15	44.3	45.5	46.8	48.2	49.3
1.4	16	44.5	45.6	47.0	48.4	49.5
1.5	17	44.7	45.8	47.2	48.6	49.7
1.6	18	44.9	46.0	47.4	48.7	49.9
1.7	19	45.0	46.2	47.5	48.9	50.0
1.8	20	45.2	46.3	47.7	49.1	50.2
1.9	21	45.3	46.4	47.8	49.2	50.4
1.10	22	45.4	46.6	48.0	49.4	50.5
1.11	23	45.6	46.7	48.1	49.5	50.7
2.0	24	45.7	46.8	48.3	49.7	50.8
2.1	25	45.8	47.0	48.4	49.8	50.9
2.2	26	45.9	47.1	48.5	49.9	51.1
2.3	27	46.0	47.2	48.6	50.0	51.2
2.4	28	46.1	47.3	48.7	50.2	51.3
2.5	29	46.2	47.4	48.8	50.3	51.4
2.6	30	46.3	47.5	48.9	50.4	51.6
2.7	31	46.4	47.6	49.0	50.5	51.7
2.8	32	46.5	47.7	49.1	50.6	51.8
2.9	33	46.6	47.8	49.2	50.7	51.9

(Contd.)

Head circumference-for-age of boys from birth to 5 years (percentiles) (Contd.)						
Year : Month	Months	3rd	15th	Median	85th	97th
2.10	34	46.6	47.8	49.3	50.8	52.0
2.11	35	46.7	47.9	49.4	50.8	52.0
3.0	36	46.8	48.0	49.5	50.9	52.1
3.1	37	46.9	48.1	49.5	51.0	52.2
3.2	38	46.9	48.1	49.6	51.1	52.3
3.3	39	47.0	48.2	49.7	51.2	52.4
3.4	40	47.0	48.3	49.7	51.2	52.4
3.5	41	47.1	48.3	49.8	51.3	52.5
3.6	42	47.2	48.4	49.9	51.4	52.6
3.7	43	47.2	48.4	49.9	51.4	52.7
3.8	44	47.3	48.5	50.0	51.5	52.7
3.9	45	47.3	48.5	50.1	51.6	52.8
3.10	46	47.4	48.6	50.1	51.6	52.8
3.11	47	47.4	48.6	50.2	51.7	52.9
4.0	48	47.5	48.7	50.2	51.7	53.0
4.1	49	47.5	48.7	50.3	51.8	53.0
4.2	50	47.5	48.8	50.3	51.8	53.1
4.3	51	47.6	48.8	50.4	51.9	53.1
4.4	52	47.6	48.9	50.4	51.9	53.2
4.5	53	47.7	48.9	50.4	52.0	53.2
4.6	54	47.7	49.0	50.5	52.0	53.3
4.7	55	47.7	49.0	50.5	52.1	53.3
4.8	56	47.8	49.0	50.6	52.1	53.4
4.9	57	47.8	49.1	50.6	52.2	53.4
4.10	58	47.9	49.1	50.7	52.2	53.5
4.11	59	47.9	49.2	50.7	52.2	53.5
5.0	60	47.9	49.2	50.7	52.3	53.5

APPENDIX XX. Head circumference-for-age of girls from birth to 5 years

Head circumference-for-age of girls from birth to 5 years (percentiles)

Year : Month	Months	3rd	15th	Median	85th	97th
0.0	0	31.7	32.7	33.9	35.1	36.1
0.1	1	34.3	35.3	36.5	37.8	38.8
0.2	2	36.0	37.0	38.3	39.5	40.5
0.3	3	37.2	38.2	39.5	40.8	41.9
0.4	4	38.2	39.3	40.6	41.9	43.0
0.5	5	39.0	40.1	41.5	42.8	43.9
0.6	6	39.7	40.8	42.2	43.5	44.6
0.7	7	40.4	41.5	42.8	44.2	45.3
0.8	8	40.9	42.0	43.4	44.7	45.9
0.9	9	41.3	42.4	43.8	45.2	46.3
0.10	10	41.7	42.8	44.2	45.6	46.8
0.11	11	42.0	43.2	44.6	46.0	47.1
1.0	12	42.3	43.5	44.9	46.3	47.5
1.1	13	42.6	43.8	45.2	46.6	47.7
1.2	14	42.9	44.0	45.4	46.8	48.0
1.3	15	43.1	44.2	45.7	47.1	48.2
1.4	16	43.3	44.4	45.9	47.3	48.5
1.5	17	43.5	44.6	46.1	47.5	48.7
1.6	18	43.6	44.8	46.2	47.7	48.8
1.7	19	43.8	45.0	46.4	47.8	49.0
1.8	20	44.0	45.1	46.6	48.0	49.2
1.9	21	44.1	45.3	46.7	48.2	49.4
1.10	22	44.3	45.4	46.9	48.3	49.5
1.11	23	44.4	45.6	47.0	48.5	49.7
2.0	24	44.6	45.7	47.2	48.6	49.8
2.1	25	44.7	45.9	47.3	48.8	49.9
2.2	26	44.8	46.0	47.5	48.9	50.1
2.3	27	44.9	46.1	47.6	49.0	50.2
2.4	28	45.1	46.3	47.7	49.2	50.3
2.5	29	45.2	46.4	47.8	49.3	50.5
2.6	30	45.3	46.5	47.9	49.4	50.6
2.7	31	45.4	46.6	48.0	49.5	50.7
2.8	32	45.5	46.7	48.1	49.6	50.8
2.9	33	45.6	46.8	48.2	49.7	50.9

(Contd.)

Head circumference-for-age of girls from birth to 5 years (percentiles) (Contd.)						
Year : Month	Months	3rd	15th	Median	85th	97th
2.10	34	45.7	46.9	48.3	49.8	51.0
2.11	35	45.8	47.0	48.4	49.9	51.1
3.0	36	45.9	47.0	48.5	50.0	51.2
3.1	37	45.9	47.1	48.6	50.1	51.3
3.2	38	46.0	47.2	48.7	50.1	51.3
3.3	39	46.1	47.3	48.7	50.2	51.4
3.4	40	46.2	47.4	48.8	50.3	51.5
3.5	41	46.2	47.4	48.9	50.4	51.6
3.6	42	46.3	47.5	49.0	50.4	51.6
3.7	43	46.4	47.6	49.0	50.5	51.7
3.8	44	46.4	47.6	49.1	50.6	51.8
3.9	45	46.5	47.7	49.2	50.6	51.8
3.10	46	46.5	47.7	49.2	50.7	51.9
3.11	47	46.6	47.8	49.3	50.7	51.9
4.0	48	46.7	47.9	49.3	50.8	52.0
4.1	49	46.7	47.9	49.4	50.9	52.1
4.2	50	46.8	48.0	49.4	50.9	52.1
4.3	51	46.8	48.0	49.5	51.0	52.2
4.4	52	46.9	48.1	49.5	51.0	52.2
4.5	53	46.9	48.1	49.6	51.1	52.3
4.6	54	47.0	48.2	49.6	51.1	52.3
4.7	55	47.0	48.2	49.7	51.2	52.4
4.8	56	47.1	48.3	49.7	51.2	52.4
4.9	57	47.1	48.3	49.8	51.3	52.5
4.10	58	47.2	48.4	49.8	51.3	52.5
4.11	59	47.2	48.4	49.9	51.4	52.6
5.0	60	47.2	48.4	49.9	51.4	52.6

APPENDIX XXI. Weight-for-length of boys from birth to 5 years

Weight-for-length of boys from birth to 2 years (percentiles)					
Length (cm)	3rd	15th	Median	85th	97th
45.0	2.1	2.2	2.4	2.7	2.9
45.5	2.1	2.3	2.5	2.8	3.0
46.0	2.2	2.4	2.6	2.9	3.1
46.5	2.3	2.5	2.7	3.0	3.2
47.0	2.4	2.5	2.8	3.1	3.3
47.5	2.4	2.6	2.9	3.1	3.4
48.0	2.5	2.7	2.9	3.2	3.5
48.5	2.6	2.8	3.0	3.3	3.6
49.0	2.7	2.9	3.1	3.4	3.7
49.5	2.7	2.9	3.2	3.5	3.8
50.0	2.8	3.0	3.3	3.7	4.0
50.5	2.9	3.1	3.4	3.8	4.1
51.0	3.0	3.2	3.5	3.9	4.2
51.5	3.1	3.3	3.6	4.0	4.3
52.0	3.2	3.4	3.8	4.1	4.5
52.5	3.3	3.6	3.9	4.3	4.6
53.0	3.4	3.7	4.0	4.4	4.7
53.5	3.5	3.8	4.1	4.5	4.9
54.0	3.6	3.9	4.3	4.7	5.0
54.5	3.8	4.0	4.4	4.8	5.2
55.0	3.9	4.2	4.5	5.0	5.4
55.5	4.0	4.3	4.7	5.1	5.5
56.0	4.1	4.4	4.8	5.3	5.7
56.5	4.3	4.6	5.0	5.4	5.9
57.0	4.4	4.7	5.1	5.6	6.0
57.5	4.5	4.8	5.3	5.8	6.2
58.0	4.6	5.0	5.4	5.9	6.4
58.5	4.8	5.1	5.6	6.1	6.5
59.0	4.9	5.2	5.7	6.2	6.7
59.5	5.0	5.4	5.9	6.4	6.9
60.0	5.1	5.5	6.0	6.5	7.0
60.5	5.3	5.6	6.1	6.7	7.2
61.0	5.4	5.8	6.3	6.8	7.4

(Contd.)

Weight-for-length of boys from birth to 2 years (percentiles) (Contd.)

Length (cm)	3rd	15th	Median	85th	97th
61.5	5.5	5.9	6.4	7.0	7.5
62.0	5.6	6.0	6.5	7.1	7.7
62.5	5.7	6.1	6.7	7.3	7.8
63.0	5.8	6.2	6.8	7.4	8.0
63.5	5.9	6.3	6.9	7.5	8.1
64.0	6.0	6.5	7.0	7.7	8.2
64.5	6.1	6.6	7.1	7.8	8.4
65.0	6.4	6.8	7.4	8.1	8.7
65.5	6.5	6.9	7.6	8.2	8.9
66.0	6.6	7.1	7.7	8.4	9.0
66.5	6.7	7.2	7.8	8.5	9.1
67.0	6.8	7.3	7.9	8.6	9.3
67.5	6.9	7.4	8.0	8.7	9.4
68.0	7.0	7.5	8.1	8.9	9.5
68.5	7.1	7.6	8.2	9.0	9.7
69.0	7.2	7.7	8.4	9.1	9.8
69.5	7.3	7.8	8.5	9.2	9.9
70.0	7.4	7.9	8.6	9.4	10.1
70.5	7.5	8.0	8.7	9.5	10.2
71.0	7.6	8.1	8.8	9.6	10.3
71.5	7.7	8.2	8.9	9.7	10.5
72.0	7.8	8.3	9.0	9.8	10.6
72.5	7.8	8.4	9.1	10.0	10.7
73.0	7.9	8.5	9.2	10.1	10.8
73.5	8.0	8.6	9.3	10.2	11.0
74.0	8.1	8.7	9.4	10.3	11.1
74.5	8.2	8.8	9.5	10.4	11.2
75.0	8.3	8.9	9.6	10.5	11.3
75.5	8.4	9.0	9.7	10.6	11.4
76.0	8.5	9.0	9.8	10.7	11.6
76.5	8.5	9.1	9.9	10.8	11.7
77.0	8.6	9.2	10.0	10.9	11.8
77.5	8.7	9.3	10.1	11.0	11.9
78.0	8.8	9.4	10.2	11.1	12.0
78.5	8.8	9.5	10.3	11.2	12.1

(Contd.)

Weight-for-height of boys from 2 to 5 years (percentiles) (Contd.)

Height (cm)	3rd	15th	Median	85th	97th
79.0	8.9	9.5	10.4	11.3	12.2
79.5	9.0	9.6	10.5	11.4	12.3
80.0	9.1	9.7	10.6	11.5	12.4
80.5	9.2	9.8	10.7	11.6	12.5
81.0	9.3	9.9	10.8	11.8	12.6
81.5	9.3	10.0	10.9	11.9	12.8
82.0	9.4	10.1	11.0	12.0	12.9
82.5	9.5	10.2	11.1	12.1	13.0
83.0	9.6	10.3	11.2	12.2	13.1
83.5	9.7	10.4	11.3	12.3	13.3
84.0	9.8	10.5	11.4	12.5	13.4
84.5	9.9	10.6	11.5	12.6	13.5
85.0	10.1	10.7	11.7	12.7	13.7
85.5	10.2	10.9	11.8	12.8	13.8
86.0	10.3	11.0	11.9	13.0	13.9
86.5	10.4	11.1	12.0	13.1	14.1
87.0	10.5	11.2	12.2	13.2	14.2
87.5	10.6	11.3	12.3	13.4	14.4
88.0	10.7	11.4	12.4	13.5	14.5
88.5	10.8	11.5	12.5	13.6	14.6
89.0	10.9	11.7	12.6	13.8	14.8
89.5	11.0	11.8	12.8	13.9	14.9
90.0	11.1	11.9	12.9	14.0	15.1
90.5	11.2	12.0	13.0	14.1	15.2
91.0	11.3	12.1	13.1	14.3	15.3
91.5	11.4	12.2	13.2	14.4	15.5
92.0	11.5	12.3	13.4	14.5	15.6
92.5	11.6	12.4	13.5	14.7	15.7
93.0	11.7	12.5	13.6	14.8	15.9
93.5	11.8	12.6	13.7	14.9	16.0
94.0	11.9	12.7	13.8	15.0	16.1
94.5	12.0	12.8	13.9	15.2	16.3
95.0	12.1	12.9	14.1	15.3	16.4
95.5	12.2	13.1	14.2	15.4	16.6
96.0	12.3	13.2	14.3	15.6	16.7
96.5	12.4	13.3	14.4	15.7	16.9
97.0	12.5	13.4	14.6	15.9	17.0
97.5	12.7	13.5	14.7	16.0	17.2
98.0	12.8	13.6	14.8	16.1	17.3
98.5	12.9	13.8	14.9	16.3	17.5

(Contd.)

Weight-for-height of boys from 2 to 5 years (percentiles) (Contd.)					
Height (cm)	3rd	15th	Median	85th	97th
99.0	13.0	13.9	15.1	16.4	17.7
99.5	13.1	14.0	15.2	16.6	17.8
100.0	13.2	14.1	15.4	16.7	18.0
100.5	13.3	14.2	15.5	16.9	18.2
101.0	13.4	14.4	15.6	17.1	18.4
101.5	13.6	14.5	15.8	17.2	18.5
102.0	13.7	14.6	15.9	17.4	18.7
102.5	13.8	14.8	16.1	17.6	18.9
103.0	13.9	14.9	16.2	17.7	19.1
103.5	14.0	15.0	16.4	17.9	19.3
104.0	14.2	15.2	16.5	18.1	19.5
104.5	14.3	15.3	16.7	18.2	19.7
105.0	14.4	15.4	16.8	18.4	19.9
105.5	14.5	15.6	17.0	18.6	20.1
106.0	14.7	15.7	17.2	18.8	20.3
106.5	14.8	15.9	17.3	19.0	20.5
107.0	14.9	16.0	17.5	19.1	20.7
107.5	15.1	16.2	17.7	19.3	20.9
108.0	15.2	16.3	17.8	19.5	21.1
108.5	15.3	16.5	18.0	19.7	21.3
109.0	15.5	16.6	18.2	19.9	21.5
109.5	15.6	16.8	18.3	20.1	21.7
110.0	15.8	16.9	18.5	20.3	22.0
110.5	15.9	17.1	18.7	20.5	22.2
111.0	16.1	17.2	18.9	20.7	22.4
111.5	16.2	17.4	19.1	20.9	22.6
112.0	16.3	17.6	19.2	21.1	22.9
112.5	16.5	17.7	19.4	21.4	23.1
113.0	16.6	17.9	19.6	21.6	23.4
113.5	16.8	18.1	19.8	21.8	23.6
114.0	17.0	18.2	20.0	22.0	23.8
114.5	17.1	18.4	20.2	22.2	24.1
115.0	17.3	18.6	20.4	22.4	24.3
115.5	17.4	18.7	20.6	22.7	24.6
116.0	17.6	18.9	20.8	22.9	24.8
116.5	17.7	19.1	21.0	23.1	25.1
117.0	17.9	19.3	21.2	23.3	25.3
117.5	18.0	19.4	21.4	23.6	25.6
118.0	18.2	19.6	21.6	23.8	25.8
118.5	18.4	19.8	21.8	24.0	26.1
119.0	18.5	20.0	22.0	24.2	26.3
119.5	18.7	20.1	22.2	24.5	26.6
120.0	18.8	20.3	22.4	24.7	26.8

APPENDIX XXII. Weight-for-length of girls from birth to 5 years

Weight-for-length of girls from birth to 2 years (percentiles)					
Length (cm)	3rd	15th	Median	85th	97th
45.0	2.1	2.2	2.5	2.7	2.9
45.5	2.2	2.3	2.5	2.8	3.0
46.0	2.2	2.4	2.6	2.9	3.1
46.5	2.3	2.5	2.7	3.0	3.2
47.0	2.4	2.6	2.8	3.1	3.3
47.5	2.4	2.6	2.9	3.2	3.4
48.0	2.5	2.7	3.0	3.3	3.5
48.5	2.6	2.8	3.1	3.4	3.7
49.0	2.7	2.9	3.2	3.5	3.8
49.5	2.8	3.0	3.3	3.6	3.9
50.0	2.8	3.1	3.4	3.7	4.0
50.5	2.9	3.2	3.5	3.8	4.1
51.0	3.0	3.2	3.6	3.9	4.3
51.5	3.1	3.4	3.7	4.0	4.4
52.0	3.2	3.5	3.8	4.2	4.5
52.5	3.3	3.6	3.9	4.3	4.7
53.0	3.4	3.7	4.0	4.4	4.8
53.5	3.5	3.8	4.2	4.6	5.0
54.0	3.6	3.9	4.3	4.7	5.1
54.5	3.7	4.0	4.4	4.9	5.3
55.0	3.9	4.1	4.5	5.0	5.4
55.5	4.0	4.3	4.7	5.2	5.6
56.0	4.1	4.4	4.8	5.3	5.8
56.5	4.2	4.5	5.0	5.5	5.9
57.0	4.3	4.6	5.1	5.6	6.1
57.5	4.4	4.8	5.2	5.7	6.2
58.0	4.5	4.9	5.4	5.9	6.4
58.5	4.6	5.0	5.5	6.0	6.5
59.0	4.8	5.1	5.6	6.2	6.7
59.5	4.9	5.2	5.7	6.3	6.9
60.0	5.0	5.4	5.9	6.5	7.0
60.5	5.1	5.5	6.0	6.6	7.2
61.0	5.2	5.6	6.1	6.7	7.3

(Contd.)

Weight-for-length of girls from birth to 2 years (percentiles) (Contd.)					
Length (cm)	3rd	15th	Median	85th	97th
61.5	5.3	5.7	6.3	6.9	7.5
62.0	5.4	5.8	6.4	7.0	7.6
62.5	5.5	5.9	6.5	7.2	7.8
63.0	5.6	6.0	6.6	7.3	7.9
63.5	5.7	6.1	6.7	7.4	8.0
64.0	5.8	6.2	6.9	7.5	8.2
64.5	5.9	6.3	7.0	7.7	8.3
65.0	6.1	6.6	7.2	8.0	8.6
65.5	6.2	6.7	7.4	8.1	8.8
66.0	6.3	6.8	7.5	8.2	8.9
66.5	6.4	6.9	7.6	8.3	9.0
67.0	6.5	7.0	7.7	8.5	9.2
67.5	6.6	7.1	7.8	8.6	9.3
68.0	6.7	7.2	7.9	8.7	9.4
68.5	6.8	7.3	8.0	8.8	9.5
69.0	6.9	7.4	8.1	8.9	9.7
69.5	7.0	7.5	8.2	9.0	9.8
70.0	7.0	7.6	8.3	9.1	9.9
70.5	7.1	7.7	8.4	9.3	10.0
71.0	7.2	7.8	8.5	9.4	10.1
71.5	7.3	7.9	8.6	9.5	10.3
72.0	7.4	7.9	8.7	9.6	10.4
72.5	7.5	8.0	8.8	9.7	10.5
73.0	7.6	8.1	8.9	9.8	10.6
73.5	7.6	8.2	9.0	9.9	10.7
74.0	7.7	8.3	9.1	10.0	10.8
74.5	7.8	8.4	9.2	10.1	10.9
75.0	7.9	8.5	9.3	10.2	11.1
75.5	8.0	8.6	9.4	10.3	11.2
76.0	8.0	8.6	9.5	10.4	11.3
76.5	8.1	8.7	9.6	10.5	11.4
77.0	8.2	8.8	9.6	10.6	11.5
77.5	8.3	8.9	9.7	10.7	11.6

(Contd.)

Weight-for-height of girls from 2 to 5 years (percentiles) (Contd.)					
Height (cm)	3rd	15th	Median	85th	97th
78.0	8.4	9.0	9.8	10.8	11.7
78.5	8.4	9.1	9.9	10.9	11.8
79.0	8.5	9.2	10.0	11.0	11.9
79.5	8.6	9.2	10.1	11.1	12.1
80.0	8.7	9.3	10.2	11.2	12.2
80.5	8.8	9.4	10.3	11.4	12.3
81.0	8.9	9.5	10.4	11.5	12.4
81.5	9.0	9.6	10.6	11.6	12.6
82.0	9.1	9.7	10.7	11.7	12.7
82.5	9.2	9.9	10.8	11.9	12.8
83.0	9.3	10.0	10.9	12.0	13.0
83.5	9.4	10.1	11.0	12.1	13.1
84.0	9.5	10.2	11.1	12.2	13.3
84.5	9.6	10.3	11.3	12.4	13.4
85.0	9.7	10.4	11.4	12.5	13.5
85.5	9.8	10.5	11.5	12.7	13.7
86.0	9.9	10.6	11.6	12.8	13.8
86.5	10.0	10.8	11.8	12.9	14.0
87.0	10.1	10.9	11.9	13.1	14.1
87.5	10.2	11.0	12.0	13.2	14.3
88.0	10.3	11.1	12.1	13.3	14.4
88.5	10.4	11.2	12.3	13.5	14.6
89.0	10.5	11.3	12.4	13.6	14.7
89.5	10.6	11.4	12.5	13.8	14.9
90.0	10.8	11.5	12.6	13.9	15.0
90.5	10.9	11.7	12.8	14.0	15.2
91.0	11.0	11.8	12.9	14.2	15.3
91.5	11.1	11.9	13.0	14.3	15.5
92.0	11.2	12.0	13.1	14.4	15.6
92.5	11.3	12.1	13.3	14.6	15.8
93.0	11.4	12.2	13.4	14.7	15.9
93.5	11.5	12.3	13.5	14.9	16.1
94.0	11.6	12.4	13.6	15.0	16.2
94.5	11.7	12.6	13.8	15.1	16.4
95.0	11.8	12.7	13.9	15.3	16.5
95.5	11.9	12.8	14.0	15.4	16.7
96.0	12.0	12.9	14.1	15.6	16.9
96.5	12.1	13.0	14.3	15.7	17.0
97.0	12.2	13.1	14.4	15.8	17.2
97.5	12.3	13.3	14.5	16.0	17.3
98.0	12.4	13.4	14.7	16.1	17.5

(Contd.)

Weight-for-height of girls from 2 to 5 years (percentiles) (Contd.)

Height (cm)	3rd	15th	Median	85th	97th
98.5	12.6	13.5	14.8	16.3	17.7
99.0	12.7	13.6	14.9	16.4	17.8
99.5	12.8	13.8	15.1	16.6	18.0
100.0	12.9	13.9	15.2	16.8	18.2
100.5	13.0	14.0	15.4	16.9	18.3
101.0	13.1	14.1	15.5	17.1	18.5
101.5	13.3	14.3	15.7	17.2	18.7
102.0	13.4	14.4	15.8	17.4	18.9
102.5	13.5	14.5	16.0	17.6	19.1
103.0	13.6	14.7	16.1	17.8	19.3
103.5	13.8	14.8	16.3	17.9	19.5
104.0	13.9	15.0	16.4	18.1	19.7
104.5	14.0	15.1	16.6	18.3	19.9
105.0	14.2	15.3	16.8	18.5	20.1
105.5	14.3	15.4	16.9	18.7	20.3
106.0	14.5	15.6	17.1	18.9	20.5
106.5	14.6	15.7	17.3	19.1	20.7
107.0	14.7	15.9	17.5	19.3	21.0
107.5	14.9	16.1	17.7	19.5	21.2
108.0	15.0	16.2	17.8	19.7	21.4
108.5	15.2	16.4	18.0	19.9	21.6
109.0	15.4	16.6	18.2	20.1	21.9
109.5	15.5	16.7	18.4	20.3	22.1
110.0	15.7	16.9	18.6	20.6	22.4
110.5	15.8	17.1	18.8	20.8	22.6
111.0	16.0	17.3	19.0	21.0	22.8
111.5	16.2	17.4	19.2	21.2	23.1
112.0	16.3	17.6	19.4	21.5	23.4
112.5	16.5	17.8	19.6	21.7	23.6
113.0	16.7	18.0	19.8	21.9	23.9
113.5	16.8	18.2	20.0	22.2	24.1
114.0	17.0	18.4	20.2	22.4	24.4
114.5	17.2	18.5	20.5	22.6	24.7
115.0	17.3	18.7	20.7	22.9	24.9
115.5	17.5	18.9	20.9	23.1	25.2
116.0	17.7	19.1	21.1	23.4	25.5
116.5	17.9	19.3	21.3	23.6	25.7
117.0	18.0	19.5	21.5	23.8	26.0
117.5	18.2	19.7	21.7	24.1	26.3
118.0	18.4	19.9	22.0	24.3	26.5
118.5	18.6	20.1	22.2	24.6	26.8
119.0	18.7	20.3	22.4	24.8	27.1
119.5	18.9	20.5	22.6	25.1	27.4
120.0	19.1	20.6	22.8	25.3	27.6

APPENDIX XXIII. WHO length/height, weight and head circumference charts of boys

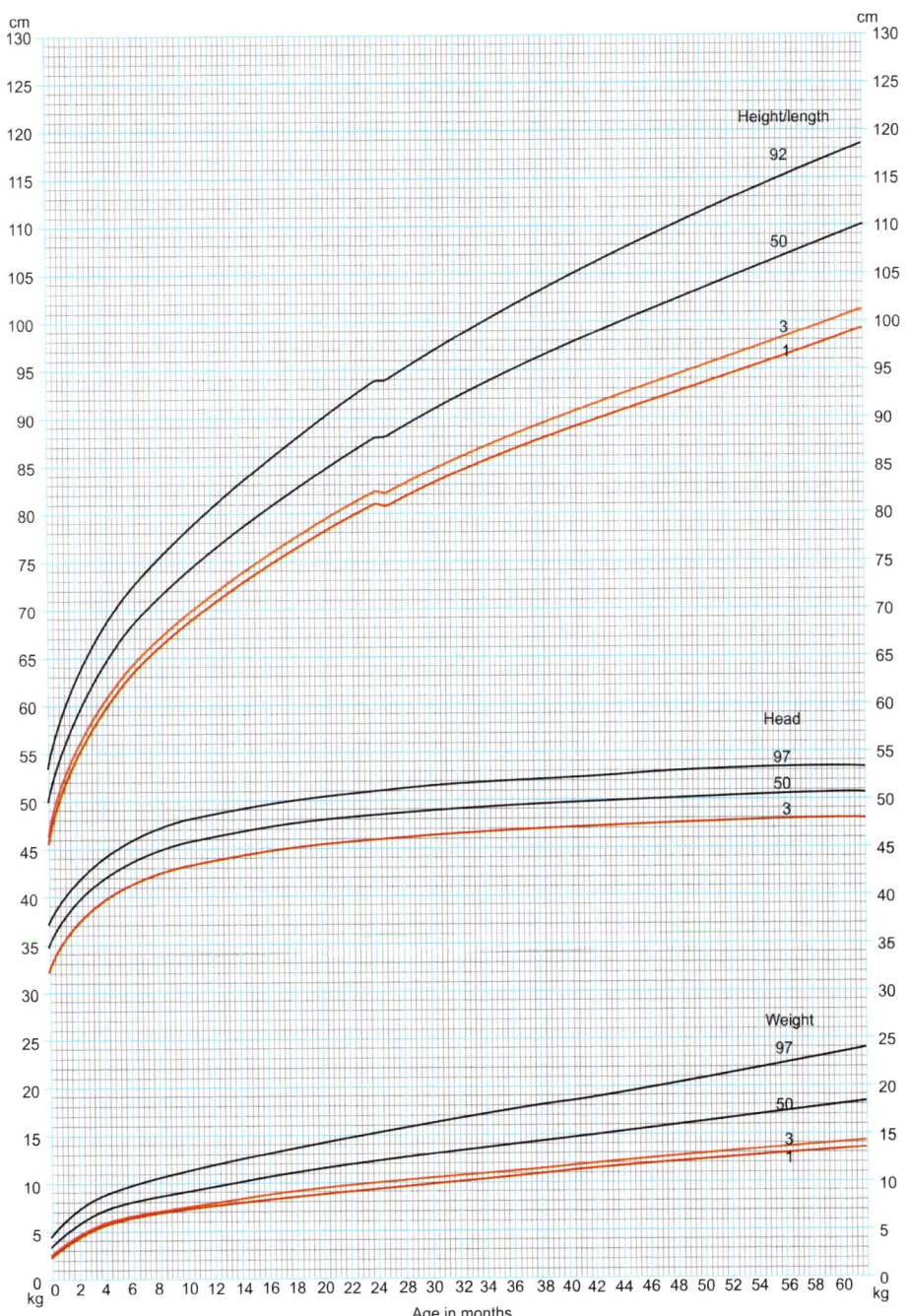

On the basis of under-5 WHO growth charts, weight below 3rd percentile is classified as under weight and below 1st percentile as severe underweight, length/height below 3rd percentile is suggestive of stunting and below 1st percentile as severely stunted; weight-for-length or height below 1st percentile is labeled as severe acute malnutrition (SAM).

Source: WHO MGRS 2006 charts; Acta Paediatrica (suppl) 2006, 450:1–110.

APPENDIX XXIV. WHO length/height, weight and head circumference charts of girls

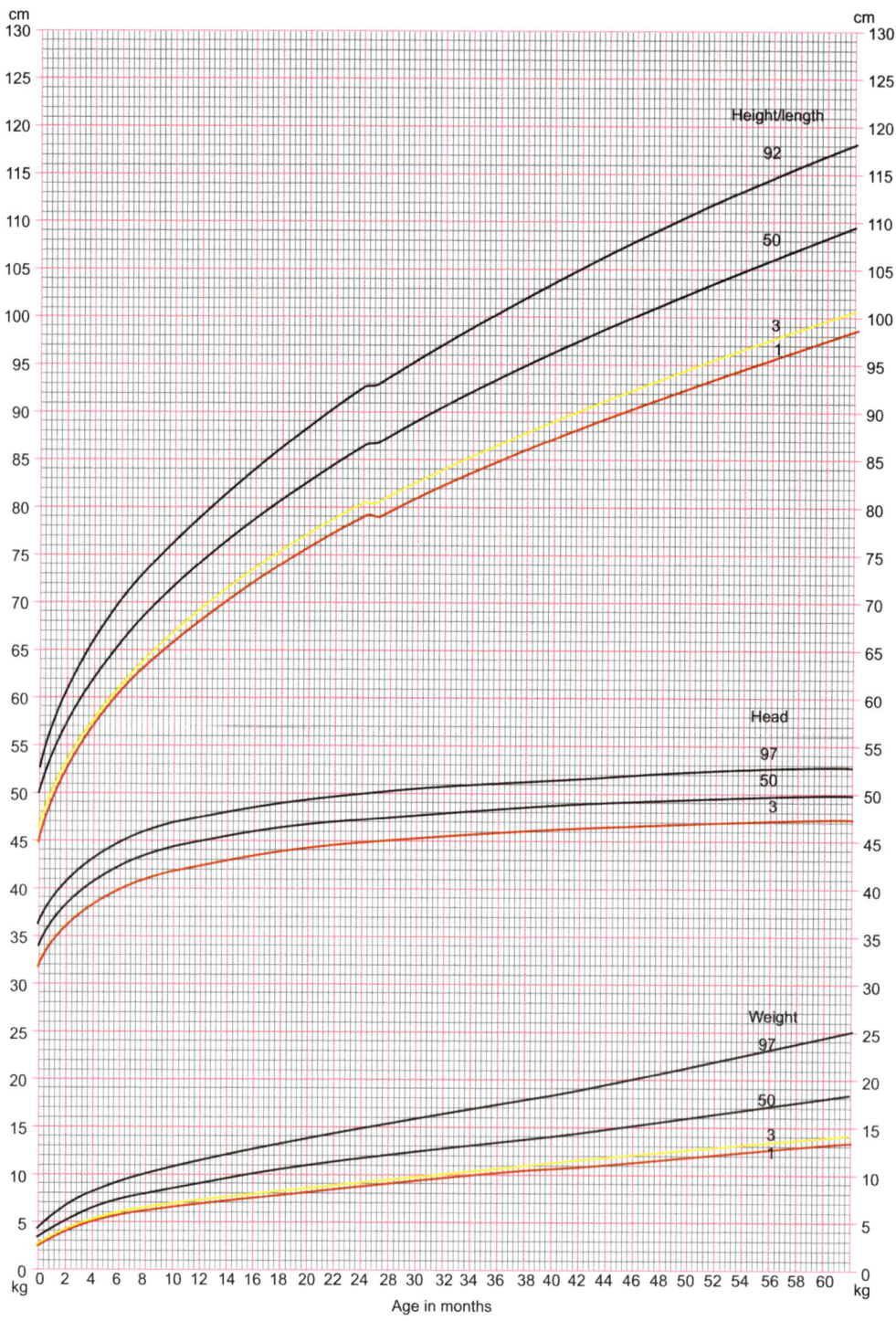

Source: WHO MGRS 2006 charts; Acta Paediatrica (Suppl.) 2006, 450:1-110

APPENDIX XXV. WHO weight-for-length/height charts of boys

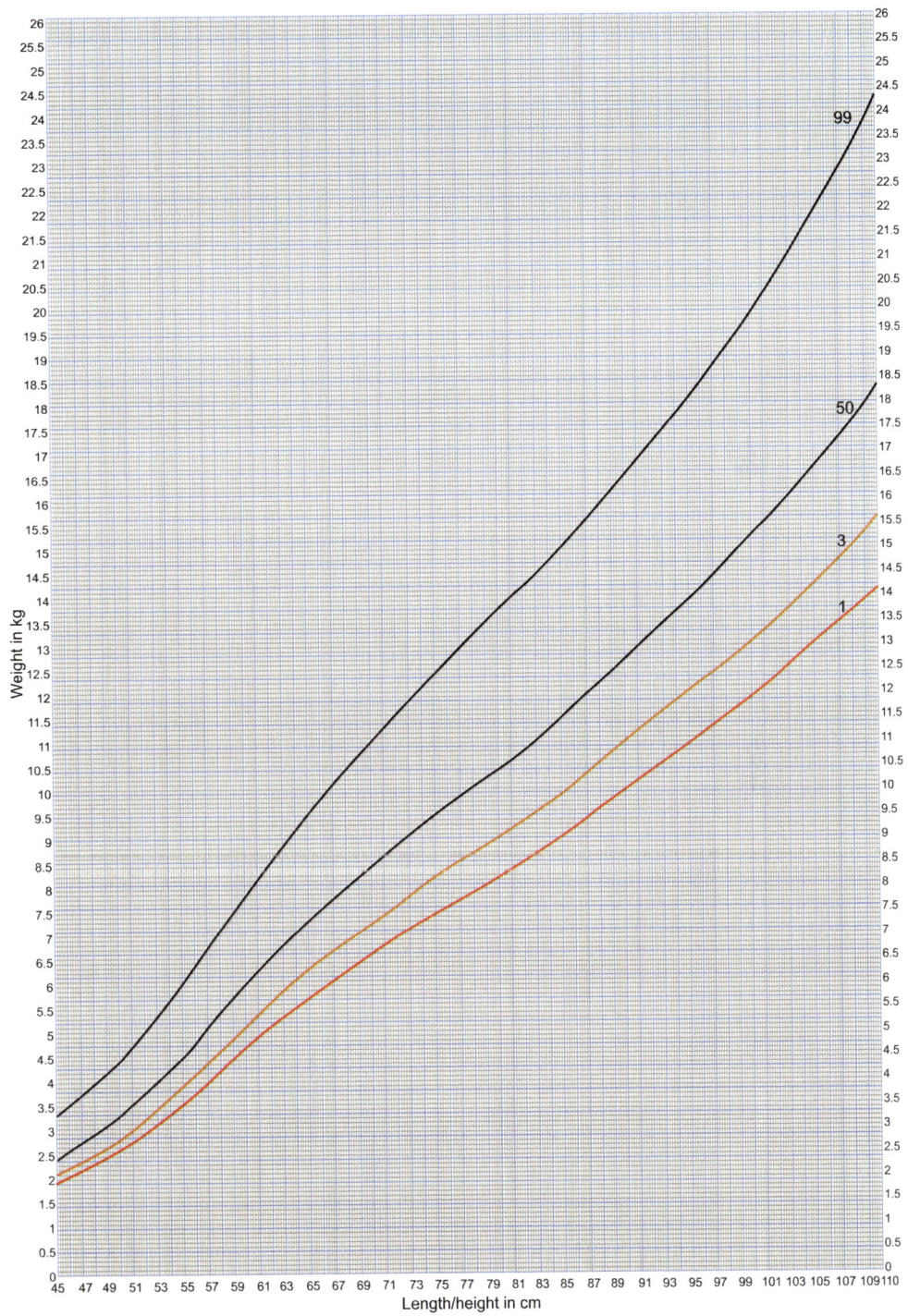

Source: WHO MGRS 2006 charts; Acta Paediatrica (suppl.) 2006, 450:1-110

APPENDIX XXVI. WHO weight-for-length/height charts of girls

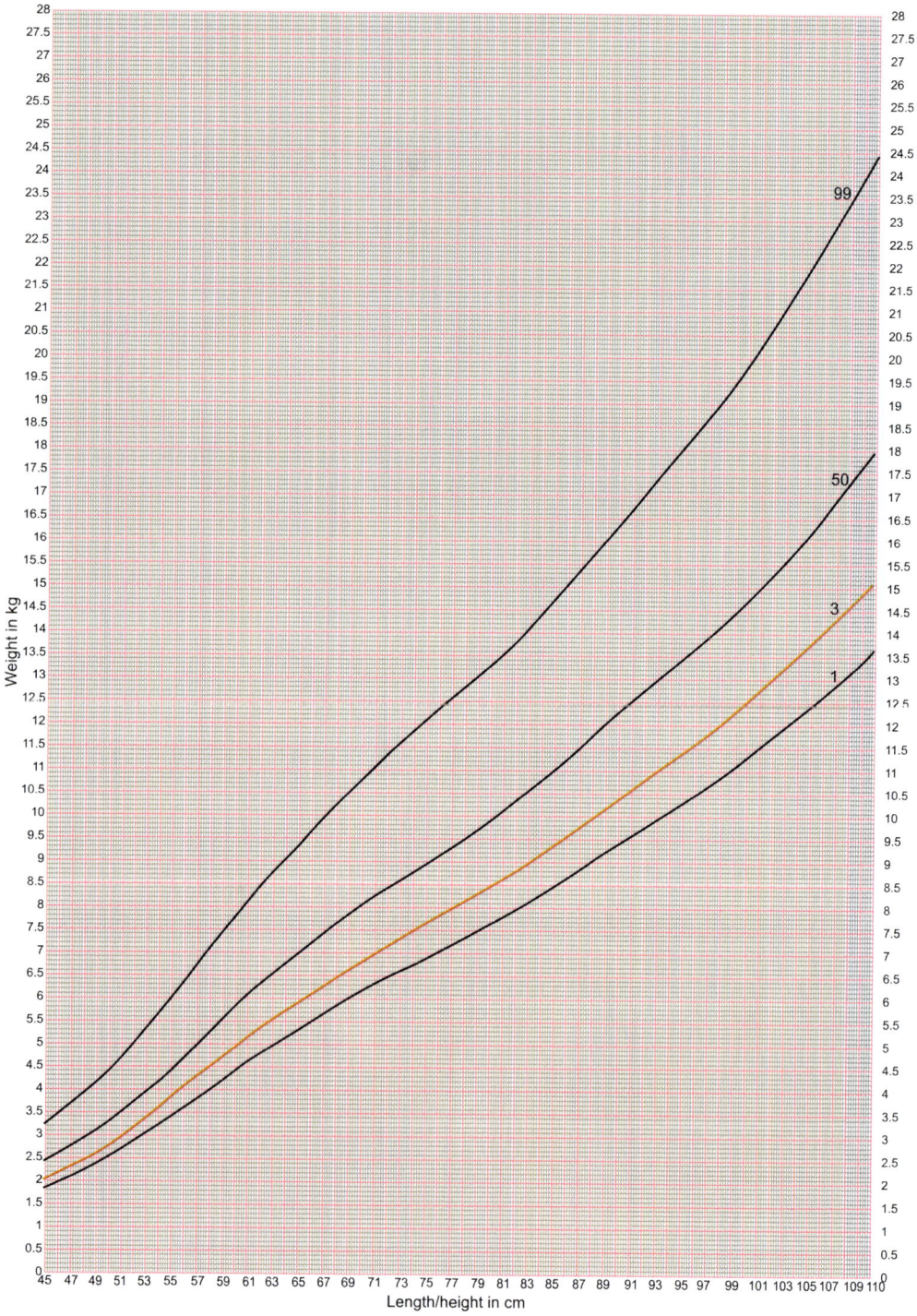

Source: WHO MGRS 2006 charts; Acta Paediatrica (Suppl.) 2006, 450:1-110

APPENDIX XXVII. IAP height and weight charts of 5-18 years boys

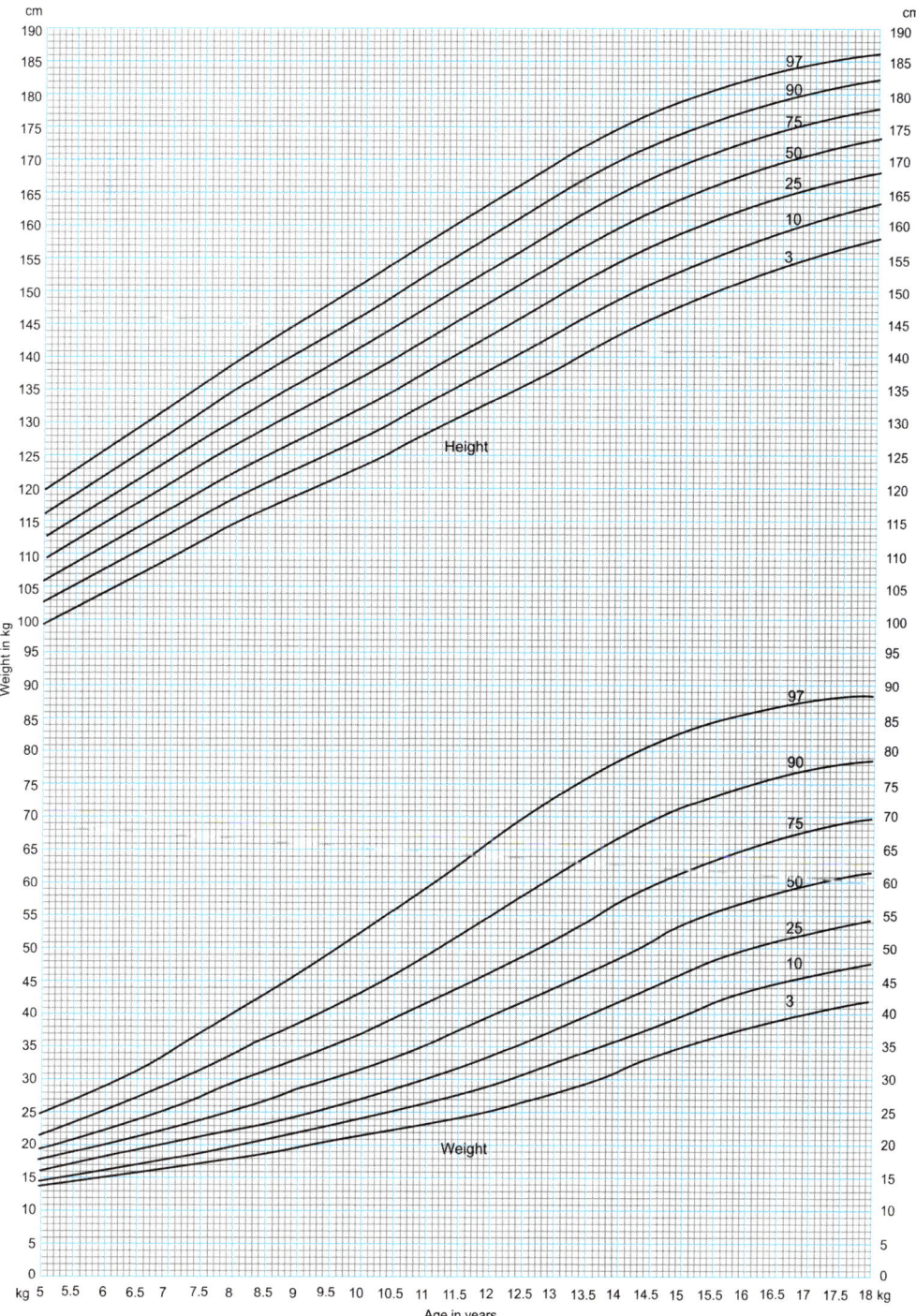

Revised IAP growth charts for height, weight and body mass index for 5 to 18-year-old Indian children.
Khadilkar V. et al. Indian Academy of Pediatrics Growth Chart Committee. Indian Pediatrics. Jan 2015, 52 : 47–55

APPENDIX XXVIII. IAP height and weight charts of 5-18 years girls

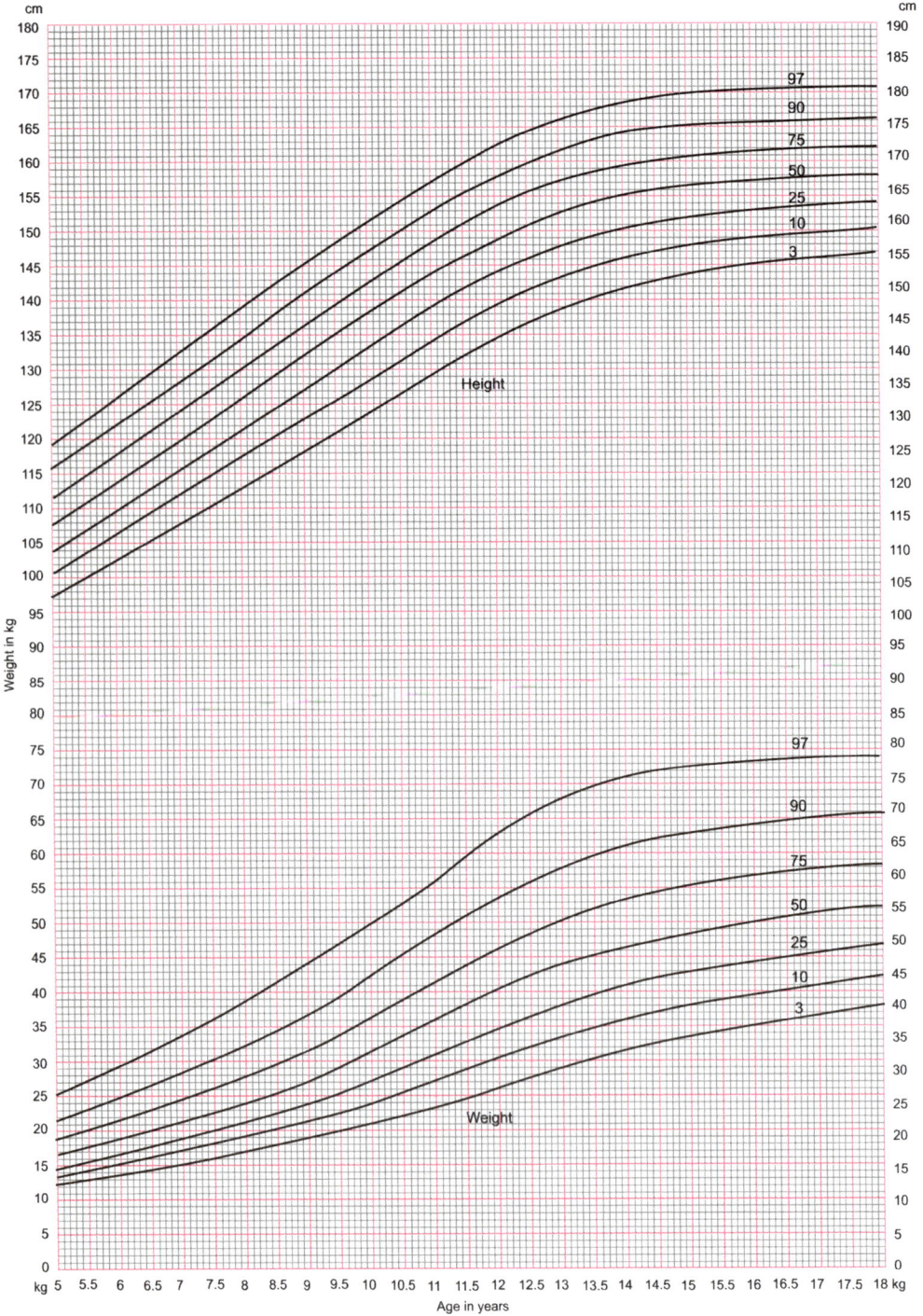

Revised IAP growth charts for height, weight and body mass index for 5 to 18-year-old Indian children.
Khadilkar V. et al. Indian Academy of Pediatrics Growth Chart Committee. Indian Pediatrics. Jan 2015, 52 : 47–55

APPENDIX XXIX. IAP BMI charts of 5-18 years boys

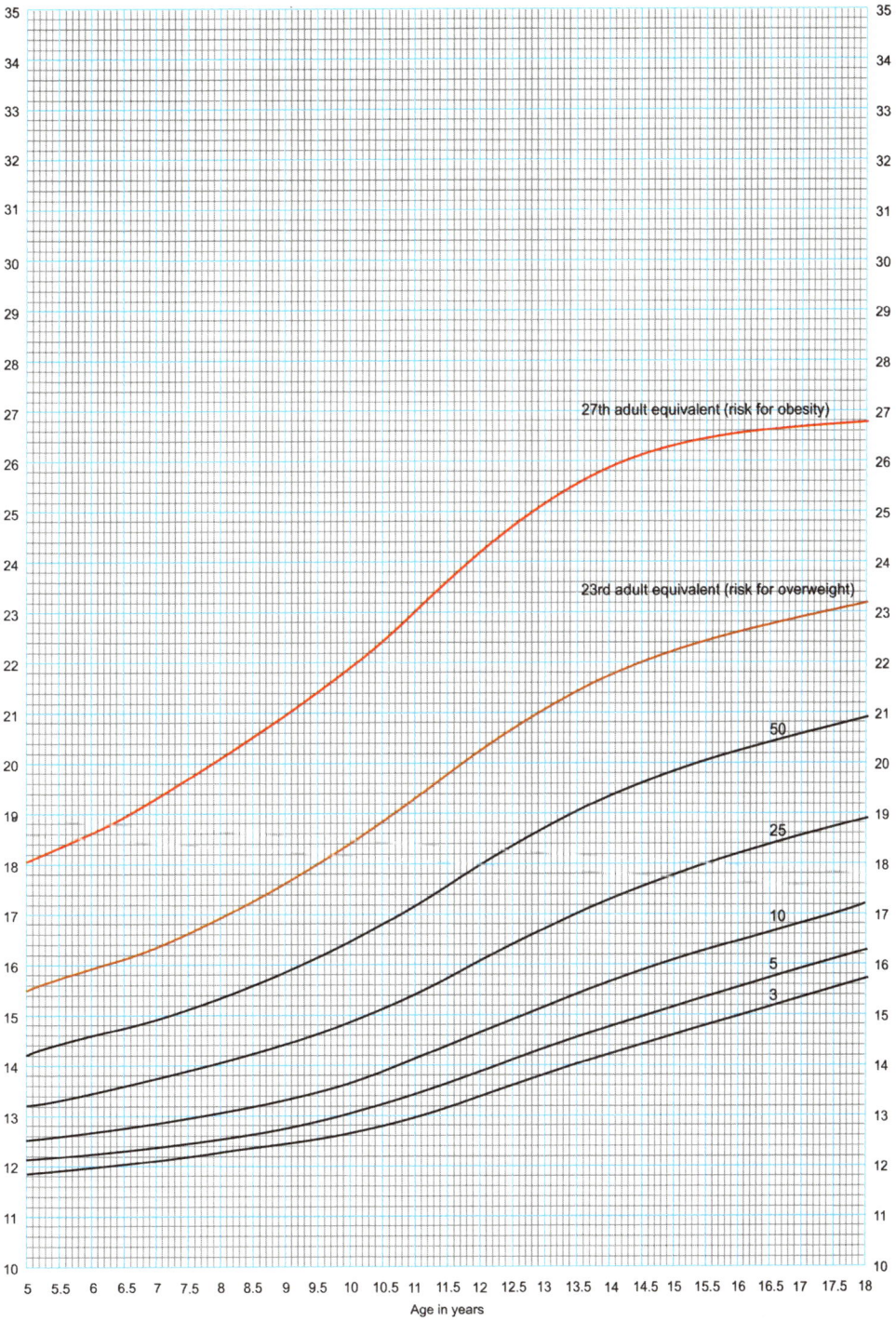

Revised IAP growth charts for height, weight and body mass index for 5 to 18-year-old Indian children.
Khadilkar V, et al. Indian Academy of Pediatrics Growth Chart Committee. Indian Pediatrics. Jan 2015, 52 : 47–55

APPENDIX XXX. IAP BMI charts of 5-18 years girls

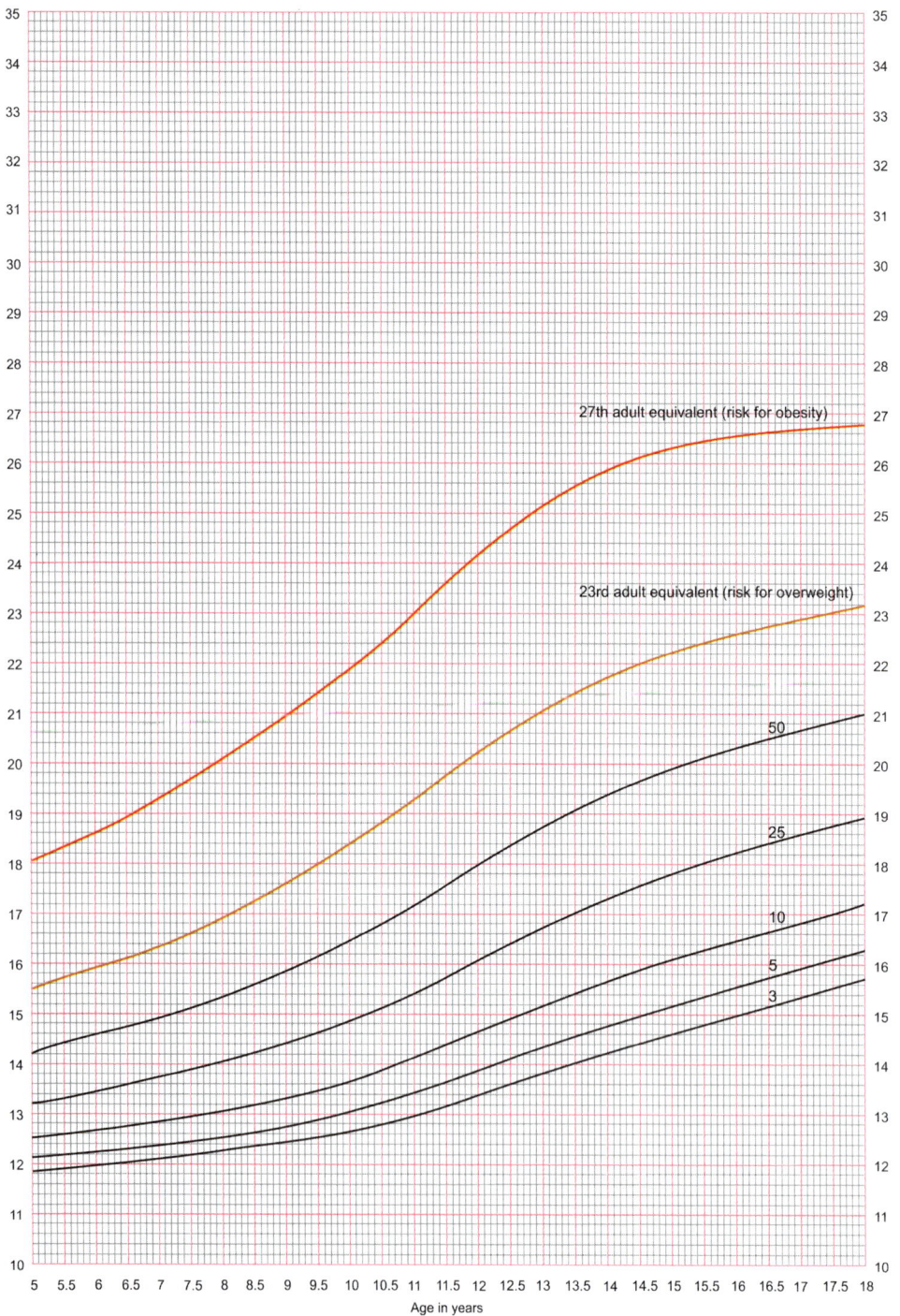

Revised IAP growth charts for height, weight and body mass index for 5 to 18-year-old Indian children.
Khadilkar V, et al. Indian Academy of Pediatrics Growth Chart Committee. Indian Pediatrics. Jan 2015, 52 : 47–55

APPENDIX XXXI. Dyslexia screener for teenagers (International Dyslexia Association)

Child's Name [   ]   **Age** [   ]   **Sex** [   ]
Date of assessment [   ]

	Yes	No
1. Do you read slowly?	☐	☐
2. Do you have trouble learning how to read?	☐	☐
3. Do you often have to read something two or three times before it makes sense?	☐	☐
4. Are you uncomfortable reading out loud?	☐	☐
5. Do you omit, transpose, or add letters when you are reading or writing?	☐	☐
6. Do you find you still have spelling mistakes in your writing even after *Spell Check*?	☐	☐
7. Do you find it difficult to pronounce uncommon multi-syllable words when you are reading?	☐	☐
8. Do you choose to read magazines or short articles rather than longer books and novels?	☐	☐
9. Do you find it extremely difficult to learn a foreign language?	☐	☐
10. Do you avoid work projects or courses that require extensive reading?	☐	☐

If you checked seven or more of these questions, this may indicate dyslexia. Consider seeking consultation from a specialist or get a formal diagnostic assessment done by a qualified examiner.
Visit International Dyslexia Association website for more details: https://dyslexiaida.org/frequently_asked_questions_2/

APPENDIX XXXII. ADHD checklist for parents

Child's Name [ ]   Age [ ]   Sex [ ]
Date of assessment [ ]
Current medications:

Tick (✓) the appropriate box

Symptoms	Severity			
	Not at all (0)	Occasional (1)	Often (2)	Very often (3)
INATTENTION*				
1. Fails to give attention to details or makes careless mistakes				
2. Difficulty in sustaining attention in tasks or fun activities				
3. Does not seem to listen when spoken to directly (ignores)				
4. Does not follow instructions and fails to finish school work				
5. Difficulty in organizing activities				
6. Avoids tasks that require sustained mental effort (easily bored)				
7. Losing things (books and stationery items)				
8. Easily distracted				
9. Forgetful in daily activities				
HYPERACTIVE/IMPULSIVE*				
1. Fidgety or squirms in seat				
2. Leaves seat when expected to sit				
3. Feels restless, runs or climbs				
4. Difficulty in doing fun activities quietly				
5. Always "on the go" or acts as if "driven by a motor"				
6. Talks excessively				
7. Blurts out answers before questions have been completed				
8. Having difficulty in awaiting one's turn				
9. Interrupting or intruding on others (conversation, games)				
OPPOSITIONAL DEFIANT BEHAVIOR**				
1. Loses temper				
2. Argues with adults				
3. Actively defies or refuses to comply with requests and rules				
4. Deliberately annoys people				
5. Blames others for his or her mistakes and misbehavior				
6. Touchy or easily annoyed by others				
7. Angry or resentful				
8. Spiteful or vindictive				

*When six or more (>6/9) of these symptoms of severity of 2 or 3 have been present for at least six months, the child is considered as inattentive, hyperactive or impulsive.

**When four or more (>4/8) of these symptoms of severity 2 or 3 have been present for at least six months, the child is considered to have oppositional defiant behavior.

APPENDIX XXXIII. Modified checklist for autism in toddlers, revised (M-CHAT-R/F)

Child's Name _____ **Age** ____ **Sex** ____

Date of assessment _____

The screening for autism can be done between 12 and 18 months in a Well Child Clinic. Parents are asked to answer the following questions, keeping in mind how the child **usually** behaves. If the behavior is rare or occasional, the answer should be No. Please tick (✓) Yes or No for every question.

1. If you point at something across the room, does your child look at it? — Yes ☐ No ☐
2. Have you ever wondered, if your child might be deaf? — Yes ☐ No ☐
3. Does your child play pretend or make-believe games? (Like feeding the doll, drinking from empty cup, talking on phone). — Yes ☐ No ☐
4. Does your child like climbing on things or enjoy playground equipment and swing? — Yes ☐ No ☐
5. Does your child make unusual finger movements near her or his eyes? — Yes ☐ No ☐
6. Does your child point with one finger to ask for something? (Snack, toy) — Yes ☐ No ☐
7. Does your child point with one finger to show you something interesting? — Yes ☐ No ☐
8. Is your child interested in other children? (Watch them or smile at them). — Yes ☐ No ☐
9. Does your child show you or share things with you? (Toy, book or flower) — Yes ☐ No ☐
10. Does your child respond when you call her or his name from behind? — Yes ☐ No ☐
11. When you smile at your child, does she or he smile back? — Yes ☐ No ☐
12. Does your child get upset or frightened by everyday noises? (Loud music, vacuum cleaner, hair dryer, banging of door, etc.) — Yes ☐ No ☐
13. Does your child walk? — Yes ☐ No ☐
14. Does your child look you in the eye when you are talking, playing and dressing her or him? — Yes ☐ No ☐
15. Does your child try to copy what you do? (Bye-bye, clap, make funny sounds) — Yes ☐ No ☐
16. If you turn your head to look at something, does your child look around to see what you are looking at? — Yes ☐ No ☐
17. Does your child try to get you to watch her or him? (Expecting praise and seeking attention) — Yes ☐ No ☐
18. Does your child understand when you tell her or him to do something? (Asking him or her to bring the toy, put the book on table) — Yes ☐ No ☐
19. If something new happens, does your child look at your face to see how you feel about it? (Strange funny noise, new person or object) — Yes ☐ No ☐
20. Does your child like movement activities? (Bouncing, swinging) — Yes ☐ No ☐

Scoring
For all items except 2, 5 and 12, the No response indicates ASD risk, while for items 2, 5 and 12 Yes is suggestive of ASD risk.
Low-risk score 0–2 score. Assess again after 24 months of age.
Medium-risk score 3–7 score. The child should be evaluated by a revised follow-up proforma (M-CHAT-R/F).
High-risk score 8–20 score. The child needs immediate diagnostic evaluation and intervention. The scoring algorithm can be downloaded from http://www.mchatscreen.com
Source: Robin DL, Casagrande K, Fein D. Validation of the modified checklist for autism in toddlers with follow-up (M-CHAT-R/F). *Pediatrics* 2014, 133(1):37–45.

Index

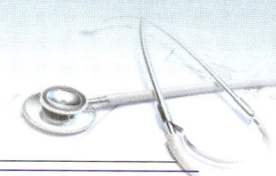

Aarskog syndrome 105
Abdomen and genitalia in a neonate 299
Abdominal diseases, common
  symptoms of 182
Abdominal distension 183
Abdominal pain 183
Abdominal reflexes 270
Abdominal viscera, surface
  anatomy of 182
Abnormal physical signs,
  differential diagnosis of 111
Abortions, recurrent 281
Abscess 45
Acne vulgaris 157
Acrocephaly 97
Acrodermatitis enteropathica 52, 159
Acuity of vision 248
Acute appendicitis 184
Acute kidney injury 186
Acute renal failure 186
Adams forward bend test 177
Adenoids 45, 200
Adenoma sebaceum 241
Adolescence 53
Adult height, prediction of 67
Adventitious sounds in the chest 211
Age-independent criteria for
  assessment of nutrition 69
Alagille syndrome 217
Alimentary system and abdomen 59, 181
Allergic "shiners" 209
Allergic rhinitis 45
Allergic salute 204
Allis sign 311
Alopecia 155
Ambiguous genitalia 194
Amniotic band disruption sequence 109
Amniotic bands 285
Amphoric breathing 210
Anal fissure 195
Anal itching 184
Anal reflex 271
Anal skin tags 195
Anasarca 38
Anemia 116
  classification of 117
  clinical evaluation of 185
Angioedema 158
Angle of Louis 198
Anhidrotic ectodermal dysplasia 155
Aniridia 184

Ankle clonus 268
Ankyloglossia 42, 186
Anomalies
  major 99
  minor 99
  types of 100
Anomalies of radial ray structures 172
Anorexia 184
Anosmia 248
Anterior fontanel 38, 120
  bulging of 120
  delayed closure of 120
Anthrax 144
Anthropometric parameters 74
Anthropometry 62
Anthropometry of neonates 287
Antimongoloid slant of eyes 127
Anuria 51
Aortic regurgitation 233
Aortic stenosis 234
Apert syndrome 109
Apex beat 226
Apgar scoring system 283
Aphasia 245
Aphthous ulcers 44, 185
Apnea test, protocol for 327
Apnea, potentially reversible causes of 327
Appendages of skin 155
Appendicitis, acute 184
Appetite, excessive 184
Apraxia 260
Arachnodactyly 172
Areas for auscultation of heart 228
Argyll-Robertson pupils 253
Arm span 74
Art and science of pediatric diagnosis 1
Art of healing 10, 12
Arthralgia 49, 173
  causes of 174
Arthritis 49, 173
  causes of 173
Arthrogryposis multiplex congenita 106
ASD secundum 234
Association defects 99
Asterixis 186, 261
Ataxia telangiectasia 104, 154, 156, 242
Atelectasis of lung 212
Athetosis 260
Atopic dermatitis 158
Atrial septal defect 234
Atrio-digital syndrome 109
Attention deficit hyperactivity disorder 93

Attributes of a
  pediatrician 2
  physician 1
Auscultatory percussion 209
Auspitz sign 151
Austin-Flint murmur 234
Autism spectrum disorders 93, 246
Automatic reflexes 246, 290, 307
Autonomic functions 276
AVPU scale for assessment of
  consciousness 244

Babinski response 271
Bacterial endocarditis 144
Balanitis 193
Barlow maneuver 309
Baroda development screening test 92
Bayley scales of infant development 78
Bazin disease 134
Beau's lines 156
Beckwith-Wiedemann syndrome 106
Beevor's sign 263
Bell tympany 212
Bell's palsy 256
Bell's phenomenon 256
Belly dancer's sign 266
Benedikt's syndrome 254
Berardinelli lipodystrophy syndrome 106
Beri-beri 51
Biot's breathing 203
Bird-headed dwarf syndrome 104
Bitot spots 51
Black ulcer 144
Bloch-Sulzberger syndrome 154
Blood pressure 36, 221
Blount disease 169
Blue dot sign 194
Blue sclerae 123
Blueberry muffins skin 191
Body mass index 72
Body odor, abnormal 139
Body proportions 114
Body ratios 71, 73
Body volume index 72
Body weight 62
Bone age 114
Bone pains 167, 172
Borborygmi 193
Bossing of skull 120
Bowed legs 50, 168
Brachycephaly 97
Bradycardia 220, 286

Brain death 325
    confirmatory tests for
    the diagnosis of 328
Brainstem reflexes 245, 326
Branchial cleft cyst 46, 298
Brazelton's 'states' of wakefulness 301
Breath-holding spells 18, 239
Breathing rates, cut offs at
    different ages 203
Breathing sounds 203
Bronchial breathing 210
Bronchophony 210
Bronchopulmonary segments of lungs 199
Brown-Sequard syndrome 269
Brudzinski's sign 248
Bruit over the hepatic area 193
Bruit over the lumbar areas 193
Build and nutrition 33
Bulbar palsy 245, 258
Bulk of muscles 261

Café au lait macules 136
Caffey disease 171
Camptodactyly 167
Candidal diaper rash 160
Candidiasis, recurrent or persistent 160
Capillary refill time 286
Caput medusae 188
Caput quadratum 97
Caput succedaneum 294
Cardiac failure 224, 300
Cardiac malformations in association
    with syndromes 217
Cardiac malformations, developmental 217
Cardiac murmurs 227, 230
    characteristics of 230
    grading of 231
    radiation of 230
    timing of 232
Cardiac silhouette 215
Cardiac thrill 226
Cardiopulmonary resuscitation 320
Cardiovascular system 60, 215, 300
Carey-Coomb murmur 233
Carnett's sign 189
Carotenemia 151
Carotid bruit 236
Carpenter syndrome 109
Carpopedal spasms 37, 241, 261
Cat's eye 126
Cataract, causes of 125
CATCH-22 syndrome 217
Caudal regression syndrome 274
Cavernous angioma 152
Cavernous breathing 210
Cavernous hemangioma 152
Central nervous system 60, 238
Central nervous system in a neonate 302
Central venous pressure 225
Cephalhematoma 294
Cerebellar signs 276

Cerebral gigantism 106
Cerebral palsy, early markers of 88
Cerebrohepatorenal syndrome 107
Cervical lymph nodes 37
Cervical lymphadenopathy 37
Chaddock's sign 271
Charcot's joints 164
Charcot-Marie-Tooth disease 169
CHARGE association 99, 217
Cherry red spot 250
Chest circumference 69
Chest pain 202, 216
Cheyne-Stokes breathing 203
Chickenpox 141
CHILD syndrome 147
Choledochal cyst 196
Chordee 194
Chorea 216, 259
    causes of 260
Chromosomal syndromes 101
Chvostek's sign 241, 261
Chylous ascites 193
Cleft palate 285
Club feet 168
Clubbing of nails 131, 186, 204, 222
Clutton's joints 164
CNS disorder
    diagnosis of 277
    localization of 277
Coarctation of aorta 235
Coffin-Lowry syndrome 108
Coffin-Siris syndrome 108
Coin test 212
Cold sores 141
Collapse of lung 212
Colle's fracture 173
Collodion baby 297
Color blindness 249
Color of skin lesions 150
Color vision 249
Coma scales 244
Coma, potentially reversible causes of 327
Common symptoms of disease 17
Communication as the key for a sound
    doctor–patient relationship 320
Compound fracture 173
Concomitant squint 41, 251
Confrontation test 249
Congenital adrenal hyperplasia 194, 300
Congenital analgia 270
Congenital blindness 249
Congenital cardiac malformations 217
Congenital dislocation of hip 168
Congenital dysplasia of hip 168
Congenital heart disease 225
Congenital malformations,
    screening for 284
Congenital phlebectasia 151
Congenital rubella syndrome 126
Congenital syphilis 164
Congenital talipes equinovarus 168

Congestive heart failure 224
    age at onset of 225
Conjunctival reflex 255, 270
Consanguinity, degree of 23
Consciousness, levels of 244
Consolidation of lung 212
Constitutional growth delay 114
Consumer protection act 314
Coordination, assessment of 264
Corneal light reflex 43
Corneal reflex 255, 270, 326
Cornelia de Lange syndrome 41, 103, 217
Corrected age 62
Corrigan's sign 233
Cortical sensations 270
Costochondral beading of ribs 51, 130, 206
Cough, different types of 19, 200
Cough and breathing difficulty, recurrent
    episodes of 201
Cover uncover test 42
Crackles on auscultation of chest 211
Cranial nerves in neonates 305
Cranial nerves, examination of 247
Craniosynostoses syndromes 109
Craniosynostosis 39, 241
Craniotabes 120, 294
Cremasteric reflex 270
Cretinism 97
Cri-du-chat syndrome 102
Critically sick child 54
Croup 201
Croup scoring system 202
Crouzon syndrome 109
Cruveilhier–Baumgarten syndrome 193
Crying child 17
Cryptorchidism 194
Cullen sign 187
Cushing syndrome 76
Cutaneous tuberculosis 164
Cutis marmorata telangiectasia
    congenita 151
Cyanosis 37, 115, 300
    causes of 116
    central 115
    differential 115, 222
    peripheral 115
Cyanotic spells 216
Cystic fibrosis 201
Cystic hygroma 298

Dactylitis 167, 172
Dandy-Walker syndrome 241
Databases for diagnosis of
    various syndromes 100
Deafness, causes of 79
Death
    clinical criteria for the diagnosis of 325
    declaration of 322
Decerebrate rigidity 244, 259
Decorticate posture 243

Index

Decorticate rigidity 259
Deep sensations 270
Deep tendon reflexes 266
    grading of 268
Deficiency of trace minerals 52
Deficiency of vitamins 51
Dehydration
    assessment of 49
    classification of 49
    hypernatremic 50
Delayed puberty 114, 135
Delusions 245
Demographic data 17
deMusset's sign 233
Dengue fever 141
Dennie–Morgan folds 204
Dentition, delayed 131
Dermatitis herpetiformis 163
Dermatoglyphics 48
Dermatographism 151
Dermatophytoses 160
Dermoid cyst 46
d'Espine sign 212
Development findings, interpretation of 92
Development
    assessment of 77
    milestones of 79
    quotient 78
    regression of 93
    screening tools for 91
    social and adaptive 86
Developmental defects 99
Developmental dysplasia of hips 309
Developmental peculiarities, minor 291
Diagnosis
    approach to 2
    art of 5
Diagnosis of death 325
Diagnostic possibilities 6, 7
Diaper rash 160
Diaphragmatic paralysis 206
Diarrhea 19
Diascopy 151
Differences between physical examination of children and adults 58
Differential cyanosis 222
Differential diagnosis of common abnormal physical signs 111
DiGeorge syndrome 217
Diplegia 264
Diplopia 251
Dislocation of hips, congenital 311
Distended urinary bladder 192, 197
Doctor–patient communication, benefits of 321
Doctor–patient relationship 320
Dolichocephaly 97
Doll's eye phenomenon 246, 326
Do-not-resuscitate orders 319
Down syndrome 101, 217

Downes scoring system 301
Drooling of saliva 138
Drug abuse 239
Drug eruptions 161
Dry oral mucosa 139
Duchenne's muscular dystrophy 217, 262
Dwarfism 112
Dying child, handling of a 322
Dysarthria 245
Dyslexia 245
Dysmorphic child 96
Dysphagia 202
Dysphonia 246
Dysplastic nails 47
Dyspnea 201
    grades of 216
Dystonia musculorum deformans 260
Dystrophic nails 157

Ebstein anomaly 235
Ecthyma gangrenosum 144
Ectodermal dysplasia 40
Eczema herpeticum 158
Edema 38, 117, 119, 186
Edema of abdominal wall 189
Edward syndrome 102, 218
Egophony 210
Eisenmenger's syndrome 235
Ellis-van Creveld syndrome 217
Emotional status 245
Empyema 212
Empyema necessitans 206
Endocardial cushion defect 234
End-of-life issues 13
ENT examination 42
Enteroviruses 141
Epicanthic folds 127
Epidermal nevus syndrome 154
Epididymitis, acute 194
Epiglottitis 201
Epispadias 194
Epistaxis 137, 216
Epulis 185
Equinus gait 179
Erb's palsy 306
Erythema induratum 134
Erythema infectiosum 141
Erythema multiforme 162
Erythema nodosum 134
Erythema of palms 149
Escobar syndrome 109
Essential tools for conducting physical examination 31
Ethical and legal issues in clinical practice 314
Ethical decisions, guidelines for making 316
Ethical practices, directives by Medical Council of India 319
Ewart's sign 212

Examination of a newborn baby 280
Exanthum subitum 141
Excessive sweating 138
Expressionless face 98

FABER test 175
FACES syndrome 146
Facial dysmorphism 39, 96
Facial palsy 98
    bilateral 256
    infranuclear 256
Facial puffiness, causes of 127
Facial response to pain 327
Facies, typical 97
Failure to thrive 111
    causes of 113
Fainting 239
Familial short stature 114
Familial versus pathological obesity, differences between 75
Family pedigree 22
Fasciculations and twitchings 261
Feeding history 25
Female genitalia 194
Fetal hydantoin syndrome 128
Fever 18
    types of 18
Fibromyalgia 178
Fibrosis of lung 214
Field of vision 249
Flapping tremors 186, 201
Flat feet 50, 169
Floppiness of muscles 178
Fluid thrill 192
Follicular hyperkeratosis 47, 161
Fontanels and sutures 38
Foster-Kennedy syndrome 250
Foville's syndrome 254
Fracture, clinical features of 173
Fragile X syndrome 105
Freeman-Sheldon syndrome 108
Friction test 212
Friedman grading of tonsils 43
Frohlich syndrome 76
Frontonasal dysplasia sequence 107
Functional cardiac murmur 236
Functional megacolon 195
Fundus examination 41, 249, 305

Gait 179, 265, 275
    abnormalities of 275
Galant reflex 308
Galeazzi sign 168
Galeazzi test 311
Gallbladder, enlargement of 196
Gallop rhythm 230
Ganglion 171
Gardner syndrome 187
Gastroesophageal reflux disease 183, 200
Gaucher's disease 196
    infantile 133
General physical examination 31, 59

Genetic diagram 22
Genu varum 168
Geographical tongue 185
German measles 141
Gestational age, assessment of 288, 291
Gilles de la Tourette syndrome 261
Gingivostomatitis 185
Glabellar tap reflex 272
Glandular fever 141
Glasgow coma scale 244
Glasgow coma scale, modified 244
Glossitis 51
Glycogen storage disease 196, 218
Goiter 46
Goldenhar syndrome 108
Gordon's sign 271
Gottron papules 149
Gower sign 262, 275
Gradenigo's syndrome 254
Graft-versus-host disease 163
Graham Steell murmur 235
Granuloma annulare 162
Grey-Turner sign 187
Growing pains 167
Growth velocity 66
Grunting 203
Gum hyperplasia 129
Gynecomastia 186

Hairy nevus 242
Halitosis 138
Hallermann-Streiff syndrome 104
Hallucinations 245
Hamman's sign 212
Hand-foot-and-mouth disease 141
Hand-Schüller-Christian disease 124
Hansen's disease 165
Harrison's sulcus 51, 206
Haverhill fever 144
Head banging 120
Head circumference 68
    growth velocity of 69
Head circumference-for-age 69
Head nodding 120
Head shape, abnormalities of 97
Healing 10
Hearing, assessment of 306
Heart sounds 227, 228
    abnormalities of 231
Height velocity 67
Height, mid-parental 68
Height-for-age 67, 72
Heiner syndrome 211
Hemangioma of infancy 152
Hematochezia 184
Hematuria 183
Hemiballismus 261
Hemihypertrophy 137, 171, 184
Hemiplegia 264
Hemolytic facies 97
Hemoptysis 202, 216

Hemoptysis vs hematemesis,
    differences between 203
Hemorrhagic disease of
    the newborn 51
Henoch-Schönlein syndrome 147
Hepatic encephalopathy 184
Hepatic facies 98
Hepatic rub 195
Hepatocellular failure 186
Hepatomegaly, isolated 195
Hepatotoxic drugs 183
Herald patch 159
Herniation of hippocampus 243
Herpangina 43
Herpenden skinfold caliper 71
Herpes simplex 141
Herpes zoster 141
Hess capillary resistance test 36
Higher mental functions 243
Hill sign 222, 234
Hips, examination of 309
Hirschsprung's disease 195
Hirsutism 156
History taking 3, 15
Hoarse cry 18, 216
Hoffmann's sign 272
Holt-Oram syndrome 218
Hoover's sign 264
Horner's syndrome 254, 307
Hospital admission, indications for 54
Hot cross bun appearance of skull 97
Hurler syndrome 218
Hutchinson's triad 164
Hydatid thrill 193
Hydrocele 193
Hydrocephalus 97
Hygroma of neck 46
Hyperextensibility of joints 173
Hyperhidrosis 139
Hypermobility of joints 173
Hyperoxia test 115
Hyperplasia of gums 129
Hyperpyrexia 18
Hypertelorism 123
Hypertension 222
    common causes of 223
    common correlates of 223
Hypertensive retinopathy 250
Hyperthermia 18
Hypertrichosis 156
Hypertrophic osteoarthropathy 131, 171
Hypertrophy of a limb 171
Hypertrophy of gums 185
Hypertrophy of muscles
    generalized 178
    localized 178
Hypoplasia of the depressor anguli oris
    muscle 284
Hypoplasia of the radius 172
Hypospadias 194
Hypotelorism 124

Hypothyroidism 52, 76
Hypotonia, generalized 178
Hypoxia, clinical features of 115
Hypoxic-ischemic encephalopathy,
    staging of 309
Hysterical coma 244
Hysterical paralysis 264
Immunization status 25
Inborn errors of metabolism,
    screening for 312
Incontinentia pigmenti 110, 154
Incoordination 276
Incurable disease, handling of
    a patient with 321
Infantile eczema 157
Infantometer 66
Infectious mononucleosis 141
Inguinal hernia 193
Inhalation of foreign body 201
Innocent murmurs 236
Integrated management of neonatal and
    childhood illnesses 9
Intolerance against doctors 323
Involuntary movements 259
Isomorphic response 149
Janeway's lesions 222
Jaundice 37, 116, 183
    causes of 118
    neonatorum 298
Jaw jerk 266
Jendrassik maneuver 267
Jeune syndrome 304
Joint pains
    fleeting 166
    migratory 166
Joint stiffness 173
Jugular venous pressure 224, 225

Kasabach-Merritt syndrome 152
Kashin–Beck disease 52
Kayser-Fleischer rings 184
Kernig's sign 245
Khamis Roche height predictor 68
Kidney mass 196
Klinefelter syndrome 76
Klippel-Trenaunay-Weber syndrome 110
Klumpke's palsy 306
Knock knees 50
Koebner phenomenon 149, 151
Koilonychia 47
Koplik's spots 43
Kuppuswamy socioeconomic
    status scale 25
Kussmaul's breathing 51, 203

Laboratory investigations 4, 317
LAMB syndrome 146
Langer-Giedion syndrome 108
Language development 86
Laron syndrome 104
Larsen syndrome 173

Laurence-Moon-Biedl syndrome 76, 105
Lazarevic's test 176
Learning disability 94
Legg-Calve-Perthés disease 176
Lejeune syndrome 102
Length or height 64
LEOPARD syndrome 110, 146, 218
Leptospirosis 144
Leukocoria 126, 306
Leukonychia 156, 186
Level of consciousness 243
Lichen planus 162
Life support, withholding or
 withdrawal of 320
Limping 179
Liver flap 186
Liver span 189
Lobar pneumonia 212
Lockjaw 132
Louis-Bar syndrome 107
Lovibond angle 132
Low set ears 128
Lower respiratory tract 198
Ludwig angina 45
Lupus vulgaris 164
Lutembacher syndrome 234
Lymphadenopathy 37, 117
 common causes of 119

Macewen's sign 38, 241
Macrocephaly 68, 97, 121
Macroglossia 129, 185
Macro-orchidism 135
Male genitalia 193
Malnutrition, classification of 66
Malpractice litigations,
 common causes of 316
Management, principles of rational 8
Mandibulofacial dysostosis 108
Marcus Gunn phenomenon 252
Marfan syndrome 172, 218
Marshall-Smith syndrome 106
Mastitis neonatorum 294
Maternal and perinatal history 280
Maternal health status 281
Maternal medications, fetal hazards of 282
McBurney point 184
McCune-Albright syndrome 137
Measles 141
Meckel-Gruber syndrome 107
Mediastinal crunch 212
Mediastinal mass 204
Megaloblastic anemia 51
Memory and orientation 245
Meningeal irritation 239
 signs of 243, 246
Meningismus 133
Meningococcemia 144
Mesenteric cyst 191
Microcephaly 68, 97, 122
Microglossia 129

Micrognathia 128
Micro-orchidism 135
Micropenis 134, 194
Mid-parental height 68
Mid-upper arm circumference 69
Migraine 239
Miliaria 160
Millard-Gubler syndrome 254
Minimally conscious state 244
Minor developmental peculiarities 291
Mitral regurgitation 233
Mitral stenosis 233
Mitral valve prolapse 233
Moebius syndrome 107, 254
Mongolian blue spots 297
Mongoloid slant of eyes 126
Monoplegia 264
Monosomy X 102, 219
Moon facies 98
Moro reflex 307
Mucopolysaccharidosis 97
Multiple pterygium syndrome 109
Murmurs 236
Murphy's sign 196
Muscle power
 assessment of 263
 grading of 264
Muscle strength, testing of 178
Muscle tone 263
 assessment of 89, 263, 289, 306
Muscular dystrophies,
 differential diagnosis of 262
Muscular hypotonia 177
Musculoskeletal developmental
 defects 168
Musculoskeletal system 166
Myalgias 178
Myocarditis 236
Myoclonus 261
Myotonic dystrophy syndrome 107

Nadas' criteria 236
Narcolepsy 239
Nasal bridge, depressed 126
Nasal speech 245
Natal teeth 130
Neck rigidity 132, 245
Neonatal pustular melanosis 298
Neonate, physical examination of a 283
Neuroblastoma 191
Neuroectodermal dysplasias 153, 241
Neurofibromatosis 110, 154
Neurogenic bladder 273
Neurological examination in neonates 302
Neuromotor development 77
 indications for assessment of 78
 methods of assessment of 78
 milestones of 79
Neuromotor retardation 77
Neutral positions of joints 174
Nevus araneus 151

Nevus flammeus 152, 297
Nevus simplex 151
Newborn baby, examination of a 280
Nikolsky's sign 151
Nocturnal cough 200
Noonan syndrome 105, 218
Nursemaid's elbow 167
Nutritional dwarfism 113
Nutritional status 185
 age-independent criteria for
  assessment of 69
 assessment of 62
Nutritional values of Indian foods 24
Nystagmus 253, 276

Obesity 75
 causes of 76
 types of 75
Objectivized structured clinical
 examination 55
Obligations of doctors towards
 their patients 317
Observation of a child 33
Observation hip 179
Obstructive uropathy 299
Obturator sign 184
Ocular movements 251
Oculocephalic reflex 326
Oligohydramnios 281
Oliguria 51
Opening snap 229
Opisthotonos 132
Oppenheim's sign 271
Optic atrophy 249
Oral cavity 185
Oral thrush 130
Organ donations, contraindications to 322
Organ transplantation 322
Oropharyngeal reflex 327
Ortolani maneuver 309
OSCE 55
OSCE stations 56
Osler nodes 222
Osteoarthropathy 204
Osteochondritis 172
Osteogenesis imperfecta 172
Ostium primum defect 234
Oxycephaly 97

Pain abdomen 20
Pain, assessment of 287
Palate, high arched 128
Palmar erythema 137, 186
Palmar grasp 308
Palmomental reflex 272
Papilledema 249
Papillitis 250
Papular urticaria 158
Parachute reflex 308
Paralysis 259
Paralytic squint 251

Parapharyngeal abscess 45
Paresthesias 269
Passive euthanasia 320
Patau syndrome 102, 218
Patellar clonus 267
Patellar tap test 177
Patent ductus arteriosus 234
Patrick test 175
Peak expiratory flow rate 204
Pectus carinatum 206
Pectus excavatum 206
Pediatric diagnosis 1
Pediatricians, attributes and
 professional qualities of 317
Pedigree chart, symbols used for
 constructing 23
PEFR, grades of 205
Pel-Ebstein fever 18
Pellagra 51
Pelvic inflammatory disease 183
Pericardial rub 233
Perinaud's syndrome 254
Peritonsillar abscess 44
Peroneal sign 37, 242
Persistent vegetative state 244
Pes cavus 169
Pes planus 169
Peutz-Jeghers syndrome 151, 185, 195
Pharyngeal sounds 211
Philtrum, abnormalities of 127
Photosensitivity skin rash 149
Phrenic nerve injury 264
Phrynoderma 47, 161
Physical examination 4
 cooperation during 32
 position of the child for 32
 sequence of 33
Physiological handicaps 58
Pica 52
Pickwikian syndrome 76
Pierre Robin sequence 107, 297
Pigeon toes 170
Pinpoint pupils 252
Pityriasis alba 159
Pityriasis rosea 159
Pityriasis versicolor 159
Plagiocephaly 97
Plantar grasp 308
Plantar reflex 271
Pleural effusion 212
Pleural friction rub 211
Pneumothorax 214
Poland syndrome 109, 206
Polycystic ovary disease 76
Polydactyly 170
Polyhydramnios 281
Pompe's disease 218
Ponderal index 72, 287
Pontine crossed paralysis 254
Porphyria erythropoietica 150
Port-wine stain 152

Position of trachea 206
Posthitis 193
Postural hypotension 222
Posture 259
Pott puffy tumor 204
Potbelly 183
Potter facies 45, 98, 100
Prader orchidometer 53, 134
Prader-Willi syndrome 75, 76, 107
Preauricular skin tags 99
Precocious puberty 53, 114
Precordial pulsations 226
Pregnancy, problems during 281
Prehn's sign 194
Preterm babies
 criteria for healthy 312
 physical parameters of 287
Pretzel test 174
Priapism 194
Prickly heat 160
Primary skin lesions 146
Primitive reflexes 290, 307
Problem-oriented medical record 28
Prognosis 12
 communication of a gloomy 322
Proptosis, causes of 124
Protein-energy malnutrition,
 classification of 72
Prune belly syndrome 188, 299
Pseudobulbar palsy 245, 256, 259
Pseudohypoparathyroidism 50, 76
Psoas sign 184, 187
Psoriasis 163
Psychogenic cough 201
Psychogenic seizures 239
Pterygium colli 132
Ptosis 252
 causes of 125
Puberty, delayed 53
Puddle sign 192
Puffiness of eyelids 127
Pulmonic stenosis 234
Pulse 35, 219
Pulse deficit 219
Pulse oximetry 115
 for screening for congenital heart
 disease 311
Pulse pressure 219
Pulsus paradoxus 204, 220
Pupillary reflex 41
Pupillary response to light 326
Pupils 252, 306
Pyknodysostosis 108
Pyloric mass 191
Pyloric tumor 191

Quac stick 71
Quadriplegia 264
Quinsy 45

Radial ray anomalies 48
Radiation of abdominal pain 183

Raised intracranial tension 239, 241
 signs of 243
Ranula 186
Rat-bite fever 144
Record keeping 27
Rectal examination 195
Rectal polyp 195
Rectal prolapse 195
Red reflex 306
Reiter's disease 167
Renal colic 183
Renal shutdown 51
Respiration, characteristics of 35
Respiratory distress in neonates,
 common causes of 303
Respiratory distress,
 assessment of 204, 301
Respiratory drive, absence of 327
Respiratory failure
 acute 205
 criteria for 205
Respiratory muscles, paralysis of 269
Respiratory system 60, 198
 in a neonate 301
Retinitis pigmentosa 250
Rett syndrome 261
Rhabdomyosarcoma 125
Rhagades 39, 164
Rhonchi 211
Rickets 51, 172
Rickety rosary 206
Rinne's test 257
Rising dullness 208
Rising test 190
Risus sardonicus 98
Romberg's sign 265
Rosary sign 149
Rose spots 145
Roseola infantum 141
Rossolimo sign 268, 271
Roth spots 224
Rothmund-Thomson syndrome 105
Rovsing sign 184
Rubella 141
Rubella syndrome 218
Rubeola 141
Rubinstein-Taybi syndrome 104
Rumpel-Leede test 36
Russell–Silver syndrome 104

Saber tibiae 53, 172
Salivary glands 39
Salmon patch 151
Sarcoma botryoides 194
Sarnat staging system 309
Scabies 157
Scalp hair, light brown 156
Scanning speech 245
Scarlet fever 144
Schamroth sign 131
Scorbutic rosary 171

Screening for inborn errors of metabolism 312
Scrofuloderma 164
Scurvy 51, 171
Seborrheic dermatitis 158
Seckel syndrome 104
Second heart sound
    abnormalities of 229
    characteristics of 229
Secondary skin lesions 147
Seizures in neonates, causes of 304
Seizures 240
    conditions mimicking 240
    differential diagnosis of 240
Sensations, assessment of 269
Setting sun sign 304
Severity of illness, assessment of 54
Sexual infantilism 114, 135
Sexual maturity rating 53, 194
Shaeffer's sign 271
Shah-Waardenburg syndrome 156
Shape of chest 205
Shifting dullness 192, 209
Shingles 141
Shock 36, 49
Short neck 132
Short stature 112
    causes of 113
Shortening of an extremity 171
Shprintzen-Goldberg syndrome 218
Silverman-Anderson score 301
Simian crease 48
    causes of 49
Single breath count 205
Single umbilical artery 284
Sinus arrhythmia 219
Sinuses, development of 204
Sinusitis
    acute 204
    chronic 204
Sjögren-Larsson syndrome 107
Skeletal dysplasia 112
Skin and its appendages 47, 140
Skin conditions, common 157
Skin lesions, morphology of 148
Skin rash
    distribution of 149
    morphology of 148
Slanting of eyes 126
Slurring speech 245
Smiling face sign 187
Smith-Lemli-Opitz syndrome 105
SOAP chart 27
Socioeconomic status 22
Sodoku 144
Sotos syndrome 106
Spastic cerebral palsy 264
Speech 86, 245
Spenic rub 196
Sphincters, abnormalities of 273
Spider nevus 151

Spine 273
Splenomegaly 196
Splinter hemorrhages 155, 222
Squint 41
Staphylococcal scalded skin syndrome 145
Staphylococcal toxic shock syndrome 145
Startle response, exaggerated 307
Steinberg sign 172
Sternal angle 224
Sternomastoid sign 207
Sternomastoid tumor 297
Stertorous breathing 211
Stevens-Johnson syndrome 161
Stickler syndrome 172
Stokes-Adams attacks 216
Straight leg raise sign 176
Strawberry nevus 152
Strawberry tongue 42, 185
Streptococcal toxic shock syndrome 145
Stridor 201, 203
Stunting 112
Sturge-Weber syndrome 110, 153, 242
Subcutaneous emphysema 207
Subcutaneous fat, measurement of thickness of 71
Subgaleal hematoma 294
Subluxation of the radial head 167
Succussion splash 193
Sunset eye sign 123
Superficial reflexes 270
Superficial sensations 270
Surface anatomy of lungs 198
Suzman sign 236
Sweating, excessive 138
Sydney line 48
Symptom review 17
Syncope 239
Syndactyly 170
Syndrome, definition of 100
Synophrys 41
System review 20
Systemic examination 59

Tache cerebrale 148
Tachycardia 220
Tachypnea 201
Tactile fremitus 207
Talipes calcaneovalgus 168, 299
Talipes equinovarus 299
Tall child, excessively 115
TAR syndrome 109, 218
Target height 68, 114
Target milestones 87
Teeth, discolored 130
Temper tantrums 18
Temperature 34
Tentorial herniation 252
Testicular size, abnormalities of 134
Testis, enlargement of 194
Tet spells 216
Tetany 52

Tetralogy of Fallot 235
Thomas test 176
Thrill 226
Thrombocytopenia with absent radius syndrome 109
Thrush 130
Thumb sign 172, 219
Thumbprint sign 201
Thyroglossal cyst 46, 298
Tics 239, 261
Tinea capitis 160
Tinea corporis 160
Tinea versicolor 159
Toad skin 161
Toeing-in 170
Toe-walking 168, 170, 179
Tongue, bald and smooth 185
Tongue-tie 42, 186, 294
Tonic neck reflex 308
TORCH infections 164
Torsion of an ovarian cyst 183
Torsion of testis 194
Torticollis 46, 133
Tourniquet test 36
Toxic epidermal necrolysis 163
Toxic erythema 297
Trace minerals, deficiencies of 52
Traction reflex 308
Trail sign 207
Transient synovitis of the hip joint 179
Transillumination of skull 38, 304
Transillumination of the chest 208
Transposition of great vessels 235
Treacher Collins syndrome 108
Tremors 259
Trendelenburg test 176
Tricuspid atresia 235
Tricuspid regurgitation 233
Trigger finger 170
Trigger thumb 170
Trignocephaly 97
Tripod sign 247
Trismus 132
Trisomy 13-15 102, 218
Trisomy 17-18 102, 218
Trisomy 21 101, 217
Trivandrum developmental screening chart 91
Trophic changes 263
Trousseau's sign 37, 241, 261
Tuberculosis cutis orificialis 165
Tuberculous verrucosa cutis 164
Tuberous sclerosis 110, 153, 155, 219
Tubular breathing 210
Turner syndrome 102, 219
Turricephaly 97
Tympanic membrane, landmarks on the 46
Typhoid fever 145
Typical facies 97

Umbilical granuloma 299
Umbilical hernia 187
Undescended testis 194
Unethical practices 318
Upper airway 198
Upper and lower motor neuron paralysis, differences between 277
Upper segment-to-lower segment body ratios 73
Urinary bladder, distended 192
Urine, discolored 183
Urticaria 158

VACTERL association 99, 219
Valsalva maneuver 231
Varicella 141
Varicoceles 194
Vascular nevi 151
Vasovagal attack 239
VATER association 99, 219
Venous hum 193, 232, 236
Venous pulsations 224
Ventricular septal defect 234
Vertigo 257
Vesicular breathing 210
Vestibulo-ocular reflex 246, 326
Violence against doctors 323
Vision, assessment of 306
Vital signs 34
  at different ages 59
  in a neonate 286
Vitamin deficiencies, clinical features of 51
Vitiligo 162
Vocal fremitus 207
Vocal resonance 210
Vomiting 19, 184
Von Hippel-Lindau disease 154
Von Recklinghausen's disease 110, 136
Vulvovaginitis 194

Waardenburg syndrome 107, 156
WAGR association 191
Waist-to-hip ratio 72
Wartenberg's sign 272
Warts 152
Weaver-Smith syndrome 106
Webbing of neck 132
Weber's syndrome 254
Weber's test 257
Weight 62
Weight-for-age 66
Weight-for-height 71
Werdnig-Hoffmann disease 258
Wheezing, unilateral 211
Whispering pectoriloquy 210
Whistling face syndrome 108
White reflex in the eye 126
Wickham's striae 162
Williams syndrome 105, 219, 234
Wilms tumor 191
Wilson disease 184
Wiskott-Aldrich syndrome 158
Wry neck 133

Xanthomata 186
Xenotransplantation 323
Xerostomia 139

Zellweger syndrome 107
Zinc deficiency, signs of 159